Clinical Principles and Analytical Techniques in Toxicology

Clinical Principles and Analytical Techniques in Toxicology

Editor: Mary Durrant

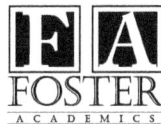

FA FOSTER
ACADEMICS

www.fosteracademics.com

www.fosteracademics.com

FA
FOSTER
ACADEMICS

Cataloging-in-Publication Data

Clinical principles and analytical techniques in toxicology / edited by Mary Durrant.
　　p. cm.
Includes bibliographical references and index.
ISBN 978-1-63242-517-1
1. Toxicology. 2. Clinical toxicology. 3. Analytical toxicology. I. Durrant, Mary.
RA1211 .C54 2018
615.9--dc23

Foster Academics,
118-35 Queens Blvd., Suite 400,
Forest Hills, NY 11375, USA

ISBN 978-1-63242-517-1 (Hardback)

Contents

Preface

The purpose of the book is to provide a glimpse into the dynamics and to present opinions and studies of some of the scientists engaged in the development of new ideas in the field from very different standpoints. This book will prove useful to students and researchers owing to its high content quality.

Toxicology is the study of the effects of toxins in living beings. It is an amalgamation of biology, pharmacology and chemistry. The field also concerns itself with the relationship and effect of dosage of particular chemicals on the organisms. This book traces the progress of the discipline and highlights some of its key concepts and applications. The text covers in detail some existent theories and innovative concepts revolving around toxicology. Scientists and students actively engaged in this field will find the text full of crucial and unexplored concepts.

At the end, I would like to appreciate all the efforts made by the authors in completing their chapters professionally. I express my deepest gratitude to all of them for contributing to this book by sharing their valuable works. A special thanks to my family and friends for their constant support in this journey.

Editor

Investigating Therapeutic Potential of *Trigonella foenum-graecum* L. as Our Defense Mechanism against Several Human Diseases

Shivangi Goyal, Nidhi Gupta, and Sreemoyee Chatterjee

Department of Biotechnology, The IIS University, Gurukul Marg, SFS, Mansarovar, Jaipur, Rajasthan 302020, India

Correspondence should be addressed to Sreemoyee Chatterjee; sreemoyee.chatterjee@iisuniv.ac.in

Academic Editor: Brad Upham

Current lifestyle, stress, and pollution have dramatically enhanced the progression of several diseases in human. Globally, scientists are looking for therapeutic agents that can either cure or delay the onset of diseases. Medicinal plants from time immemorial have been used frequently in therapeutics. Of many such plants, fenugreek is one of the oldest herbs which have been identified as an important medicinal plant by the researchers around the world. It is potentially beneficial in a number of diseases such as diabetes, hypercholesterolemia, and inflammation and probably in several kinds of cancers. It has industrial applications such as synthesis of steroidal hormones. Its medicinal properties and their role in clinical domain can be attributed to its chemical constituents. The 3 major chemical constituents which have been identified as responsible for principle health effects are galactomannan, 4-OH isoleucine, and steroidal saponin. Numerous experiments have been carried out *in vivo* and *in vitro* for beneficial effects of both the crude chemical and of its active constituent. Due to its role in health care, the functional food industry has referred to it as a potential nutraceutical. This paper is about various medicinal benefits of fenugreek and its potential application as therapeutic agent against several diseases.

1. Introduction

Many chemicals are encountered by human either accidentally because they are in the atmosphere or by contact during occupational and recreational activities or by ingestion of food additives. It is conceivable that some chemicals may be inadvertently released into the environment and therefore be injurious to human health. With the increasing rate of use of industrialization and diesel exhaust emission and cigarette smoke; it is obvious that the chemicals are capable of producing undesirable effects on biological tissues. The air pollution index correlated with respiratory and digestive tract and urogenital, blood and skin cancer. Air pollution was estimated to account for 80% of premature deaths, while 14% of death rate was due to chronic diseases according to data provided by World Health Organization (WHO). Evaluation by WHO's International Agency for Research on Cancer (IARC) in 2013 found out the close connection between outdoor air pollution, specifically particulate matter, and increased cancer incidence.

A number of environmental chemicals, both man-made and of natural occurrence, are under strong suspicion as carcinogens, which are important in the etiology of the cancer. Polycyclic aromatic hydrocarbons (PAHs) are ubiquitous environmental pollutants and represent one of the few clearly defined classes of chemicals responsible for the development of skin cancers. Humans are constantly exposed to PAHs through polluted air, cigarette smoke, automobile exhaust, and other airborne pollutants [1]. Polycyclic hydrocarbons vary in their carcinogenic potencies; for example, the compound dibenz[a,c]anthracene has very little carcinogenic activity [2]. Among the most potent hydrocarbon carcinogens are 3-methylcholanthrene and 7,12-dimethylbenz[a]anthracene (DMBA) [3]. DMBA serves as a tumor initiator by making necessary mutations in chemically induced skin tumors in mice. This DMBA, a polycyclic aromatic hydrocarbon, is currently the most frequently utilized initiating agent but additional agents can serve as chemical initiators. Systemic exposure of DMBA is generally effective; however, it is often applied topically to induce skin carcinogenesis in two-stage skin papillomagenesis murine models [4].

Among several different types of cancers known, skin cancer is found to be the most uncommon malignancy in the world; however, the rate of increase in skin cancer over the years has been observed to be progressive [5]. According to the survey, there has been a 65% rise in the incidence since 1980. In the United States, more than 33% of the cancers are skin cancers, while statistics in India account for 1-2% of diagnosed cancers. Researchers have reported basal cell carcinoma as the common form of skin cancer worldwide, while squamous cell carcinoma is known to be the most prevalent form of skin cancer in India. Skin cancer can be divided into two forms: nonmelanoma skin cancers (NMSCs) and melanoma skin cancers (MSCs). Both squamous cell carcinoma (SCC) and basal cell carcinoma (BCC) come under the heading of NMSCs [6].

Various studies have been done by researchers around the world to find out strategies for preventing and treating cancers. Traditional therapies such as radiation, chemotherapy, and surgery have been in use but severe side effects often force patients not to opt for these. For incidence, treatment against breast cancer utilized systemic chemotherapy and failed to give satisfying results [7]. Similarly, usage of doxorubicin as a chemotherapeutic agent against breast cancer treatment not only was less effective but also was toxic to normal tissues [8]. Thus chemoprevention provides a promising strategy to combat dreadful diseases like cancer, several adverse effects such as osteoporosis, and degenerative diseases [9]. Prevention, inhibition of progression and reversal of the normal physiological conditions by the use of natural products, biological products, or synthetic agents, is called chemoprevention. These natural products/extracts in form of day-today dietary components possess the potential of reducing the toxic effects rendered by chemotherapy. According to the epidemiological study, consumption of fruits and vegetables resulted in 50% decrease in cancer development and incidence. F'guyer in his study suggested phytochemicals such as curcumin, green tea extracts, gingerol, and quercetin which could fight against the reactive oxygen species (ROS) of skin and can help in treatment against skin carcinogenesis [10]. With onset of wider research involving preclinical and clinical observations in chemoprevention, valuable data have been generated. This could be beneficial in preventing the onset of disease and suppressing its progress and developing an outlook towards chemoprevention as a challenging and rational strategy of future. Earlier discoveries involved isolation of anticancer drugs from plants such as *Catharanthus roseus, Camptotheca acuminate, and Taxus brevifolia*. Some of these are presently used as potential anticancer drugs like Taxol, Vincristine, Vinblastine, and Camptothecin [11]. Citrus peel extract containing phenolic and flavonoid compounds has been known to be potential natural antioxidant [12]. Multipurpose approaches of the plants offering antioxidant, anti-inflammatory, antidiabetic, and other roles have thus rendered them as the potential and indispensable candidate for the drug discovery without harming the normal physiology of the human body.

One of the traditionally known plants is *Trigonella foenum-graecum* (L.) (fenugreek). It grows once a year and is a self-pollinating plant. Species of *Trigonella* are widely distributed throughout the world. The plant has been mainly found on the continents of Asia (India and China), parts of Europe, Africa, Australia, and North and South America [13]. It bears two cotyledons and belongs to subfamily Papilionaceae, family Leguminosae (Fabaceae). The genus, *Trigonella*, is a Greek word which means "three angled" and the word fenugreek which is derived from *foenum-graecum* means Greek hay. Presence of complex array of important phytochemicals renders fenugreek as one of the important medicinal plants. The leaves and seeds of methi (Indian name) have been used extensively to prepare extracts and powders for medicinal uses [14]. Scientists have reported several medicinal uses of fenugreek seeds such as remedies for diabetes and hypercholesterolemia, hepatoprotective protection against free radicals, and protection against breast and colon cancer [15]. These protective roles are possible due to the nonnutritive secondary metabolites also known as phytochemicals. The major constituents that are present in fenugreek seeds are carbohydrates, proteins, lipids, alkaloids, flavonoids, fibers, saponins, steroidal saponins, vitamins, and minerals, nitrogen compounds which can be categorized under nonvolatile and volatile constituents [16].

2. Fenugreek as Potential Therapeutic Agent against Several Diseases

Apart from the usage in bakery products, frozen dairy products, condiments, spices, pickles, and beverages, fenugreek is known to have numerous beneficial health effects. Gastric ulcers can easily be treated by fenugreek seeds. The seed oil acts as an emollient and makes skin smoother and soft. The cleansing action of fenugreek makes it a valuable plant as it helps purify blood, cleaning lymphatic system, and detoxify the body. In diseases like hay fever and sinusitis it can be used. The seeds are considered useful in heart disease and aphrodisiac and as a galactogogue promoting lactation [17]. Different regions in the world use fenugreek for different purposes; for example, in China, seeds are used to treat cervical cancer and for kidney problems. The aerial parts of plant are used to treat abdominal cramps during diarrhea in the Middle East and the Balkans. In southern India, roasted seeds are used as a treatment for dysentery. The smallpox patients are also given an infusion of seeds as a cooling agent. Being a natural health product, it is capable of treating and curing diseases, thus providing medical and health benefits. As a result of which, it has been considered a potential nutraceutical [18]. Apart from the traditional medicinal uses, fenugreek is found to have many pharmacological properties such as antidiabetic, antinociceptive, anticarcinogenic, antioxidant, anti-inflammatory, and hypocholesterolemic which are discussed below in detail. Tables 1(a) and 1(b) show different activities *in vivo* and *in vitro*, respectively.

2.1. Antidiabetic Activity. One of the chronic metabolic diseases is diabetes mellitus which occurs as a result of

TABLE 1: (a) Different pharmacological activities *in vivo*. (b) Different pharmacological activities *in vitro*.

(a)

Activity	Dose	Content	Mode of application	Vehicle	Parameters	Reference
Anticancer	200 mg/kg b.wt	Flavonoids	—	Aqueous and olive oil	Inhibition of the mammary hyperplasia	[35]
	100 mg/kg and 200 mg/kg b.wt	—	Intraperitoneal	Ethanolic	Alterations of ascites cells	[36]
	25–800 mg/kg b.wt	Saponins, flavonoids, alkaloids, and galactomannans	Oral	Methanol	General: tumor incidence; biochemical: liver GSH and LPO	[39]
	2 g/kg b.wt	Saponins, flavonoids, and fiber	Oral	—	Inhibition of colon carcinogenesis by modulating glucuronidase and mucinase activity	[41]
Antidiabetic	0.44–1.74 g/kg·d	—	Oral	Aqueous	Reduction in blood glucose and improvement of hemorheological properties	[20]
	50 mg/kg b.wt and 100 mg/kg b.wt	—	Oral	Water	Decrease in blood glucose	[23]
	0.5 g/kg b.wt	—	Oral	Alcoholic	Reduction of blood glucose level	[62]
	1 g/kg b.wt	—	Oral	Aqueous and methanolic	Hypoglycemic effect	[63]
Anticholesterol/ hypocholesterolemic	0.44–1.74 g/kg·d	—	Oral	Aqueous	Reduction in blood lipid levels	[20]
	100 mg/kg b.wt	—	Oral	Water	Decrease in serum lipids	[23]
	0.5 g/kg	—	—	—	Decrease in triglycerides and total cholesterol	[43]
	30 or 50 g ethanol extract/kg b.wt	Saponins	Oral	Ethanol	Reductions in plasma cholesterol levels	[62]
Anti-inflammatory	50–200 mg/kg b.wt	—	—	Aqueous	Stimulatory effect on immune system	[64]
	150 mg/kg b.wt	—	—	Ethanolic	Effective against acute and chronic inflammation	[65]
Antioxidant	0.4 g/kg b.wt	—	Oral	—	Reduction in the level of serum MDA	[66]
	0.11 g/kg b.wt	—	—	—	Decrease in SOD activity	[67]
	0.4 g/kg b.wt	Flavonoids and polyphenols	Oral	Aqueous	Decrease in the level of MDA	[68]
Antimicrobial		Flavonoids		Aqueous	Inhibition of *E. coli* and *M. furfur*	[55]
				Aqueous, methanolic, and ethanolic	Methanolic and ethanolic extracts were effective against *E. coli*, *S. typhi*, and *S. aureus*	[69]

(b)

Activity	Dose	Constituent	Vehicle	Parameters	Reference
Antioxidant	20–100 μg/mL	Polyphenols	Methanol	Scavenging hydroxyl radical, DPPH, abts, changes in LPO, SOD, and inhibition of H_2O_2 induced lipid peroxidation	[27]
	25–200 mg/mL	Flavonoids and alkaloids	Ethanolic	Scavenging DPPH and inhibition of lipid peroxidation	[65]
Anticancer				Induction of apoptosis in HT-29 human colon cancer cells	[30]
		Diosgenin		Inhibition of cell proliferation in the human osteosarcoma 1547 cell line	[38]
		Diosgenin	Chloroform	Killed MCF-7 human immortalized breast cells	[40]
			Ethanolic	Cytotoxic to breast cancer cell line and prostate cancer cell line	

(b) Continued.

Activity	Dose	Constituent	Vehicle	Parameters	Reference
Antidiabetic	0.33 and/or 3.3 mg/mL	Saponin, sapogenin, diosgenin, and trigonelline	Ethanolic	Inhibition of glucose uptake	[70]
	1 gm/day	4-Hydroxyisoleucine	Hydro-alcoholic	Direct pancreatic β-cell stimulation, delayed gastric emptying, and inhibition of glucose transport	[71]
	5–20 mM	—	Aqueous	Reduction in v_{max} of d(+)-glucose uptake	[72]
Anti-inflammatory		Saponin	Methanolic	Inhibition of TNF-α in THP-1 cell lines and restrained synthesis of melanin in murine melanoma B16F-1 cells	[48]
		Steroidal saponin	Aqueous	Peroxyl radical scavenging effects and reduction of release of ROS from inflamed mucosa	[73]
Antimicrobial	16–128 mg/mL	Essential oil	Methanolic and acetone	Antimicrobial activity against *Pseudomonas* spp. and *E. coli*	[53]
	100 mg	Defensin		Inhibits the mycelial spread of *Rhizoctonia solani*	[57]

disordered metabolism of carbohydrates, proteins, and lipids. Though several forms of treatments are available in terms of medications and injectable insulin, they are accompanied with side effects. Diabetes mellitus can be regulated by the food habits which not only offer an economical approach but also are rich in chemical constituents that will help in maintaining blood glucose level. One of the well-studied herbal plants is fenugreek which has been quite researched with respect to its effect on diabetes. In one of the published studies by Raju et al., it is documented that seeds, leaves, and its extracts are a good agent in our fight against diabetes [19]. Xue et al., induced diabetes by streptozotocin in rats and effect of fenugreek water seed extract was determined via three different dose levels by intragastric intubation. It was observed that there was a weight gain in fenugreek treated mice as compared to the group that received only streptozotocin. In addition, blood glucose level decreased to a greater extent as compared to the group that received streptozotocin only [20]. Similar results were obtained in the study done by another group of researchers who found that there was an increase in the body weight of rabbits that were supplemented with fenugreek as compared to the alloxan monohydrate induced diabetic rabbits. Plasma glucose level was reduced by the oral administration of fenugreek seed powder not only in the diabetic rabbits but also in nondiabetic rabbits [21]. Ramesh et al. studied the effect of fenugreek seeds on alloxan induced diabetic rats. Histopathological analysis of pancreas of placebo controls was done in which normal acini and cytosol in the islets of Langerhans was observed. But there was an extensive damage to islets of Langerhans and reduced dimensions of islets in alloxan induced diabetes. Islets of Langerhans in diabetic rats that were treated with fenugreek extract were found to be restored [22].

An active compound can also be isolated from the crude extract which can perform a beneficial role against the glucose level. One such study was done by Moorthy et al. who isolated GII from the aqueous extract of fenugreek seeds. This isolated compound was able to reduce blood glucose in glucose tolerance test in subdiabetic and moderately diabetic rabbits. This isolated compound even showed better results than the standard tolbutamide [23].

Even in Egyptian folk medicine, fenugreek held an important place as a hypoglycemic agent. In an *in vitro* study being done by Gad et al., the extract of fenugreek in a dose-dependent manner was able to inhibit α-amylase activity. A further *in vivo* study concluded and confirmed *in vitro* inhibition as it showed suppression of starch digestion and absorption in normal rats, suggesting that the hypoglycemic effect of the used plant extract was mediated through insulin-mimetic effect [24].

Sharma observed the effects on the human patients who had reduced blood glucose concentration after the consumption of either the seeds or the leaves. Greater amount of reduction was observed using the whole seed followed by the gum isolated from cooked or uncooked seeds [25]. In another study by the same group, it was observed that, on consecutive consumption of fenugreek seeds, serum total cholesterol, LDL and VLDL cholesterol, and triglycerides were significantly reduced but no effect on HDL cholesterol levels was found [26]. The important constituents that are found to be responsible for generating the antidiabetic effects are galactomannan rich soluble fiber fraction, saponin, and an amino acid called 4-hydroxyleucine which helped in increasing insulin in hyperglycemic rats and humans [27].

2.2. Antioxidant Activity. Free radicals are being studied by the researchers for a long time as radicals are a source of ROS that hamper the structure of lipid membrane and thus initiate cascade of events leading to various diseases. To suppress generation of free radicals, natural products have been found as safe and effective remedy. One of the herbal extracts which is known to have antioxidant potential is fenugreek. Various studies have been done by the researchers to determine the antioxidant potential of fenugreek. Kaviarasan et al. conducted experiments on rat liver to evaluate the antioxidant potential of fenugreek seeds and it was found that methanolic seed extract was able to quench the free radicals [28]. This group in another set of experiments investigated the protective effect of fenugreek seed polyphenol extract. Rat liver was damaged using ethanol but when treated with fenugreek seed polyphenol extract ($200 \, mg \, kg^{-1} \, day^{-1}$) there was a significant reduction in the levels of lipid peroxidation products and protein carbonyl content. Also there was an increase in the activities of antioxidant enzymes along with restoration of the levels of thiol groups [29]. Similar study was conducted by Thirunavukkarasu et al. in rats by using aqueous extract of fenugreek seeds. Ethanol was fed for 60 days to induce toxicity in rats which resulted in enhancement in the activities of serum aspartate transaminase, alanine transaminase, and alkaline phosphatase. However, simultaneously administrating aqueous extract of fenugreek seeds resulted in an increase of antioxidant level and prevented further rise in lipid peroxidation. The administration of aqueous seed extract could result in prevention of the enzymatic leakage and the rise in lipid peroxidation and enhancement of the antioxidant potential. Histopathological studies related to the rat liver and brain revealed the protective role of the seed extract against ethanol induced toxicity [30].

The constituents that are understood to be responsible were flavonoids and phenolic compounds which generally marks their presence in the polar solvent system due to their self-polar nature. Thus, due to the ability of fenugreek extracts to quench the radicals, it can be a useful candidate to alleviate the harmful effects of various diseases and thus can be used for treatment purposes.

2.3. Antitumor and Anticarcinogenic Activity. The chemical constituents of fenugreek possessing anticancer activity are phytoestrogens and saponins [31]. Saponins selectively inhibit cell division in tumor cells and also can activate apoptotic programs which can lead to programmed cell death [32]. In an *in vivo* study that was carried out on rats, azoxymethane was used to induce colon cancer. The effect of fenugreek seed powder along with its bioactive compound diosgenin was checked and it was observed that both the crude extract and diosgenin were able to inhibit the formation of aberrant crypt foci (ACF) which can be observed as preneoplastic lesion. After the positive response of the extract in *in vivo* experiment, anticancer potential of diosgenin was explored in *in vitro* experiments. HT-29 human colon cancer cells were used and it was seen that diosgenin inhibited the proliferation of cells along with the induction of apoptosis. The effect on apoptosis can be validated by observing the effect on apoptotic proteins. Diosgenin suppressed the expression of proapoptotic protein bcl-2 and there was an increase in the expression of caspase-3, an antiapoptotic protein [31].

Shishodia and Aggarwal reported diosgenin to have anticancer activity in bone cancer. It suppressed cell proliferation and development of bone cells through inhibition of tumor necrosis factor [33]. Protodioscin, a furostanol saponin isolated from fenugreek, also induces apoptotic changes leading to death in a leukemic cell line (HL-60) [34]. Several studies on anticancer properties of chemical constituents of fenugreek have been done and have shown positive results. Some constituent of alkaloids, called "trigonelline," has revealed potential for use in cancer therapy [35].

In vivo cytostatic and cytotoxic effect of fenugreek seed extract was studied. Breast cancer in the mammalian model, that is, female Wistar rats, was induced by DMBA, a polycyclic aromatic hydrocarbon. Inhibition of the mammary hyperplasia and decrease in its incidence were seen after aqueous seed extract of fenugreek was given daily to the rats at a dose of 200 mg/kg b.wt for 120 days. Diosgenin was shown to suppress osteoclastogenesis which was induced by a cytokine, RANKL, through activation of NF-$\kappa\beta$. An increasing dose of diosgenin inhibited TNF-α activated transcription factors such as NF-$\kappa\beta$ and Akt. Thus decrease in the cell proliferation by diosgenin was due to its inhibition on NF-$\kappa\beta$ regulated gene products. The cell line used in the experiment was human chronic myelogenous leukemia (KBM-5) cells [36]. The ethanolic seed extract showed the antineoplastic effect against Ehrlich Ascites Carcinoma cells in mice. Intraperitoneal administration of the extract resulted in change in number and growth pattern of ascites cells and tumor growth was also seemed to be significantly inhibited [37].

In vitro studies of the ethanolic seed extract revealed its cytotoxic effect on a number of cancer cell lines such as breast cancer cell lines, prostate cancer cell lines, and pancreatic cancer cell lines [38]. Yet another study by Moalic et al. was done on diosgenin which showed its inhibitory effect on the human osteosarcoma cell line, that is, 1547 cell line [39]. The underlying mechanism was the arrest of cell cycle at G1 phase and the induction of apoptosis. Chemomodulatory effect of fenugreek seed extract was evaluated by Chatterjee et al. on two-stage mice skin carcinogenesis. DMBA and TPA were used to induce the skin tumor in mice which was inhibited by methanolic seed extract [40]. Chloroform seed extract also showed the effective killing of MCF-7 human immortalized breast cells through induction of apoptosis [41].

Devasena and Menon observed that fenugreek seeds in the diet inhibited colon carcinogenesis by modulating the activities of β-glucuronidase and mucinase [42]. The seed powder in the diet decreased the activity of β-glucuronidase significantly and prevented the free carcinogens from acting on colonocytes. Mucinase helped in hydrolyzing the protective mucin. This was attributed to the presence of fiber, flavonoids, and saponins.

2.4. Hypocholesterolemic Activity. Anticholesterol activity of fenugreek extracts has been well studied by the researchers all over the world. Studies have been performed *in vivo* and were not limited to the rats and mice as they were also performed on different species of rabbits. Singhal et al. studied that the inclusion of fenugreek seeds as a diet component for the mice aided in reducing cholesterol level up to 42% and 58% both in control group and in hypocholesterolemic group, respectively [43]. Another study was done to test the effects of fenugreek leaves on the cholesterol level. There was a reduction in total blood cholesterol, LDL, VLDL level, and triglycerides and there was an increase in HDL cholesterol level after the consumption of dried fenugreek leaves in Albino rabbits [44]. Presence of cholesterol in plasma is an indicator of coronary heart disease. Researchers have studied the effect of fenugreek seed extract on the lipid profile of plasma. Fenugreek seed administration and its extracts significantly decreased plasma cholesterol, triglyceride, and LDL cholesterol. However, HDL cholesterol level was found to be constant; that is, no effect was registered on it [45].

Isolation of a compound named GII from the seed extract of fenugreek with water was found to alter the level of serum lipids in diabetic induced rabbits. GII was able to reduce the total cholesterol level and increase HDL cholesterol which is an indicator of good cholesterol. There was a reduction in triacylglycerols, phospholipids, and free fatty acids [23]. The chemical constituents responsible for the activity are saponins, specifically diosgenin, galactomannan, and fiber.

2.5. Antigenotoxic Activity.

Some researchers have used plant systems to examine the antigenotoxic effect of fenugreek. Chromosomal aberration assay in the *Allium* root is one of the most established assays to monitor the toxicity at the gene level. Root tip meristem cells of onion were treated with toxic chromium trioxide. Methanolic extract of the leaves of fenugreek showed dose-dependent decrease in chromosomal aberration in *Allium cepa* roots. Studies have also been done in microbial systems to observe the antimutagenic effect of fenugreek. Aqueous extract of fenugreek seeds inhibited the mutagenic activity of the direct acting mutagens against *Salmonella typhimurium* [46].

2.6. Anti-Inflammatory Activity.

Fenugreek for past many years has been in use as a traditional medicine in several countries like Iran, southern India, and African countries as a remedy for inflammation and its related effects. The main chemical constituents responsible for the anti-inflammatory activity are alkaloids, saponins, and flavonoids. Sharififara et al. studied the *in vivo* effect of methanolic extract using cream based system. Inflammation in terms of edema was induced in Wistar rats using careegenan and anti-inflammatory effect was observed both by intraperitoneal administration and by the topical application in form of the cream [47].

Kawabata et al. studied the anti-inflammatory and antimelanogenic effect in *in vitro* system using human monocytic cell line (THP-1) [48]. Production of inflammatory cytokines such as IL-1, IL-6, and TNF-α was initiated using phorbol myristate acetate. Inhibitory action of fenugreek extract with methanol as a solvent system was observed with suppression in TNF-α production. The extract was further subjected to the isolation of bioactive compounds such as saponin and two other compounds which were also found to inhibit other cytokines like IL-1 and IL-6 along with TNF-α. The inhibitory effects were concentration dependent. Some contrasting results as compared to *in vitro* study were also evident in *in vivo* system as studied by Raju and others. TNF-α protein levels in the liver and plasma of obese rats were found to be upregulated when fenugreek was orally consumed. This is an indicator of opposing activity of fenugreek seed on the production of TNF-α. There are some complex mechanisms (e.g., digestion, uptake, and metabolism) by which orally administered substance(s) can modulate biological mediators *in vivo*. The opposing results in the production of TNF-α by fenugreek could be understood in terms of the difference between *in vitro* and *in vivo* systems [48]. Another study carried out by Sumanth et al. involved observing the anti-inflammatory effect against the ulcer production. Immersion stress and indomethacin were used to induce ulcer in rats. The aqueous extract of fenugreek seeds showed the antiulcer effect as calculated by the ulcer index [49]. The protective activity of the extract against ulcer could be attributed to its known

antioxidant activity. Not only seeds but also antipyretic and anti-inflammatory activity of the leaves of *T. foenum-graecum* have been reported [50]. On similar lines, Ravichandiran and Jayakumari compared the anti-inflammatory activity of a bioactive compound isolated from fenugreek seed and leaves extracts and its aqueous extracts both in *in vivo* and in *in vitro* systems. It was observed that chloroform fraction of seeds and aqueous extract of leaves of fenugreek were effective against anti-inflammatory activity [51].

In a recent study, it was observed that when fenugreek was administered to diabetic mice, macrophage infiltration into adipose tissue was inhibited. Moreover, mRNA expression levels of inflammatory genes were also reduced. It is also suggested that fenugreek accelerates the wound healing process in rats injured in the posterior neck area due to its antioxidant potential [52].

2.7. Antimicrobial Activity.

For past many years, scientists have been working on natural extracts to evaluate the antimicrobial properties for the development of novel therapeutics. Several plant systems such as *Coriandrum sativum*, *Curcuma longa*, *Citrus lemon*, and *Ocimum sanctum* have been studied by the scientists which exhibited antimicrobial action. Among various varieties of herbal extracts, fenugreek is also one of the candidates that have been tested for its activity against wide variety of microorganisms like bacteria, virus, and fungus [53–56].

Sensitivity of the extracts towards bacteria is dependent not only on the solvent system but also on the type of microorganisms as can be understood by the study done by Dash et al. [53]. A different strategy was employed to prepare the aqueous extract of fenugreek by Sheikhlar et al. Along with his coworkers, study was conducted on both the methanolic extract and aqueous extract against Gram-positive and Gram-negative bacteria. Contrary to the results obtained by other scientists, this study revealed performance by the methanolic extract, while the aqueous extract showed no activity at all concentrations. This study provided an insight into the dependence of antibacterial activity on the solvent system being chosen for the extract preparation [54]. Chandra et al. prepared the aqueous extract of fenugreek seeds and employed disc diffusion method to study the antibacterial effect on three bacteria, namely, *E. coli*, *P. putida*, and *M. furfur*. The extract was found to be effective against *E. coli* and *M. furfur* but showed no response against *P. putida* [55]. Crude extract of fenugreek seeds using methanol and acetone was tested against the four Gram-negative bacteria and it was observed that though the methanolic extract showed the broad range specificity towards various species, *S. typhi* showed resistance towards the acetonic extract. Also among all the four different strains *E. coli* was found to show the highest sensitivity towards acetonic extract, while methanolic extract showed an elevated response against *Pseudomonas* spp. It is also suggested that sprouted or the germinated seeds had enhanced antimicrobial activity specifically against *H. pylori* [56].

Secondary metabolites found in fenugreek seed extract possessed the antimicrobial activity as could be understood by various studies done by scientists. Similarly, these

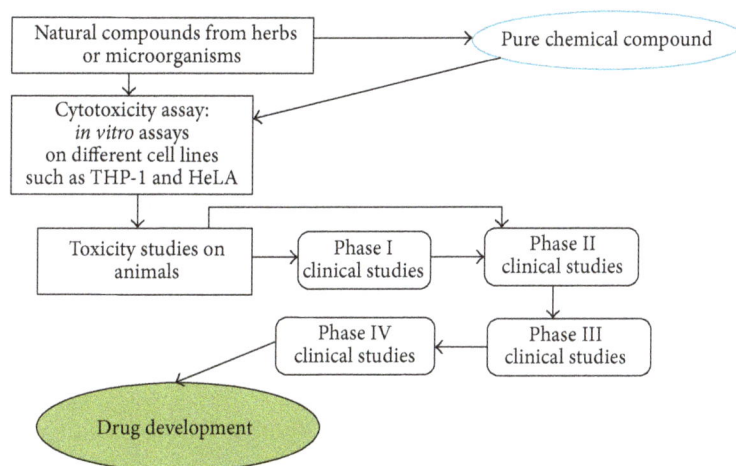

FIGURE 1: Herbal product as phytopharmaceutical: steps involved in the process of drug development.

constituents can be found in the leaves of the fenugreek herb which can also exhibit the same property. Fungus being one of the microorganisms has also shown its sensitivity towards one of the proteins called defensin extracted from fenugreek leaves. Defensin not only inhibited the mycelial spread of *Rhizoctonia solani* but also inhibited spore germination and consequential hyphal growth of *Phaeoisariopsis* [57].

2.8. Gastroprotective Effect. In addition to various kinds of extracts, researchers have tried to extract oil from fenugreek seed which also possesses pharmacological properties. One such property is gastroprotective activity observed in oil extracted from fenugreek seed. The incidence of gastric ulceration, mean ulcer score, and ulcer index were found be significantly decreased in a group of mice subjected to indomethacin to induce ulcer. The decrease in the gastric ulcer can be attributed to phytic acid, saponins, and trigonelline found in the essential oil of fenugreek [58]. One of the studies reveals protective effect of aqueous extract of fenugreek seed against reflux esophagitis (RE) in rats and thus its potential to be used in clinical trial studies [59].

Pharmacological Profile. See Tables 1(a) and 1(b).

3. Discussion

With the onset of industrialization and progressive development, humans' reliability on machine has increased tremendously. But all this has come up with a very heavy cost of pollution and sedentary life style which resulted in rise in incidences of several diseases. Globally, cancer is one such disease that has become a big menace to humans. As per Indian population census data, the rate of mortality due to cancer in India was high and alarming with about 806,000 existing cases by the end of the last century [60]. After cardiovascular diseases, it is the most common cause of deaths among patients in India, responsible for mortality of about 300,000 deaths per year [61]. Lack of treatment and timely diagnosis along with poor availability of preventive methods and awareness are the major reasons for such high

morbidity and mortality associated with cancer. Among the population in India, generally all types of cancers have been studied though the prevalence rate is highly variable. The types of cancer observed in Indian patients include the cancers of skin, lungs, breast, rectum, stomach, prostate, liver, cervix, esophagus, bladder, blood, and mouth. Both internal and external factors seem to be responsible for the cause of cancer. The internal factors are genetic mutations and hormonal, poor immune conditions and external or environmental factors include food habits, industrialization, over growth of population, pollution of air, water, and soil, excessive use of insecticides and pesticides, and many more. Since India is a growing economy, it cannot bear excessive burden of expensive treatment of such diseases and hence needs special attention on preventive natural and herbal treatment methods.

Natural products derived from herbs and microorganisms have played a crucial role in numerous sectors for many centuries, one of them being treatment of diseases and health management. In spite of their widespread usage, some loopholes are there which need to be filled in. The crude extract of the herbs is a complex mixture of many compounds which makes it difficult to unravel the property of a specific compound. Therefore isolating a bioactive compound can act as a starting point for the drug development. Furthermore, emphasis should be given on the safety, efficacy, and toxicity of the preparation derived from medicinal plants. Amount of dose is also an important factor in toxicity and hence should be taken into consideration. As a result, the ultimate effect can be maximized and it will act as a boon for the health care industry. Figure 1 can help us in understanding the process of drug development.

4. Conclusion

In this review, attempts have been made to describe the reported phytochemistry of fenugreek and its pharmacological uses. Because of its medicinal effects, many scientists consider fenugreek as a potential nutraceutical. The clinical uses of fenugreek can be attributed to the rich chemical constituents it possesses. These chemicals make it a strong candidate in every domain as they help in alleviating dependence on synthetic drugs as well as other expensive treatments to cure diseases. Further research and investigations can be done to isolate the bioactive compound from crude extract for drug development as it holds a promising future in the field of natural products to cure diseases. Proper research studies along with planned clinical trials are theneed of the hour so that the natural product from the plant can produce fruitful results for mankind.

Conflict of Interests

The authors declare that there is no conflict of interests regarding the publication of this paper.

References

[1] H. Mukhtar, H. F. Merk, and M. Athar, "Skin chemical carcinogenesis," *Clinics in Dermatology*, vol. 7, no. 3, pp. 1–10, 1989.

[2] C. Heidelberger, "Chemical carcinogenesis, chemotherapy: cancer's continuing core challenges," *Cancer Research*, vol. 30, no. 6, pp. 1549–1569, 1970.

[3] J. W. Flesher and K. L. Sydnor, "Carcinogenicity of derivatives of 7,12-dimethylbenz(a) anthracene," *Cancer Research*, vol. 31, no. 12, pp. 1951–1954, 1971.

[4] L. Vellaichamy, S. Balakrishnan, K. Panjamurthy, S. Manoharan, and L. M. Alias, "Chemopreventive potential of piperine in 7,12-dimethylbenz[a]anthracene-induced skin carcinogenesis in Swiss albino mice," *Environmental Toxicology and Pharmacology*, vol. 28, no. 1, pp. 11–18, 2009.

[5] S. V. Deo, S. Hazarika, N. K. Shukla, S. Kumar, M. Kar, and A. Samaiya, "Surgical management of skin cancers: experience from a regional cancer centre in North India," *Indian Journal of Cancer*, vol. 42, no. 3, pp. 145–150, 2005.

[6] S. Panda, "Non-melanoma skin cancer in India: current scenario," *Indian Journal of Dermatology*, vol. 55, no. 4, pp. 373–378, 2010.

[7] S. K. Wattanapitayakul, L. Chularojmontri, A. Herunsalee, S. Charuchongkolwongse, S. Niumsakul, and J. A. Bauer, "Screening of antioxidants from medicinal plants for cardioprotective effect against doxorubicin toxicity," *Basic & Clinical Pharmacology & Toxicology*, vol. 96, no. 1, pp. 80–87, 2005.

[8] C. Fimognari, M. N. Nüsse, M. Lenzi, D. Sciuscio, G. Cantelli-Forti, and P. Hrelia, "Sulforaphane increases the efficacy of doxorubicin in mouse fibroblasts characterized by p53 mutations," *Mutation Research*, vol. 601, no. 1-2, pp. 92–101, 2006.

[9] A. Uliasz and J. M. Spencer, "Chemoprevention of skin cancer and photoaging," *Clinics in Dermatology*, vol. 22, no. 3, pp. 178–182, 2004.

[10] B. H. Youn and H. J. Yang, "Chemoprevention of skin cancer with dietary phytochemicals," in *Skin Cancer Overview*, Y. Xi, Ed., chapter 8, InTech, 2011.

[11] N. Merina, K. J. Chandra, and K. Joben, "Medicinal plants with potential anticancer activity: a review," *International Research Journal of Pharmacy*, vol. 3, no. 6, pp. 26–30, 2012.

[12] B. B. Li, B. Smith, and M. M. Hossain, "Extraction of phenolics from citrus peels: I. Solvent extraction method," *Separation and Purification Technology*, vol. 48, no. 2, pp. 182–188, 2006.

[13] S. N. Acharya, J. E. Thomas, and S. K. Basu, "Fenugreek: an 'old world' crop for the 'new world'," *Biodiversity*, vol. 7, no. 3-4, pp. 27–30, 2006.

[14] E. Basch, C. Ulbricht, G. Kuo, P. Szapary, and M. Smith, "Therapeutic applications of fenugreek," *Alternative Medicine Review*, vol. 8, no. 1, pp. 20–27, 2003.

[15] M. M. Al-Oqail, N. N. Farshori, E. S. Al-Sheddi, J. Musarrat, A. A. Al-Khedhairy, and M. A. Siddiqui, "*In vitro* cytotoxic activity of seed oil of fenugreek against various cancer cell lines," *Asian Pacific Journal of Cancer Prevention*, vol. 14, no. 3, pp. 1829–1832, 2013.

[16] H. S. Snehlata and D. R. Payal, "Fenugreek (*Trigonella foenum graecum* L.): an overview," *International Journal of Current Pharmaceutical Review and Research*, vol. 2, no. 4, pp. 169–187, 2012.

[17] D. Tiran, "The use of fenugreek for breast feeding women," *Complementary Therapies in Nursing and Midwifery*, vol. 9, no. 3, pp. 155–156, 2003.

[18] E. K. Kalra, "Nutraceutical-definition and introduction," *American Association of Pharmaceutical Sciences*, vol. 5, no. 3, pp. 27–28, 2003.

[19] J. Raju, D. Gupta, A. R. Rao, P. K. Yadava, and N. Z. Baquer, "*Trigonella foenum graecum* (fenugreek) seed powder improves glucose homeostasis in alloxan diabetic rat tissues by reversing the altered glycolytic, gluconeogenic and lipogenic enzymes," *Molecular and Cellular Biochemistry*, vol. 224, no. 1-2, pp. 45–51, 2001.

[20] W.-L. Xue, X.-S. Li, J. Zhang, Y.-H. Liu, Z.-L. Wang, and R.-J. Zhang, "Effect of *Trigonella foenum-graecum* (Fenugreek) extract on blood glucose, blood lipid and hemorheological properties in streptozotocin-induced diabetic rats," *Asia Pacific Journal of Clinical Nutrition*, vol. 16, no. 1, pp. 422–426, 2007.

[21] A. M. Abdelatif, M. Y. Ibrahim, and A. S. Mahmoud, "Antidiabetic effects of fenugreek (*Trigonella foenum-graecum*) seeds in the domestic rabbit (*Oryctolagus cuniculus*)," *Research Journal of Medicinal Plant*, vol. 6, no. 6, pp. 449–455, 2012.

[22] B. K. Ramesh, Yogesh, H. L. Raghavendra, S. M. Kantikar, and K. B. Prakash, "Antidiabetic and histopathological analysis of fenugreek extract on alloxan induced diabetic rats," *International Journal of Drug Development and Research*, vol. 2, no. 2, pp. 356–364, 2010.

[23] R. Moorthy, K. M. Prabhu, and P. S. Murthy, "Anti-hyperglycemic compound (GII) from fenugreek (*Trigonella foenum-graecum linn.*) seeds, its purification and effect in diabetes mellitus," *Indian Journal of Experimental Biology*, vol. 48, no. 11, pp. 1111–1118, 2010.

[24] M. Z. Gad, M. M. El-Sawalhi, M. F. Ismail, and N. D. El-Tanbouly, "Biochemical study of the anti-diabetic action of the egyptian plants fenugreek and balanites," *Molecular and Cellular Biochemistry*, vol. 281, no. 1-2, pp. 173–183, 2006.

[25] R. D. Sharma, "Effect of fenugreek seeds and leaves on blood glucose and serum insulin responses in human subjects," *Nutrition Research*, vol. 6, no. 12, pp. 1353–1364, 1986.

[26] R. D. Sharma, T. C. Raghuram, and N. S. Rao, "Effect of fenugreek seeds on blood glucose and serum lipids in type I diabetes," *European Journal of Clinical Nutrition*, vol. 44, no. 4, pp. 301–306, 1990.

[27] M. Al-Habori and A. Raman, "Antidiabetic and hypocholesterolemic effects of fenugreek," *Phytotherapy Research*, vol. 12, no. 4, pp. 233–242, 1998.

[28] S. Kaviarasan, G. H. Naik, R. Gangabhagirathi, C. V. Anuradha, and K. I. Priyadarsini, "*In vitro* studies on antiradical and

antioxidant activity of (*Trigonella foenum graecum*) fenugreek seeds," *Food Chemistry*, vol. 103, pp. 31–37, 2007.

[29] S. Kaviarasan, R. Sundarapandiyan, and C. V. Anuradha, "Protective action of fenugreek (*Trigonella foenum graecum*) seed polyphenols against alcohol-induced protein and lipid damage in rat liver," *Cell Biology and Toxicology*, vol. 24, no. 5, pp. 391–400, 2008.

[30] V. Thirunavukkarasu, C. V. Anuradha, and P. Viswanathan, "Protective effect of fenugreek (*Trigonella foenum graecum*) seeds in experimental ethanol toxicity," *Phytotherapy Research*, vol. 17, no. 7, pp. 737–743, 2003.

[31] J. Raju, J. M. R. Patlolla, M. V. Swamy, and C. V. Rao, "Diosgenin, a steroid saponin of *Trigonella foenum graecum* (Fenugreek), inhibits azoxymethane-induced aberrant crypt foci formation in F344 rats and induces apoptosis in HT-29 human colon cancer cells," *Cancer Epidemiology Biomarkers and Prevention*, vol. 13, no. 8, pp. 1392–1398, 2004.

[32] G. Francis, Z. Kerem, P. S. Makkar, and K. Becker, "The biological action of saponins in animals systems: a review," *British Journal of Nutrition*, vol. 88, pp. 587–605, 2002.

[33] S. Shishodia and B. B. Aggarwal, "Diosgenin inhibits osteoclastogenesis, invasion, and proliferation through the downregulation of Akt, IκB kinase activation and NF-κB-regulated gene expression," *Oncogene*, vol. 25, no. 10, pp. 1463–1473, 2006.

[34] H. Hibasami, H. Moteki, K. Ishikawa et al., "Protodioscin isolated from fenugreek (*Trigonella foenumgraecum* L.) induces cell death and morphological change indicative of apoptosis in leukemic cell line H-60, but not in gastric cancer cell line KATO III," *International Journal of Molecular Medicine*, vol. 11, no. 1, pp. 23–26, 2003.

[35] R. D. Bhalke, S. J. Anarthe, K. D. Sasane, S. N. Satpute, S. N. Shinde, and V. S. Sangle, "Antinociceptive activity of *Trigonella foenum graecum* leaves and seeds (Fabaceae)," *International Journal of Pharmacy and Technology*, vol. 8, no. 2, pp. 57–59, 2009.

[36] A. Amin, A. Alkaabi, S. Al-Falasi, and S. A. Daoud, "Chemopreventive activities of *Trigonella foenum graecum* (Fenugreek) against breast cancer," *Cell Biology International*, vol. 29, no. 8, pp. 687–694, 2005.

[37] A. Ardelean, G. Pribac, A. Hermenean et al., "Cytostatic and cytotoxic effects of *Trigonella foenum graecum* (fenugreek) seed extract," *Studia Universitatis Vasile Goldiş Seria Ştiinţele Vieţii*, vol. 20, no. 1, pp. 25–29, 2010.

[38] S. Shabbeer, M. Sobolewski, R. K. Anchoori et al., "Fenugreek: a naturally occurring edible spice as an anticancer agent," *Cancer Biology and Therapy*, vol. 8, no. 3, pp. 272–278, 2009.

[39] S. Moalic, B. Liagre, C. Corbière et al., "A plant steroid, diosgenin, induces apoptosis, cell cycle arrest and COX activity in osteosarcoma cells," *FEBS Letters*, vol. 506, no. 3, pp. 225–230, 2001.

[40] S. Chatterjee, M. Kumar, and A. Kumar, "Chemomodulatory effect of *Trigonella foenum graecum* (L.) seed extract on two stage mouse skin carcinogenesis," *Toxicology International*, vol. 19, no. 3, pp. 287–294, 2012.

[41] K. K. Khoja, G. Shafi, T. N. Hasan et al., "Fenugreek, a naturally occurring edible spice, kills MCF-7 human breast cancer cells via an apoptotic pathway," *Asian Pacific Journal of Cancer Prevention*, vol. 12, no. 12, pp. 3299–3304, 2011.

[42] T. Devasena and V. P. Menon, "Fenugreek affects the activity of β-glucuronidase and mucinase in the colon," *Phytotherapy Research*, vol. 17, no. 9, pp. 1088–1091, 2003.

[43] P. C. Singhal, R. K. Gupta, and L. D. Joshi, "Hypocholesterolmic effect of seeds," *Current Science*, vol. 51, pp. 136–137, 1982.

[44] J. M. A. Hannan, B. Rokeya, O. Faruque et al., "Effect of soluble dietary fibre fraction of *Trigonella foenum graecum* on glycemic, insulinemic, lipidemic and platelet aggregation status of Type 2 diabetic model rats," *Journal of Ethnopharmacology*, vol. 88, no. 1, pp. 73–77, 2003.

[45] S. Chatterjee, N. Goswami, P. Bhatnagar, M. Kumar, and A. Kumar, "Antimutagenic and chemopreventive potentialities of fenugreek (*Trigonella foenum graecum*) graecum seed extract," *Oxidants and Antioxidants in Medical Science*, vol. 2, no. 1, pp. 45–53, 2013.

[46] A. Sharma, M. Kumar, M. Chandel, and S. J. Kaur, "Modulation of chromium trioxide induced genotoxicity by methanol extract of leaves of *Trigonella foenum-graecum* L.," *Journal of Experimental and Integrative Medicine*, vol. 29, no. 1, pp. 77–83, 2012.

[47] F. Sharififara, P. Khazaelia, and N. Alli, "Evaluation of anti-inflammatory activity of topical preparations from Fenugreek (*Trigonella foenum graecum* L.) seeds in a cream base," *Iranian Journal of Pharmaceutical Sciences: Summer*, vol. 5, no. 3, pp. 157–162, 2009.

[48] T. Kawabata, M.-Y. Cui, T. Hasegawa, F. Takano, and T. Ohta, "Anti-inflammatory and anti-melanogenic steroidal saponin glycosides from fenugreek (*Trigonella foenum graecum* L.) seeds," *Planta Medica*, vol. 77, no. 7, pp. 705–710, 2011.

[49] J. Raju and R. P. Bird, "Alleviation of hepatic steatosis accompanied by modulation of plasma and liver TNF-α levels by *Trigonella foenum graecum* (fenugreek) seeds in Zucker obese (fa/fa) rats," *International Journal of Obesity*, vol. 30, no. 8, pp. 1298–1307, 2006.

[50] M. Sumanth, P. Kapil, and P. Mihir, "Screening of aqueous extract of *Trigonella foenum graecum* seeds for its antiulcer activity," *International Journal of Research in Pharmaceutical and Biomedical Sciences*, vol. 2, no. 3, pp. 1085–1089, 2011.

[51] A. Ahmadiani, M. Javan, S. Semnanian, E. Barat, and M. Kamalinejad, "Anti-inflammatory and antipyretic effects of *Trigonella foenum-graecum* leaves extract in the rat," *Journal of Ethnopharmacology*, vol. 75, no. 2-3, pp. 283–286, 2001.

[52] V. Ravichandiran and S. Jayakumari, "Comparative study of bioactive fraction of *Trigonella foenum graecum* L. leaf and seed extracts for inflammation," *International Journal of Frontiers in Science and Technology*, vol. 1, no. 2, pp. 128–148, 2013.

[53] B. K. Dash, S. Sultana, and N. Sultana, "Antibacterial activities of methanol and acetone extracts of Fenugreek (*Trigonella foenum*) and Coriander (*Coriandrum sativum*)," *Life Sciences and Medicine Research*, vol. 2011, pp. 1–8, 2011.

[54] A. Sheikhlar, A. R. Alimon, H. M. Daud, C. R. Saad, and H. Shanagi, "Screening of *Morus alba*, *Citrus limon* and *Trigonella foenum-graecum* extracts for antimicrobial properties and phytochemical compounds," *Journal of Biological Sciences*, vol. 13, no. 5, pp. 386–392, 2013.

[55] R. Chandra, V. Dwivedi, K. Shivam, and A. K. Jha, "Detection of antimicrobial activity of *Oscimum sanctum* (Tulsi) & *Trigonella foenum graecum* (Methi) against some selected bacterial & fungal strains," *Research Journal of Pharmaceutical, Biological and Chemical Sciences*, vol. 2, no. 4, pp. 809–813, 2011.

[56] N. Moradi and K. Moradi, "Physiological and pharmaceutical effects of fenugreek (*Trigonella foenum graecum* L.) as a multipurpose and valuable medicinal plant," *Global Journal of Medicinal Plant Research*, vol. 1, no. 2, pp. 199–206, 2013.

[57] S. Olli and P. B. Kirti, "Cloning, characterization and antifungal activity of defensin Tfgd1 from *Trigonella foenum graecum* L.,"

Journal of Biochemistry and Molecular Biology, vol. 39, no. 3, pp. 278–283, 2006.

[58] M. A. Kamel, R. Z. Hamza, N. E. Abdel-Hamid, and F. A. Mahmoud, "Anti-ulcer and gastro protective effects of fenugreek, ginger and peppermint oils in experimentally induced gastric ulcer in rats," *Journal of Chemical and Pharmaceutical Research*, vol. 6, no. 2, pp. 451–468, 2014.

[59] R. Kheirandish, O. Azari, and S. Shojaeepour, "Protective effect of Fenugreek (*Trigonella foenum graecum*) seed extract on experimental reflux esophagitis in rat," *Iranian Journal of Veterinary Surgery*, vol. 8, no. 2, pp. 49–56, 2013.

[60] D. N. Rao and B. Ganesh, "Estimate of cancer incidence in India in 1991," *Indian Journal of Cancer*, vol. 35, no. 1, pp. 10–18, 1998.

[61] F. Bray and B. Møller, "Predicting the future burden of cancer," *Nature Reviews Cancer*, vol. 6, no. 1, pp. 63–74, 2006.

[62] A. Stark and Z. Madar, "The effect of an ethanol extract derived from fenugreek (*Trigonella foenum-graecum*) on bile acid absorption and cholesterol levels in rats," *British Journal of Nutrition*, vol. 69, no. 1, pp. 277–287, 1993.

[63] T. Zia, S. N. Hasnain, and S. K. Hasan, "Evaluation of the oral hypoglycaemic effect of *Trigonella foenum-graecum* L. (methi) in normal mice," *Journal of Ethnopharmacology*, vol. 75, no. 2-3, pp. 191–195, 2001.

[64] B. Bin-Hafeez, R. Haque, S. Parvez, S. Pandey, I. Sayeed, and S. Raisuddin, "Immunomodulatory effects of fenugreek (*Trigonella foenum graecum* L.) extract in mice," *International Immunopharmacology*, vol. 3, no. 2, pp. 257–265, 2003.

[65] N. Subhashini, G. Nagarajan, and S. Kavimani, "Anti-inflammatory and *in vitro* antioxidant property of *Trigonella foenum graecum* seeds," *Journal of Pharmacology and Toxicology*, vol. 6, no. 4, pp. 371–380, 2011.

[66] S. A. Sakr, H. A. Mahran, and S. M. Abo-El-Yazid, "Effect of fenugreek seeds extract on cyclophosphamide-induced histomorphometrical, ultrastructural and biochemical changes in testes of albino mice," *Toxicology and Industrial Health*, vol. 28, no. 3, pp. 276–288, 2012.

[67] S. Panda, P. Tahiliani, and A. Kar, "Inhibition of triiodothyronine production by fenugreek seed extract in mice and rats," *Pharmacological Research*, vol. 40, no. 5, pp. 405–409, 1999.

[68] H. A. Lamfon, "Effect of fenugreek seed extract on carbendazim inhibited spermatogenesis in albino rats," *Journal of Applied Pharmaceutical Science*, vol. 2, no. 4, pp. 9–13, 2010.

[69] M. Ayesha, P. Ahmed, V. C. Gupta et al., "A study of antimicrobial activity of few medicinally important herbal single drugs extracted in ethanol, methanol and aqueous solvents," *Pharmacognosy Journal*, vol. 2, no. 10, pp. 351–356, 2010.

[70] M. Al-Habori, A. Raman, M. J. Lawrence, and P. Skett, "*In vitro* effect of fenugreek extracts on intestinal sodium-dependent glucose uptake and hepatic glycogen phosphorylase A," *International Journal of Experimental Diabetes Research*, vol. 2, no. 2, pp. 91–99, 2001.

[71] A. Gupta, R. Gupta, and B. Lal, "Effect of *T. foenum graecum* (fenugreek) seeds on glycemic control and insulin resistance in type 2 diabetes mellitus: a double blind placebo controlled study," *Journal of the Association of Physicians of India*, vol. 49, pp. 1057–1061, 2001.

[72] M. M. Patel and S. Mishra, "A kinetic study for *in-vitro* intestinal uptake of monosaccharide across rat everted gut sacs in the presence of some antidiabetic medicinal plants," *The Internet Journal of Alternative Medicine*, vol. 7, no. 1, pp. 1–7, 2009.

[73] L. Langmead, C. Dawson, C. Hawkins, N. Banna, S. Loo, and D. S. Rampton, "Antioxidant effects of herbal therapies used by patients with inflammatory bowel disease: an in vitro study," *Alimentary Pharmacology and Therapeutics*, vol. 16, no. 2, pp. 197–205, 2002.

2

Biomonitoring with Micronuclei Test in Buccal Cells of Female Farmers and Children Exposed to Pesticides of Maneadero Agricultural Valley, Baja California, Mexico

Idalia Jazmin Castañeda-Yslas,[1] María Evarista Arellano-García,[1] Marco Antonio García-Zarate,[2] Balam Ruíz-Ruíz,[3] María Guadalupe Zavala-Cerna,[4] and Olivia Torres-Bugarín[4]

[1]*Facultad de Ciencias, Universidad Autónoma de Baja California, 22800 Ensenada, BC, Mexico*
[2]*Centro de Investigación Científica y de Educación Superior de Ensenada, 22800 Ensenada, BC, Mexico*
[3]*Escuela de Ciencias de la Salud, Universidad Autónoma de Baja California, 22800 Ensenada, BC, Mexico*
[4]*School of Medicine, Universidad Autónoma de Guadalajara, 44100 Guadalajara, JAL, Mexico*

Correspondence should be addressed to María Guadalupe Zavala-Cerna; g_zavala_78@hotmail.com
and Olivia Torres-Bugarín; oliviatorres@hotmail.com

Academic Editor: Anthony DeCaprio

Feminization of the agricultural labor is common in Mexico; these women and their families are vulnerable to several health risks including genotoxicity. Previous papers have presented contradictory information with respect to indirect exposure to pesticides and DNA damage. We aimed to evaluate the genotoxic effect in buccal mucosa from female farmers and children, working in the agricultural valley of Maneadero, Baja California. Frequencies of micronucleated cells (MNc) and nuclear abnormalities (NA) in 2000 cells were obtained from the buccal mucosa of the study population ($n = 144$), divided in four groups: (1) farmers ($n = 37$), (2) unexposed ($n = 35$), (3) farmers' children ($n = 34$), and (4) unexposed children ($n = 38$). We compared frequencies of MNc and NA and fitted generalized linear models to investigate the interaction between these variables and exposition to pesticides. Differences were found between farmers and unexposed women in MNc ($p < 0.0001$), CC ($p = 0.3376$), and PN ($p < 0.0001$). With respect to exposed children, we found higher significant frequencies in MNc ($p < 0.0001$), LN ($p < 0.0001$), CC ($p < 0.0001$), and PN ($p < 0.004$) when compared to unexposed children. Therefore working as a farmer is a risk for genotoxic damage; more importantly indirectly exposed children were found to have genotoxic damage, which is of concern, since it could aid in future disturbances of their health.

1. Introduction

Health risk associated with different labors is related to contact with corrosive, infectious, carcinogen, cytotoxic, mutagenic, or genotoxic agents. Research around genetic toxicology and risk assessment or workplace exposure is important since exposure to several hazardous agents is common and could aid in health issues; agricultural activity is often associated with exposure to high volumes of pesticides, mainly organochlorines, organophosphorus, carbamates, pyrethroids, and various inorganic compounds, which are used to control pests in the agriculture zone of Baja California, Mexico [1]. Such chemical agents are an important source of soil and water contamination that will have an impact on living organisms' health, including humans. Pesticides can enter the body by three routes: oral and respiratory routes and contact with skin and mucosal tissue. Pesticide exposure can cause acute poisoning with nausea, vomiting, headache, chest pain, eye, skin, and throat irritation and additionally can cause potential long term health effect with allergies, cancer, nervous system damage, birth defects, and infertility [2]. Adverse effects of pesticides depend on the dose, route, and type; since some can have metabolites that accumulate and persist in living organisms, additionally toxic effects of these compounds are associated with malnutrition and dehydration [3]. Furthermore some pesticides have been tested individually by *in vitro* genotoxicity testing methods and considered as potential chemical mutagens [4].

Women that work as farmers in the agricultural valley in Maneadero, Baja California, usually are coming from the south of the country, most of them from indigenous ancestors with scarce education, and most of them are not provided with medical insurance or social security, even though they are continuously exposed to pesticides [5, 6]. Hazardous exposition to pesticides has been previously documented in the valley of Salinas located in Baja California [7].

In Maneadero valley children are indirectly exposed to pesticides through contact with their farmer mothers and the environment, since most of them live less than 500 m from the agricultural areas. Children are especially vulnerable to adverse effects from pesticides, from conception through birth, due to their constant growth and excessive proliferation rate. Furthermore, early in life exposure to pesticides may be particularly detrimental given that children do not have adult level of enzymes to detoxify until after age of 7 [8], especially for organophosphate pesticides. Additionally during this age there is a rapid and formative brain development which can result affected after pesticide exposure if there are genetic variants that result in decreased PON1, an enzyme related to detoxification [9].

Several studies have evaluated pesticides effects in offspring from farmers and described the presence of neurological damage, respiratory affection, birth defects, diabetes, cardiovascular diseases, hormonal problems, and genotoxicity [10–13]. To evaluate genotoxic damage, the methodology frequently used is expensive and complicated and usually involves invasion; opposite to this, the micronuclei test (MN test) performed in buccal mucosa cells is a precise, inexpensive, noninvasive, and easy method for measuring DNA damage and cell death in the oral epithelium not requiring cell cultures [14–17]. Furthermore, an increased frequency of MN is an efficient biomarker used for the diagnosis of genomic instability, since MN presence represents fragments or whole chromosomes that failed to join the nucleus during cell division and are considered excellent markers of genotoxicity [15, 18].

Nuclear abnormalities (NA) are additional biomarkers that can be recognized through the performance of the MN test; these abnormalities can occur during cell differentiation, indicating DNA damage, cytotoxicity, or cell death when observed in high frequencies [19–21]. Such NA can be identified in the cytoplasm or in the nuclei itself; they consist of binucleated cells (BN), lobulated nuclei (LN), karyorrhexis (KR), condensed chromatin (CC), pyknotic nuclei (PN), and karyolysis (KL). Molecular mechanisms that drive the presence of each of these NA are not well understood, neither is their biological significance in terms of cell function.

There has been a clear association between pesticide exposure and genotoxic damage previously; nonetheless most studies did not evaluate genotoxicity through the MN test; we believe that since this is a more practical methodology

especially for children, our results can be replicated to search for genotoxicity in farmers and their children working in different countries, without the requirement of expensive, more elaborated, and invasive techniques [17–19, 21].

The purpose of the present study was to evaluate the genotoxic effect through the MN test and nuclear abnormalities (NA) in buccal mucosal cells of farmers who work at the agricultural valley of Maneadero and children living in close proximity to the fields.

2. Methods

2.1. Ethical Considerations. This study was approved by the research and bioethics committee of Universidad Autonoma de Baja California with registry number 5-031-074-07-001. The study complied with Mexican Research Regulations and the Declaration of Helsinki. Each participant gave their informed consent before sampling.

2.2. Study Population. Study subjects were selected in an intentional nonprobabilistic way, and only after acceptance via informed consent they were included in the study; cases were all encountered, working in the agricultural fields of Maneadero, Baja California, being constantly exposed to several groups of pesticides. Controls were unexposed women selected from a distant population (16 km) in Ensenada, Baja California, who were healthy housewives or black coated workers. We divided the study population into four groups: (1) farmers, (2) unexposed, (3) farmers' children, and (4) unexposed children. Study subjects were interviewed to obtain personal and clinical information according to predesigned questioner, including the following: age, alimentary habits, smoking, alcohol intake, and time of exposure to pesticides. Subjects with history of cancer, radiotherapy, current infections, and dental procedures within the previous month were excluded from the study.

2.3. Cell Collection and Staining. Each participant rinsed their mouth with water to keep it clean and exfoliated buccal mucosal cells were collected through a smear of the inside lining of the subjects' oral mucosa of both cheeks. The smears were directly transferred to slides previously coded and dried at room temperature. Afterwards, these slides were fixed with 80% ethanol for 48 h and stained with acetoorcein for 2 h and fast green for 10 minutes as previously described [15, 19, 21–23].

2.4. MN and NA in Exfoliated Buccal Cells. The cells in the oral mucosa samples were analyzed using a Carl Zeiss IVFL Axiostar Plus microscope with the objective 100x/1.25. The MNC score was quantified manually and blindly by the same observer, for a total of 2000 cells in order to identify both normal cells and abnormal MN or other NA, using the HUMNxl scoring criteria [17–19, 21], briefly described in here: *Normal cells* (NC) with the nucleus are uniformly stained, oval- or circle-shaped, and smaller than the cytoplasm. There is absence of any other structure besides the nucleus that contains DNA; these cells are considered as completely differentiated cells. *Micronucleated cells* (MNc) are characterized by the presence of a main nucleus and smaller structures denominated micronuclei (MN). One MN has circle or oval shape and its length is between 1/3 and 1/16 of the main nucleus; the intensity of the stain, texture, and plane is equal in both structures. MN characteristics are as follows: rounded smooth perimeter suggestive of a membrane, less than a third the diameter of the associated nucleus, but large enough to discern shape and color; staining intensity similar to that of the nucleus; similar texture to that of nucleus; same focal plane as nucleus; and absence of overlap with, or bridge to, the nucleus. *Binucleated cells* (BN) are cells with two main nuclei, and usually both nuclei are in close proximity or even in contact, both with similar shape and stain to a normal nucleus. BN formation seems to be related to interference during the procedures at the end of cell division. Karyorrhexis (KR) is characterized by nuclear chromatin aggregation and fragmented cell membrane, visualized as a denominated nuclear spotted pattern, indicative of nuclear fragmentation which will lead to nuclear disintegration. Condensed chromatin (CC) is when the nuclei look intensively stained, with chromatin aggregates and intact cell membrane, a denominated nuclear spotted or nuclear striated pattern. It is evident that chromatin is aggregated in some nucleus regions, while other areas lack the presence of chromatin. When the condensation is extended, it appears like a fragmented nucleus; these just like karyorrhexis cells end up with nuclear fragmentation, which leads to eventual disintegration of the nucleus. Cells with pyknotic nuclei (PN) have a nucleus diameter of approximately 1/3 of normal nucleus, with high density of nuclear material which is uniformly distributed, but highly stained. Karyolysis (KL) is when the nucleus has complete lack of DNA which probably represents an advanced stage of cellular death. *Nuclear Buds* (NBUDs): the nucleus presents a strong constriction in one extreme, suggestive of nuclear elimination material process by budding formation. The lobule has similar characteristics in morphology to the nucleus but it is smaller (1/3 to 1/4 of the main nucleus).

2.5. Statistical Analysis. For descriptive purposes about age and exposure years results are expressed as mean (standard deviation); indigenous language, education, daily income, time of exposition, smoking, drinking, and diet habits are expressed as percentages; MNc and NA counts are expressed as mean (standard deviation) and reported as the number of occurrences per 2000 cells. Except for age, the distribution of the variables was not able to pass normality test (Shapiro-Wilks test $p > 0.01$); after this and in order to establish inferences about the risk of farmers to develop MNc and NA we used the Mann-Whitney U tests. To analyze factors that can be associated with increased MNc we determined the OR and performed Fisher exact test. A p value of <0.05 was considered to be statistically significant. All statistical analyses were conducted with the Statistical Program GraphPad Prism V5.

3. Results and Discussion

3.1. Demographics and General Characteristics of Study Population. Maneadero valley is located 10 km at the south of Ensenada with parcel extension of 4,200 hectares in

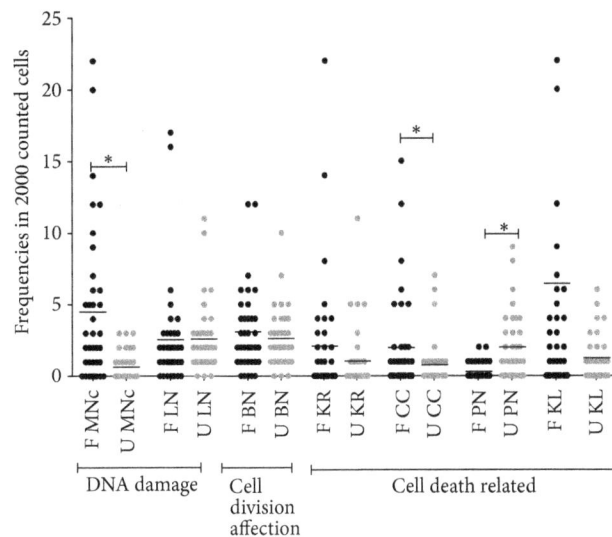

FIGURE 1: Frequencies of micronucleated cells and nuclear abnormalities in farmers and unexposed women. F = farmers; U = unexposed; MNc = micronucleated cells; LN = cells with lobulated nucleus; BN = binucleated cells; KR = karyorrhexis; CC = cells with condensed chromatin; PN = pyknotic cells; and KL = karyolysis. *$p < 0.05$.

which 40% of the obtained products are produced the entire year and 60% are seasonal. Main commercial activity in this region is agriculture and products obtained from this region include tomatoes, potatoes, zucchinis, cilantro, lettuce, onions, grapes, strawberry, olive, asparagus, green tomatillo, barley, alfalfa, rye, and flowers. Different pesticides are used in this zone and are described in Table 1.

In the present study a total of 144 women and their offspring were included; mean age of farmers ($n = 37$) was 35.5 ± 12.4 years, and that of unexposed women ($n = 35$) was 31.9 ± 10.6. For their children, mean age of farmer's children ($n = 34$) was 7.8 ± 3.2 years and that of children from unexposed women ($n = 38$) was 10.3 ± 3.4 years. There was significant difference between ages of exposed and unexposed groups; this is an important consideration since it has been documented that aging is associated with increased frequencies of MN [14]. Farmers' years of exposure were 7.7 ± 8.7, ranging from 1 to 25 years; other characteristics of the examined population are represented in Table 2.

3.2. Frequency of MNc and NA in Farmers. We compared frequencies of MNc and NA between farmers and unexposed women and found significant differences in MNc ($p < 0.0001$), CC ($p = 0.0376$), and PN ($p < 0.0001$) represented in Table 3; more detailed information about dispersion of values is evident in Figure 1; as noticed the dispersion is bigger in the farmers group when compared to unexposed women, except for the nuclear abnormality PN, which is cell death related. Furthermore values obtained from farmers represent the highest frequencies in MNc and NA, when compared to all other groups, except for PN which was more frequently found in the unexposed group.

TABLE 1: Main pesticides used in Baja California, Mexico.

Mechanism of action	Uses	Chemical group	Concentration %, EPA classification[a] (toxicity[b])
		Organophosphate	
		Diazinon	25–90, not likely (IV)
		Azinphos-methyl	35, not likely (I)
Inhibits acetylcholinesterase and is a DNA alkylating agent, classified as carcinogenic, mutagenic, and teratogenic	Insecticide	Malathion	90, evidence (IV)
		Dimethoate	40, C (II)
		Methamidophos	39.6–48.3, E (IB)
	Herbicide	Bensulide	12.5, not likely (III)
		Glyphosate	48, E (IV)
		Carbamate	
	Insecticide	Methomyl	90, E (IB)
Rapid onset; inhibits acetylcholinesterase and other enzymes	Insecticide	Oxamyl	24–42, E (IA)
	Fungicide	Mancozeb	56.4–80, B2 (III)
	Fungicide	Maneb	75–80, B2 (III)
		Organochlorines	
GABA receptor antagonist inhibits Ca^{2+}, Mg^{2+} channels.	Insecticide	Endosulfan	25–48, not likely (I)
		Pyrethroid	
Affects Na^+ channels	Insecticide	Permethrin	34–48, C (IB)
		Bifenthrin	10, C (II)
		Biperidiles	
Interferes in electrons transference and inhibits the reduction of NADP to NADPH during photosynthesis, with superoxide radical formation	Herbicide	Paraquat	24, C (IA)
		Others	
Mechanism of action not clearly stablished	Fungicide	Copper oxychloride	85.0, D (III)
	Fungicide	Chlorothalonil	54, likely (IV)

[a]Chemicals Evaluated for Carcinogenic Potential, Science Information Management Branch, Health Effects Division, Office of Pesticide Program, US Environmental Protection Agency (2006) [35]. A, human carcinogen; B, probable human carcinogen; B1, limited evidence of carcinogenicity from epidemiological studies; B2, sufficient evidence from animal studies; C, possible human carcinogen; D, not classifiable as to human carcinogenicity; E, evidence of noncarcinogenicity for humans; nd, no data available; evidence, suggestive evidence of carcinogenicity, but not sufficient to assess human carcinogenic potential; likely, likely to be carcinogenic to humans; not likely, not likely to be carcinogenic to humans. [b]World Health Organization Classification of Pesticides by Hazard: IA—extremely hazardous; IB—highly hazardous; II—moderately hazardous; III—slightly hazardous [36].

The presence of MNc in the exposed group reflects both genotoxic damage and cell death. With respect to NA, some authors suggest that the presence of binucleated cells (BN) is indicative of genotoxic damage, while pyknosis, condensed chromatin, karyorrhexis, and karyolysis are originated after cytotoxic damage [17].

Even though the clinical significance of NA presence has not been fully elucidated, an honest attempt has been made by previous researchers to try to understand their biological meaning; all of these NA have been associated with the presence of diverse chronic and degenerative diseases, as well as with exposition to hazardous chemicals. In general, the presence of BN is a reflection of failure of cytokinesis due to either defects in formation of the microfilament ring or cell cycle arrest due to malsegregation of chromosomes or telomere dysfunction [17]. The presence of MNc and LN is related to chromosomal instability or DNA damage, while CC, KR, PN, and KL are associated with cell death.

Previous studies in Mexico evaluating genotoxic damage after pesticide exposure were mostly performed in lymphocytes, and significant increased frequencies of MNc were found in exposed subjects [1, 24–26]. Only a few studies have evaluated buccal mucosa cells, and results were contradictory [27, 28]. Internationally, Bolognesi et al. performed a literature review to analyze the association between MN presence and pesticide exposure; they found 18 studies performed in lymphocytes of which 9 had positive results and 9 could not sustain an association; additionally 13 studies were performed in buccal mucosa cells, of which only 5 demonstrated an association between MNc and pesticide exposure [4].

During the present study we were interested in a small subgroup of farmers that were found to have >5 MNc (14 out of 37 women); this subgroup could be at risk of developing health related issues. Because of this, we searched for other factors that could be responsible for higher MNc frequencies, such as alcohol consumption and tobacco use, living in

TABLE 2: Social and demographic characteristics of farmers from the Maneadero valley and unexposed women.

		Farmers ($n = 37$)	Unexposed ($n = 34$)
		%	%
Indigenous language	Yes	27	24
	Not	73	76
Education	None	58	5
	Basic	23	19
	Middle	4	14
	Higher	15	62
Daily income	MXP	$115.5	$189.5
Time of residence in sampled locations	1 to 5 years	30	36
	6 to 10 years	5	9
	10 or more years	61	55
Years of exposition to pesticides	1 to 5 years	51	
	6 to 10 years	22	NA
	10 to 25 years	27	
Smoke	Yes	6	0
	Not	94	100
Alcohol	Yes	6	9
	Not	94	91
Fruit intake (per week)		3.00 ± 2.27	5.09 ± 1.30
Vegetable intake (per week)		2.63 ± 2.67	5.18 ± 1.94
Additional supplements (vitamins)	Yes	24	0
	Not	15	100
	Unanswered	3	—

MXP: Mexican pesos; NA: nonapplicable.

TABLE 3: Frequencies of micronuclei and nuclear abnormalities in farmers from the Maneadero valley and children.

	Women ($n = 71$)			Children ($n = 72$)		
	Farmers ($n = 37$)	Unexposed ($n = 34$)	p value	Farmers ($n = 34$)	Unexposed ($n = 38$)	p value
Age	35.5 ± 12.4	27.7 ± 9.4	0.0047	7.8 ± 3.2	10.3 ± 3.4	0.0111
MNc	4.5 ± 5.5	0.7 ± 0.9	<0.0001	2.5 ± 2.5	0.1 ± 0.2	<0.0001
LN	2.5 ± 3.7	2.6 ± 2.5	0.3512	3.7 ± 5.3	0.7 ± 2.3	<0.0001
BN	3.1 ± 2.9	2.6 ± 2.1	0.7317	2.2 ± 2.0	2.3 ± 2.0	0.2833
KR	2.1 ± 4.4	1.0 ± 2.3	0.2480	3.0 ± 5.1	1.0 ± 1.2	0.9863
CC	2.0 ± 3.4	0.8 ± 1.7	0.0376	2.4 ± 4.2	0.1 ± 0.3	<0.0001
PN	0.3 ± 0.6	2.0 ± 2.3	<0.0001	0.3 ± 0.5	1.4 ± 1.8	0.0043
KL	6.4 ± 12.1	1.2 ± 1.6	0.0558	4.4 ± 6.4	4.3 ± 3.1	0.0617

MNc = micronucleated cells; LN = lobulated nucleus; BN = binucleated cells; PN = pyknotic cells; CC = condensed chromatin; KR = karyorrhexis; KL = karyolysis. Results are presented as mean ± SD from number of occurrences per 2000 counted cells. p value was obtained with the Mann-Whitney U test.

close proximity to the fields (<500 mts^2), time of exposition to pesticides (>5 years), and increased age (>35 years); we found that none of these factors, previously associated with increased MNc frequency, was significantly associated with higher frequencies of MNc; results from this analysis are represented in Table 4.

There are only a few studies that assess the distances where people involved in farming are living; one of these studies was carried out by Lee and colleagues [29] after reviewing agricultural activity in 11 states of the USA; they concluded that farmers as well as people who live in close proximity to the fields (<400 m^2) are at risk of suffering

from the adverse events of pesticides due to contamination of the air, water, and soil. Although a significant association between living in close proximity to the field and high MNc frequencies was not observed in the present study, during sampling we found families living very close to the Maneadero agricultural valley, right outside the fields, which is of concern, since most of these subjects will suffer in the future from several types of affection that have been consistently implicated with pesticides.

When we evaluated frequencies of MNc in association with time of exposure to pesticides, we found that there was a slight increase in MNc frequencies after acute exposition

TABLE 4: Risk factors that could increase MNc frequency in farmers ($n = 37$).

Variable	Samples n (%)	>5 MNc n (%)	<5 MNc n (%)	OR (CI 95%)	p value
Alcohol consumption and tobacco use	5 (14)	3 (8)	2 (5)	5.36 (0.74–38.70)	0.1102
Living in close proximity to fields (<400 m^2)	21 (57)	7 (19)	14 (38)	2.17 (0.46–10.20)	0.4613
Time of exposition to pesticides (>5 years)	18 (49)	5 (14)	13 (34)	1.07 (0.25–4.59)	1.000
Age (>35 years of age)	11 (30)	5 (14)	6 (16)	3.50 (0.75–16.27)	0.1249

MNc: micronucleated cells, CI: confidence interval. Fisher's exact test (two-sided); a p value < 0.05 would have been considered significant.

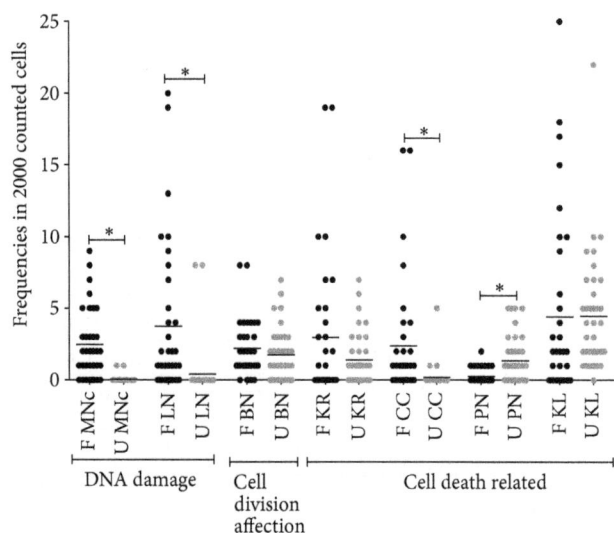

FIGURE 2: Micronuclei and nuclear abnormalities frequencies in indirectly exposed children and unexposed children. MNc = micronucleated cells; LN = cells with lobulated nucleus; BN = binucleated cells; KR = karyorrhexis; CC = cells with condensed chromatin; PN = pyknotic cells; and KL = karyolysis. $^*p$ < 0.05.

<5 years (5.0 ± 6.7) when compared to subjects with >5 years of exposition to pesticides (3.9 ± 4.1). Even though this difference was nonsignificant, this finding could reflect the natural history of pesticide exposure, with an exacerbated response during the acute exposition, and later, during a chronic low level exposure to pesticides, the induction of an adaptive response related to an increase in apoptosis sensitivity and/or a more extended cell cycle delay enables appropriate DNA repair and therefore a decrease in MNc frequency [30].

3.3. Frequency of MNc and NA in Children. With respect to children, the highest frequencies of MNc were found in farmers' children (p < 0.0001), when we analyzed NA and increased frequency of some of them was also evident: LN (p < 0.0001), CC (p < 0.0001), and PN (p = 0.0043). These differences can be found in Table 3 and the dispersion of values in Figure 2. In accordance with our findings, other studies in Mexico and South America with children being exposed to pesticides found increased frequency of MNc, even though NA can differ in results [31–33].

The induction of MNc formation after indirect exposure to pesticides might be due to the fact that farmers' homes are located in close proximity to the fields and additionally by contact with clothes or personal objects impregnated with pesticides. Children are especially susceptible to genotoxic damage due to differences in the mutagens metabolism, distribution, and excretion, when compared to adults [34]. Additionally we should consider, as suggested by Holland et al., that in children cell division dynamics are different when compared to adults, since it has been demonstrated that cellular migration occurs in a different rate influenced by the age and hormonal differences [12].

Our findings suggest that in farmers' children there is a chromosomal instability represented by increased frequencies of MNc and NL; additionally they could suffer from cytotoxicity, since CC represents cells that are no longer transcriptionally active and undergoing apoptosis. The presence of PN represents an irreversible condensation of chromatin; this NA is often found with CC and KR although their biological significance is not clear [17].

In order to clearly identify the genotoxic damage that these children are exposed to, future research is needed, where information about the degree of exposition is registered, including lifestyle, nutrition, and immune function in order to be able to elucidate mechanisms for micronuclei generation during childhood and adult life.

4. Concluding Remarks

Farmers are at risk of developing genotoxic damage secondary to pesticide exposition; more importantly their children who are living in close proximity to the fields demonstrate this genotoxic damage. Children can be easily monitored for genotoxic damage through the MN test; it would be of extreme importance to develop more studies with prospective design in order to obtain information about relative risks and even more important to design strategies directed towards the prevention of future genotoxic damage of the identified population with higher MNc and NA frequencies, given the fact that they are susceptible to health related issues.

Conflict of Interests

The authors declare that there is no conflict of interests regarding the publication of this paper.

References

[1] E. Zuñiga-Violante, E. Arellano-García, L. Camarena-Ojinaga et al., "Daño genético y exposición a plaguicidas en trabajadores agricolas del valle de san quintin, Baja California, Mexico," *Revista de Salud Ambiental*, vol. 12, no. 2, pp. 93–101, 2012.

[2] A. S. Gaikwad, P. Karunamoorthy, S. J. Kondhalkar, M. Ambikapathy, and R. Beerappa, "Assessment of hematological, biochemical effects and genotoxicity among pesticide sprayers in grape garden," *Journal of Occupational Medicine and Toxicology*, vol. 10, p. 11, 2015.

[3] J. A. Patil, A. J. Patil, A. V. Sontakke, and S. P. Govindwar, "Occupational pesticides exposure of sprayers of grape gardens in Western Maharashtra (India): effects on liver and kidney function," *Journal of Basic and Clinical Physiology and Pharmacology*, vol. 20, no. 4, pp. 335–355, 2009.

[4] C. Bolognesi, A. Creus, P. Ostrosky-Wegman, and R. Marcos, "Micronuclei and pesticide exposure," *Mutagenesis*, vol. 26, no. 1, pp. 19–26, 2011.

[5] B. García, "Reestructuración económica y feminización del mercado de trabajo en México," *Papeles de Población*, vol. 27, pp. 45–61, 2001.

[6] L. Camarena Ojinaga, C. von Glascoe, C. Martínez Valdés, and E. Arellano García, "Occupational risks and health: perceptions of indigenous female agricultural workers in northwestern Mexico," *Salud Colectiva*, vol. 9, no. 2, pp. 247–256, 2013.

[7] J. Moreno-Mena, "Los valles agricolas de Baja California: espacios de agricultura para la exportacion," in *Migración Poder y Procesos Rurales*, pp. 66–77, Plaza y Valdés Editores, San Rafael, Mexico, 2008.

[8] K. Huen, K. Harley, J. Brooks et al., "Developmental changes in PON1 enzyme activity in young children and effects of PON1 polymorphisms," *Environmental Health Perspectives*, vol. 117, no. 10, pp. 1632–1638, 2009.

[9] B. Eskenazi, K. Kogut, K. Huen et al., "Organophosphate pesticide exposure, PON1, and neurodevelopment in school-age children from the CHAMACOS study," *Environmental Research*, vol. 134, pp. 149–157, 2014.

[10] B. Eskenazi, J. Chevrier, S. A. Rauch et al., "In utero and childhood polybrominated diphenyl ether (PBDE) exposures and neurodevelopment in the CHAMACOS study," *Environmental Health Perspectives*, vol. 121, no. 2, pp. 257–262, 2013.

[11] J. Chevrier, B. Eskenazi, N. Holland, A. Bradman, and D. B. Barr, "Effects of exposure to polychlorinated biphenyls and organochlorine pesticides on thyroid function during pregnancy," *American Journal of Epidemiology*, vol. 168, no. 3, pp. 298–310, 2008.

[12] N. Holland, A. Fucic, D. F. Merlo, R. Sram, and M. Kirsch-Volders, "Micronuclei in neonates and children: effects of environmental, genetic, demographic and disease variables," *Mutagenesis*, vol. 26, no. 1, pp. 51–56, 2011.

[13] J. T. Efird, E. A. Holly, S. Preston-Martin et al., "Farm-related exposures and childhood brain tumours in seven countries: results from the search international brain tumour study," *Paediatric and Perinatal Epidemiology*, vol. 17, no. 2, pp. 201–211, 2003.

[14] M. Fenech, N. Holland, W. P. Chang, E. Zeiger, and S. Bonassi, "The HUman MicroNucleus Project—an international collaborative study on the use of the micronucleus technique for measuring DNA damage in humans," *Mutation Research/Fundamental and Molecular Mechanisms of Mutagenesis*, vol. 428, no. 1-2, pp. 271–283, 1999.

[15] S. Bonassi, E. Coskun, M. Ceppi et al., "The HUman MicroNucleus project on eXfoLiated buccal cells (HUMN XL): the role of life-style, host factors, occupational exposures, health status, and assay protocol," *Mutation Research/Reviews in Mutation Research*, vol. 728, no. 3, pp. 88–97, 2011.

[16] O. Torres-Bugarin, M. G. Zavala-Cerna, A. Flores-Garcia, and M. L. Ramos-Ibarra, "Procedimientos básicos de la prueba de micronúcleos y anormalidades nucleares en células exfoliadas de mucosa oral," *El Residente*, vol. 1, pp. 4–11, 2013.

[17] C. Bolognesi, S. Knasmueller, A. Nersesyan, P. Thomas, and M. Fenech, "The HUMNxl scoring criteria for different cell types and nuclear anomalies in the buccal micronucleus cytome assay—an update and expanded photogallery," *Mutation Research*, vol. 753, no. 2, pp. 100–113, 2013.

[18] P. E. Tolbert, C. M. Shy, and J. W. Allen, "Micronuclei and other nuclear anomalies in buccal smears: methods development," *Mutation Research/Environmental Mutagenesis and Related Subjects*, vol. 271, no. 1, pp. 69–77, 1992.

[19] P. E. Tolbert, C. M. Shy, and J. W. Allen, "Micronuclei and other nuclear anomalies in buccal smears: a field test in snuff users," *American Journal of Epidemiology*, vol. 134, no. 8, pp. 840–850, 1991.

[20] P. Thomas, N. Holland, C. Bolognesi et al., "Buccal micronucleus cytome assay," *Nature Protocols*, vol. 4, no. 6, pp. 825–837, 2009.

[21] O. Torres-Bugarín, M. G. Zavala-Cerna, A. Nava, A. Flores-García, and M. L. Ramos-Ibarra, "Potential uses, limitations, and basic procedures of micronuclei and nuclear abnormalities in buccal cells," *Disease Markers*, vol. 2014, Article ID 956835, 13 pages, 2014.

[22] O. Torres-Bugarín, R. Covarrubias-Bugarín, A. L. Zamora-Perez, B. M. G. Torres-Mendoza, M. García-Ulloa, and F. G. Martínez-Sandoval, "Anabolic androgenic steroids induce micronuclei in bucca mucosa cells of bodybuilders," *British Journal of Sports Medicine*, vol. 41, no. 9, pp. 592–596, 2007.

[23] O. Torres-Bugarín, A. Ventura-Aguilar, A. Zamora-Perez et al., "Evaluation of cisplatin + 5-FU, carboplatin + 5-FU, and ifosfamide + epirubicine regimens using the micronuclei test and nuclear abnormalities in the buccal mucosa," *Mutation Research—Genetic Toxicology and Environmental Mutagenesis*, vol. 539, no. 1-2, pp. 177–186, 2003.

[24] S. Gomez-Arroyo, Y. Diaz-Sanchez, M. A. Meneses-Perez et al., "Cytogenetic biomonitoring in a Mexican floriculture worker group exposed to pesticides," *Mutation Research*, vol. 466, no. 1, pp. 117–124, 2000.

[25] M. C. O. Arellano, C. Von-Glascoe, B. Ruiz, E. Zuñiga, and T. Monraño, "Daño genotóxico en mujeres y hombres expuestos en cuatro localidades de Baja California," in *Instituto Nacional de Ecología. Secretaría de Medio Ambiente y Recursos Naturales (SEMARNAT)*, pp. 95–113, Género, Ambiente y Contaminación por Sustancias Químicas, 2012.

[26] T. Montaño-Soto, E. Arellano-García, L. Camarena-Ojinaga et al., "Genotoxic biomonitoring and exposure to pesticides in women laborers at maneadero valley in Baja California, Mexico," *International Journal of Applied and Natural Sciences*, vol. 3, no. 2, pp. 89–96, 2014.

[27] C. Martinez-Valenzuela and S. Gomez-Arroyo, "Riesgo genotóxico por exposición a plaguicidas en trabajadores agrícolas," *La Revista Internacional de Contaminación Ambiental*, vol. 23, pp. 185–200, 2007.

[28] R. Castro, V. Ramírez, and P. Cuenca, "Micronúcleos y otras anormalidades nucleares en el epitelio oral de mujeres expuestas

ocupacionalmente a plaguicidas," *Revista de Biología Tropical*, vol. 1, no. 2, pp. 611–621, 2014.

[29] S.-J. Lee, L. Mehler, J. Beckman et al., "Acute pesticide illnesses associated with off-target pesticide drift from agricultural applications: 11 states, 1998–2006," *Environmental Health Perspectives*, vol. 119, no. 8, pp. 1162–1169, 2011.

[30] M. Kirsch-Volders and M. Fenech, "Inclusion of micronuclei in non-divided mononuclear lymphocytes and necrosis/apoptosis may provide a more comprehensive cytokinesis block micronucleus assay for biomonitoring purposes," *Mutagenesis*, vol. 16, no. 1, pp. 51–58, 2001.

[31] L. S. Benitez, M. L. Macchi, V. Fernández et al., *Daño Celular en una Población Infantil Potencialmente Expuesta a Pesticidas*, vol. 131, BASE Investigaciones Sociales, 2010.

[32] S. Gómez-Arroyo, C. Martínez-Valenzuela, S. Calvo-González et al., "Assessing the genotoxic risk for Mexican children who are in residential proximity to agricultural areas with intense aerial pesticide applications," *Revista Internacional de Contaminacion Ambiental*, vol. 29, no. 3, pp. 217–225, 2013.

[33] N. Bernardi, N. Gentile, F. Mañas, Á. Méndez, N. Gorla, and D. Aiassa, "Assessment of the level of damage to the genetic material of children exposed to pesticides in the province of Cordoba," *Archivos Latino-Americanos de Pediatría*, vol. 113, no. 2, pp. 126–131, 2015.

[34] M. Neri, A. Fucic, L. E. Knudsen, C. Lando, F. Merlo, and S. Bonassi, "Micronuclei frequency in children exposed to environmental mutagens: a review," *Mutation Research—Reviews in Mutation Research*, vol. 544, no. 2-3, pp. 243–254, 2003.

[35] Health Effects Division, Office of Pesticide Programs, and US Environmental Protection Agency, "Chemicals Evaluated for Carcinogenic Potential, Science Information Management Branch," 2006, http://www.fluoridealert.org/wp-content/pesticides/pesticides.cancer.potential.2006.pdf.

[36] WHO, *World Health Organization Classification of Pesticides by Hazard*, World Health Organization, Geneva, Switzerland, 2010.

3

Chronic Exposure to Arsenic in Drinking Water Causes Alterations in Locomotor Activity and Decreases Striatal mRNA for the D2 Dopamine Receptor in CD1 Male Mice

Claudia Leticia Moreno Ávila, Jorge H. Limón-Pacheco, Magda Giordano, and Verónica M. Rodríguez

Departamento de Neurobiología Conductual y Cognitiva, Instituto de Neurobiología, Universidad Nacional Autónoma de México, Boulevard Juriquilla 3001, 76230 Querétaro, QRO, Mexico

Correspondence should be addressed to Verónica M. Rodríguez; vermire@yahoo.com

Academic Editor: Brad Upham

Arsenic exposure has been associated with sensory, motor, memory, and learning alterations in humans and alterations in locomotor activity, behavioral tasks, and neurotransmitters systems in rodents. In this study, CD1 mice were exposed to 0.5 or 5.0 mg As/L of drinking water for 6 months. Locomotor activity, aggression, interspecific behavior and physical appearance, monoamines levels, and expression of the messenger for dopamine receptors D1 and D2 were assessed. Arsenic exposure produced hypoactivity at six months and other behaviors such as rearing and on-wall rearing and barbering showed both increases and decreases. No alterations on aggressive behavior or monoamines levels in striatum or frontal cortex were observed. A significant decrease in the expression of mRNA for D2 receptors was found in striatum of mice exposed to 5.0 mg As/L. This study provides evidence for the use of dopamine receptor D2 as potential target of arsenic toxicity in the dopaminergic system.

1. Introduction

Arsenic (As) is a natural occurring element widely found in the environment, due to its ubiquitous presence in the earth's crust and to its high usage in several anthropogenic activities such as fabrication of computer chips, glass manufacturing, mining waste, agrochemicals (insecticides, rodenticides, herbicides, plant desiccants, and fertilizers), and wood preservatives [1]. The main route of As exposure is via drinking water (DW), which in several regions of the world exceeds the World Health Organization (WHO) permitted level of 0.010 mg As/L. For example, levels as high as 0.2 mg As/L were found in Argentina [2], 2.97 mg As/L in Bangladesh [3], 0.5 mg As/L in Chile [4], 0.4 mg As/L in Mexico [5], and 0.8 mg As/L in Taiwan [6]. There are also reports of accidental exposure through drinks or foods tainted with As. An example of such events was the ingestion of contaminated milk powder produced by the Morinaga Milk Industry Company in Japan during the 1950s, when infants were exposed to doses of 4.2–7.0 mg As/L of milk [7].

Ingestion of DW contaminated with As is associated with several adverse effects on human health [8–15]. Effects on the central nervous system include memory deficits [11, 16], reduced intellectual functions (decreased verbal IQ) [12], epilepsy, minimal brain damage, mental retardation, and IQ less than 85 [7], and mood changes including depression, easy irritability, anxiety disorder, or lack of concentration [17].

Behavioral studies have primarily used the rat model of As exposure and have found that locomotor activity is altered depending on the dose of As administered, route and time of exposure, and specific strain used [18]. Studies using the mouse as a model have also found changes in locomotor activity, both increases and decreases, related to dose, duration of exposure, strain, and gender [19, 20]. These and other studies also assessed the effects of As exposure on the dopaminergic system and have found that As exposure either reduced striatal levels of the dopamine (DA) metabolites [19], increased DA content in striatal homogenates [21], or decreased striatal DA in female mice in a dose-dependent manner [20].

One of the advantages of using mice instead of rats is that mouse red blood cells do not sequester As by binding it to the sulfhydryl groups of hemoglobin as the rat does, which explains why the rat is not a good toxicokinetic model of As exposure [22–24]. In addition, the availability of transgenic mouse strains could contribute to understanding the mechanisms of action of As. However, mouse strains show substantial behavioral variability, and as Adams et al. suggest [25] the choice of host strain in transgenic research must be made carefully. Outbred strains like the CD1 are robust, easy to breed, and resistant to diseases, mimic genetically heterogenous populations [25], and exhibit a more variable phenotype [26]. In contrast, "inbred strains like the C57Bl/6J are considered to be nearly homozygous (genetically identical) and are usually chosen for their relatively restricted genetic variability and reliable behavioral profile" [26]. Also, earlier studies suggest that the C57Bl/6 strain may have lowered dopaminergic function, as evidenced by its increased susceptibility to the effects of haloperidol and to the neurotoxin MPTP [27].

Previous studies from our laboratory and from others have demonstrated that the dopaminergic system is a target of As toxicity altering its functions at several levels of regulation including DA synthesis and signaling. These include disturbance in DA levels in a gender-specific manner, accompanied by changes in mRNA expression of genes related to dopaminergic and antioxidant systems in the striatum of different rodent models such as DA receptors D1, D2, D3, and D4 [20, 28, 29]. According to those studies DA receptors seem to be good candidates to evaluate alterations caused by chronic ingestion of As via drinking water in the dopaminergic system in rodents. To support its potential use as biomarkers, the expression of DA receptors D1a and D2 was evaluated together with the locomotor activity and aggressive behavior, levels of DA, and its metabolites in striatal tissue of CD1 mice exposed to 0.5 and 5.0 mg As/L of DW for six months. Then, we compared the results with those of previous studies using C57BL/6J mice, an inbred strain, and those described in rats, and discuss the potential use of DA receptor D2 as a potential biomarker of As toxicity in the dopaminergic system.

2. Experimental Design

2.1. Animals. Forty-five, two-month-old male CD1 mice were acquired from the vivarium of the Instituto de Neurobiología, UNAM and kept under a 12-hour inverted dark/light cycle (lights on at 20:00) with constant temperature (23 ± 2°C). Experiments were carried out according to the Norma Oficial Mexicana de la Secretaría de Agricultura (SAGARPA NOM-062-ZOO-1999), which complies with the guidelines in the Institutional Animal Care and Use Committee Guidebook (NIH Publication 80-23, Bethesda, MD, USA, 1996), and were approved by the local committee on Bioethics.

2.2. Chemicals. Sodium arsenite (99.6% purity) was acquired from J.T. Baker (Phillipsburg, NJ, USA); reagents for high

performance liquid chromatography with electrochemical detection (HPLC-ED) were acquired from Sigma-Aldrich (St. Louis, MO, USA), unless otherwise is stated. Of the inorganic As compounds, sodium arsenite is one of the most common trivalent compounds used in toxicological studies and resembles the presence of this form in wells of contaminated areas.

2.3. Materials and Methods. Fifteen mice per group received 0.5 or 5.0 mg As/L of DW for six months. The As-containing DW solutions were prepared daily from a 1000 mg As/L solution in deionized water, and the pH was adjusted to 7.0 in order to minimize the oxidation of arsenite to arsenate. Control groups received deionized water adjusted to pH = 7.0. Three separate groups of animals were used, and intermediate doses of As were chosen based on the results obtained in mice [20] or rats [30–32]. In order to achieve comparable levels of As in humans, mice have to be exposed to greater concentrations than those found in the environment. In this respect, mice metabolize and clear As and its metabolites from tissues more efficiently than humans (for more details, see [33]).

Body weight and the presence of body lesions and those not classified as lesions (whisker trimming, hair barbering, and disheveled coat) were evaluated weekly throughout the duration of the experiment. The locomotor activity, the presence of aggressive behaviors, and typical rodent behaviors such as rearing and grooming were evaluated monthly from the first to the sixth month of As exposure. After six months of exposure, mice were euthanized by cervical decapitation, brain was extracted, and both left and right striatum and frontal cortex were dissected on ice and frozen at −80°C; striatum and frontal cortex from one hemisphere were used to measure DA and serotonin and their metabolites, while the striatum from the other hemisphere was used to evaluate the expression of the genes for DA receptors (*Drd1* and *Drd2*).

2.4. Behavioral Tests

2.4.1. Spontaneous Locomotor Activity. Once a month mice were individually placed in an automated locomotor activity chamber equipped with horizontal and vertical infrared beams (Accuscan Instruments Inc., Columbus, OH, USA). Locomotor activity was recorded, and data were collected over the course of a 25-hour session. The first hour, which is usually when the highest activity is displayed, was evaluated separately, form the remaining 24 h (12 h light : 12 h dark). The locomotor activity parameters evaluated included total distance (the distance in cm traveled by the animal) and horizontal activity (activity that blocks sensors on the chamber's horizontal axis). Food and water were available *ad libitum* during this session.

2.4.2. On- and Off-Wall Rearing Behavior. Mice were placed individually in an acrylic box and were allowed to explore this box for 8 minutes. After this acclimation period, stereotyped behaviors such as on- and off-wall rearing were recorded. Rearing behavior was defined as any vertical movement that raised the mouse forepaws above the height of the mouse standing on four paws. On-wall rearing was recorded when mice touched the wall anytime during the incorporation.

TABLE 1: Primer sets used for SYBR green-based qPCR analysis of dopamine receptors.

Target	Abbreviation	Primer	Primer sequence	Primer length (nt)	Amplicon size (bp)	Gene bank accession number
Dopamine receptor D1a	Drd1	Forward	5′ CAG TCC ATG CCA AGA ATT GCC AGA 3′	24	255	NM_010076.3
		Reverse	5′ AAT CGA TGC AGA ATG GCT GGG TCT 3′	24		
Dopamine receptor D2	Drd2	Forward	5′ TGA ACA GGC GGA GAA TGG 3′	18	70	NM_010077.2
		Reverse	5′ CTG GTG CTT GAC AGC ATC TC 3′	20		
Beta-actin	Bact	Forward	5′ CCA GGT CAT CAC TAT TGG CAA CGA G 3′	25	141	NM_007393.3
		Reverse	5′ TCT TTA CGG ATG TCA ACG TCA CAC T 3′	25		

nt: nucleotide, bp: base pair.

Rearing behavior had to be maintained for at least five seconds to be recorded. These criteria were based on a modification of the protocol by Russell et al. [34]. The analysis of these behaviors was done using the Observer software (version 3.0, Noldus, Wageningen, Netherlands), and the cumulative time spent on these behaviors was evaluated.

2.4.3. Aggression Test (Intruder-Resident Paradigm). In order to evaluate the presence of antagonist behavior due to As exposure, we followed a modified version of the resident-intruder test by Koolhaas et al. [35]. Briefly, a single mouse of each experimental group (control, 0.5 or 5.0 mg As/L in DW) remained in a neutral cage for 300 s; subsequently a male intruder was introduced into the resident's cage for 300 s. The confrontations were terminated after the first attack-bite; additional 300 s were added if no attack-bite by the resident occurred. The behavioral repertoire was videotaped and later analyzed using the Observer software. The events evaluated were latency to first attack, frequency and total duration of attacks, boxing, and tail rattling [36]. Encounters that included biting and that were at least three seconds apart were considered an attack [37].

2.5. Determination of DA, Serotonin, and Their Metabolites. DA, its metabolites 3,4-dihydroxyphenylacetic acid (DOPAC) and homovanillic acid (HVA), and serotonin (5-HT) were measured using HPLC with electrochemical detection as described elsewhere [20]. Briefly, a portion of striatum or frontal cortex was collected separately and disrupted by sonication in a solution of 0.1 M perchloric acid. The resulting homogenates were centrifuged at 10,000 ×g for 40 min, supernatants were frozen at −80°C, and pellets were digested in 0.5 M NaOH for protein determination by the Bradford technique. Briefly, a PerkinElmer pump series 200 (Waltham, MA, USA) was joined to a chromatographic column (Grace Davison Discovery Sciences, Deerfield, IL, USA) packed with a catecholamine adsorbosphere (3 μm particle size, 100 × 4.8 mm). An electrochemical detector bioanalytical system, LC-4C (West Lafayette, IN, USA) was coupled to the system, the amperometric potential was set at 850 mV relative to the silver/silver chloride electrode, and the sensitivity of the detector was set at 5 (striatum) or 2 (frontal cortex) ηA. The mobile phase consisted of 0.1 M monobasic phosphate solution containing 0.5 mM sodium octyl sulfate, 0.03 mM

EDTA, and 13% (vol/vol) methanol. The results were analyzed with the TotalChrom Navigator version 6.3.1.0504 (PerkinElmer) and are expressed in ng/mg tissue protein. DA turnover was expressed as the ratio of DOPAC to DA, an index of DA utilization.

2.6. Analysis of mRNA Expression of DA Receptors by qPCR. Total RNA was isolated from striatum tissue samples using the TRIzol reagent (Invitrogen, Carlsbad, CA) and treated with RNase-free DNase (Promega, Madison, WI) to remove potential contamination by genomic DNA. RNA purity was determined from the ratio of absorbance readings at 260/280 nm with a NanoDrop ND-1000 (Thermo Scientific, Wilmington, DE, USA). Total RNA (0.5 μg) from each sample was used for the cDNA synthesis using the M-MLV reverse transcriptase (Promega), Oligo dT (Invitrogen), and random hexamers primers following the manufacturer's instructions. Real-time PCR was performed with a LightCycler instrument version 1.5 (Roche, Mannheim, Germany) using the Light-Cycler FastStart DNA master SYBR Green I (Roche). The primers used in this experiment (Table 1) corresponded to DA receptor 1a (Drd1), DA receptor 2 (Drd2), and beta-actin (Bact). The cDNA samples previously prepared were diluted 1 : 5 and used as the template for the real-time PCR. Thermal conditions were 10 min denaturation, followed by 50 cycles at 95°C for 1 sec, 60°C for 10 sec, and 72°C for 12 sec. PCR amplifications were repeated in triplicate. At the end of each PCR reaction, a melting curve analysis was performed to confirm that a single product had been amplified. In addition, the expected size of the amplicon was verified by sequencing and electrophoresis of the PCR product in 1% EtBr agarose gels. Housekeeping gene β-actin was used as endogenous control of expression and the relative expression of the transcripts of each DA receptor of interest was calculated by using the $2^{-\Delta\Delta Ct}$ method [38].

2.7. Statistical Analysis. For the body weight gain and locomotor activity recorded for 24 hours, we used a two-way analysis of variance with repeated-measures in one factor (RMANOVA; treatment × time of day) followed by Fisher's LSD test in the case of significant main effects or interactions. Levels of 5-HT, DA, and their metabolites in brain regions were analyzed using one-way ANOVA with post hoc assessment in the event of main effects of treatment (Fisher's LSD tests). Data from aggression test, Drd1 and Drd2 mRNA

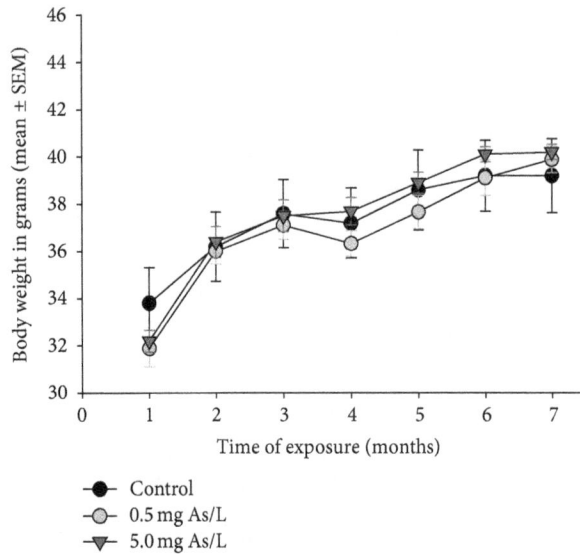

FIGURE 1: Growth rate of mice exposed to 0.5 or 5.0 mg As/L of drinking water for six months.

levels, were analyzed using the Kruskall-Wallis test with Mann-Whitney U test as post hoc assessment in the event of main effects of treatment. The presence of body lesions was evaluated using chi-square test. Statistical significance was defined as $p < 0.05$

3. Results

3.1. Body Weight and General Appearance. Mice exposed to 0.5 or 5.0 mg As/L of DW did not differ from control group in body weight evaluated monthly, although all groups gained weight overtime as shown in Figure 1.

Regarding the general appearance, As treatment did not increase the number of body lesions, or those changes not classified as lesions (whisker trimming, hair barbering, or disheveled coat) on mice treated with As. Mice treated with 5.0 mg As/L showed transitory increases in hair barbering at months 1 and 2 of As treatment, in comparison to control group.

3.2. Spontaneous Locomotor Activity. During the initial 1 h of recording, no significant effects of As treatment or interaction were found on horizontal activity, total distance, or stereotypy counts (data not shown).

No treatment effects were found from months 1 to 5 on 24-hour locomotor activity. Locomotor activity (total distance and horizontal activity) was significantly different between treated and control animals at six months of As exposure. For total distance, there was only a significant interaction ($F(14, 203) = 2.09$, $p = 0.0138$) and sample effects ($F(7, 203) = 20.89$, $p < 0.0001$). Post hoc analyses showed a biphasic effect of As treatment; mice treated with 5.0 mg As/L travelled less distance during the dark phase of the cycle but travelled more distance in comparison to the control group during the light phase of the dark-light cycle

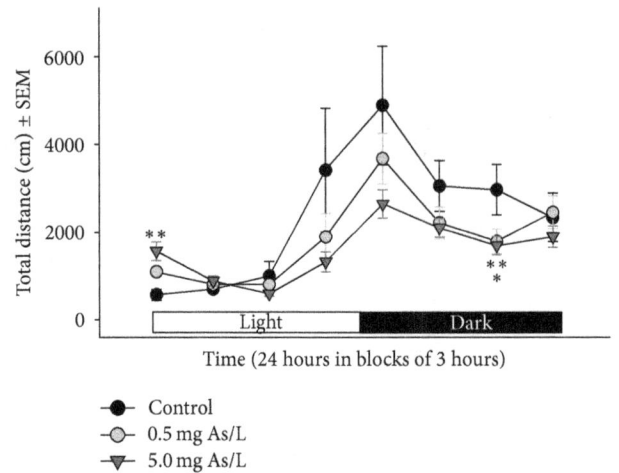

(a)

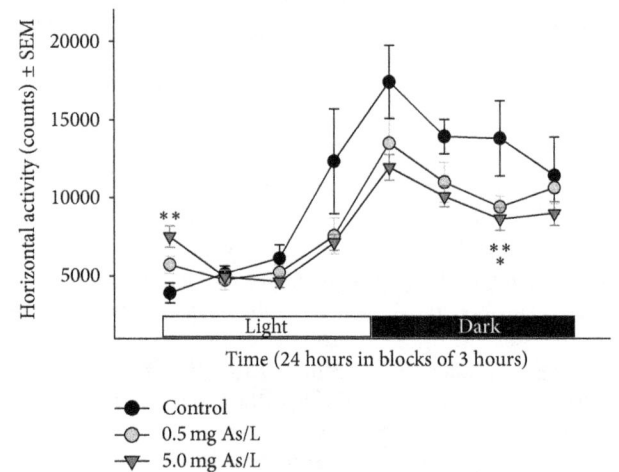

(b)

FIGURE 2: Effect of the chronic exposure to 0.5 or 5.0 mg As/L of drinking water on total distance (a) and horizontal activity (b). Spontaneous locomotor activity was recorded over the course of a 24-hour dark/light cycle at six months of As exposure. * and ** denote differences between the 0.5 and 5.0 mg As/L groups, respectively, from the control group, $p < 0.05$.

as shown in Figure 2. Regarding the horizontal activity, there was a significant effect of treatment ($F(2, 29) = 6.683$, $p = 0.0041$), sample ($F(7, 203) = 28.736$, $p < 0.0001$), and interaction ($F(14, 203) = 2.023$, $p = 0.0177$). Post hoc analyses showed similar changes in both groups exposed to As, that is, hyperactivity at the beginning of the light part of the cycle and hypoactivity during the dark part of the cycle, as shown in Figure 2.

3.3. On- and Off-Wall Rearing Behavior. Regarding the on-wall rearing behavior, a significant effect of As treatment was observed at two and three months ($H(2, 33) = 6.166$–8.569, $p < 0.05$) of As exposure. Post hoc analyses showed a higher frequency of on-wall rearing in the group treated with 5.0 mg As/L in comparison to the control group, on the second month of As exposure ($U = 22.500$, $p = 0.0326$).

TABLE 2: On- and off-wall rearing behavior.

Time of exposure	Control	0.5 mg As/L	5.0 mg As/L
	On-wall rearing		
Month 1	2.50 (6.00)	3.50 (8.00)	7.00 (7.50)
Month 2	2.50 (3.50)	1.50 (5.50)	**5.00 (5.50)***
Month 3	5.00 (6.00)	**0 (2.50)***	7.00 (11.50)
Month 4	5.00 (7.50)	5.50 (7.50)	4.00 (3.50)
Month 5	0.50 (7.50)	5.50 (10.50)	7.00 (7.75)
Month 6	3.00 (9.00)	3.50 (4.00)	6.00 (10.25)
	Off-wall rearing		
Month 1	1.50 (7.00)	3.00 (2.50)	**10.00 (6.75)***
Month 2	7.50 (7.50)	1.00 (4.50)	8.00 (9.75)
Month 3	4.00 (6.50)	0.50 (3.50)	8.00 (11.25)
Month 4	3.50 (7.50)	1.50 (6.00)	4.00 (5.00)
Month 5	3.00 (8.00)	2.50 (8.50)	3.00 (9.75)
Month 6	4.00 (9.00)	3.00 (4.00)	8.00 (11.00)

Values are median and interquartile range of cumulative spent time on these behaviors ($n = 7$–13).
* denotes differences from the control group, $p < 0.05$.

On the third month of As treatment, the group exposed to 0.5 mg As/L ($U = 22.000$, $p = 0.0449$) showed less frequency of on-wall rearing compared to the control group. The subsequent analyses at 4, 5, or 6 months of As treatment did not reveal differences in the frequency of this behavior (Table 2).

For the off-wall rearing behavior, there was a significant group effect ($H(2, 33) = 10.158$, $p = 0.0062$) at one month of As exposure. Post hoc analyses showed that the group treated with 5.0 mg As/L displayed this behavior more than the control group ($U = 22.000$, $p = 0.0298$). Subsequent analyses at 2, 3, 4, 5, or 6 months of As treatment did not show any alteration in this behavior (Table 2).

3.4. Aggression Test (Intruder-Resident Paradigm). At two months of exposure the group exposed to 5.0 mg As/L has shown decreases in the latency to attack and in tail rattling in comparison to control group. No more differences were found between As-treated and control group in the latency to first attack, frequency and total duration of attacks, boxing, and tail rattling during the six months of As treatment (Table 3).

3.5. Determination of DA and Its Metabolites and 5-HT. No significant As effects on the content of monoamines and their metabolites were found on striatum and frontal cortex of mice sacrificed after six months of As treatment, as shown in Table 4.

3.6. mRNA Levels of DA Receptors. Exposure to As caused a significant downregulation of *Drd2* mRNA in the striatum ($H = (2, N = 24) = 6.180$, $p = 0.045$) at the dose of 5.0 mg As/L (U's = 8, $p = 0.011$) (Figure 3). In contrast, no significant changes on *Drd1* mRNA expression were observed in the striatum of groups treated with As in comparison to the control group ($H = (2, N = 24) = 0.261$, $p = 0.878$).

TABLE 3: Aggression test (intruder-resident paradigm).

Time of exposure	Control	0.5 mg As/L	5.0 mg As/L
	Latency to first attack (time)		
Month 1	382.25 (554.90)	600.00 (487.60)	600.00 (378.02)
Month 2	154.80 (538.55)	446.10 (447.10)	**600.00 (0.00)**
Month 3	178.75 (401.35)	600.00 (473.85)	600.00 (216.30)
Month 4	600.00 (283.00)	450.00 (503.90)	516.20 (371.32)
Month 5	600.00 (424.50)	600.00 (311.40)	600.00 (297.10)
Month 6	600.00 (294.55)	600.00 (419.75)	600.00 (133.27)
	Frequency (counts)		
Month 1	1.00 (2.50)	0 (1.50)	0 (1.00)
Month 2	1.00 (2.00)	0.50 (2.50)	0 (0)
Month 3	1.00 (0.50)	0 (1.50)	0 (1.00)
Month 4	0 (0.50)	0.50 (1.50)	1.00 (1.00)
Month 5	0 (1.50)	0 (1.00)	0 (1.25)
Month 6	0 (0.50)	0 (1.0)	0 (1.25)
	Total duration of attacks (time)		
Month 1	23.80 (1213.15)	0 (22.85)	0 (22.49)
Month 2	32.20 (46.20)	6.70 (99.50)	0 (0)
Month 3	11.75 (30.25)	0 (57.40)	0 (5.24)
Month 4	0 (6.80)	5.6 (22.60)	0.76 (22.37)
Month 5	0 (12.25)	0 (11.45)	0 (13.40)
Month 6	0 (8.30)	0 (11.35)	0 (3.17)
	Boxing (counts)		
Month 1	0 (0)	0 (2.00)	0 (1.00)
Month 2	0 (1.00)	0 (0.50)	0 (0)
Month 3	0.50 (1.00)	0 (1.00)	0 (0.25)
Month 4	0 (0)	0 (0.50)	0 (1.25)
Month 5	0 (0)	0.50 (1.00)	0 (0.25)
Month 6	0 (1.50)	0.50 (1.50)	0 (0)
	Tail rattling (counts)		
Month 1	0 (9.00)	0 (3.00)	0 (1.00)
Month 2	1.00 (9.50)	0.50 (4.00)	**0 (0)**
Month 3	4.50 (10.00)	0 (2.50)	0 (0.50)
Month 4	0 (1.50)	1.00 (3.00)	1.00 (3.25)
Month 5	0 (11.00)	0.50 (4.00)	0 (2.75)
Month 6	0 (8.00)	1.50 (9.50)	0 (2.00)

Values are median and interquartile range ($n = 7$–13).

4. Discussion

From a toxicological perspective, there is considerable interest in finding essential biomarkers to evaluate the effects of environmental toxicants in the nervous system and in the dopaminergic neurotransmission system in particular. We found that chronic As exposure may alter targets other than the tissue levels of monoamines. In this regard, we found that chronic As exposure causes hypoactivity accompanied by decreases in mRNA expression of the *Drd2* receptor; we also found transitory and biphasic alterations on the on- and off-wall rearing behavior which could be due to transient alterations in the monoaminergic systems.

TABLE 4: Regional brain content of monoamines (ng/mg protein) in striatum and frontal cortex of mice exposed to 0.5 or 5.0 mg As/L of drinking water for six months.

Brain region	Treatment	DA	DOPAC	HVA	5-HT	5-HIAA	DOPAC/DA
	Control	80.60 ± 13.00	5.29 ± 1.56	4.22 ± 0.95	5.71 ± 1.26	2.87 ± 0.57	0.06 ± 0.01
Striatum	0.5 mg As/L	91.22 ± 19.37	2.86 ± 0.04	4.20 ± 0.70	5.19 ± 1.36	2.58 ± 0.48	0.06 ± 0.01
	5.0 mg As/L	55.70 ± 6.83	3.70 ± 0.83	3.35 ± 0.46	5.80 ± 1.05	2.29 ± 0.35	0.07 ± 0.01
	Control	1.17 ± 0.31	ND	ND	4.37 ± 1.51	2.42 ± 0.72	—
Frontal cortex	0.5 mg As/L	1.86 ± 0.39	ND	ND	6.18 ± 1.16	1.88 ± 0.42	—
	5.0 mg As/L	1.53 ± 0.23	ND	ND	8.06 ± 2.17	2.22 ± 0.35	—

Values are mean ± SEM (n = 7–13) and are reported as ng/mg of protein. DA, dopamine; DOPAC, 3,4-dihydroxyphenylacetic acid; HVA, homovanillic acid; 5-HT, serotonin; 5-HIAA, 5-hydroxyindoleacetic acid. ND: not detected.

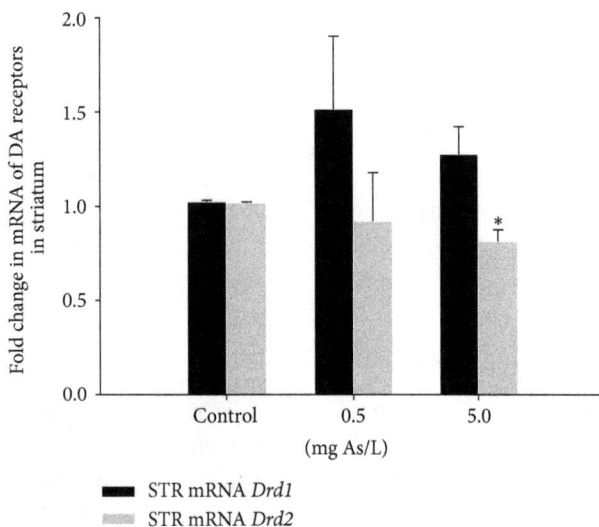

FIGURE 3: Dopamine receptors D1 (*Drd1*) and D2 (*Drd2*) mRNA expression in the striatum of male CD1 mice exposed chronically to 0.5 or 5.0 mg As/L of As in drinking water. Data was normalized to *Bact* and is presented as fold change relative to control group (mean ± SEM). * denotes differences from the control group, $p <$ 0.05.

4.1. Body Weight and General Appearance. Chronic exposure to doses as low as 0.5 mg As/L or moderate doses such as 5.0 mg As/L of drinking water did not cause alterations in body weight compared to control group for the duration of the treatment which agrees with previous studies in rodents exposed to this metalloid [20, 28]. Previous studies of our group and others have demonstrated that in CD1 mice As enters and is distributed into brain regions after a short time exposure (9 days) [39, 40], and this is also observable in other chronic models [20, 28]. The transitory hairless patches found in the group exposed to 5.0 mg As/L at months 1 and 2 are in accordance with Nagaraja and Desiraju [41] who reported temporary hairless patches on male rats at day 20 of exposure to 5.0 mg As/kg BW as sodium arsenate, while Rodríguez et al. [42] also reported hair loss mainly during As exposure in the group of male rats treated with 20 mg As/kg BW.

4.2. As Exposure Produces Alterations in Locomotor Activity. The long-term exposure to As produces biphasic alterations in both total distance traveled and horizontal activity of the CD1 male mice locomotor activity. The alterations found in locomotor activity were not due to malaise by As exposure, since no changes in body weight or general appearance were found during As treatment.

Hypoactivity was found during the dark phase and hyperactivity was present at the beginning (initial 3 hours) of the light phase of the dark/light cycle on the group exposed to 5.0 mg As/L, while the group exposed to 0.5 mg As/L showed only the hypoactivity during the dark phase. These results are not in agreement with a previous study by Bardullas et al. [20] with the C57Bl/6J mouse strain where they reported that exposure to 0.5 mg As/L for 4 months produced hyperactivity during the light phase of the cycle, while no effects were reported in the group exposed to 5.0 mg As/L. The different responses to As exposure could be due to inherent variations between mice strains. Indeed, CD1 and C57BL/6J strains have been shown to differ in their susceptibility to the neurotoxin MPTP, the C57Bl/6J mouse strain being much more susceptible [43] since this strain has less midbrain DA neurons [44] and lower DA function in striatum [45]. On the other hand for hyperbaric oxygen-induced convulsions, the CD1 strain is more sensitive [46]. The same group reported increased striatal norepinephrine levels in CD1 in comparison to the C57Bl/6J mouse strain [47]. At the neuroanatomical level, the C57Bl/6J mice have larger cerebral cortex and ventricular compartments than age-matched CD1 mice, but the volume of the striatum is bigger in the CD1 strain [48].

Decreases in motor activity due to As exposure have already been shown in studies using rats [19, 28, 42, 49]. In these studies the decreases in locomotor activity were found when doses above 10 mg As/L were used. It is important to mention that the pattern of hypoactivity due to the exposure of 0.5 or 5.0 mg As/L found in this study is similar to the one found by Rodríguez et al. [28] using male rats treated with the high dose of 50 mg As/L for twelve months. These observations suggest that male CD1 mice may be more sensitive to As intoxication in comparison to the male Sprague-Dawley rat that needs doses as high as 50 mg As/L of DW but less sensitive than the C57Bl/6J male mice which need only four months of exposure to show changes in locomotor activity [20].

4.3. On- and Off-Wall Rearing Behavior. The transitory and biphasic alterations observed at months 1 and 2 of As treatment on the on- and off-wall rearing behavior could be due to alterations in the monoaminergic systems. It has been shown that the administration of amphetamine to adult male rats increases both on- and off-wall rearing [34] whereas the lesion of noradrenergic or dopaminergic systems decreases rearing in mice [50]. In the present study we verified the content of monoamines only at the end of the six months of As treatment.

4.4. Aggressive Behavior. The protocol and doses of As exposure used in this study do not evidence increased aggressive behavior in CD1 male mice. The As-treated mice only showed aggressive behavioral components necessary to establish a social hierarchy inside a group, such as grooming, chasing, and barbering [51].

4.5. Monoamine Levels. Chronic As exposure did not cause alterations in monoamine content in striatum or prefrontal cortex of CD1 male mice. This explains in part the lack of aggressive behavior in mice exposed to As. The absence of alterations in brain monoamine levels in this study is in agreement with a previous study that reported no changes in DA or its metabolites in striatum of C57Bl/6J male mice exposed to similar doses of As used in this study [20].

According to several studies As exposure causes alterations in several neurotransmitter systems including the monoaminergic systems only when rodents are exposed to high doses of this metalloid [19–21, 28, 41, 42, 52]. In addition to the differences in As doses, the discrepancies between this study and those present in the literature could be due to differences in the species or strain used, the duration of treatments, the mode of administration, and the source of As (sodium arsenite, sodium arsenate, or arsenic trioxide).

Earlier studies had suggested that hypoactivity could be due to alterations in the dopaminergic system [53], but from the data presented here we can conclude that the hypoactivity observed in these rodents after six months of As exposure is not due to alterations in brain monoamine levels. Our finding however does not discard the involvement of changes at the level of dopaminergic signaling, DA release, or DA receptors, as we discuss below, since it is well known that As can stimulate or inhibit several signaling routes [54, 55] or affect different levels of DA system regulation which could be involved in movement control.

4.6. mRNA of DA Receptors Drd1 and Drd2. In this study, we found that only the *Drd2* was downregulated in the striatum of mice chronically exposed to 5.0 mg As/L; this finding is important because it involves changes at postsynaptic level. Whereas activation of presynaptic DA D2 receptors generally causes a decrease in DA release that in turn results in decreased locomotor activity, activation of postsynaptic receptors stimulates locomotion [56]. This result could explain in part why we observed hypoactivity in mice exposed to 5.0 mg As/L and agrees with a previous study in which mRNA expression of *Drd2* was observed to be downregulated in a dose-dependent manner by chronic exposure to As in the nucleus accumbens of the rat [28]. It must be noted that other studies have shown the opposite effect in mRNA expression

of D2 in the striatum of rats postnatally exposed to 2 or 4 mg As/kg of BW [29] and in striatum of mice exposed to 1–100 mg As/L DW for three weeks [57].

The fact that in this study mice presented the above stated alterations at six months of As exposure is particularly relevant, since similar alterations were developed only by male Sprague-Dawley rats treated with the high dose of 50 mg As/L and only after one year of treatment. Locomotion is primarily controlled by the ventral striatum through activation of Drd1 and Drd2 and Drd3 receptors [58]; and synergistic interactions are necessary to produce complete locomotor stimulation [59]. The finding of downregulation of *Drd2* in striatum in this study is highly relevant since mutant animals lacking Drd2 are akinetic and bradykinetic, with significantly reduced spontaneous movement that resembles the extrapyramidal symptoms of Parkinson's disease [60]. In the present study, we must be cautious with the interpretation of the downregulation of *Drd2*, because the locomotor hypokinesia was observed only in the dark phase and appears not to be a constant condition. But we emphasize that it is possible that the locomotor hypoactivity seen in the mice exposed to As may be the result of downregulation of striatal *Drd2*.

It remains a challenge to correlate the changes in behavior with neurochemical alterations or disruptions in expression of genes related to the dopaminergic system from a classical toxicological point of view. Moreover, in the case of DA receptors, their specific participation in behavioral paradigms is still a matter of debate. Alternative explanations to our results in relation to DA content and *Drd2* expression in chronic As exposure must consider the complexity of the dopaminergic system. DA receptors are regulated at several levels including transcription and synthesis, internalization and transport, and changes in affinity.

As mentioned earlier, chronic As exposure has been shown to change DA neurochemistry as evidenced by gender-specific alterations in locomotor activity and molecular alterations related to tyrosine hydroxylase (TH) and antioxidant mRNA expression in mice [20], changes in mRNA expression of DA receptors D1 (*Drd1*) and D2 (*Drd2*) in striatum and nucleus accumbens of male rats [28], increased mRNA expression of DA receptors D1 (*Drd1*), D2 (*Drd2*), D3 (*Drd3*), and D4 (*Drd4*) together with decreased TH in striatum and cerebral cortex of adult C57Bl/6 mice [57], increased binding and mRNA expression of D2 receptors, and increased expression of TH protein levels in striatum of Wistar rats [29].

DA receptors regulate the expression of their own genes; for instance, disruption of the nigrostriatal dopaminergic pathway with 6-OHDA increases *Drd2* mRNA expression in striatonigral and striatopallidal neurons [61]. Similarly, chronic treatment with haloperidol increases *Drd2* mRNA expression in the caudate putamen [62]. In this study, it is possible that As exposure impaired DA receptor-dependent signaling resulting in *Drd2* mRNA downregulation. Another possibility is that dopaminergic transmission could have been increased by As treatment. This would not necessarily depend on the de novo synthesis of DA but on alterations in its transporter, as is the case of mice lacking dopamine transporter (DAT). These mice show overactive dopaminergic transmission and downregulation in the mRNA of *Drd1* and *Drd2* [63]. Further studies are necessary to evaluate this hypothesis in the model of chronic exposure to As.

In conclusion, exposure to 0.5 or 5.0 mg As/L for six months in CD1 male mice did not alter the typical intraspecific behaviors necessary to establish a social hierarchy, nor did it alter normal monoamine levels. Mice treated with the highest dose of As displayed hypoactivity and decreases in *Drd2* mRNA in the striatum at the end of treatment. The fact that these changes were detected after six months of As exposure is of particular relevance, since similar alterations were observed in male Sprague-Dawley rats treated with a high dose of As (50 mg As/L) only after one year of treatment. Based on these findings, we can conclude that the CD1 male mouse is more sensitive to As exposure than the Sprague-Dawley male rat and may represent a better model of As neurotoxicity. Although the interpretation and prediction of the effects of environmental toxicants on the dopaminergic system remain a complex issue, from a toxicological perspective the contribution of this study is the hypothesis that DA receptors, particularly *Drd2*, may be a potential target for the effects of As exposure in rodents.

Disclosure

The views expressed in this paper are the authors' and do not reflect official policy of position of the institution of funders.

Competing Interests

The authors declare that there is no conflict of interests regarding this research paper.

Acknowledgments

The authors acknowledge Dr. Dorothy Pless for critical review of this paper and M. C. Adriana González Gallardo at the Unidad de Proteogenómica of the Instituto de Neurobiología, Biól. Maria Soledad Mendoza Trejo, and Fernando Rodríguez for their technical assistance. This paper was supported by CONACYT Grant nos. 60662 and 152842 to Verónica M. Rodríguez and DGAPA-UNAM PAPIIT Grant nos. 214608 and 202013 to Verónica M. Rodríguez. Jorge H. Limón-Pacheco (no. 43533) and Claudia Leticia Moreno Ávila (270233) received a fellowship from CONACYT.

References

[1] R. U. Ayres, "Toxic heavy metals: materials cycle optimization," *Proceedings of the National Academy of Sciences of the United States of America*, vol. 89, no. 3, pp. 815–820, 1992.

[2] G. Concha, B. Nermell, and M. Vahter, "Metabolism of inorganic arsenic in children with chronic high arsenic exposure in northern Argentina," *Environmental Health Perspectives*, vol. 106, no. 6, pp. 355–359, 1998.

[3] M. M. H. Khan, F. Sakauchi, T. Sonoda, M. Washio, and M. Mori, "Magnitude of arsenic toxicity in tube-well drinking water in bangladesh and its adverse effects on human health including cancer: evidence from a review of the literature," *Asian Pacific Journal of Cancer Prevention*, vol. 4, no. 1, pp. 7–14, 2003.

[4] A. H. Smith, M. Goycolea, R. Haque, and M. L. Biggs, "Marked increase in bladder and lung cancer mortality in a region of Northern Chile due to arsenic in drinking water," *American Journal of Epidemiology*, vol. 147, no. 7, pp. 660–669, 1998.

[5] M. E. Cebrian, A. Albores, M. Aguilar, and E. Blakely, "Chronic arsenic poisoning in the North of Mexico," *Human Toxicology*, vol. 2, no. 1, pp. 121–133, 1983.

[6] A. H. Smith, C. Hopenhayn-Rich, M. N. Bates et al., "Cancer risks from arsenic in drinking water," *Environmental Health Perspectives*, vol. 97, pp. 259–267, 1992.

[7] M. Dakeishi, K. Murata, and P. Grandjean, "Long-term consequences of arsenic poisoning during infancy due to contaminated milk powder," *Environmental Health: A Global Access Science Source*, vol. 5, article 31, 2006.

[8] R. Jackson and J. W. Grainge, "Arsenic and cancer," *Canadian Medical Association Journal*, vol. 113, no. 5, pp. 396–401, 1975.

[9] C.-J. Chen, S.-L. Wang, J.-M. Chiou et al., "Arsenic and diabetes and hypertension in human populations: a review," *Toxicology and Applied Pharmacology*, vol. 222, no. 3, pp. 298–304, 2007.

[10] J. L. Rosado, D. Ronquillo, K. Kordas et al., "Arsenic exposure and cognitive performance in Mexican Schoolchildren," *Environmental Health Perspectives*, vol. 115, no. 9, pp. 1371–1375, 2007.

[11] S.-Y. Tsai, H.-Y. Chou, H.-W. The, C.-M. Chen, and C.-J. Chen, "The effects of chronic arsenic exposure from drinking water on the neurobehavioral development in adolescence," *NeuroToxicology*, vol. 24, no. 4-5, pp. 747–753, 2003.

[12] J. Calderón, M. E. Navarro, M. E. Jimenez-Capdeville et al., "Exposure to arsenic and lead and neuropsychological development in Mexican children," *Environmental Research*, vol. 85, no. 2, pp. 69–76, 2001.

[13] J. D. Hamadani, F. Tofail, B. Nermell et al., "Critical windows of exposure for arsenic-associated impairment of cognitive function in pre-school girls and boys: a population-based cohort study," *International Journal of Epidemiology*, vol. 40, no. 6, pp. 1593–1604, 2011.

[14] M. Rodríguez-Barranco, F. Gil, A. F. Hernández et al., "Postnatal arsenic exposure and attention impairment in school children," *Cortex*, vol. 74, pp. 370–382, 2016.

[15] S. Vibol, J. H. Hashim, and S. Sarmani, "Neurobehavioral effects of arsenic exposure among secondary school children in the Kandal Province, Cambodia," *Environmental Research*, vol. 137, pp. 329–337, 2015.

[16] A. Franzblau and R. Lilis, "Acute arsenic intoxication from environmental arsenic exposure," *Archives of Environmental Health*, vol. 44, no. 6, pp. 385–390, 1989.

[17] S. C. Mukherjee, M. M. Rahman, U. K. Chowdhury et al., "Neuropathy in arsenic toxicity from groundwater arsenic contamination in West Bengal, India," *Journal of Environmental Science and Health—Part A Toxic/Hazardous Substances and Environmental Engineering*, vol. 38, no. 1, pp. 165–183, 2003.

[18] V. M. Rodríguez, M. E. Jiménez-Capdeville, and M. Giordano, "The effects of arsenic exposure on the nervous system," *Toxicology Letters*, vol. 145, no. 1, pp. 1–18, 2003.

[19] I. Tadanobu, Y. F. Zhang, M. Shigeo et al., "The effect of arsenic trioxide on brain monoamine metabolism and locomotor activity of mice," *Toxicology Letters*, vol. 54, no. 2-3, pp. 345–353, 1990.

[20] U. Bardullas, J. H. Limón-Pacheco, M. Giordano, L. Carrizales, M. S. Mendoza-Trejo, and V. M. Rodríguez, "Chronic low-level arsenic exposure causes gender-specific alterations in

locomotor activity, dopaminergic systems, and thioredoxin expression in mice," *Toxicology and Applied Pharmacology*, vol. 239, no. 2, pp. 169–177, 2009.

[21] J. J. Mejía, F. Díaz-Barriga, J. Calderón, C. Ríos, and M. E. Jiménez-Capdeville, "Effects of lead-arsenic combined exposure on central monoaminergic systems," *Neurotoxicology and Teratology*, vol. 19, no. 6, pp. 489–497, 1997.

[22] M. Vahter, "Biotransformation of trivalent and pentavalent inorganic arsenic in mice and rats," *Environmental Research*, vol. 25, no. 2, pp. 286–293, 1981.

[23] S. Chong, K. Dill, and E. McGown, "The interaction of phenyldichloroarsine with erythrocytes," *Journal of Biochemical Toxicology*, vol. 4, no. 1, pp. 39–45, 1989.

[24] Y. Shiobara, Y. Ogra, and K. T. Suzuki, "Animal species difference in the uptake of dimethylarsinous acid (DMA^{III}) by red blood cells," *Chemical Research in Toxicology*, vol. 14, no. 10, pp. 1446–1452, 2001.

[25] B. Adams, T. Fitch, S. Chaney, and R. Gerlai, "Altered performance characteristics in cognitive tasks: comparison of the albino ICR and CD1 mouse strains," *Behavioural Brain Research*, vol. 133, no. 2, pp. 351–361, 2002.

[26] J. L. Short, J. Drago, and A. J. Lawrence, "Comparison of ethanol preference and neurochemical measures of mesolimbic dopamine and adenosine systems across different strains of mice," *Alcoholism: Clinical and Experimental Research*, vol. 30, no. 4, pp. 606–620, 2006.

[27] S. C. Fowler, T. J. Zarcone, and E. Vorontsova, "Haloperidol-induced microcatalepsy differs in CD-1, BALB/c, and C57BL/6 mice," *Experimental and Clinical Psychopharmacology*, vol. 9, no. 3, pp. 277–284, 2001.

[28] V. M. Rodríguez, J. H. Limón-Pacheco, L. Carrizales, M. S. Mendoza-Trejo, and M. Giordano, "Chronic exposure to low levels of inorganic arsenic causes alterations in locomotor activity and in the expression of dopaminergic and antioxidant systems in the albino rat," *Neurotoxicology and Teratology*, vol. 32, no. 6, pp. 640–647, 2010.

[29] L. P. Chandravanshi, R. K. Shukla, S. Sultana, A. B. Pant, and V. K. Khanna, "Early life arsenic exposure and brain dopaminergic alterations in rats," *International Journal of Developmental Neuroscience*, vol. 38, pp. 91–104, 2014.

[30] S. Shila, V. Kokilavani, M. Subathra, and C. Panneerselvam, "Brain regional responses in antioxidant system to α-lipoic acid in arsenic intoxicated rat," *Toxicology*, vol. 210, no. 1, pp. 25–36, 2005.

[31] J.-H. Luo, Z.-Q. Qiu, W.-Q. Shu, Y.-Y. Zhang, L. Zhang, and J.-A. Chen, "Effects of arsenic exposure from drinking water on spatial memory, ultra-structures and NMDAR gene expression of hippocampus in rats," *Toxicology Letters*, vol. 184, no. 2, pp. 121–125, 2009.

[32] S. Jiang, J. Su, S. Yao et al., "Fluoride and arsenic exposure impairs learning and memory and decreases mGluR5 expression in the hippocampus and cortex in rats," *PLoS ONE*, vol. 9, no. 4, Article ID e96041, 2014.

[33] V. M. Rodríguez, J. H. Limón-Pacheco, L. M. Del Razo, and M. Giordano, "Effects of inorganic arsenic exposure on glucose transporters and insulin receptor in the hippocampus of C57BL/6 male mice," *Neurotoxicology and Teratology*, vol. 54, pp. 68–77, 2016.

[34] K. H. Russell, M. Giordano, and P. R. Sanberg, "Amphetamine-induced on- and off-wall rearing in adult laboratory rats," *Pharmacology, Biochemistry and Behavior*, vol. 26, no. 1, pp. 7–10, 1987.

[35] J. M. Koolhaas, T. Schuurman, and P. R. Wiepkema, "The organization of intraspecific agonistic behaviour in the rat," *Progress in Neurobiology*, vol. 15, no. 3, pp. 247–268, 1980.

[36] K. A. Miczek and J. M. O'Donnell, "Intruder-evoked aggression in isolated and nonisolated mice: effects of psychomotor stimulants and L-Dopa," *Psychopharmacology*, vol. 57, no. 1, pp. 47–55, 1978.

[37] S. Ogawa, J. Chan, A. E. Chester, J.-A. Gustafsson, K. S. Korach, and D. W. Pfaff, "Survival of reproductive behaviors in estrogen receptor β gene- deficient (βERKO) male and female mice," *Proceedings of the National Academy of Sciences of the United States of America*, vol. 96, no. 22, pp. 12887–12892, 1999.

[38] K. J. Livak and T. D. Schmittgen, "Analysis of relative gene expression data using real-time quantitative PCR and the 2-ΔΔCT method," *Methods*, vol. 25, no. 4, pp. 402–408, 2001.

[39] V. M. Rodríguez, L. M. Del Razo, J. H. Limón-Pacheco et al., "Glutathione reductase inhibition and methylated arsenic distribution in Cd1 mice brain and liver," *Toxicological Sciences*, vol. 84, no. 1, pp. 157–166, 2005.

[40] L. C. Sánchez-Peña, P. Petrosyan, M. Morales et al., "Arsenic species, AS3MT amount, and AS3MT gen expression in different brain regions of mouse exposed to arsenite," *Environmental Research*, vol. 110, no. 5, pp. 428–434, 2010.

[41] T. N. Nagaraja and T. Desiraju, "Regional alterations in the levels of brain biogenic amines, glutamate, GABA, and GAD activity due to chronic consumption of inorganic arsenic in developing and adult rats," *Bulletin of Environmental Contamination and Toxicology*, vol. 50, no. 1, pp. 100–107, 1993.

[42] V. M. Rodríguez, L. Carrizales, M. E. Jiménez-Capdeville, L. Dufour, and M. Giordano, "The effects of sodium arsenite exposure on behavioral parameters in the rat," *Brain Research Bulletin*, vol. 55, no. 2, pp. 301–308, 2001.

[43] P. K. Sonsalla and R. E. Heikkila, "The influence of dose and dosing interval on MPTP-induced dopaminergic neurotoxicity in mice," *European Journal of Pharmacology*, vol. 129, no. 3, pp. 339–345, 1986.

[44] B. Hitzemann, K. Dains, S. Kanes, and R. Hitzemann, "Further studies on the relationship between dopamine cell density and haloperidol-induced catalepsy," *The Journal of Pharmacology and Experimental Therapeutics*, vol. 271, no. 2, pp. 969–976, 1994.

[45] S. R. George, T. Fan, G. Y. Ng, S. Y. Jung, B. F. O'Dowd, and C. A. Naranjo, "Low endogenous dopamine function in brain predisposes to high alcohol preference and consumption: reversal by increasing synaptic dopamine," *Journal of Pharmacology and Experimental Therapeutics*, vol. 273, no. 1, pp. 373–379, 1995.

[46] P. Mialon, C. Cann-Moisan, L. Barthélémy, J. Caroff, P. Joanny, and J. Steinberg, "Effect of one hyperbaric oxygen-induced convulsion on cortical polyamine content in two strains of mice," *Neuroscience Letters*, vol. 160, no. 1, pp. 1–3, 1993.

[47] P. Joanny, P. Mialon, C. Cann-Moisan, C. Caroff, and J. Steinberg, "Regional brain bioamine levels under hyperbaric oxygen in two unequally susceptible strains of mice," *Aviation, Space, and Environmental Medicine*, vol. 71, no. 9, pp. 929–934, 2000.

[48] X. J. Chen, N. Kovacevic, N. J. Lobaugh, J. G. Sled, R. M. Henkelman, and J. T. Henderson, "Neuroanatomical differences between mouse strains as shown by high-resolution 3D MRI," *NeuroImage*, vol. 29, no. 1, pp. 99–105, 2006.

[49] H. Schulz, L. Nagymajtényi, L. Institoris, A. Papp, and O. Siroki, "A study on behavioral, neurotoxicological, and immunotoxicological effects of subchronic arsenic treatment in rats," *Journal*

of Toxicology and Environmental Health—Part A, vol. 65, no. 16, pp. 1181–1193, 2002.

[50] T. Archer and A. Fredriksson, "Influence of noradrenaline denervation on MPTP-induced deficits in mice," *Journal of Neural Transmission*, vol. 113, no. 9, pp. 1119–1129, 2006.

[51] K. A. Miczek, E. W. Fish, J. F. De Bold, and R. M. De Almeida, "Social and neural determinants of aggressive behavior: pharmacotherapeutic targets at serotonin, dopamine and γ-aminobutyric acid systems," *Psychopharmacology*, vol. 163, no. 3-4, pp. 434–458, 2002.

[52] N. Tripathi, G. M. Kannan, B. P. Pant, D. K. Jaiswal, P. R. Malhotra, and S. J. S. Flora, "Arsenic-induced changes in certain neurotransmitter levels and their recoveries following chelation in rat whole brain," *Toxicology Letters*, vol. 92, no. 3, pp. 201–208, 1997.

[53] K. Svensson, A. Carlsson, R. M. Huff, T. Kling-Petersen, and N. Waters, "Behavioral and neurochemical data suggest functional differences between dopamine D2 and D3 receptors," *European Journal of Pharmacology*, vol. 263, no. 3, pp. 235–243, 1994.

[54] Y. Kumagai and D. Sumi, "Arsenic: signal transduction, transcription factor, and biotransformation involved in cellular response and toxicity," *Annual Review of Pharmacology and Toxicology*, vol. 47, pp. 243–262, 2007.

[55] I. L. Druwe and R. R. Vaillancourt, "Influence of arsenate and arsenite on signal transduction pathways: an update," *Archives of Toxicology*, vol. 84, no. 8, pp. 585–596, 2010.

[56] J.-M. Beaulieu and R. R. Gainetdinov, "The physiology, signaling, and pharmacology of dopamine receptors," *Pharmacological Reviews*, vol. 63, no. 1, pp. 182–217, 2011.

[57] M. Kim, S. Seo, K. Sung, and K. Kim, "Arsenic exposure in drinking water alters the dopamine system in the brains of C57BL/6 mice," *Biological Trace Element Research*, vol. 162, no. 1–3, pp. 175–180, 2014.

[58] C. Missale, S. R. Nash, S. W. Robinson, M. Jaber, and M. G. Caron, "Dopamine receptors: from structure to function," *Physiological Reviews*, vol. 78, no. 1, pp. 189–225, 1998.

[59] J. K. Dreher and D. M. Jackson, "Role of D1 and D2 dopamine receptors in mediating locomotor activity elicited from the nucleus accumbens of rats," *Brain Research*, vol. 487, no. 2, pp. 267–277, 1989.

[60] J.-H. Baik, R. Picetti, A. Saiardi et al., "Parkinsonian-like locomotor impairment in mice lacking dopamine D2 receptors," *Nature*, vol. 377, no. 6548, pp. 424–428, 1995.

[61] C. R. Gerfen, T. M. Engber, L. C. Mahan et al., "D1 and D2 dopamine receptor-regulated gene expression of striatonigral and striatopallidal neurons," *Science*, vol. 250, no. 4986, pp. 1429–1432, 1990.

[62] V. Bernard, C. le Moine, and B. Bloch, "Striatal neurons express increased level of dopamine D2 receptor mRNA in response to haloperidol treatment: a quantitative in situ hybridization study," *Neuroscience*, vol. 45, no. 1, pp. 117–126, 1991.

[63] B. Giros, M. Jaber, S. R. Jones, R. M. Wightman, and M. G. Caron, "Hyperlocomotion and indifference to cocaine and amphetamine in mice lacking the dopamine transporter," *Nature*, vol. 379, no. 6566, pp. 606–612, 1996.

4

Cement Dust Exposure and Perturbations in Some Elements and Lung and Liver Functions of Cement Factory Workers

Egbe Edmund Richard, Nsonwu-Anyanwu Augusta Chinyere, Offor Sunday Jeremaiah, Usoro Chinyere Adanna Opara, Etukudo Maise Henrieta, and Egbe Deborah Ifunanya

Department of Medical Laboratory Science, Faculty of Allied Medical Sciences, College of Medical Sciences, University of Calabar, Calabar 543000, Nigeria

Correspondence should be addressed to Nsonwu-Anyanwu Augusta Chinyere; austadechic@yahoo.com

Academic Editor: Steven J. Bursian

Background. Cement dust inhalation is associated with deleterious health effects. The impact of cement dust exposure on the peak expiratory flow rate (PEFR), liver function, and some serum elements in workers and residents near cement factory were assessed. *Methods.* Two hundred and ten subjects (50 workers, 60 residents, and 100 controls) aged 18–60 years were studied. PEFR, liver function {aspartate and alanine transaminases (AST and ALT) and total and conjugated bilirubin (TB and CB)}, and serum elements {lead (Pb), copper (Cu), manganese (Mn), iron (Fe), cadmium (Cd), selenium (Se), chromium (Cr), zinc (Zn), and arsenic (As)} were determined using peak flow meter, colorimetry, and atomic absorption spectrometry, respectively. Data were analysed using ANOVA and correlation at $p = 0.05$. *Results.* The ALT, TB, CB, Pb, As, Cd, Cr, Se, Mn, and Cu were significantly higher and PEFR, Fe, and Zn lower in workers and residents compared to controls ($p < 0.05$). Higher levels of ALT, AST, and Fe and lower levels of Pb, Cd, Cr, Se, Mn, and Cu were seen in cement workers compared to residents ($p < 0.05$). Negative correlation was observed between duration of exposure and PEFR ($r = -0.416$, $p = 0.016$) in cement workers. *Conclusions.* Cement dust inhalation may be associated with alterations in serum elements levels and lung and liver functions while long term exposure lowers peak expiratory flow rate.

1. Introduction

Deleterious effects of exposure to constituents of cement dust on organ system in humans have been described. Molecules of primary importance in cement dust in terms of content and potential health effects basically include 60–67% calcium oxide, 17–25 silicon oxide (SiO_2), and 3–5% aluminium (Al) oxide, with some amount of iron oxide, chromium (Cr), potassium, sodium, sulphur, and magnesium oxide [1, 2]. Occupational exposures to aluminum (Al), iron (Fe), calcium (Ca), and silicon (Si) have been associated with decreased lung function indicators in exposed workers [3, 4]. Hepatosplenic silicosis and hepatic porphyria, with associated changes in liver function parameters, have also been described as some of the systemic effects of silica. Lipid peroxidation, oxidative damage, and immunologic mechanisms have been described as pathologic mechanisms of cement

dust induced toxicities [5, 6]. Some essential elements necessary for normal physiologic functions are also constituents of cement dust. Toxicity from these essential trace elements occurs only when the exposure is above the range which can be accommodated by homeostatic mechanisms [7].

Studies on effects of cement dust exposure on lung and liver functions in occupationally exposed individuals in Nigeria have been documented [2, 8, 9]; however, information on the levels of some essential and nonessential elements and their relative or absolute contribution to lung and liver toxicities among individuals occupationally exposed to cement dust is still uncertain. This study therefore estimates the lung and liver functions and levels of some essential and nonessential elements in residents and workers in cement factory sites to determine their possible contribution to impairment of lung and liver functions in these individuals.

2. Materials and Methods

2.1. Study Design. This study was conducted at the United Cement Company (UNICEM) at Mfamosing, Akamkpa local government area, Cross River State, Nigeria. The Mfamosing limestone deposit serves as the major source of raw materials used by UNICEM for the production of ordinary Portland cement (OPC). Since July 2009, the Mfamosing cement plant produces approximately 2.5 million metric tons of cement per annum and currently employs about 350 permanent workers. The factory has four major departments: Production (Crusher, Raw Mill, Kiln, Cement Mill, and Packing Section), Engineering and Maintenance (Mechanical and Electrical Section), Mining, and Administration (Cashier, Administrative Officer, Security, and Marketing Section). The site is close to 200 m west to Mbebui village at coordinates 05.04493°N, 008.298995°E, 500 m south to Abifan community at coordinates 05.07591°N, 008.52192°E, and 200 m east to Mfamosing community and 100 m east to main quarry site at coordinates 05.06993°N, 008.53908°E [10].

2.2. Selection of Subjects. Two hundred and ten male subjects aged 18–60 years who fulfilled the inclusion criteria were randomly selected for this study. This study population comprised fifty regular cement factory workers, sixty residents of the communities surrounding the UNICEM factory, and one hundred apparently healthy individuals residing in Calabar metropolis 45 km away from the factory, not exposed to cement dust, who served as control subjects. Informed consent was obtained from them and ethical approval was obtained from The Center of Clinical Governance, Research and Training, Ministry of Health, Cross River State. This study was carried out in accordance with the Ethical Principles for Medical Research Involving Human Subjects as outlined in the Helsinki Declaration in 1975 (revised in 2000). Test subjects of the study were selected from the production section of the cement factory. This comprises permanent employees of the factory who are occupationally exposed to cement dust daily for not less than 2 years in the course of their work. Host community resident subjects were also individuals that had been resident in the communities proximal to the cement factory for not less than 2 years, while control subjects were individuals who had never been occupationally exposed to cement dust and are resident in Calabar metropolis.

Participants were notified several days before the commencement of the study and were given appropriate instructions. The physical characteristics of the subjects included weight and height measured with the use of weighing scale and stadiometer, respectively. Systolic and diastolic blood pressure were taken using sphygmomanometer. All subjects of the study were interviewed to establish their level of literacy and were assisted in filling the questionnaire to minimize errors. Sociodemographic data were collected by an interviewer-administered structured questionnaire aiming to determine age, educational levels, socioeconomic status, years of exposure as deduced from date of employment, site or position at the workplace, and use and nonuse of safety gadgets such as dust masks. Information on general health and history of past disease(s) and habits such as smoking, consumption of alcoholic beverages, and addictions were collected according to the British Medical Research Council questionnaire (BMRC, 1960). Individuals with a history of cigarette smoking, tobacco sniffing or chewing, liver disease or pulmonary disorders, chronic organ or systemic illness, and long term medication were excluded from the study.

2.3. Sample Collection. Blood samples were collected from midmorning to noon for both subjects and controls. Seven milliliters of blood was collected by venipuncture under aseptic conditions into a dry, clean plain sample container. The blood was allowed to clot and was centrifuged at 3,500 revolutions per minute for 5 minutes. After centrifuging, the serum was separated with the aid of a Pasture pipette and dispensed into dry chemically clean serum container, after which the samples were analysed immediately or stored at −20°C for subsequent analysis.

2.4. Laboratory Methods

2.4.1. Estimation of Alanine Aminotransferase (ALT) [11]. Consider

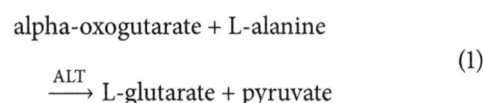

$$
\begin{aligned}
&\text{alpha-oxogutarate + L-alanine} \\
&\xrightarrow{\text{ALT}} \text{L-glutarate + pyruvate}
\end{aligned}
\tag{1}
$$

Alanine aminotransferase catalyzes the transfer of amino group from L-alanine to α-ketoglutarate forming pyruvate and L-glutamate. Pyruvate reacts with 2,4-dinitrophenylhydrazine to form 2,4-dinitrophenylhydrazone whose concentration is proportional to the ALT activity.

2.4.2. Estimation of Aspartate Aminotransferase (AST), Reitman and Frankel [11]. Consider

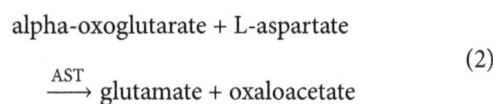

$$
\begin{aligned}
&\text{alpha-oxoglutarate + L-aspartate} \\
&\xrightarrow{\text{AST}} \text{glutamate + oxaloacetate}
\end{aligned}
\tag{2}
$$

Aspartate aminotransferase (AST) catalyses the transfer of amino acid group from aspartate to ketoglutarate, forming oxaloacetate and glutamate. The oxaloacetate reacts with 2,4-dinitrophenylhydrazine to form 2,4-dinitrophenylhydrazone which in alkaline pH is reddish brown and whose concentration is proportional to the AST activity.

2.4.3. Estimation of Bilirubin by Modified Valley's Method [12]. Serum bilirubin is present in two forms: conjugated which is mostly with glucuronic acid and unconjugated which is known as free bilirubin. Both react with diazotized sulphanilic acid to give a rose-purple azobilirubin. Conjugated bilirubin reacts in aqueous solution (direct reaction) whereas the unconjugated bilirubin requires an accelerator or solubilizer such as benzoate urea as in this method or alcohol which is used in other methods (indirect reaction).

TABLE 1: Mean age, anthropometric indices (weight, height, and BMI), systolic BP, diastolic BP, some liver function tests, peak expiratory flow rate, and serum elements levels in cement workers, residents near cement factory, and controls.

Parameter	Cement workers $n = 50$	Residents $n = 60$	Controls $n = 100$	F-value	p value
Age (years)	39.98 ± 5.56	38.32 ± 4.03	37.67 ± 5.32	0.453	0.636
Weight (kg)	61.04 ± 13.53	62.04 ± 12.55	61.90 ± 13.35	0.204	0.816
Height (meters)	1.67 ± 0.10	1.68 ± 0.09	1.72 ± 0.06	0.055	0.747
BMI (kg/m^2)	23.35 ± 2.56	23.95 ± 2.32	23.10 ± 2.11	2.574	0.079
Sys. BP (mmHg)	128.80 ± 8.80	127.80 ± 8.83	128.80 ± 7.86	0.166	0.847
Diast. BP (mmHg)	84.20 ± 13.10	82.33 ± 10.14	82.50 ± 10.76	0.476	0.622
ALT (IU)	29.78 ± 2.58	11.25 ± 0.96	8.72 ± 0.41	76.53	0.000*
AST (IU)	37.00 ± 2.61	17.41 ± 1.70	9.46 ± 0.64	84.29	0.000*
TB (μmol/L)	18.26 ± 0.91	18.18 ± 0.81	13.82 ± 0.62	12.80	0.000*
CB (μmol/L)	7.57 ± 0.58	7.33 ± 0.52	5.84 ± 0.27	5.66	0.004*
PEFR (L/min)	324.96 ± 10.40	340.25 ± 10.38	400.17 ± 9.10	16.97	0.000*
Fe (μg/dL)	102.08 ± 1.78	96.13 ± 1.43	150.99 ± 1.35	447.99	0.000*
Zn (μg/dL)	80.94 ± 2.01	78.25 ± 1.86	106.52 ± 0.70	147.64	0.000*
Pb (μg/dL)	15.93 ± 0.42	20.09 ± 0.64	10.33 ± 0.60	70.32	0.000*
As (μg/dL)	0.011 ± 0.002	0.011 ± 0.005	0.003 ± 0.002	183.45	0.000*
Cd (μg/dL)	0.042 ± 0.008	1.950 ± 0.212	0.022 ± 0.001	102.20	0.000*
Cr (μg/dL)	0.033 ± 0.003	1.60 ± 0.125	0.012 ± 0.000	200.39	0.000*
Se (μg/dL)	0.022 ± 0.004	1.75 ± 0.127	0.044 ± 0.015	217.479	0.000*
Mn (μg/L)	2.970 ± 0.074	3.346 ± 0.062	2.579 ± 0.038	56.101	0.000*
Cu (μg/dL)	216.64 ± 6.93	234.62 ± 7.16	173.06 ± 3.662	37.83	0.000*

*Significant at $p < 0.05$; Sys. BP = systolic blood pressure; Diast. BP = diastolic blood pressure.

2.4.4. Estimation of Trace Element by Atomic Absorption Spectrophotometer [13]. An extract of the physiological sample is deproteinized and the filtrate is treated as lanthanum. This is aspirated in AAS which measures the absorbance of trace metals at various wavelengths corresponding to its bandwidth. The absorbance is proportional to the concentration of trace element in the sample.

2.4.5. Estimation of Peak Expiratory Flow Rate by Peak Expiratory Flow Meter. The PEFR test is done with a peak expiratory flow meter: Spiroflow by Spirometrics, USA (originally described by Wright and McKerrow [14]). This is a simple handheld instrument with a mouthpiece on one end and a scale on the other. A small plastic arrow moves when air is blown into the mouthpiece, measuring the airflow speed. The subject breathes in deeply to full lung saturation and then blows into the mouthpiece as quickly and as hard as possible. The reading is taken and the procedure repeated two additional times. The highest record of the three is noted. If the subject coughs or sneezes while breathing out, the procedure will be repeated again. The PEFR readings were taken during break hour of 12 noon to 1 pm for the cement workers and for other subjects of the study.

2.5. Statistical Analysis. Data analysis was done using the statistical package for social sciences (SPSS version 20.0). Student's *t*-test analysis was used to determine mean differences between variables. Analysis of variance (ANOVA) was used to test significance of variations within and among group means and Fisher's least significant difference (LSD) post hoc test was used for comparism of multiple group means. Pearson correlation analysis was employed to determine relationship between variables. A two-sided probability value $p < 0.05$ was considered statistically significant

3. Results

Mean age, anthropometric indices (weight, height, and body mass index), systolic and diastolic blood pressure, some liver function tests (ALT, AST, TB, and CB), peak expiratory flow (PEFR), and serum elements levels (Fe, Zn, Pb, As, Cd, Cr, Se, Mn, and Cu) in cement workers, residents near the cement factory, and controls were shown in Table 1. Significant variations ($p < 0.05$) were observed in liver function test, peak expiratory flow, and serum elements levels in cement workers, residents living near the cement factory, and controls. No variations were observed in the levels of other indices studied ($p > 0.05$).

Table 2 shows comparison of some liver function test and PEFR of cement workers, residents near cement factory, and controls using post hoc analysis. The ALT, AST, TB, and CB were significantly higher and PEFR was lower in cement workers and residents near cement factory compared to controls ($p < 0.05$). The ALT and AST levels were

TABLE 2: Comparison of some liver function tests and peak expiratory flow in cement workers, residents near cement factory, and controls using post hoc analysis.

Parameter	Cem. workers $n = 50$	Controls $n = 100$	Mean diff.	p value
	Groups			
ALT (IU)	29.78 ± 2.57	8.72 ± 0.41	21.06 ± 1.75	0.000^*
AST (IU)	37.00 ± 2.61	9.46 ± 0.64	27.540 ± 2.12	0.000^*
TB (μmol/L)	18.26 ± 0.91	13.82 ± 0.62	4.44 ± 1.09	0.000^*
CB (μmol/L)	7.57 ± 0.58	5.84 ± 0.27	1.73 ± 0.60	0.004^*
PEFR (L/min)	324.96 ± 10.40	400.17 ± 9.10	-75.21 ± 14.58	0.000^*
	Residents $n = 60$	Controls $n = 100$		
ALT (IU)	11.25 ± 0.96	8.72 ± 0.41	2.53 ± 0.55	0.000^*
AST (IU)	17.41 ± 1.70	9.46 ± 0.64	$7.95.90 \pm 2.00$	0.000^*
TB (μmol/L)	18.18 ± 0.81	13.82 ± 0.62	4.36 ± 0.18	0.000^*
CB (μmol/L)	7.33 ± 0.52	5.84 ± 0.27	1.49 ± 0.26	0.004^*
PEFR (L/min)	340.25 ± 10.38	400.17 ± 9.10	-59.92 ± 0.13	0.000^*
	Cem. workers $n = 50$	Residents $n = 60$		
ALT (IU)	29.78 ± 2.58	11.25 ± 0.96	18.53 ± 1.94	0.000^*
AST (IU)	37.00 ± 2.61	17.41 ± 1.70	19.58 ± 2.35	0.000^*
TB (μmol/L)	18.264 ± 0.91	18.18 ± 0.81	$.081 \pm 1.204$	0.947
CB (μmol/L)	7.57 ± 0.58	7.33 ± 0.52	$.24 \pm 0.67$	0.723
PEFR (L/min)	324.96 ± 10.40	340.25 ± 10.38	-15.29 ± 16.12	0.344

*Significant at $p < 0.05$.

significantly higher in cement workers compared to residents ($p < 0.05$). No significant differences were observed in TB, CB, and PEF levels in cement workers and residents ($p > 0.05$).

Comparison of serum elements levels in cement workers, residents near the cement factory, and controls using post hoc analysis was shown in Table 3. Cement workers and residents have significantly higher levels of Pb, As, Cd, Cr, Se, Mn, and Cu and lower levels of Fe and Zn compared to the controls ($p < 0.05$). Higher levels of Fe and lower levels of Pb, Cd, Cr, Se, Mn, and Cu were seen in cement workers compared to residents ($p > 0.05$). No significant differences were seen in Zn and As levels of cement workers and residents ($p > 0.05$).

Figure 1 shows the correlation plot of duration of exposure to cement dust against peak expiratory flow rate in cement workers. A significant negative correlation ($r = -0.416$, $p = 0.001$) was observed between duration of exposure and peak expiratory flow rate in cement workers.

4. Discussion

The lung and liver function and some serum elements levels in occupationally exposed cement workers and residents near cement factories were studied. Decreased peak expiratory flow rate (PEFR) was observed in cement workers and residents living near cement factory when compared to unexposed controls. Similar findings have also been reported in cement workers in other developing countries [4, 15, 16]. Association of cement dust exposure with chronic

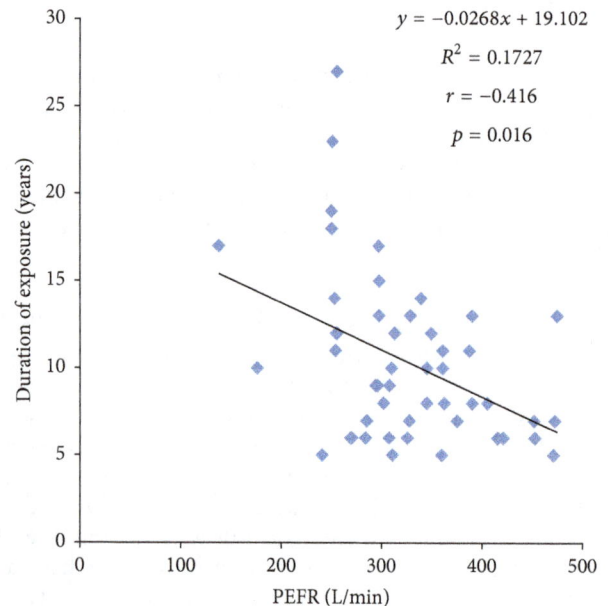

FIGURE 1: Correlation plot of duration of exposure to cement dust against peak expiratory flow rate in cement workers.

impairment of lung function and respiratory symptoms such as cough, phlegm, and chest tightness and lung function indices has been described [17]. Accumulation of cement

TABLE 3: Comparison of serum elements level in cement workers, residents near cement factory, and controls using post hoc analysis.

Parameter	Groups		Mean diff.	p value
	Cem. workers	Controls		
	n = 50	n = 100		
Fe (μg/dL)	102.08 ± 1.78	150.99 ± 1.35	−48.92 ± 2.19	0.000*
Zn (μg/dL)	80.95 ± 2.01	106.52 ± 0.70	−25.58 ± 1.97	0.000*
Pb (μg/dL)	15.93 ± 0.42	10.33 ± 0.60	5.60 ± 0.89	0.000*
As (μg/dL)	0.011 ± 0.002	0.003 ± 0.002	0.008 ± 0.001	0.000*
Cd (μg/dL)	0.042 ± 0.008	0.022 ± 0.001	0.035 ± 0.005	0.000*
Cr (μg/dL)	0.033 ± 0.013	0.012 ± 0.000	0.021 ± 0.002	0.000*
Se (μg/dL)	0.023 ± 0.004	0.044 ± 0.015	−0.010 ± 0.002	0.000*
Mn (μg/L)	2.97 ± 0.074	2.58 ± 0.038	0.39 ± 0.078	0.000*
Cu (μg/dL)	216.65 ± 6.93	173.07 ± 3.66	43.58 ± 7.917	0.000*
	Residents	Controls		
	n = 60	n = 100		
Fe (μg/dL)	96.13 ± 1.429	150.99 ± 1.35	−54.86 ± 0.08	0.000*
Zn (μg/dL)	78.25 ± 1.863	106.52 ± 0.70	−28.28 ± 1.16	0.000*
Pb (μg/dL)	20.091 ± 0.643	10.33 ± 0.60	9.76 ± 0.04	0.000*
As (μg/dL)	0.011 ± 0.005	0.003 ± 0.002	0.007 ± 0.003	0.000*
Cd (μg/dL)	1.95 ± 0.21	0.022 ± 0.001	1.93 ± 0.143	0.000*
Cr (μg/dL)	1.60 ± 0.13	0.012 ± 0.000	1.60 ± 0.08	0.000*
Se (μg/dL)	1.75 ± 0.13	0.044 ± 0.015	1.71 ± 0.09	0.000*
Mn (μg/L)	3.35 ± 0.06	2.58 ± 0.038	0.77 ± 0.07	0.000*
Cu (μg/dL)	234.62 ± 7.17	173.07 ± 3.66	61.56 ± 0.50	0.000*
	Cem. workers	Residents		
	n = 50	n = 60		
Fe (μg/dL)	102.08 ± 1.78	96.13 ± 1.43	5.945 ± 2.422	0.015*
Zn (μg/dL)	80.95 ± 2.007	78.25 ± 1.86	2.69 ± 2.19	0.219
Pb (μg/dL)	15.93 ± 0.42	20.09 ± 0.64	−4.16 ± 0.98	0.000*
As (μg/dL)	0.011 ± 0.002	0.011 ± 0.005	.0002 ± 0.0005	0.693
Cd (μg/dL)	0.042 ± 0.008	1.95 ± 0.212	−1.91 ± 0.168	0.000*
Cr (μg/dL)	0.033 ± 0.013	1.60 ± 0.125	−1.57 ± 0.10	0.000*
Se (μg/dL)	0.023 ± 0.004	1.75 ± 0.127	−1.73 ± 0.103	0.000*
Mn (μg/L)	2.97 ± 0.074	3.35 ± 0.062	−.38 ± 0.09	0.000*
Cu (μg/dL)	216.65 ± 6.93	234.62 ± 7.17	−17.97 ± 8.75	0.041*

*Significant at $p < 0.05$.

dust particles on upper and lower airways of the trachea-bronchial region of the lungs results in shortness of breath, chest tightness, sneezing, and coughing. Interaction between cement dust particles and the mast cell or basophil surface results in their degranulation and release of a variety of pharmacological active agents, including histamine and serotonin; the effect of these amines on tissues such as bronchial smooth muscles and vascular endothelium produces many of the symptoms of atopic conditions observed [18].

Prolonged duration of exposure to cement dust was associated with decreased peak expiratory flow. Similar observations have been reported by other studies [15, 16, 19, 20]. Bioaccumulation of some specific components as chromium and silica present in the cement dust in the respiratory tract may lead to delayed hypersensitivity reaction and chronic inflammation and hence impaired respiratory function. Contrary to our findings, a study by Fell et al. [1] reported no

association between duration of cement dust exposure and decreased peak expiratory flow.

Increased levels of serum alanine aminotransferase, aspartate aminotransferase, and total and conjugated bilirubin were observed in cement workers compared to controls. The higher levels of aminotransferase observed in the cement workers are still within normal range for the liver enzyme in circulation and hence are not indicative of liver impairment. The liver has a high functional reserve capacity and only shows dysfunction when about 50% of the hepatocytes are affected. However, this increase may be an indication of potential for future development of hepatotoxic complications in occupationally exposed individuals. Our findings are in agreement with reports from other studies [8, 21]. Contrary to our findings, elevated serum levels of alanine aminotransferase, aspartate aminotransferase, and alkaline phosphatase above the normal ranges have been reported in cement workers by Al Salhen [22]. Cement dust inclusion particles, diffuse swelling, proliferation of hepatic sinusoidal lining cells, sarcoid granulomas, and perisinusoidal and portal fibrosis have been described in the hepatocytes of cement mill workers. These changes have been associated with hepatic lesions produced by inhaled cement dust [23].

Increased serum lead, arsenic, cadmium, chromium, selenium, manganese, and copper levels and lower iron and zinc levels were observed in cement workers and residents living near cement factory when compared to unexposed controls. Increased levels of chromium, copper, manganese, and selenium have also been demonstrated in cement factory workers and had been attributed to their exposure to cement dust [6, 24]. The toxic effect of most elements depends principally on the absorption, concentration, and persistence of the element at its site of action. These elements react with the endogenous target molecule such as receptors, enzymes, DNA, proteins, and lipids and critically alter their biologic functions, producing structural and functional changes that result in toxic damage [25]. Zinc and copper are components of antioxidant enzyme copper-zinc superoxide dismutase (Cu-Zn SOD). The increased demand on the antioxidant system to buffer the deleterious effects of heavy metal accumulation may account for lower zinc levels and a compensatory increase in copper levels seen in cement factory workers compared to unexposed controls. The body tends to retain copper to combat heavy antioxidant demands [6]. Decreased iron levels seen in cement workers may be associated with increased copper levels. Copper is a component of ceruloplasmin which catalyzes the oxidation of iron to ferric forms for binding to its transport protein transferrin and subsequent storage in tissues and synthesis of haemoglobin. Therefore, increased copper implies increased conversion and removal of circulating iron and hence decreased serum levels seen in cement factory workers [6].

Cement workers had higher levels of ALT, AST, and Fe and lower levels of Pb, Cd, Cr, Se, Mn, and Cu compared to residents of communities near the cement factory. The observation of higher serum levels of ALT, AST, and Fe and lower Cu seen has been discussed above. Contrary to our findings, no significant difference was reported in serum blood lead levels of cement workers and residents of neighboring community in a cement factory [26]. Lower levels of Pb, Cd, Cr, Se, and Mn in cement workers compared to residents may be attributed to the observation that cement factory workers are mandated to observe the laid down protective and safety precaution of the use of dust masks at factory site. Residents, on the other hand, do not observe such precautionary measures. Higher elements levels in residents compared to cement workers may also be attributed to duration of exposure which is also a determining factor in serum elements concentration. Cement workers are mere employees of the cement factory whose exposure to cement dust is dependent on duration of employment. Residents on the other hand spend almost all their life time in their community and are therefore exposed to cement dust on daily basis. The continuous inhalation or ingestion makes even the smallest concentration of such toxic elements a concern to their health. This is because the effects of

exposure to any hazardous substance depend on the route of the exposure, concentration of substance, and duration of exposure. The level of toxicity found in short term exposure may be remedied, but the long term toxicity is associated with undesirable health consequences.

The findings of this study have shown that occupational exposure to cement dust may be associated with changes in the homeostasis of some essential and toxic elements resulting in higher levels of Pb, As, Cd, Cr, Se, Mn, and Cu and lower levels of Fe and Zn which may be implicated in impaired peak expiratory flow rate with potentials for future development of hepatotoxicity. These observations emphasize the need for adequate safety and precautionary measures among cement factory workers.

Conflict of Interests

The authors declare that there is no conflict of interests regarding the publication of this paper.

References

[1] A. K. M. Fell, T. R. Thomassen, P. Kristensen, T. Egeland, and J. Kongerud, "Respiratory symptoms and ventilatory function in workers exposed to Portland cement dust," *Journal of Occupational and Environmental Medicine*, vol. 45, no. 9, pp. 1008–1014, 2003.

[2] A. M. Gbadebo and O. D. Bankole, "Analysis of potentially toxic metals in airborne cement dust around Sagamu, Southwestern Nigeria," *Journal of Applied Sciences*, vol. 7, no. 1, pp. 35–40, 2007.

[3] A. A. Baccarelli, Y. Zheng, X. Zhang et al., "Air pollution exposure and lung function in highly exposed subjects in Beijing, China: repeated-measure study," *Particle and Fibre Toxicology*, vol. 11, pp. 51–60, 2014.

[4] Z. K. Zeleke, B. E. Moen, and M. Bråtveit, "Cement dust exposure and acute lung function: a cross shift study," *BMC Pulmonary Medicine*, vol. 10, article 19, 2010.

[5] N. Zawilla, F. Taha, and Y. Ibrahim, "Liver functions in silica-exposed workers in Egypt: possible role of matrix remodeling and immunological factors," *International Journal of Occupational and Environmental Health*, vol. 20, no. 2, pp. 146–156, 2014.

[6] J. O. Ogunbileje and O. M. Akinosun, "Biochemical and haematological profile in nigerian cement factory workers," *Research Journal of Environmental Toxicology*, vol. 5, no. 2, pp. 133–140, 2011.

[7] Health Risk Assessment Guidance for Metals (HERAG), "Assessment of occupational dermal exposure and dermal absorption for metals and inorganic compounds," HERAG fact sheet 12007, 2007.

[8] J. O. Ogunbileje, O. M. Akinosun, O. G. Arinola, and P. Akinduti, "Immunological classes (IgG, IgA, IgM and IgE) and liver function tests in Nigerian cement factory workers," *Researcher*, vol. 2, no. 4, pp. 55–58, 2010.

[9] W. Alakija, V. I. Iyawe, L. N. Jarikre, and J. C. Chiwuzie, "Ventilatory function of workers at Okpella cement factory in Nigeria," *West African Journal of Medicine*, vol. 9, no. 3, pp. 187–192, 1990.

[10] G. A. Lameed, "Environmental impact assessment of cement factory production on biodiversity: a case study of UNICEM,

Calabar Nigeria," *World Journal of Biological Research*, vol. 1, pp. 1–7, 2008.

[11] S. Reitman and S. Frankel, "A colorimetric method for the determination of serum glutamic oxalacetic and glutamic pyruvic transaminases," *American Journal of Clinical Pathology*, vol. 28, no. 1, pp. 56–63, 1957.

[12] D. Watson, "Analytic methods for bilirubin in blood plasma," *Clinical Chemistry*, vol. 7, pp. 603–625, 1961.

[13] M. E. Everson, "Spectrophotometric techniques," in *Tietz Textbook of Clinical Chemistry*, C. A. Burtis and E. R. Ashwood, Eds., pp. 75–93, W. B. Saunders, Philadelphia, Pa, USA, 3rd edition, 1999.

[14] B. M. Wright and C. B. McKerrow, "Maximum forced expiratory flow rate as a measure of ventilatory capacity: with a description of a new portable instrument for measuring it," *British Medical Journal*, vol. 2, no. 5159, pp. 1041–1046, 1959.

[15] S. Shaikh, A. A. Nafees, V. Khetpal, A. A. Jamali, A. M. Arain, and A. Yousuf, "Respiratory symptoms and illnesses among brick kiln workers: a cross sectional study from rural districts of Pakistan," *BMC Public Health*, vol. 12, article 999, 2012.

[16] A. Mandal (Majee) and R. Majumder, "Assessment of pulmonary function of cement industry workers from," *Progress in Health Sciences*, vol. 3, no. 1, pp. 65–71, 2013.

[17] H. Noor, C. L. Yap, O. Zolkepli, and M. Faridah, "Effect of exposure to dust on lung function of cement factory workers," *Medical Journal of Malaysia*, vol. 55, no. 1, pp. 51–58, 2000.

[18] J. G. Ayres, "The effects of inhaled materials on the lung and other target organs," in *Occupational Hygiene*, K. Gardiner and J. M. Harrington, Eds., vol. 2, pp. 7–13, Wiley-Blackwell, 3rd edition, 2005.

[19] O. G. Akanbi, O. Ismaila, W. Olaoniye, K. T. Oriolowo, and A. Odusote, "Assessment of post-work peak expiratory flow rate of workers in cement company," *Sigurnost*, vol. 56, no. 4, pp. 315–322, 2014.

[20] S. A. Meo, A. M. Al-Drees, A. A. Al Masri, F. Al Rouq, and M. A. Azeem, "Effect of duration of exposure to cement dust on respiratory function of non-smoking cement mill workers," *International Journal of Environmental Research and Public Health*, vol. 10, no. 1, pp. 390–398, 2013.

[21] F. B. Mojiminiyi, I. A. Merenu, M. T. Ibrahim, and C. H. Njoku, "The effect of cement dust exposure on haematological and liver function parameters of cement factory workers in Sokoto, Nigeria," *Nigerian Journal of Physiological Sciences*, vol. 23, no. 1-2, pp. 111–114, 2008.

[22] K. S. Al Salhen, "Assessment of oxidative stress, haematological, kidney and liver function parameters of Libyan cement factory workers," *Journal of American Science*, vol. 10, no. 5, pp. 58–65, 2014.

[23] J. C. Pimentel and A. P. Menezes, "Pulmonary and hepatic granulomatous disorders due to the inhalation of cement and mica dusts," *Thorax*, vol. 33, no. 2, pp. 219–227, 1978.

[24] J. O. Ogunbilege, O. M. Akinosun, P. A. Akinduti, L. A. Nwaobi, and O. A. Ejilude, "Serum levels of some trace metals and leucocyte differential count in Nigeria cement factory workers; Possible toxicityimplications," *Florida Int. J.*, vol. 2, pp. 55–58, 2010.

[25] L. J. Langman and B. M. Kapur, "Toxicology: then and now," *Clinical Biochemistry*, vol. 39, no. 5, pp. 498–510, 2006.

[26] O. O. Babalola and S. O. Babajide, "Selected heavy metals and electrolyte levels in blood of workers and residents of industrial communities," *African Journal of Biochemistry Research*, vol. 3, no. 3, pp. 37–40, 2009.

5

Comparative Hepatotoxicity of Fluconazole, Ketoconazole, Itraconazole, Terbinafine, and Griseofulvin in Rats

Star Khoza,[1] **Ishmael Moyo,**[1] **and Denver Ncube**[2]

[1]*Department of Clinical Pharmacology, College of Health Sciences, University of Zimbabwe, Harare, Zimbabwe*
[2]*Department of Anatomy, College of Health Sciences, University of Zimbabwe, Harare, Zimbabwe*

Correspondence should be addressed to Star Khoza; skhoza@medsch.uz.ac.zw

Academic Editor: Brad Upham

Oral ketoconazole was recently the subject of regulatory safety warnings because of its association with increased risk of inducing hepatic injury. However, the relative hepatotoxicity of antifungal agents has not been clearly established. The aim of this study was to compare the hepatotoxicity induced by five commonly prescribed oral antifungal agents. Rats were treated with therapeutic oral doses of griseofulvin, fluconazole, itraconazole, ketoconazole, and terbinafine. After 14 days, only ketoconazole had significantly higher ALT levels ($p = 0.0017$) and AST levels ($p = 0.0008$) than the control group. After 28 days, ALT levels were highest in the rats treated with ketoconazole followed by itraconazole, fluconazole, griseofulvin, and terbinafine, respectively. The AST levels were highest in the rats treated with ketoconazole followed by itraconazole, fluconazole, terbinafine, and griseofulvin, respectively. All drugs significantly elevated ALP levels after 14 days and 28 days of treatment ($p < 0.0001$). The liver enzyme levels suggested that ketoconazole had the highest risk in causing liver injury followed by itraconazole, fluconazole, terbinafine, and griseofulvin. However, histopathological changes revealed that fluconazole was the most hepatotoxic, followed by ketoconazole, itraconazole, terbinafine, and griseofulvin, respectively. Given the poor correlation between liver enzymes and the extent of liver injury, it is important to confirm liver injury through histological examination.

1. Introduction

In 2013, the United States Food and Drug Administration (US FDA) and the European Medicines Agency's Committee on Medical Products for Human Use (EMA-CHMP) concurrently issued safety warnings and limited the use of oral ketoconazole because of its association with increased risk of inducing hepatic injury, risk of drug interactions, and increased risk of adrenal insufficiency [1, 2]. The two agencies recommended that ketoconazole should be used "only when alternative antifungal therapies are not available or tolerated." In addition to the safety warning, the FDA issued another directive recommending that drug companies and researchers should avoid using oral ketoconazole in drug interaction studies [3]. The regulatory safety warnings on oral ketoconazole have serious implications on its use in the clinical and drug development settings. Ketoconazole has been widely used for more than three decades in the treatment of fungal infections and has been the principal prototype human cytochrome P450 3A inhibitor in drug interaction studies and drug metabolism research during drug development [4–6].

The link between ketoconazole and hepatotoxicity is well established [7–10]. However, for a long time the evidence suggested that the hepatotoxicity was mild, rarely fatal, and reversible upon discontinuation of the drug [7, 8, 10]. An estimated prevalence of serious hepatotoxicity of one in 15,000 patients was reported in the United Kingdom in the first decade of oral ketoconazole market authorization [10]. Incidence data on ketoconazole induced hepatotoxicity is scarce. In a randomized controlled study, subclinical hepatic dysfunction was observed in 17.5% of patients treated with ketoconazole while none of the patients treated with griseofulvin had evidence of hepatic dysfunction [11]. By contrast, a recent meta-analysis of 204 studies reported an overall incidence of ketoconazole-associated hepatotoxicity of between 3.6% and 4.2% [12].

Although the hepatotoxicity of antifungal agents is well established [9, 13–19], their relative hepatotoxicity has not been extensively evaluated [20]. Two epidemiological studies reported contrasting findings regarding the relative hepatotoxicity of antifungal agents [21, 22]. One of the studies cited by the FDA in its regulatory decision reported that ketoconazole was associated with the highest relative risk (RR = 228; 95% CI: 33.9–933.0) when compared to nonusers, followed by itraconazole (RR = 17.7; 95% CI: 2.6–72.6) and terbinafine (RR = 4.2; 95% CI: 0.2–24.9) [21]. This study included a cohort of 69,830 patients in the United Kingdom who had received at least one prescription for fluconazole, griseofulvin, itraconazole, ketoconazole, or terbinafine between 1991 and 1996. Of the 69,830 patients included in the study, only 1052 received ketoconazole. The incidence rates of hepatotoxicity were highest in patients treated with ketoconazole (19.0 per 10,000), followed by itraconazole (1.0 per 10,000) and terbinafine (0.7 per 10,000) [21]. In contrast to the study by García Rodríguez et al. (1999), Kao and associates reported the highest incidence rate of drug-induced liver injury of 31.6 per 10,000 patients in individuals who received fluconazole, compared to 4.9 for ketoconazole, 4.3 for griseofulvin, 3.6 for itraconazole, and 1.6 for terbinafine [22]. The study included 90,847 patients in Taiwan who received oral antifungal agents between 2002 and 2008. Of these patients, 57,321 received oral ketoconazole [22].

Based on the currently available evidence, it is uncertain which antifungal agent poses the greatest risk of hepatotoxicity. The small number of cases in the two epidemiological studies that reported on the relative hepatotoxicity of antifungal agents limits the interpretation of their findings [21, 22]. The findings by García Rodríguez et al. (1999) were based on 16 cases of acute liver injury [21]. Of these 16 cases, five occurred during current use of oral antifungal agents: two were using ketoconazole, two were using itraconazole, and one was using terbinafine. Out of the ten remaining cases, only one had a history of using an antifungal agent while the other nine cases occurred before the use of any antifungal agent. Similarly, the study by Kao et al. (2014) was based on only 52 cases of drug-induced liver injury [22]. Of the 52 cases, 28 used ketoconazole, 14 were of fluconazole, 8 were of griseofulvin, 3 were of itraconazole, and 2 were of terbinafine. In addition to the failure by these two epidemiologic studies to provide conclusive evidence regarding the antifungal agent with the greatest risk of hepatotoxicity, few head-to-head experimental studies have evaluated the relative hepatotoxicity of oral antifungal agents in clinical settings or using animal models [11, 23–25]. Furthermore, the higher number of cases of liver injury reported with ketoconazole than fluconazole might be related to the higher number of prescriptions for ketoconazole than fluconazole. Given the implications of the safety warnings issued in 2013 on the use of ketoconazole in clinical settings and during drug development research, there is need for experimental studies that evaluate the relative hepatotoxicity of azole antifungal agents. The objective of this study was to compare the hepatotoxicity effects of the five commonly prescribed oral antifungal agents (ketoconazole, fluconazole, itraconazole, terbinafine, and griseofulvin). We hypothesized that fluconazole is more hepatotoxic than ketoconazole based on histological examination.

2. Materials and Methods

2.1. Materials. All biochemical kits for alanine aminotransferase (ALT), aspartate amino transferases (AST), and alkaline phosphatase (ALP) were sourced from Beckman Coulter Inc. (California, USA). Terbinafine (Lamisil®; batch number U0638; marketed by Novartis Pharma Ltd., United Kingdom), itraconazole (Canditral®; batch number 01141282; marketed by Glenmark Pharmaceuticals Ltd., India), griseofulvin (Griseon®; batch number 178046; marketed by Plus Five Pharmaceuticals Ltd., Zimbabwe), fluconazole (Flumyc-200®; batch number AHP054014; marketed by Ipca Laboratories Ltd., India), and ketoconazole (Nizol®; batch number 13312; marketed by Intas Pharmaceuticals Ltd., India) were all sourced from a local pharmaceutical wholesaler. Standard diet pellets were obtained from National Foods Pvt. Ltd., Zimbabwe. Formaldehyde (37% solution), paraffin wax, haematoxylin, eosin, and other standard laboratory chemicals were sourced from Sigma-Aldrich (United Kingdom). Blood collection tubes (Vacuette® Z serum clot activator tubes) were sourced from Greiner Bio-One (United Kingdom). Microcentrifuge tubes (LW2075; batch number 110488) were sourced from Alpha Laboratories (Hampshire, United Kingdom).

2.2. Animals and Dosing Procedures. Sixty-six 6-week-old male Sprague Dawley rats weighing 180–200 g were adapted to laboratory conditions for five days before experimentation. The rats were housed in plastic cages in groups of six with wood shavings as bedding under a 12-hour light/12-hour dark cycle. The rats were maintained in a conventional animal house with an ambient temperature of 25 ± 2°C and were given commercial standard diet rat pellets and tap water ad libitum. Ethical clearance to conduct the study was obtained from the Joint Parirenyatwa Hospital and College of Health Sciences Research Ethics Committee (approval number: JREC/328/14). The animals were handled and treated following the principles outlined in the "Guide for the Care and Use of Laboratory Animals" prepared by the National Academy of Sciences and published by the National Institutes of Health (NIH publication 86-23 Rev. 1985).

The rats were divided into eleven groups (each group with six rats) including the control group. The rats in the control group were sacrificed one day before drug administration (day 0) in the active treatment groups. Five groups of rats received a daily single oral antifungal agent dose for 14 days. The other five groups of rats received a daily single oral antifungal agent dose for 28 days. The intragastric method (oral gavage) was used during drug administration. The treatment interventions were 20 mg/kg fluconazole, 50 mg/kg griseofulvin, 20 mg/kg ketoconazole, 20 mg/kg itraconazole, and 25 mg/kg terbinafine. Antifungal agents are frequently prescribed for two weeks or four weeks for most systemic and topical fungal infections. The equivalent doses in rats for common adult dose ranges for systemic and topical infections

TABLE 1: Effect of the five oral antifungal agents (griseofulvin, fluconazole, ketoconazole, itraconazole, and terbinafine) on serum activities of AST, ALT, and ALP in rats after 14 days of treatment.

Groups	AST/IU mean ± SEM	ALT/IU mean ± SEM	ALP/IU mean ± SEM
Control	58.50 ± 5.40^a	60.17 ± 6.30^a	152.17 ± 5.57^a
Griseofulvin	124.33 ± 25.17^a	86.33 ± 8.06^a	$370.50 \pm 19.81^{b,c}$
Fluconazole	$275.83 \pm 69.45^{a,b}$	$178.33 \pm 42.85^{a,b}$	$409.50 \pm 29.78^{b,c}$
Ketoconazole	431.17 ± 101.89^b	283.17 ± 61.96^b	324.67 ± 18.33^b
Itraconazole	$272.00 \pm 48.10^{a,b}$	$172.17 \pm 44.18^{a,b}$	$414.50 \pm 17.19^{b,c}$
Terbinafine	135.67 ± 34.98^a	88.67 ± 6.10^a	420.33 ± 26.30^c

AST: aspartate aminotransferase, ALT: alanine aminotransferase, and ALP: alkaline phosphatase
[a–e]Tukey's post hoc analysis: like letters (a–e) indicate nonsignificant differences.

for the antifungal agents are as follows: fluconazole (10–20 mg/kg), griseofulvin (25–50 mg/kg), ketoconazole (10–20 mg/kg), itraconazole (10–40 mg/kg), and terbinafine (10–25 mg/kg). A suspension of each drug in distilled water was prepared two hours prior to administration. The doses were calculated using the formula provided by the US FDA (i.e., animal dose = clinical human dose × conversion factor for rats [6.2]) [26].

2.3. Sampling and Biochemical Assays. Blood samples were collected on three different occasions on days 0, 15, and 29, using the cardiac puncture method. Day 0 was the day before initial drug administration. Blood samples collected from rats sacrificed on day 0 were for the determination of baseline liver enzyme levels in the clan of the rats. Day 15 was defined as the day after the rats had completed 14-day courses of drug treatment, that is, 24 hours after last dose. Day 29 was defined as the day after the rats had completed 28-day courses of treatment. Blood samples (4.0 ml) were collected using red top (black ring) vacutainers (6.0 ml Vacuette® Z serum clot activator tubes; Greiner Bio-One Ltd., UK) and were left to clot for 30 minutes before being spun down. Blood samples were spun down at 1200 rpm for 10 minutes and the serum transferred to 1.5 ml plastic microcentrifuge tubes (Alpha Laboratories, UK). The serum was then stored at −18°C up to the day of analysis (at most 7 days). The Beckman AU680® chemistry analyser was used to determine plasma levels of ALP, AST, and ALT. Aspartate transaminase (AST) and alanine transaminase (ALT) activity in serum were assayed using a procedure based on the method developed by Wróblewski and Ladue [27–29]. Alkaline phosphatase (ALP) activity in serum was assayed by a procedure based on the method developed by Bowers Jr. and McComb [30].

2.4. Histological Examination. All the animals were sacrificed humanly under chloroform anaesthesia at the end of each treatment period. Livers were removed and fixed in 10% formalin for 24 hours. The whole liver tissue samples were then put in an automated tissue processer Leica TP10202 for 24 hours for dehydration using alcohol and clearing using xylol. The liver samples were then embedded in paraffin wax and cut into sections of 5 μm thickness, mounted on clean glass slides coated with Mayer's egg albumin, and were stained with hematoxylin and eosin (H&E). Liver sections containing the central venule were used to make comparisons across treatment groups. Light microscopy (Motic BA210®) was used to generate photomicrographs during histological examinations. All histologic examinations were performed by the same histologist (DN).

2.5. Statistical Analysis. Data are presented as the mean value ± standard error of the mean (SEM). Comparisons among multiple groups were done using one way ANOVA followed Tukey's post hoc test as appropriate. Two group comparisons were done using Student's t-test. Kruskal-Wallis test and Mann–Whitney test were used as appropriate whenever the normality assumption was violated. The significance level was set at $\alpha = 0.05$. Statistical analysis was carried out using Graph Pad® Prism Version 6.0 for Windows (California, USA).

3. Results

3.1. Biochemical Findings. After 14 days of treatment, only ketoconazole had significantly higher ALT levels ($p = 0.0017$) and AST levels ($p = 0.0008$) than the control group. The ALT and AST levels were highest in rats treated with ketoconazole, followed by fluconazole, itraconazole, terbinafine, and griseofulvin. ALT levels in rats treated with ketoconazole were significantly higher than the levels in rats treated with griseofulvin ($p = 0.0066$) and terbinafine ($p = 0.0074$). Similarly, AST levels in rats treated with ketoconazole were significantly higher than the levels in rats treated with griseofulvin ($p = 0.0076$) and terbinafine ($p = 0.0109$). However, no significant differences in ALT and AST levels were observed between ketoconazole and fluconazole and between ketoconazole and itraconazole ($p > 0.05$). All drugs had significantly higher ALP levels than the control group after 14 days of treatment ($p < 0.0001$). Rats treated with terbinafine had the highest ALP levels, followed by those treated with itraconazole, fluconazole, griseofulvin, and ketoconazole, respectively. Table 1 shows the effect of the antifungal agents on liver enzymes in rats after 14 days of treatment.

After 28 days of treatment, all the drugs had significantly higher AST levels compared to the control group ($p < 0.001$). The AST levels were highest in the rats treated with ketoconazole followed by itraconazole, fluconazole,

TABLE 2: Effect of the five oral antifungal agents (griseofulvin, fluconazole, ketoconazole, itraconazole, and terbinafine) on serum activities of AST, ALT, and ALP in rats after 28 days of treatment.

Groups	AST/IU mean ± SEM	ALT/IU mean ± SEM	ALP/IU mean ± SEM
Control	58.50 ± 5.40[a]	60.17 ± 6.30[a]	152.17 ± 5.57[a]
Griseofulvin	172.83 ± 11.48[b]	114.50 ± 6.06[b]	418.17 ± 8.07[b]
Fluconazole	323.67 ± 19.49[c]	243.00 ± 16.43[c]	566.33 ± 15.46[c]
Ketoconazole	608.17 ± 24.78[d]	400.00 ± 14.73[d]	446.00 ± 14.13[b,d]
Itraconazole	440.17 ± 12.98[e]	296.67 ± 13.62[e]	554.33 ± 24.40[c,d]
Terbinafine	179.67 ± 13.89[b]	105.83 ± 4.24[a,b]	499.17 ± 16.77[d]

AST: aspartate aminotransferase, ALT: alanine aminotransferase, and ALP: alkaline phosphatase
[a–e] Tukey's post hoc analysis: like letters (a–e) indicate nonsignificant differences.

terbinafine, and griseofulvin, respectively. All drugs, except terbinafine, had significantly higher ALT levels compared to the control group after 28 days of treatment ($p < 0.05$). The ALT levels were highest in the rats treated with keto-conazole followed by itraconazole, fluconazole, griseofulvin, and terbinafine, respectively. All drugs had significantly higher ALP levels than the control group after 28 days of treatment ($p < 0.001$). Fluconazole caused the highest ALP levels, followed by itraconazole, terbinafine, ketoconazole, and griseofulvin, respectively. Table 2 shows the effect of the antifungal agents on liver enzymes in rats after 28 days of treatment.

AST levels after 28 days of treatment with itraconazole were significantly higher than the levels after 14 days of treatment ($p = 0.0071$). Similarly, treatment with itraconazole ($p = 0.0226$), terbinafine ($p = 0.0434$), and griseofulvin ($p = 0.0190$) for 28 days resulted in higher ALT levels than treatment for 14-day courses, respectively. Furthermore, there were significant duration-dependent elevations in ALP levels after treatment with fluconazole ($p = 0.0009$), ketoconazole ($p = 0.0004$), itraconazole ($p = 0.0009$), and terbinafine ($p = 0.0300$) for 28 days compared with treatments for 14 days. Figure 1 shows a comparison of liver enzymes after 14 days and 28 days of treatment.

3.2. Histopathological Findings. There were no gross pathological changes observed by naked eye examination. Figure 2 shows photomicrographs of the livers of the control and after treatment with the antifungal agents. Light microscopic examination of livers of control rats showed normal lobulation with clear outlines, normal Kupffer cells with distinct cell boundaries and clearly visible nuclei, no infiltration of central venules by leukocytes, and lack of mitotic figures (Figure 2(a)). Treatment with fluconazole resulted in the most severe damage compared to all the groups. A reduction in cell nuclear density in centrilobular, severe hepatocyte degeneration, severe inflammation and necrosis, granuloma, and bile duct hyperplasia were observed after fluconazole treatment (Figure 2(b)). Although there was no significant difference in cell death between the 14- and 28-day courses, in the 28-day course the tissue exhibited minor indications of recovery with the normal lobulation appearing. Infiltration of central venules by leukocytes and nuclei of Kupffer cell were less after 28 days of treatment.

Ketoconazole caused the same level of hepatocyte degeneration, inflammation, and necrosis as that observed with fluconazole (Figure 2(c)). However, there were fewer granulomas and less severe bile duct hyperplasia during treatment with ketoconazole than with fluconazole. Venular infiltration and hepatic parenchymal invasion, in addition to centrilobular degeneration, was observed during treatment with ketoconazole. By contrast, mitotic figures, cell atrophy, and fewer nuclei were more profound compared to other groups. The severity of hepatic damage increased slightly during the 28-day course with more necrotic cells being observed than during the 14-day course. However, leukocyte infiltration was moderately less after 28 days of treatment than over the 14-day course.

In the group treated with itraconazole, most notable features were leukocytes infiltration of the central venules and mitotic figures, which worsened after 28 days of treatment compared to 14 days of treatment (Figure 2(d)). Terbinafine caused mild hepatic damage during both courses, with few mitotic figures and minor central venule infiltration by leukocytes observed (Figure 2(e)). No significant duration-dependent cell damage was observed during treatment with terbinafine. Griseofulvin caused mild hepatic damage, inflammation, centrilobular necrosis, and central venule infiltration by leukocytes (Figure 2(f)). No significant duration-dependent cell damage was observed during treatment with griseofulvin and this group caused the least hepatic damage. Based on the histological observations, fluconazole caused the worst hepatic damage followed by ketoconazole, itraconazole, terbinafine, and griseofulvin, respectively. The summary of histopathological findings is presented in Table 3.

4. Discussion

The purpose of the present study was to compare the hepatotoxicity of clinically used doses of fluconazole, grise-ofulvin, itraconazole, ketoconazole, and terbinafine. The pattern of liver enzyme levels indicated that ketoconazole, fluconazole, and itraconazole caused mixed hepatic injury (i.e., cholestatic-hepatocellular injury) while griseofulvin and terbinafine appear to have predominantly resulted in cholestatic injury. Azole antifungal agents have been reported to cause both hepatocellular and cholestatic injury [18]. The increase in liver enzymes with longer treatment duration

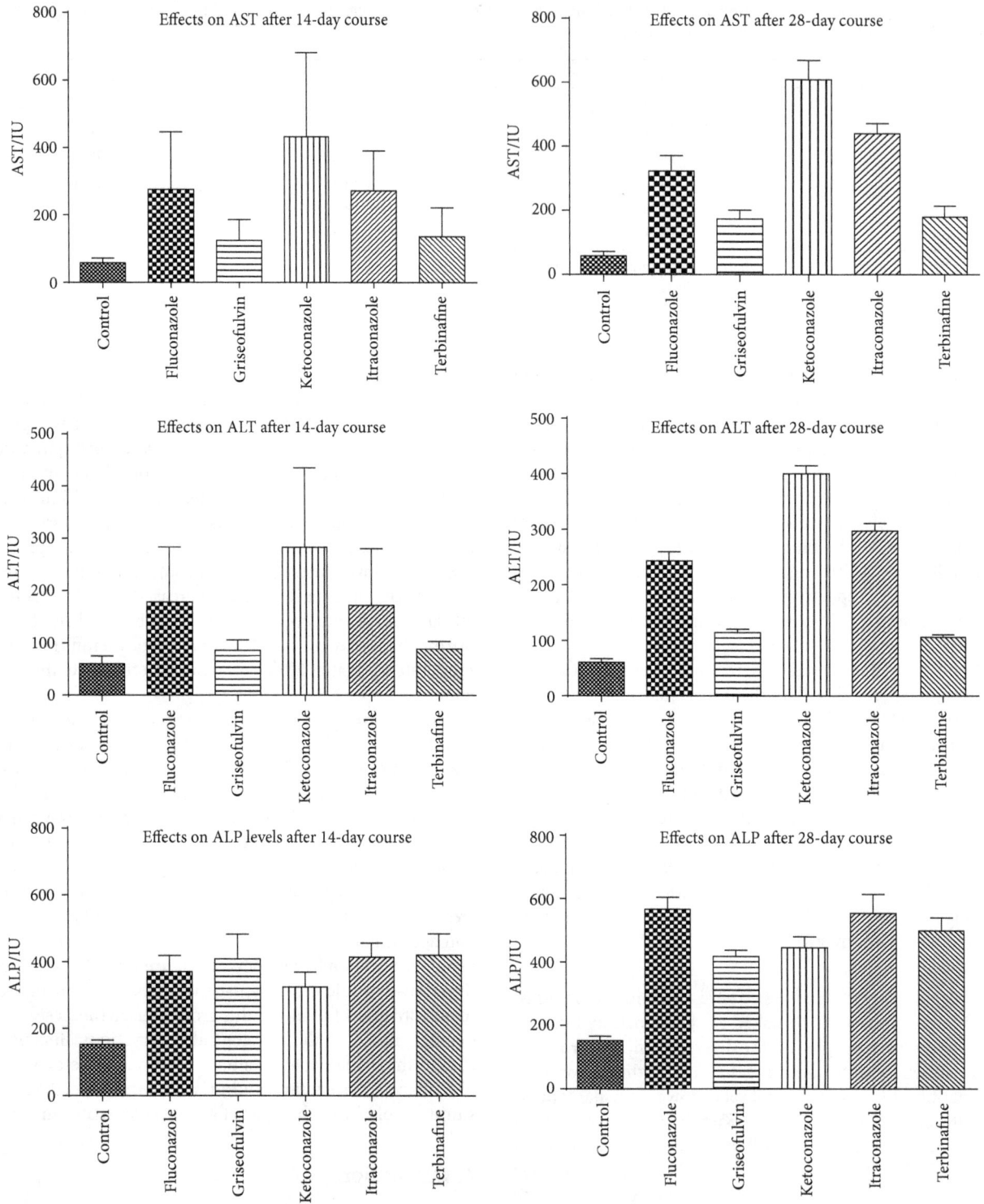

FIGURE 1: Serum levels of AST, ALT, and ALP, for the control group and the groups that received 14- and 28-day courses of fluconazole, griseofulvin, ketoconazole, itraconazole, and terbinafine.

was noted with all antifungal agents, with itraconazole and terbinafine recording the highest changes in liver enzymes. In contrast, significant histological changes were observed with itraconazole while only slight worsening in hepatic damage was observed with ketoconazole treatment. The increase in the risk of hepatotoxicity during longer treatment with antifungal agents has been reported in several studies [22–24, 31] and regular monitoring of liver enzymes in patients that require long treatment with antifungal agents is standard practice.

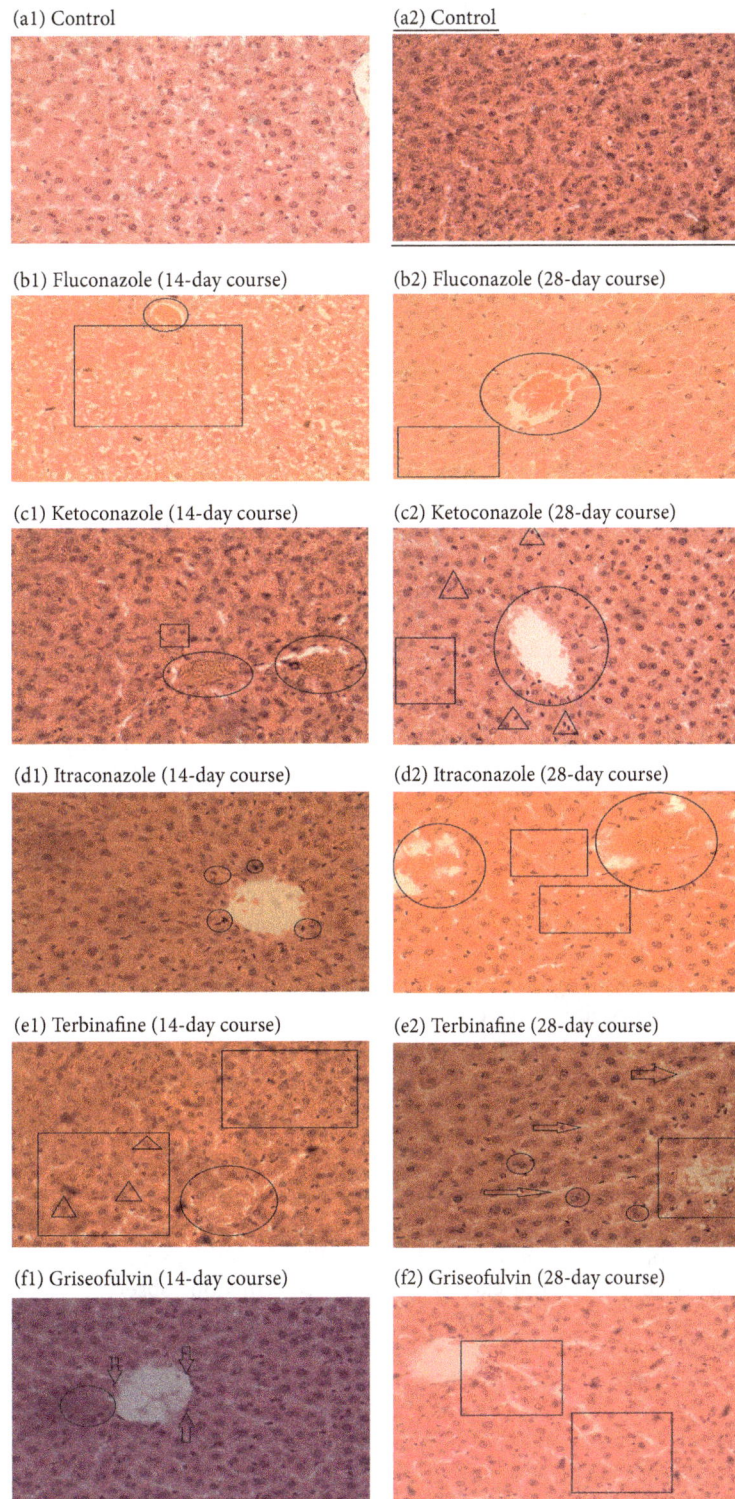

FIGURE 2: Photomicrographs of liver sections of the control group (a) and after 14- and 28-day courses of fluconazole (b), ketoconazole (c), itraconazole (d), terbinafine (e), and griseofulvin (f). (a) Normal lobulation with clear outlines, normal cells with visible outlines, and single nuclei. (b) In 14-day plate the rectangular area shows a marked reduction of cell numbers in the perivenular area. Circular areas indicate infiltration of venules by leukocytes. 28-day course plate shows reduced cellular density similar to 14-day plate. (c) Rectangular area indicates reduced cell density; circular areas indicate perivenular region with minor necrotic figures, that is, dark spots on plate. Triangular region indicates scattered necrotic foci (28-day course). (d) Minor venular distortion indicated by the circular demarcations here; triangular areas show apoptotic cells. Rectangular area shows reduced cell density. (e) Rectangular area shows paucity of cells; circular areas show clustering of cells which is a possible indication of stress. (f) Rectangular areas show a reduction in cell numbers and tissue striations (28 d). Perivenular cell paucity is hedicated by the circular area on the plate (14 d). Also apparent are necrotic foci around the central venue (arrows). All plates are ×200 magnification.

TABLE 3: Histopathological findings in livers of treatment with antifungal agents.

Treatment group	Histological findings in the liver			
	Hepatocyte degeneration	Necrosis	Inflammation	Bile duct hyperplasia and granuloma
Ketoconazole	+++	+++	+++	++
Fluconazole	+++	+++	+++	+++
Itraconazole	++	++	++	+
Griseofulvin	+	+	+	+
Terbinafine	+	+	+	++

Normal (<4 lesions); + mild (4–7 lesions); ++ moderate (8–11 lesions); +++ severe lesions (≥12 lesions per slide); inflammation was determined based on the presence of macrophages and scattered neutrophils and eosinophils in central venules.

Based on liver enzyme levels observed in this study, ketoconazole had the highest risk in causing liver injury followed by itraconazole, fluconazole, terbinafine, and griseofulvin. The relative hepatotoxicity of antifungal agents based on liver enzymes is consistent with several studies. The higher ALT levels during treatment with ketoconazole than during treatment with fluconazole observed in this study is consistent with an in vitro study that reported that ketoconazole significantly increased the levels of ALT and lactate dehydrogenase (LDH) in cultured rat hepatocytes while fluconazole had minimal effects on both biomarkers [23]. Hepatotoxicity produced by ketoconazole and its main metabolite (N-deacetyl ketoconazole) presents as elevation of ALT or lactate dehydrogenase (Rodriguez and Acosta Jr., 1997) [32, 33]. Similarly, in concordance with the present study, an in vivo study reported that itraconazole treatment resulted in significantly higher ALT and ALP levels than fluconazole in rats treated for 14 days [24]. An in vitro study using rat hepatocyte cultures also reported similar findings regarding the relative hepatotoxicity of itraconazole and fluconazole [34]. More recently, a meta-analysis of 39 studies incorporating more than 8,000 patients reported that 17.4% of patients treated with itraconazole had elevated serum liver enzymes compared to 2.0% of fluconazole users [19]. Griseofulvin has also been observed to have a lower risk of causing hepatotoxicity than ketoconazole in clinical studies [11].

The observation that fluconazole causes more hepatic damage than ketoconazole based on histological examinations is not consistent with an in vitro study which reported that ketoconazole caused more hepatotoxicity than fluconazole in cultured rat hepatocytes (Rodriguez and Acosta Jr. 1995) [23]. Another in vitro study reported that itraconazole caused more hepatic damage than fluconazole in rat hepatocyte cultures while the present study observed that fluconazole causes more hepatic damage than itraconazole based on histology examinations [34]. Similarly, in an in vivo study by Somchit et al. (2004), hepatocellular necrosis, degeneration of periacinar and midzonal hepatocytes, bile duct hyperplasia, biliary cirrhosis, and giant cell granuloma were observed in rats treated with itraconazole while mild degenerative changes of centrilobular hepatocytes were observed in the rats treated with fluconazole [24]. However, the study by Somchit et al. (2004) used doses that ranged between 7 and 70 times higher than the recommended daily

human doses in humans while the present study used doses equivalent to human therapeutic doses [24]. Similarly, the hepatocytes in the in vitro studies were exposed to doses that were higher than those used therapeutically. Therefore, the difference between observations made in the present study and the study by Somchit et al. (2004) and the in vitro studies may be explained by the differences in the hepatotoxicity mechanisms at therapeutic doses compared to toxic doses. Secondly, the different routes of administration in the present study and the study by Smochit et al. (2004) may also explain the differences in the findings. In the study by Somchit et al. (2004), drugs were administered intraperitoneally while the oral route was used in the present study [24].

The observation during histological examination that fluconazole is more hepatotoxic than ketoconazole and itraconazole is consistent with the results from a large population-based study of 90,847 users of antifungal agents in Taiwan [22]. In this Taiwanese population, the incidence rate of drug-induced liver injury in patients treated with fluconazole was more than sixfold higher than in patients treated with ketoconazole, griseofulvin, itraconazole, and terbinafine. In addition, fatality after acute liver injury was associated with fluconazole. Out of six fatal drug-induced liver injury cases, five were current users of fluconazole while one was using both fluconazole and ketoconazole [22]. In contrast to the observations made in our study using histology reports and the study by García Rodríguez et al. (2014), an epidemiologic study of 69,830 patients in the United Kingdom observed that the incidence rate of acute liver injury was more than 13-fold higher in patients treated ketoconazole than in patients treated with itraconazole and terbinafine [21]. In this population of patients who filled prescriptions for oral antifungal agents between 1991 and 1996, ketoconazole had the highest risk for causing acute liver injury followed by itraconazole, terbinafine, fluconazole, and griseofulvin. None of the 35,833 current users of fluconazole experienced acute liver injury while one case was associated with past use of fluconazole [21].

In the present study, biochemical assays revealed that ketoconazole was the most hepatotoxic antifungal agent while histological examinations indicated that fluconazole was the most hepatotoxic. Similarly, a population-based study that used biochemical assays as the only diagnostic tool reported that ketoconazole was the most hepatotoxic while the study that used a combination of biochemical assays, biopsy, and tissue pathology reported that fluconazole was the most hepatotoxic [21, 22]. The discrepancy between histological examinations and biochemical assays in this study and the difference between the two epidemiological studies that used different diagnostic approaches for acute liver injury suggests that relative hepatotoxicity of antifungal agents may depend on the diagnostic tests used. Furthermore, the fact that most of the drug-induced liver hepatotoxicity cases in clinical use are usually based on liver enzymes and not histological examinations may explain the higher incidence of ketoconazole-associated hepatotoxicity reports than those reported during fluconazole use. Despite their lack of specificity and poor correlation with the degree of liver injury, biochemical assays remain the cornerstone of identifying drug-induced liver injury because they are the most feasible, least-invasive, and cheapest diagnostic tests. However, given the low correlation between liver enzymes and the degree of hepatic damage [35], histology assessments provide better information in deciding the relative hepatotoxicity of chemical agents, including antifungal agents.

5. Conclusions

Liver enzyme levels suggested that ketoconazole is likely to cause liver injury than fluconazole while histopathological examinations revealed that fluconazole is more hepatotoxic than ketoconazole. The diagnostic criteria used in the evaluation of hepatotoxicity of antifungal agents should be taken into consideration when reviewing the evidence on their relative hepatotoxicity. Given the poor correlation between liver enzymes and the extent of liver injury, it is important to confirm liver injury through histological examination before a diagnosis of hepatotoxicity can be made in clinical settings.

Ethical Approval

Ethical clearance to conduct the study was obtained from the Joint Parirenyatwa Hospital and College of Health Sciences Research Ethics Committee (approval number: JREC/328/14). The animals were handled and treated following the principles outlined in the "Guide for the Care and Use of Laboratory Animals" prepared by the National Academy of Sciences and published by the National Institutes of Health (NIH publication 86-23 Rev. 1985).

Competing Interests

The authors declare that there are no competing interests.

Authors' Contributions

Star Khoza was involved in the conception and design of the study, data analysis and interpretation, and drafting of the manuscript. Ishmael Moyo was involved in the design of the study, dosing of rats, biochemical analysis, data analysis and interpretation, and revision of the manuscript. Denver Ncube participated in the design of the study, interpretation

of histology slides, and revising of the manuscript. All authors read and approved the final manuscript.

Acknowledgments

The authors are grateful to Mr. Charles Mudzingwa from the Department of Anatomy at the University of Zimbabwe for the assistance in the preparation of the plates for histopathological examinations.

References

[1] Food and Drug Administration Drug Safety Communication, *FDA Limits Usage of Nizoral (ketoconazole) Oral Tablets Due to Potentially Fatal Liver Injury and Risk of Drug Interactions and Adrenal Gland Problems*, FDA, Silver Spring, Md, USA, 2013, http://www.fda.gov/drugs/drugsafety/ucm362415.htm.

[2] European Medicines Agency's Committee on Medicinal Products for Human Use (EMA-CHMP), European Medicines Agency Recommends Suspension of Marketing Authorisations for Oral Ketoconazole, EMA July 2013, http://www.ema.europa.eu/ema/index.jsp?curl=pages/news_and_events/news/2013/07/news_detail_001855.jsp&mid=WC0b01ac058004d5c1.

[3] Food and Drug Administration Drug Safety Communication, *FDA Advises Against Using Oral Ketoconazole in Drug Interaction Studies Due to Serious Potential Side Effects*, FDA, Silver Spring, Md, USA, 2013, http://www.fda.gov/Drugs/DrugSafety/ucm371017.htm.

[4] B. Han, J. Mao, J. Y. Chien, and S. D. Hall, "Optimization of drug-drug interaction study design: comparison of minimal physiologically based pharmacokinetic models on prediction of CYP3A inhibition by ketoconazole," *Drug Metabolism and Disposition*, vol. 41, no. 7, pp. 1329–1338, 2013.

[5] I. Fuchs, V. Hafner-Blumenstiel, C. Markert et al., "Effect of the CYP3A inhibitor ketoconazole on the PXR-mediated induction of CYP3A activity," *European Journal of Clinical Pharmacology*, vol. 69, no. 3, pp. 507–513, 2013.

[6] Z. Yang, B. Vakkalagadda, G. Shen et al., "Inhibitory effect of ketoconazole on the pharmacokinetics of a multireceptor tyrosine kinase inhibitor BMS-690514 in healthy participants: assessing the mechanism of the interaction with physiologically-based pharmacokinetic simulations," *Journal of Clinical Pharmacology*, vol. 53, no. 2, pp. 217–227, 2013.

[7] J. H. Lewis, H. J. Zimmerman, G. D. Benson, and K. G. Ishak, "Hepatic injury associated with ketoconazole therapy. Analysis of 33 cases," *Gastroenterology*, vol. 86, no. 3, pp. 503–513, 1984.

[8] B. H. C. Stricker, A. P. R. Blok, F. B. Bronkhorst, G. E. Van Parys, and V. J. Desmet, "Ketoconazole-associated hepatic injury. A clinicopathological study of 55 cases," *Journal of Hepatology*, vol. 3, no. 3, pp. 399–406, 1986.

[9] K. N. Buchi, P. D. Gray, and K. G. Tolman, "Ketoconazole hepatotoxicity: an in vitro model," *Biochemical Pharmacology*, vol. 35, no. 16, pp. 2845–2847, 1986.

[10] G. Lake-Bakaar, P. J. Scheuer, and D. S. Sherlock, "Hepatic reactions associated with ketoconazole in the United Kingdom," *British Medical Journal*, vol. 294, no. 6569, pp. 419–422, 1987.

[11] R.-N. Chien, L.-J. Yang, P.-Y. Lin, and Y.-F. Liaw, "Hepatic injury during ketoconazole therapy in patients with onychomycosis: a controlled cohort study," *Hepatology*, vol. 25, no. 1, pp. 103–107, 1997.

[12] J. Y. Yan, X. L. Nie, Q. M. Tao, S. Y. Zhan, and Y. D. Zhang, "Ketoconazole associated hepatotoxicity: a systematic review and meta-analysis," *Biomedical and Environmental Sciences*, vol. 26, no. 7, pp. 605–610, 2013.

[13] A. Srebrnik, S. Levtov, R. Ben-Ami, and S. Brenner, "Liver failure and transplantation after itraconazole treatment for toenail onychomycosis," *Journal of the European Academy of Dermatology and Venereology*, vol. 19, no. 2, pp. 205–207, 2005.

[14] Z. Perveze, M. W. Johnson, R. A. Rubin et al., "Terbinafine-induced hepatic failure requiring liver transplantation," *Liver Transplantation*, vol. 13, no. 1, pp. 162–164, 2007.

[15] K. R. Reddy and E. R. Schiff, "Hepatotoxicity of antimicrobial, antifungal, and antiparasitic agents," *Gastroenterology Clinics of North America*, vol. 24, no. 4, pp. 923–936, 1995.

[16] R. O. Chiprut, A. Viteri, C. Jamroz, and W. P. Dyck, "Intrahepatic cholestasis after griseofulvin administration," *Gastroenterology*, vol. 70, no. 6, pp. 1141–1143, 1976.

[17] S. A. Linnebur and B. L. Parnes, "Pulmonary and hepatic toxicity due to nitrofurantoin and fluconazole treatment," *Annals of Pharmacotherapy*, vol. 38, no. 4, pp. 612–616, 2004.

[18] M. Thiim and L. S. Friedman, "Hepatotoxicity of antibiotics and antifungals," *Clinics in Liver Disease*, vol. 7, no. 2, pp. 381–399, 2003.

[19] J.-L. Wang, C.-H. Chang, Y. Young-Xu, and K. A. Chan, "Systematic review and meta-analysis of the tolerability and hepatotoxicity of antifungals in empirical and definitive therapy for invasive fungal infection," *Antimicrobial Agents and Chemotherapy*, vol. 54, no. 6, pp. 2409–2419, 2010.

[20] C.-H. Chang, Y. Young-Xu, T. Kurth, J. E. Orav, and A. K. Chan, "The safety of oral antifungal treatments for superficial dermatophytosis and onychomycosis: a meta-analysis," *The American Journal of Medicine*, vol. 120, no. 9, pp. 791–798.e3, 2007.

[21] L. A. García Rodríguez, A. Duque, J. Castellsague, S. Pérez-Gutthann, and B. H. C. Stricker, "A cohort study on the risk of acute liver injury among users of ketoconazole and other antifungal drugs," *British Journal of Clinical Pharmacology*, vol. 48, no. 6, pp. 847–852, 1999.

[22] W.-Y. Kao, C.-W. Su, Y.-S. Huang et al., "Risk of oral antifungal agent-induced liver injury in Taiwanese," *British Journal of Clinical Pharmacology*, vol. 77, no. 1, pp. 180–189, 2014.

[23] R. J. Rodriguez and D. Acosta Jr., "Comparison of ketoconazole- and fluconazole-induced hepatotoxicity in a primary culture system of rat hepatocytes," *Toxicology*, vol. 96, no. 2, pp. 83–92, 1995.

[24] N. Somchit, A. R. Norshahida, A. H. Hasiah, A. Zuraini, M. R. Sulaiman, and M. M. Noordin, "Hepatotoxicity induced by antifungal drugs itraconazole and fluconazole in rats: a comparative in vivo study," *Human and Experimental Toxicology*, vol. 23, no. 11, pp. 519–525, 2004.

[25] M. S. Zakaria, "Comparative study between Griseofulvin and Fluconazole hepatotoxic effects and the protective role of Silymarin," *El-Minia Medical Bulletin*, vol. 16, no. 1, pp. 274–285, 2005.

[26] Center for Drug Evaluation and Research (CDER), *Guidance for Industry Estimating the Maximum Safe Starting Dose in Initial Clinical Trials for Therapeutics in Adult Healthy Volunteer*, U.S. Department of Health and Human Services Food and Drug Administration, 2005, http://www.fda.gov/downloads/Drugs/.../Guidances/UCM078932.pdf.

[27] F. Wróblewski and J. S. Ladue, "Serum glutamic pyruvic transaminase in cardiac and hepatic disease," *Proceedings of the Society for Experimental Biology and Medicine*, vol. 91, no. 4, pp. 569–571, 1956.

[28] A. Karmen, F. Wroblewski, and J. S. Ladue, "Transaminase activity in human blood," *The Journal of clinical investigation*, vol. 34, no. 1, pp. 126–131, 1955.

[29] H. U. Bergmeyer and M. Horder, "International federation of clinical chemistry. Scientific committee. Expert panel on enzymes. IFCC document stage 2, draft 1; 1979-11-19 with a view to an IFCC recommendation. IFCC methods for the measurement of catalytic concentration of enzymes. Part 3. IFCC method for alanine aminotransferase," *Journal of Clinical Chemistry and Clinical Biochemistry*, vol. 18, no. 8, pp. 521–534, 1980.

[30] G. N. Bowers Jr. and R. B. McComb, "Measurement of total alkaline phosphatase activity in human serum," *Clinical Chemistry*, vol. 21, no. 13, pp. 1988–1995, 1975.

[31] M. E.-H. A. Kemeir, "Hepatotoxic effect of itraconazole in experimental rats," *American Journal of Animal and Veterinary Sciences*, vol. 9, no. 1, pp. 46–52, 2014.

[32] R. J. Rodriguez and D. Acosta Jr, "Metabolism of ketoconazole and deacetylated ketoconazole by rat hepatic microsomes and flavin-containing monooxygenases," *Drug Metabolism and Disposition*, vol. 25, no. 6, pp. 772–777, 1997.

[33] R. J. Rodriguez and D. Acosta Jr., "N-Deacetyl ketoconazole-induced hepatotoxicity in a primary culture system of rat hepatocytes," *Toxicology*, vol. 117, no. 2-3, pp. 123–131, 1997.

[34] N. Somchit, S. M. Hassim, and S. H. Samsudin, "Itraconazole and fluconazole-induced toxicity in rat hepatocytes: a comparative in vitro study," *Human and Experimental Toxicology*, vol. 21, no. 1, pp. 43–48, 2002.

[35] D. E. Amacher, "A toxicologist's guide to biomarkers of hepatic response," *Human and Experimental Toxicology*, vol. 21, no. 5, pp. 253–262, 2002.

6

Histopathological Study of Cyclosporine Pulmonary Toxicity in Rats

Said Said Elshama,[1,2] **Ayman El-Meghawry EL-Kenawy,**[2,3]
and Hosam-Eldin Hussein Osman[2,4]

[1]*Department of Forensic Medicine and Clinical Toxicology, College of Medicine, Suez Canal University, P.O. Box 3457, Ismailia, Egypt*
[2]*Taif University, Taif, Saudi Arabia*
[3]*Department of Molecular Biology, GEBRI, University of Sadat City, P.O. Box 79, Sadat City, Egypt*
[4]*Department of Anatomy, College of Medicine, Al-Azhar University, P.O. Box 345, Cairo, Egypt*

Correspondence should be addressed to Said Said Elshama; saidelshama@yahoo.com

Academic Editor: Samir Lutf Aleryani

Cyclosporine is considered one of the common worldwide immunosuppressive drugs that are used for allograft rejection prevention. However, articles that address adverse effects of cyclosporine use on the vital organs such as lung are still few. This study aims to investigate pulmonary toxic effect of cyclosporine in rats by assessment of pulmonary histopathological changes using light and electron microscope examination. Sixty male adult albino rats were divided into three groups; each group consists of twenty rats. The first received physiological saline while the second and third groups received 25 and 40 mg/kg/day of cyclosporine, respectively, by gastric gavage for forty-five days. Cyclosporine reduced the lung and body weight with shrinkage or pyknotic nucleus of pneumocyte type II, degeneration of alveoli and interalveolar septum beside microvilli on the alveolar surface, emphysema, inflammatory cellular infiltration, pulmonary blood vessels congestion, and increase of fibrous tissues in the interstitial tissues and around alveoli with negative Periodic Acid-Schiff staining. Prolonged use of cyclosporine induced pulmonary ultrastructural and histopathological changes with the lung and body weight reduction depending on its dose.

1. Introduction

Cyclosporine A (CsA) is considered one of the common immunosuppressive agents which are used during organ transplantation preventing allograft rejection and increasing the rates of patients' survival and as a treatment for autoimmune diseases. It is a cyclic endecapeptide whereas it is extracted from the fungus called *Tolypocladium inflatum* [1].

Recent studies reported that long-term use of cyclosporine A may lead to many systemic toxic effects such as nephrotoxicity, hepatotoxicity, and cardiovascular affection based on its oxidative stress mechanism that generates free radicals inducing lipid peroxidation in the different organs [2]. Other studies referred that oxidative damage may develop pulmonary disorders during systemic or local administration of cyclosporine; therefore the safety of its use is still considered a controversial issue [3].

Organ transplantation such as a lung transplantation is a lifesaving procedure whereas the rate of its use is increasing in the different countries such as the United States and Japan and then the rate of cyclosporine use is also rising [4] although the incidence risk of bronchogenic carcinoma and pulmonary fibrosis development with the use of cyclosporine A is ranging from 2 to 4% in some cases [5].

So, the present study aims to investigate the toxic effect of cyclosporine on the lung tissues in rats via assessment of pulmonary histopathological changes by using light and electron microscope examination.

2. Material and Methods

Sixty healthy male adult albino rats weighing 200 ± 20 g were obtained from the animal house of King Abdulaziz University, Jeddah, exposed to 12 hr day and night cycles with a free access to water and the standard rat pellet during the experimental period. They were divided into three groups; each group consists of twenty rats. The first group (control) received physiological saline only while the second received 25 mg/kg/day of cyclosporine dissolved in physiological saline [6], whereas the third group received 40 mg/kg/day of cyclosporine dissolved in physiological saline [7]. Daily administration of physiological saline and cyclosporine was done for forty-five days by using gastric gavage whereas cyclosporine was available in a soft gelatin capsule (50 mg) that was manufactured by R. P. Scherer GmbH & Co. KG, Eberbach/Baden, Germany, for Novartis Pharma AG, Basel, Switzerland.

2.1. Histopathological Studies. Rats were weighed and then they were sacrificed under diethyl ether anesthesia after 24 hours from the last administration of cyclosporine. An incision was carried out in the chest for a lung excision that was weighed and washed several times with a normal saline and then fixed by an intratracheal instillation of 10% neutral buffered formalin. The preserved tissues were dehydrated, embedded in paraffin, sectioned at 3-4 μm thickness, and stained by haematoxylin and eosin, Periodic Acid-Schiff (PAS), and Mallory stain [8]. The pulmonary histological slides were examined and scored under a light microscope by a blinded pathologist to the experimental groups for quantifying the extent of lung histopathological changes using a scoring scale of 0 to 4 for each lung damage parameter (oedema, hemorrhage, cell infiltration, and alveolar septal thickening) with total score of 0–16 [9, 10].

Ultrastructural studies on the lung cells were carried out by using an electron microscope whereas the lung tissue specimens were prepared via fixation in 2.7% glutaraldehyde solution in 0.1 M phosphate buffer for 1.5 hours at 4°C and then they were washed in 0.15 M phosphate buffer (pH 7.2) and postfixed in 2% osmic acid solution in 0.15 M phosphate buffer for one hour at 4°C. Dehydration was carried out in acetone while the inclusion was in the epoxy embedding resin Epon 812. The blocks were cut with an ultramicrotome type LKB at 70 nm thickness. The sections were doubly contrasted with the solutions of uranyl acetate and lead citrate for analysis by using an electron microscope [11].

2.2. Ethical Considerations. The most appropriate animal species was chosen for this research. Promotion of the high standard of the care and animal well-being at all times was done. Appropriate sample size was calculated by using the fewest number of animals to obtain the valid results statistically. Painful procedures were performed under anesthesia to avoid distress and pain. Our standards of the animal care and administration met those required by applicable international laws and regulations [12].

2.3. Statistical Analysis. Statistical analysis was performed by using SPSS version 17. Variability of the results was expressed as mean ± SD. Results were analyzed by using one-way ANOVA and *post hoc* multiple comparisons test (TUKEY) to investigate the difference among groups. A P value of 0.05 was considered statistically significant.

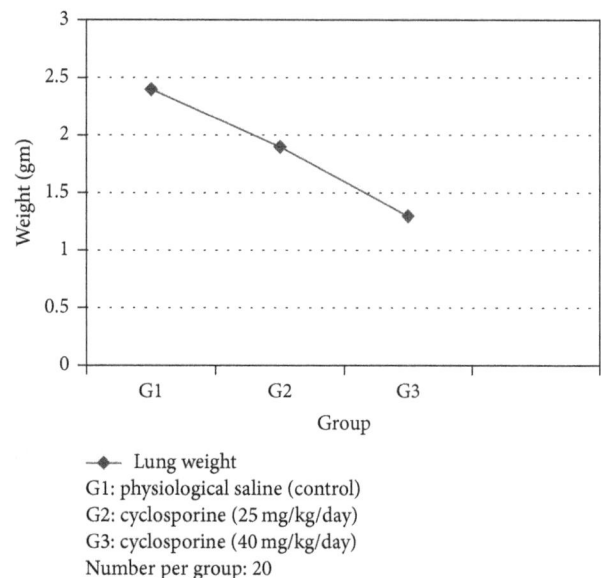

Lung weight
G1: physiological saline (control)
G2: cyclosporine (25 mg/kg/day)
G3: cyclosporine (40 mg/kg/day)
Number per group: 20

FIGURE 1: The effect of cyclosporine different doses on the rats' lung weight.

3. Results

3.1. Effect of Cyclosporine Different Doses on the Rats' Lung Weight, Body Weight, and the Lung/Body Weight Ratio. There is a significant decrease in the rats' lung and body weight of second group which received 25 mg/kg/day of cyclosporine in comparison with the control group while there is a significant decrease in the rats' lung and body weight of third group which received 40 mg/kg/day of cyclosporine in comparison with the second and control groups.

Figure 1 shows that mean + SD values of the rats' lung weight in control, second, and third groups are 2.4 ± 0.18; 1.9±0.19; and 1.3±0.24, respectively, whereas F value is 86.473 indicating a difference between groups which is statistically significant ($P < 0.001$).

Table 1 shows that mean + SD values of the rats' body weight in control, second, and third groups are 210.9 ± 15.11; 155.35±12.15; and 99.55±10.26, respectively. The value of F is 179.85 indicating the difference between the groups while the value of P is <0.001 indicating that the difference between the groups is statistically significant. The lung/body weight ratio in control, second, and third groups is 1.14%, 1.22%, and 1.31%, respectively.

3.2. Histopathological Findings

3.2.1. Pulmonary Histopathological Findings by Using a Light Microscope. Examination of the lung tissues in the first group rats (control) which received physiological saline showed a normal lung architecture, thin interalveolar septa, folded columnar epithelial cells of bronchiole, clearly seen alveolar sacs, normal pulmonary vessels with positive stain of Periodic Acid-Schiff (PAS), and normal fibrous tissues distribution (Figures 2(a), 3(a), and 4(a)). Rats of the second group which received 25 mg/kg/day of cyclosporine showed thickened wall

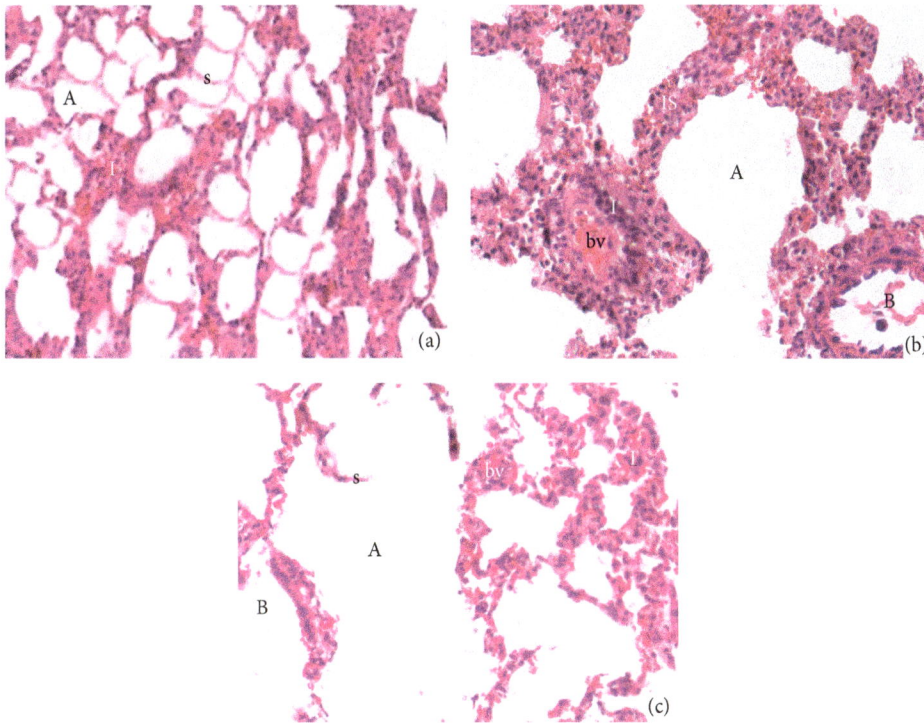

FIGURE 2: (a) A photomicrograph of transverse section in the control rat lung shows normal architecture of alveoli (A) with thin interalveolar septa (s) and normal interstitial tissues (I) (H&E ×400). (b) A photomicrograph of transverse section in the second group rat lung shows marked thickening of interstitial tissues (IS) with numerous areas of cellular infiltration (I), congested blood capillaries (bv), and bronchiole (B) with widening alveoli (A) (H&E ×400). (c) A photomicrograph of transverse section in the third group rat lung shows loss of normal architecture, cellular infiltration (I), fragmentation and degeneration of alveoli and interalveolar septum (s) with a subsequent compensatory dilatation of alveoli (A), thickened and congested pulmonary blood vessels (bv), and degenerated bronchiolar wall (B) (H&E ×400).

TABLE 1: Comparison between effects of cyclosporine different doses on the rats' lung weight, body weight, and the lung/body weight ratio.

| Parameter | Group | | |
| | First | Second | Third |
	M ± SD	M ± SD	M ± SD
Body weight (gm)	210.9 ± 15.11	155.35 ± 12.15*	99.55 ± 10.26**
Lung weight (gm)	2.4 ± 0.18	1.9 ± 0.19*	1.3 ± 0.24**
Lung/body weight ratio %	1.14	1.22*	1.31**

First group: physiological saline (control).
Second group: cyclosporine (25 mg/kg/day).
Third group: cyclosporine (40 mg/kg/day).
M ± SD: mean ± standard deviation. Number per group: 20
*$P < 0.001$: significant difference in comparison with the control group
**$P < 0.001$: significant difference in comparison with the second group.

of bronchiole with moderately congested blood capillaries, macrophages infiltration in the alveolar spaces, degenerated and thickened interalveolar septa with moderate positive Periodic Acid-Schiff (PAS) stain, and mild fibrous tissues distribution (Figures 2(b), 3(b), and 4(b)). The lung tissues in the third group rats which received 40 mg/kg/day of cyclosporine showed degeneration of alveoli and interalveolar septum, emphysema, marked thinning of interstitial tissues, aggregations areas of inflammatory cellular infiltration beside thickened and congested pulmonary blood vessels, negative Periodic Acid-Schiff (PAS) stain, and the increase of fibrous tissues in the interstitial tissues and around alveoli (Figures 2(c), 3(c), and 4(c)).

Table 2 showed the severity of pulmonary histopathological changes according to scoring scale, whereas a statistical significant difference in the overall scores of the lung histopathological parameters (oedema, hemorrhage, cell infiltration, and alveolar septal thickening) was observed in the second group in comparison with the control group and in the third group in comparison with the second and control groups.

3.2.2. Pulmonary Histopathological Findings by Using an Electron Microscope. The ultrastructure of lung cells in the first group rats (control) which received physiological saline showed a rounded nucleus of pneumocyte type II that is surrounded by lamellar bodies with normal mitochondria and normal microvilli on the alveolar surface (Figure 5(a)). But the ultrastructure of lung cells in the second group rats showed a shrinkage nucleus of pneumocyte type II which is surrounded by vacuoles and congested blood capillaries filled with the blood in cytoplasm with degenerated microvilli on

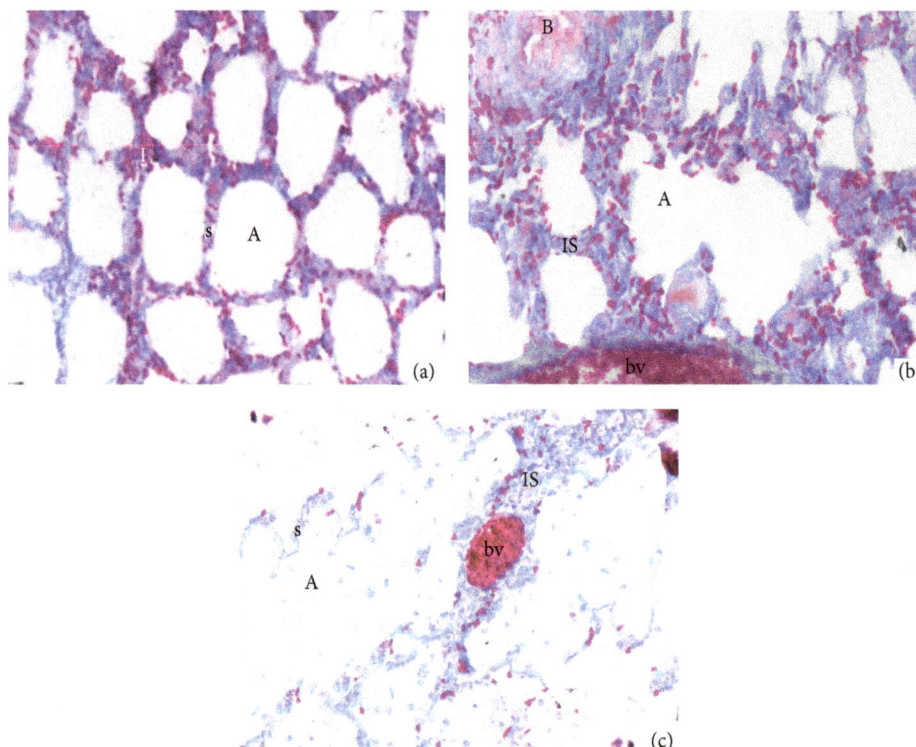

FIGURE 3: (a) A photomicrograph of transverse section in the control rat lung shows normal distribution of fibrous tissues and architecture of alveoli (A) with thin interalveolar septa (s) and normal interstitial tissues (I) (Mallory ×400). (b) A photomicrograph of transverse section in the second group rat lung shows mild distribution of fibrous tissues around alveoli (A) with thickening of the interalveolar septa (IS) and bronchiole (B) (Mallory ×400). (c) A photomicrograph of transverse section in the third group rat lung shows loss of normal architecture, increase of fibrous tissues around alveoli (A), subsequent compensatory dilatation of other alveoli, marked thinning of the interalveolar septum (s) with an increase of fibrous tissues in the areas of interstitial tissues (IS), and thickened and congested pulmonary blood vessels which contain hemorrhagic blood cells (bv) (Mallory ×400).

TABLE 2: Comparison between effects of cyclosporine different doses on the rats' lung histopathological parameters.

Parameter	Group		
	First	Second	Third
	M ± SD	M ± SD	M ± SD
Oedema	0.1 ± 0.1	1.1 ± 0.5*	1.7 ± 0.5**
Hemorrhage	0.4 ± 0.8	2.0 ± 0.9*	3.3 ± 0.4**
Cell infiltration	0.2 ± 0.8	4.1 ± 0.5*	5.6 ± 0.3**
Alveolar septal thickening	0.1 ± 0.3	2.9 ± 0.5*	2.4 ± 0.3**
Total score	0.2 ± 0.4	2.52 ± 0.6*	3.25 ± 0.4**

First group: physiological saline (control).
Second group: cyclosporine (25 mg/kg/day).
Third group: cyclosporine (40 mg/kg/day).
M ± SD: mean ± standard deviation. Number per group: 20
*$P < 0.001$: significant difference in comparison with the control group
**$P < 0.001$: significant difference in comparison with the second group.

the surface of alveoli (Figure 5(b)). The ultrastructure of lung cells in the third group rats showed a pyknotic nucleus of pneumocyte type II that is surrounded by vacuoles which are variable in the amount and size with more congested blood capillaries filled with the blood in cytoplasm with degenerated microvilli in the alveolar surface (Figure 5(c)).

4. Discussion

Many previous studies indicated that there is a correlation between the prolonged use of cyclosporine among transplant organ patients and vital organs toxicity development. However, its adverse effects on vital organ such as lung are still obscure because of the paucity of researches that focus on it. So, our study tries to investigate pulmonary toxicity of cyclosporine by assessment of the probable histopathological changes via using light and electron microscope examination.

The current study showed that lung and body weights are significantly decreased in the second group which received 25 mg/kg/day of cyclosporine in comparison with the control group while the lung and body weights of third group which received 40 mg/kg/day of cyclosporine showed a significant decrease in comparison with the second group; thus the lung/body weight ratio is also affected. This is in agreement with Wongmekiat et al. [13], who indicated that cyclosporine toxicity affects the appetite beside its catabolic effect inducing the body weight loss, and in consistency also with Chakravarthi et al. [14], who referred to the fact that

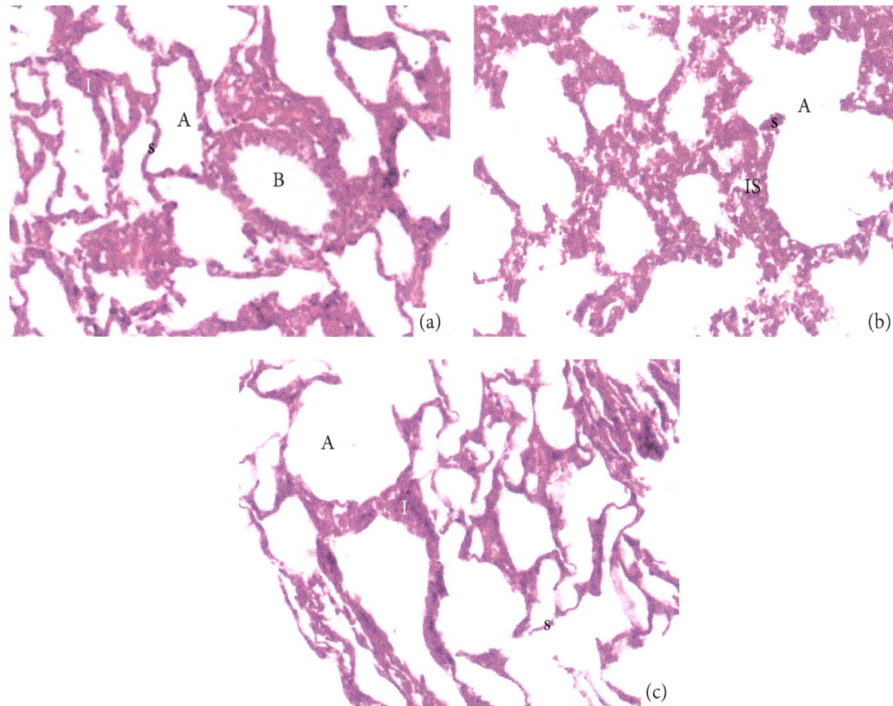

FIGURE 4: (a) A photomicrograph of transverse section in the control rat lung shows positive PAS staining with normal architecture of alveoli (A) with thin interalveolar septa (s) and normal interstitial tissues (I) (PAS ×400). (b) A photomicrograph of transverse section in the second group rat lung shows moderate positive PAS staining with nearly normal architecture of alveoli (A), thick interalveolar septa (s), and interstitial tissues (I) (PAS ×400). (c) A photomicrograph of transverse section of third group rat lung shows negative PAS staining, accumulation of inflammatory cells near the blood vessels with abnormal architecture of alveoli (A), and destruction of the interalveolar septa (s) and interstitial tissues (I) (PAS ×400).

cyclosporine induces cell apoptosis which is correlated with the affected organ weight reduction and this is in contrast with Sato et al. [15], who confirmed that normal pulmonary cells are protected from cyclosporine induced apoptosis.

Our results revealed that the third group which received 40 mg/kg/day of cyclosporine induced marked pulmonary histopathological abnormalities such as a pyknotic nucleus of pneumocyte type II, degeneration of alveoli with its microvilli, and emphysema with inflammatory cellular infiltration and pulmonary vessels congestion in consistency with Yousef and ALRajhi [16] while the second group which received 25 mg/kg/day of cyclosporine showed mild pulmonary ultrastructures and histopathological changes such as a shrinkage nucleus of pneumocyte type II, degenerated microvilli on the alveolar surface, thickened wall of bronchiole with moderately congested blood capillaries and macrophages infiltration in the alveolar spaces, and nearly normal architecture of alveoli with thickened interalveolar septa. Furthermore, the overall lung lesion severity scores were differed significantly between the second and third groups indicating that the severity of cyclosporine induced pulmonary histological changes depending on its dose.

Most of the published articles focused on a fact which shows that generation of free radicals inducing oxidative stress leads to molecular and cellular damage which are considered the cause of cyclosporine toxic effects on the different body organs [17]. The effects of released reactive oxygen species (ROS) by normal respiratory system are counteracted by glutathione and antioxidants enzymes such as catalase and peroxidase; therefore more generation of ROS via cyclosporine leads to the balance disturbance with antioxidants defense mechanism inducing toxic cellular substances which lead to histopathological changes [18].

The present study showed that cyclosporine increases fibrous tissues formation in the lung interstitial tissues and around alveoli depending on its dose in consistency with Katrin et al. [19], who referred to the fact that cyclosporine can be trigger to stimulate fibroblast proliferation via mediators which are induced by the epithelial cells of airway passages. According to Esposito et al. [20], there is a correlation between cyclosporine cytotoxicity and mitochondrial enzyme activity disturbance and its ability to react with the nucleus receptors to prevent genetic transcription of proteins that are secreted by fibroblasts, macrophages, monocytes, and endothelial cells. Therefore, cyclosporine affects the cell of lung tissues as a result of multiple effects such as carbohydrates depletion in the cytoplasm of lung cell that leads to the lung structure disturbance which is supported in the current study by a negative stain of Periodic Acid-Schiff.

5. Conclusion

The prolonged use of cyclosporine may induce pulmonary histopathological and ultrastructural changes such as shrinkage or pyknotic nucleus of pneumocyte type II, degeneration

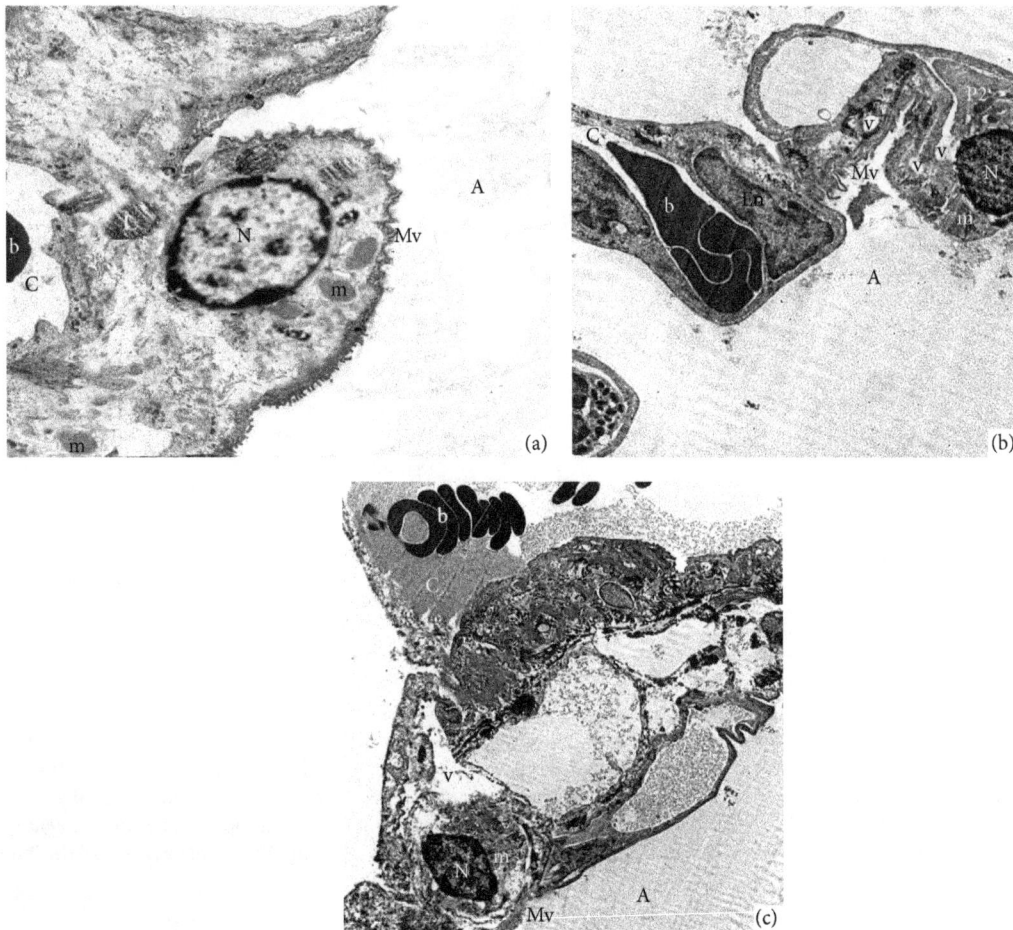

FIGURE 5: (a) Electronic microscopic picture of the control rat lung shows rounded nucleus (N) of pneumocyte type II, lamellar bodies (L) around the nucleus, and mitochondria (m) in cytoplasm with microvilli (Mv) on the surface of alveoli (A) (×10000). (b) Electronicmicroscopic picture of the second group rat lung shows a shrinkage nucleus (N) of pneumocyte type II, vacuoles and congested blood capillaries (C) filled with the blood (b) in the cytoplasm and around the nucleus, degenerated mitochondria (m) in cytoplasm with degenerated microvilli (Mv) on the surface of alveoli (A) (×10000). (c) Electronic microscopic picture of the third group rat lung shows pyknotic nucleus (N) of pneumocyte type II, a variable number of vacuoles (v) and more congested blood capillaries (C) filled with the blood (b) around the nucleus, and degenerated mitochondria (m) in cytoplasm with degenerated microvilli (Mv) on the surface of alveoli (A) (×10000).

of alveoli, emphysema with an inflammatory cellular infiltration, pulmonary vessels congestion, and lung and body weight reduction depending on its dose and based on reactive oxygen species generation. Therefore, further researches on human should be done in the future to verify our results and confirm pulmonary toxicity of cyclosporine prolonged use.

Conflict of Interests

The authors declare that there is no conflict of interests regarding the publication of this paper.

References

[1] J. R. Chapman and B. J. Nankivell, "Nephrotoxicity of ciclosporin A: short-term gain, long-term pain?" *Nephrology Dialysis Transplantation*, vol. 21, no. 8, pp. 2060–2063, 2006.

[2] R. Rezzani, "Exploring cyclosporine A-side effects and the protective role-played by antioxidants: the morphological and immunohistochemical studies," *Histology and Histopathology*, vol. 21, no. 1–3, pp. 301–316, 2006.

[3] D. M. Lyu and M. R. Zamora, "Medical complications of lung transplantation," *Proceedings of the American Thoracic Society*, vol. 6, no. 1, pp. 101–107, 2009.

[4] T. Shiraishi, Y. Okada, Y. Sekine et al., "Registry of the Japanese society of lung and heart-lung transplantation: the official Japanese lung transplantation report 2008," *General Thoracic and Cardiovascular Surgery*, vol. 57, no. 8, pp. 395–401, 2009.

[5] J. Mathew and R. A. Kratzke, "Lung cancer and lung transplantation: a review," *Journal of Thoracic Oncology*, vol. 4, no. 6, pp. 753–760, 2009.

[6] A. J. Cologna, L. V. D. S. Lima, S. Tucci Jr. et al., "Cyclosporine action on kidneys of rats submitted to normothermic ischaemia and reperfusion," *Acta Cirúrgica Brasileira*, vol. 23, no. 1, pp. 36–41, 2008.

[7] Uz. Ebru, Uz. Burak, A. Kaya et al., "Protective effect of erdosteine on cyclosporine induced chronic nephrotoxicity in rats," *Nephro-Urology*, vol. 3, no. 4, pp. 280–284, 2011.

[8] J. D. Bancroft and M. Gamble, *Theory and Practice Histological Techniques*, Churchill Livingstone, New York, NY, USA, 5th edition, 2002.

[9] R. Akcılar, A. Akcılar, H. Şimşek et al., "Hyperbaric oxygen treatment ameliorates lung injury in paraquat intoxicated rats," *International Journal of Clinical and Experimental Pathology*, vol. 8, no. 10, pp. 13034–13042, 2015.

[10] L. Yamanel, U. Kaldirim, Y. Oztas et al., "Ozone therapy and hyperbaric oxygen treatment in lung injury in septic rats," *International Journal of Medical Sciences*, vol. 8, no. 1, pp. 48–55, 2011.

[11] L. Graham and J. M. Orenstein, "Processing tissue and cells for transmission electron microscopy in diagnostic pathology and research," *Nature Protocols*, vol. 2, no. 10, pp. 2439–2450, 2007.

[12] M. M. Naderi, A. Sarvari, A. Milanifar, S. B. Boroujeni, and M. M. Akhondi, "Regulations and ethical considerations in animal experiments: international laws and islamic perspectives," *Avicenna Journal of Medical Biotechnology*, vol. 4, no. 3, pp. 114–120, 2012.

[13] O. Wongmekiat, N. Leelarugrayub, and K. Thamprasert, "Beneficial effect of shallot (*Allium ascalonicum* L.) extract on cyclosporine nephrotoxicity in rats," *Food and Chemical Toxicology*, vol. 46, no. 5, pp. 1844–1850, 2008.

[14] S. Chakravarthi, C. Fu Wen, and N. Haleagrahara, "Apoptosis and expression of bcl-2 in cyclosporine induced renal damage and its reversal by beneficial effects of 4′, 5′, 7′- trihydroxyflavone," *Journal of Analytical Bio-Science*, vol. 32, no. 4, pp. 320–327, 2009.

[15] M. Sato, I. Tsujino, M. Fukunaga et al., "Cyclosporine A induces apoptosis of human lung adenocarcinoma cells via caspase-dependent pathway," *Anticancer Research*, vol. 31, no. 6, pp. 2129–2134, 2011.

[16] O. M. Yousef and W. I. ALRajhi, "The probable protective role of vitamin C against cyclosporine an induced pulmonary changes in mice," *Journal of Life Sciences and Technologies*, vol. 1, no. 1, pp. 1–6, 2013.

[17] H. Argani, A. Ghorbanihaghjo, N. Rashtchizadeh, S. Seifirad, and Y. Rahbarfar, "Effect of cyclosporine-a on paraoxonase activity in wistar rats," *International Journal of Organ Transplantation Medicine*, vol. 2, no. 1, pp. 25–31, 2011.

[18] J. Lee, "Use of antioxidants to prevent cyclosporine a toxicity," *Toxicological Research*, vol. 26, no. 3, pp. 163–170, 2010.

[19] E. Katrin, R. Michael, K. Janette, R. Peter, and A. R. Glanville, "Cyclosporine A mediates fibroproliferation through epithelial cell," *Transplantation*, vol. 77, no. 12, pp. 1886–1893, 2004.

[20] C. Esposito, A. Fornoni, F. Cornacchia et al., "Cyclosporine induces different responses in human epithelial, endothelial and fibroblast cell cultures," *Kidney International*, vol. 58, no. 1, pp. 123–130, 2000.

7

Microcystin-LR Induced Immunotoxicity in Mammals

Yaqoob Lone, Mangla Bhide, and Raj Kumar Koiri

Department of Zoology, Dr. Harisingh Gour Central University, Sagar, Madhya Pradesh 470003, India

Correspondence should be addressed to Raj Kumar Koiri; rkkoiri@gmail.com

Academic Editor: William Valentine

Microcystins are toxic molecules produced by cyanobacterial blooms due to water eutrophication. Exposure to microcystins is a global health problem because of its association with various other pathological effects and people all over the world are exposed to microcystins on a regular basis. Evidence shows that microcystin-LR (MC-LR) may adversely affect the immune system, but its specific effects on immune functions are lacking. In the present review, immunotoxicological effects associated with MC-LR in animals, humans, and *in vitro* models have been reported. Overall, the data shows that chronic exposure to MC-LR has the potential to impair vital immune responses which could lead to increased risk of various diseases including cancers. Studies in animal and *in vitro* models have provided some pivotal understanding into the potential mechanisms of MC-LR related immunotoxicity suggesting that further investigation, particularly in humans, is required to better understand the relationship between development of disease and the MC-LR exposure.

1. Introduction

The frequent occurrence of cyanobacterial blooms with increasing water eutrophication has become a worldwide concern. Cyanobacterial blooms are often coupled with the production of different ranges of bioactive and toxic metabolites with microcystins (MCs) being the most widely studied [1]. More than 90 microcystin isoforms have been detected, among which microcystin-leucine arginine (MC-LR, Figure 1(a)) is the most abundant and the most toxic variant of microcystin [2]. MC-LR is a potential carcinogen for animal and humans, and the International Agency for Research on Cancer has classified MC-LR as a possible human carcinogen due to its potential carcinogenic activity via inhibition of protein phosphatases, which leads to the hyperphosphorylation of cellular proteins [3]. The provisional guideline set by the World Health Organization for MC-LR in drinking water is $1 \mu g/L$, but the concentration of MCs in many water bodies is far beyond that guideline; for example, in Sagar lake water (India, Figure 1(b)) MC-LR was found to be $0.67 \mu g/mL$ [4]. MC-LR, which is a well-known hepatotoxin, also induces damage in other organs as was supported by evidence of kidney impairment, gastrointestinal disorder, reproductive toxicity, immune intruders, and embryo toxicity [5–7]. There are reports which suggest that microcystin can alter the immune system through several mechanisms like lymphocyte proliferation reduction, modulation of phagocytic activity, adaptation of natural killer cell activity, and disturbance of cytokine synthesis [8, 9]. This lethal effect of MCs on human being and livestock considerably depends on the stimulation of their immune system; thus MCs alter the immunomodulatory activities [10]. In this review, an attempt has been made to figure out the information regarding conditions and mechanisms of immunotoxic activity of MCs.

2. Role of Hematological Parameters in Microcystin Mediated Immunotoxicity

Cyanobacteria produce a range of bioactive and toxic metabolites, which have been reported to bioaccumulate in aquatic food chains and have been reported to impact human health indirectly due to the presence of toxins in edible fish [11]. Various documented toxic effects of microcystins include chronic hepatocarcinogenicity and oxidative stress as well as modulations of hepatological parameters and immunosuppression via inhibition of IFN production and synthesis of cytokines [11]. Thus the immune system is prone to exposure and is sensitive to toxic agents. Previous studies have

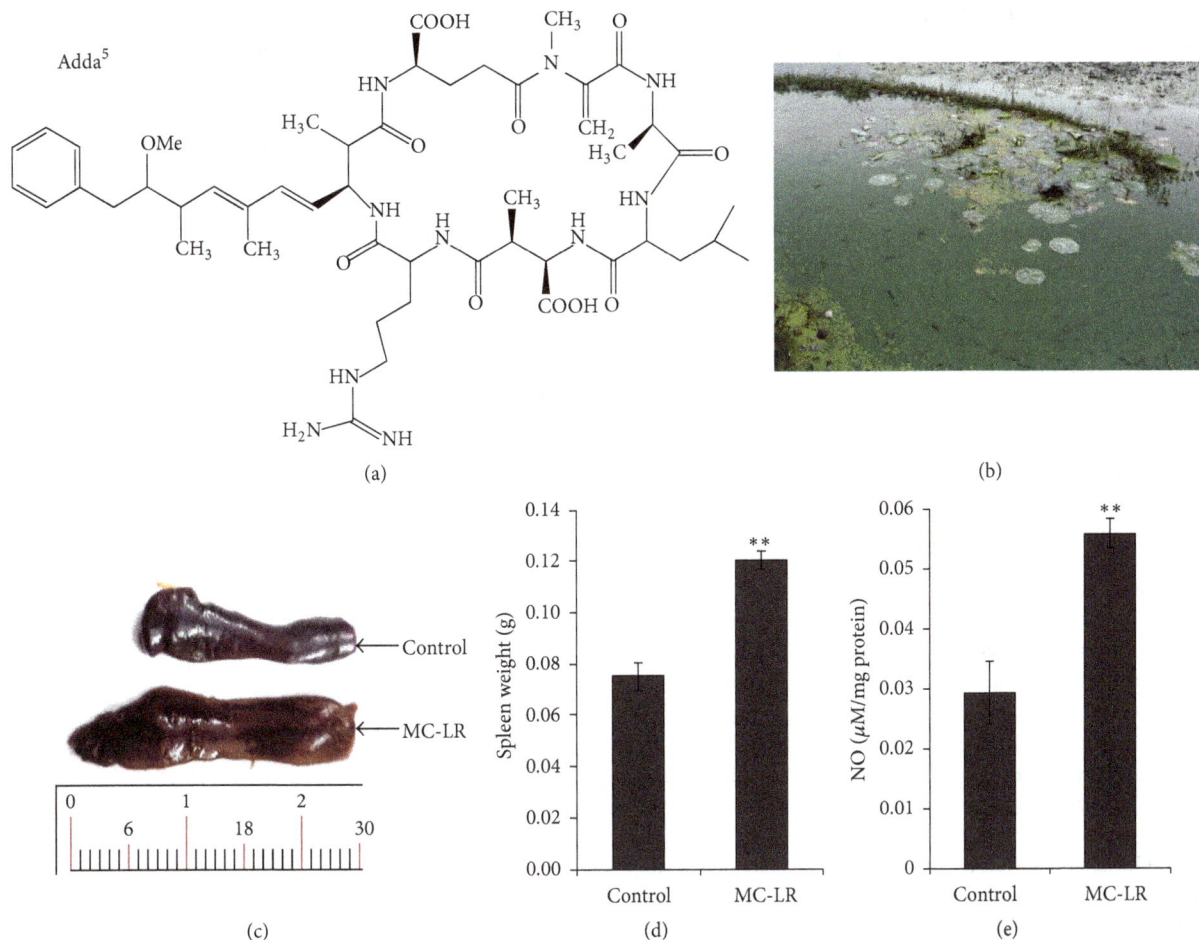

(a)

(b)

(c)

(d)

(e)

FIGURE 1: Structure of microcystin-LR (a) and *Microcystis aeruginosa* bloom in Sagar lake water (b) and MC-LR treatment of mice for 14 days shows splenomegaly (c) and causes a significant increase in the weight of spleen (d) and NO level in spleen (e). Values represent mean ± SD, where $n = 3$. $**p < 0.01$ (control versus MC-LR treated mice).

observed thrombocytopenia (platelet deficiency) in animals treated with MCs or cyanobacteria bloom extracts entirely containing MCs [12, 13]. Early investigations of mice treated with MCs have found thrombocytopenia, pulmonary thrombi, and hepatic congestion and it has been reported that rats treated with an acute dose of MC-LR (125 μg/kg, i.p.) showed a significant decrease in WBC and mean corpuscular volume and a significant increase in platelets [12, 14]. Palikova et al. observed that mice fed with different concentration of cyanobacterial bloom extract for 28 days showed significant differences in RBC count, hematocrit value, MCH, MCV, and MCHC in comparison with the control group [11]. Previous results from the comet assay in mice leukocytes have shown that MC-LR (37.5 μg/kg bw/day, i.p.) induced a 2-fold transient increase in the level of DNA breaks after 30 min exposure [15]. *In vivo* studies by Kujbida et al. suggested that topical application of MC-LR (1000 nM) for 4 hours to male rats caused an improvement of the number of rolling and adhered leukocytes in the endothelium of postcapillary mesenteric venules [16].

Yuan et al. reported that, after the administration of MC-LR (50 μg/kg bw), when blood was collected at 0, 1, and 3 hours and with 12 μg/kg bw, when blood was collected at 0, 1, 3, 12, 24, 48, and 168 hours, respectively, significant increase in plasma white blood cells was observed [17]. Takahashi et al. reported that rats treated with MC-LR (100 and 200 μg/kg, i.p.) for one hour showed dose dependent reductions in leukocyte count, erythrocyte count, hemoglobin (Hb) concentration, coagulation parameters, and hematocrit (Ht) [13]. Recently we investigated the effect of MC-LR (15 μg/kg bw, i.p.) for 14 days on mice and observed that the treatment caused a significant elevation of hemoglobin and RBC, whereas it significantly declined WBC (Table 1, $p < 0.005$). Grabow et al. revealed that erythrocytes exposed to MC-LR had significant morphological changes [18]. Incubation of human erythrocytes with MC-LR concentrations of 1–1000 nM for 1, 6, 12, and 24 hours resulted in hemolysis and echinocytes and conversion of oxyhemoglobin to methemoglobin and a decrease in membrane fluidity [19]. Further in the treated erythrocytes activities of glutathione reductase and superoxide dismutase declined, while ROS and lipid peroxidation increased. Zhou et al. reported that when mice were exposed to MC-LR at the doses of 0.5, 2, and 8 μg/kg bw

TABLE 1: Hematological parameters in blood of control and MC-LR treated mice for 14 days.

Hematological parameters	Control	Microcystin-LR
RBC (10^6/mm^3)	7.25 ± 0.72	$3.12 \pm 0.12^{**}$
WBC (10^3/mm^3)	4.21 ± 0.29	$5.73 \pm 0.26^{**}$
Hb (g/dL)	9.21 ± 0.25	$6.23 \pm 0.48^{**}$

Values are mean $\pm$ SD ($n = 3$), $^{**}p < 0.01$ (control versus MC-LR treated groups).

every 48 h for 30 days, prominent decrease in RBC, Hb, and Ht was observed as compared to control [20].

3. Microcystins Activate Neutrophils and Macrophages

Neutrophils play significant role in regulation of cancer development and spontaneous tumorigenesis [21]. Activated neutrophils release ROS and play an important role in host defense system and removal of debris but they can also cause damage and injury to tissues [22]. Neutrophils have been reported to be involved in the liver injury induced by MC-LR [23]. Kujbida et al. had shown that MC-LR and [Asp^3]-MC-LR increase migration of human neutrophils and ROS formation and its killing capacity [24]. Treatment of both rat and human neutrophils with MC-LA and MC-LR (1 and 1000 nM) for 24 hours has been observed to cause loss of membrane integrity as well an increase in percentage of cells with fragmented DNA in rats whereas in humans an increase in neutrophil viability and decrease in percentage of cells with fragmented DNA was observed [25]. Previous reports have suggested that MCs have a chemotactic effect [16, 26] and can attract neutrophil as well as enhance their migration, as the cells are induced to produce additional amounts of chemokine [16]. *In vitro* studies have shown that all the three MCs cause neutrophil chemotaxis by increasing intracellular calcium levels [25].

Macrophages play an important role in immunity and foreign particles like microorganisms, macromolecules, and injured or apoptotic tissues [27] and other antigens are phagocytosed by macrophages [28]. Stimulated macrophages produce a number of enzymes, NO, and chemokines like IL-1β, TNFα, and GM-CSF for the primary protection of the host [29, 30]. In our studies, we have observed that concentration of NO in spleen increases significantly in mice treated with MC-LR (15 μg/kg bw, i.p.) for 14 days (Figure 1(e)). Alterations in the level of cytokines or chemokines are considered as a marker of immunomodulation. Shen et al. examined the function of MCs on the phagocytosis of peritoneal cells in mice exposed to sublethal doses (16, 32, 64 mg/kg bw, i.p.) for 14 days and observed that MCs reduced phagocytic index of peritoneal phagocyte [31]. Microcytins also produced the inhibition of lipopolysaccharide induced lymphocyte proliferation and the dose dependent decrease of the numbers of antibody forming cells in mice that were immunized by using T-dependent antigen sheep red blood cells. *In vitro* studies of mice macrophages incubated with MC-LR at dose of 1, 10, 100, and 1000 nmol/L for 24 hours were studied by Chen

et al. during which he observed the downregulation of NO production and mRNA levels of iNOS, IL-1β, and TNFα in peritoneal macrophages [32].

4. Microcystins Alter and Activate Lymphocyte

Using human and chicken peripheral blood lymphocytes treated with 1, 10, and 25 μg/mL for 12, 24, 48, and 72 hours, Lankoff et al. showed that MC-LR influences the production of IL-2 and IL-6 and decreases the proliferation of T as well as B lymphocytes [33]. Human lymphocytes pretreated with MC-LR (1 μg/mL) have been reported to increase the level of DNA damage as a function of time which might be due to apoptosis [33]. When mouse splenocytes were exposed to 7.5 μg/mL of MC-LR for 4 and 24 hours, apoptosis was observed only in B cells whereas T cells were not affected [34]. We have also observed that treatment of mice with MC-LR (15 μg/kg bw) for 14 days results in splenomegaly and significant increase in weight of spleen (Figures 1(c) and 1(d)) and cotreatment with nitrate was observed to potentiate this MC-LR induced toxicity in mice [35]. Flow cytometric analysis of nonstimulated lymphocytes treated with MC-LR (7.5 μg/mL) for 4 and 24 hours has shown that MC-LR induces apoptosis in the B cell subpopulation via the B cell antigen receptor pathway, but not in T cells [34].

When mice were treated with three doses of MCs equivalent (4.97, 9.94, and 19.88 μg/kg bw/i.p.) for 14 days, it was found that B cell was more susceptible, maybe due to the depression of B cell surface markers or B cell growth cytokines or their receptors by MCs [31]. Mice exposed at four doses of 7, 12, 24, and 36 mg/kg body weight for 8 hours resulted in a significant decrease of mRNA levels of TNFα, IL-1β (proinflammatory cytokines), and IL-4, IL-2, and IL-10 (Th1/Th2 related cytokines), while IL-6 level was unaffected [36]. In mice, prolonged exposure of MC-LR has been reported to cause DNA damage and inhibition of proliferation of bone marrow cells and changes of hematopoietic factors, which is an indicator of severe damage in bone marrow cells [20].

5. Conclusions

MC-LR is one of the most toxic cyanotoxins that has been extensively studied. However there are only few studies elucidating the possible connection between observed immunomodulating activities of MCs or other cyanotoxins. In the present review, an attempt has been made to comprehensively address the impact of MC-LR toxicity on immune system. In this paper, we have mainly described the *in vitro* and *in vivo* effect of MC-LR on both acute and chronic immune system of mice and an attempt has been made to describe the possible pathways and molecules which might be implicated in MC-LR induced immunotoxicity in mice.

Abbreviations

GM-CSF: Granulocyte macrophage
         colony-stimulating factor
Hb: Hemoglobin

Ht: Hematocrit
IL: Interleukin
iNOS: Inducible nitric oxide synthase
MCH: Mean cell hemoglobin
MCHC: Mean corpuscular hemoglobin concentration
MC-LR: Microcystin-LR
MCs: Microcystins
MCV: Mean corpuscular volume
RBC: Red blood cells
ROS: Reactive oxygen species
TNF: Tumor necrosis factor
WBC: White blood cells.

Conflict of Interests

The authors declare that there is no conflict of interests.

Acknowledgments

Yaqoob Lone thanks Dr. Harisingh Gour Central University, Sagar, for fellowship. This work was financially supported by a project from UGC Faculty Research Promotion Scheme (F.30-12/2014/BSR) and SERB (SERB/LS-816/2013), Govt. of India, sanctioned to Raj Kumar Koiri. The authors are grateful to Department of Zoology, Dr. Harisingh Gour Central University, Sagar, for providing infrastructural facilities and financial support.

References

[1] M. Welker and H. von Döhren, "Cyanobacterial peptides—nature's own combinatorial biosynthesis," *FEMS Microbiology Reviews*, vol. 30, no. 4, pp. 530–563, 2006.

[2] D. Dietrich and S. Hoeger, "Guidance values for microcystins in water and cyanobacterial supplement products (blue-green algal supplements): a reasonable or misguided approach?" *Toxicology and Applied Pharmacology*, vol. 203, no. 3, pp. 273–289, 2005.

[3] H. Fan, Y. Cai, P. Xie et al., "Microcystin-LR stabilizes c-myc protein by inhibiting protein phosphatase 2A in HEK293 cells," *Toxicology*, vol. 319, no. 1, pp. 69–74, 2014.

[4] Y. Lone, R. K. Koiri, and M. Bhide, "An overview of the toxic effect of potential human carcinogen Microcystin-LR on testis," *Toxicology Reports*, vol. 2, pp. 289–296, 2015.

[5] V. R. Beasley, W. O. Cook, A. M. Dahlem, S. B. Hooser, R. A. Lovell, and W. M. Valentine, "Algae intoxication in livestock and waterfowl," *The Veterinary Clinics of North America: Food Animal Practice*, vol. 5, no. 2, pp. 345–361, 1989.

[6] X. Zhang, P. Xie, W. Wang et al., "Dose-dependent effects of extracted microcystins on embryonic development, larval growth and histopathological changes of southern catfish (*Silurus meridionalis*)," *Toxicon*, vol. 51, no. 3, pp. 449–456, 2008.

[7] Y. Zhou, J. Yuan, J. Wu, and X. Han, "The toxic effects of microcystin-LR on rat spermatogonia in vitro," *Toxicology Letters*, vol. 212, no. 1, pp. 48–56, 2012.

[8] M. A. Cooper, T. A. Fehniger, and M. A. Caligiuri, "The biology of human natural killer-cell subsets," *Trends in Immunology*, vol. 22, no. 11, pp. 633–640, 2001.

[9] M. Vitale, A. Bassini, P. Secchiero et al., "NK-active cytokines IL-2, IL-12, and IL-15 selectively modulate specific protein kinase C (PKC) isoforms in primary human NK cells," *The Anatomical Record*, vol. 266, no. 2, pp. 87–92, 2002.

[10] S. S. Yea, H. M. Kim, H.-M. Oh, K.-H. Paik, and K.-H. Yang, "Microcystin-induced down-regulation of lymphocyte functions through reduced IL-2 mRNA stability," *Toxicology Letters*, vol. 122, no. 1, pp. 21–31, 2001.

[11] M. Palikova, P. Ondrackova, J. Mares et al., "In vivo effects of microcystins and complex cyanobacterial biomass on rats (*Rattus norvegicus* var. *alba*): changes in immunological and haematological parameters," *Toxicon*, vol. 73, pp. 1–8, 2013.

[12] D. N. Slatkin, R. D. Stoner, and W. H. Adams, "Atypical pulmonary thrombosis caused by a toxic cyanobacterial peptide," *Science*, vol. 220, no. 4604, pp. 1383–1385, 1983.

[13] O. Takahashi, S. Oishi, and M. F. Watanabe, "Defective blood coagulation is not causative of hepatic haemorrhage induced by microcystin-LR," *Pharmacology & Toxicology*, vol. 76, no. 4, pp. 250–254, 1995.

[14] J. Ravindran, D. Kumar, and P. V. Lakshmanarao, "Protective effect of rifampicin on microcystin-LR induced physiological and haematological changes in rats," *Journal of Cell and Tissue Research*, vol. 11, no. 1, pp. 2451–2458, 2011.

[15] E. Dias, H. Louro, M. Pinto et al., "Genotoxicity of microcystin-LR in *in vitro* and *in vivo* experimental models," *BioMed Research International*, vol. 2014, Article ID 949521, 9 pages, 2014.

[16] P. Kujbida, E. Hatanaka, M. A. R. Vinolo et al., "Microcystins - LA, -YR, and -LR action on neutrophil migration," *Biochemical and Biophysical Research Communications*, vol. 382, no. 1, pp. 9–14, 2009.

[17] G. Yuan, P. Xie, X. Zhang et al., "*In vivo* studies on the immunotoxic effects of microcystins on rabbit," *Environmental Toxicology*, vol. 27, no. 2, pp. 83–89, 2012.

[18] W. O. K. Grabow, W. C. Du Randt, O. W. Prozesky, and W. E. Scott, "Microcystis aeruginosa toxin: cell culture toxicity, hemolysis and mutagenicity assays," *Applied and Environmental Microbiology*, vol. 43, no. 6, pp. 1425–1433, 1982.

[19] P. Sicińska, B. Bukowska, J. Michałowicz, and W. Duda, "Damage of cell membrane and antioxidative system in human erythrocytes incubated with microcystin-LR in vitro," *Toxicon*, vol. 47, no. 4, pp. 387–397, 2006.

[20] W. Zhou, X. Zhang, P. Xie, H. Liang, and X. Zhang, "The suppression of hematopoiesis function in Balb/c mice induced by prolonged exposure of microcystin-LR," *Toxicology Letters*, vol. 219, no. 2, pp. 194–201, 2013.

[21] K. E. De Visser, A. Eichten, and L. M. Coussens, "Paradoxical roles of the immune system during cancer development," *Nature Reviews Cancer*, vol. 6, no. 1, pp. 24–37, 2006.

[22] H. Jaeschke, G. J. Gores, A. I. Cederbaum, J. A. Hinson, D. Pessayre, and J. J. Lemasters, "Mechanisms of hepatotoxicity," *Toxicological Sciences*, vol. 65, no. 2, pp. 166–176, 2002.

[23] US EPA, "Toxicological reviews of cyanobacterial toxins: microcystins LR, RR, YR and LA (external review draft)," DC EPA/600/R-06/139, US Environmental Protection Agency, Washington, DC, USA, 2006.

[24] P. Kujbida, E. Hatanaka, A. Campa, P. Colepicolo, and E. Pinto, "Effects of microcystins on human polymorphonuclear leukocytes," *Biochemical and Biophysical Research Communications*, vol. 341, no. 1, pp. 273–277, 2006.

[25] P. Kujbida, E. Hatanaka, A. Campa, R. Curi, S. H. P. Farsky, and E. Pinto, "Analysis of chemokines and reactive oxygen species formation by rat and human neutrophils induced by microcystin-LA, -YR and -LR," *Toxicon*, vol. 51, no. 7, pp. 1274–1280, 2008.

[26] M. Hernández, M. Macia, C. Padilla, and F. F. Del Campo, "Modulation of human polymorphonuclear leukocyte adherence by cyanopeptide toxins," *Environmental Research*, vol. 84, no. 1, pp. 64–68, 2000.

[27] F. Takizawa, S. Tsuji, and S. Nagasawa, "Enhancement of macrophage phagocytosis upon iC3b deposition on apoptotic cells," *FEBS Letters*, vol. 397, no. 2-3, pp. 269–272, 1996.

[28] M. Ichinose, M. Asai, K. Imai, and M. Sawada, "Enhancement of phagocytosis in mouse macrophages by Pituitary Adenylate Cyclase Activating Polypeptide (PACAP) and related peptides," *Immunopharmacology*, vol. 30, no. 3, pp. 217–224, 1995.

[29] C. Kawagishi, K. Kurosaka, N. Watanabe, and Y. Kobayashi, "Cytokine production by macrophages in association with phagocytosis of etoposide-treated P388 cells in vitro and in vivo," *Biochimica et Biophysica Acta (BBA)—Molecular Cell Research*, vol. 1541, no. 3, pp. 221–230, 2001.

[30] L. C. Mongan, T. Jones, and G. Patrick, "Cytokine and free radical responses of alveolar macrophages in vitro to asbestos fibres," *Cytokine*, vol. 12, no. 8, pp. 1243–1247, 2000.

[31] P. P. Shen, S. W. Zhao, W. J. Zheng, Z. C. Hua, Q. Shi, and Z. T. Liu, "Effects of cyanobacteria bloom extract on some parameters of immune function in mice," *Toxicology Letters*, vol. 143, no. 1, pp. 27–36, 2003.

[32] T. Chen, X. Zhao, Y. Liu, Q. Shi, Z. Hua, and P. Shen, "Analysis of immunomodulating nitric oxide, iNOS and cytokines mRNA in mouse macrophages induced by microcystin-LR," *Toxicology*, vol. 197, no. 1, pp. 67–77, 2004.

[33] A. Lankoff, Ł. Krzowski, J. Glab et al., "DNA damage and repair in human peripheral blood lymphocytes following treatment with microcystin-LR," *Mutation Research*, vol. 559, no. 1-2, pp. 131–142, 2004.

[34] I. Teneva, R. Mladenov, N. Popov, and B. M. Dzhambazov, "Cytotoxicity and apoptotic effects of microcystin-LR and anatoxin-a in mouse lymphocytes," *Folia Biologica*, vol. 51, no. 3, pp. 62–67, 2005.

[35] Y. Lone, R. K. Koiri, and M. Bhide, "Nitrate enhances microcystin-LR induced toxicity in mice," *Austin Journal of Molecular and Cellular Biology*, vol. 2, no. 1, p. 1006, 2015.

[36] Q. Shi, J. Cui, J. Zhang, F. X. Kong, Z. C. Hua, and P. P. Shen, "Expression modulation of multiple cytokines in vivo by cyanobacteria blooms extract from Taihu Lake, China," *Toxicon*, vol. 44, no. 8, pp. 871–879, 2004.

8

A 90-Day Oral Toxicological Evaluation of the Methylurate Purine Alkaloid Theacrine

Amy Clewell,[1] Gábor Hirka,[2] Róbert Glávits,[2] Philip A. Palmer,[1] John R. Endres,[1] Timothy S. Murbach,[1] Tennille Marx,[1] and Ilona Pasics Szakonyiné[2]

[1]AIBMR Life Sciences, Inc., 2800 East Madison Street, Suite 202, Seattle, WA 98112, USA
[2]Toxi-Coop Zrt., Magyar Jakobinusok tere 4/B, Budapest 1122, Hungary

Correspondence should be addressed to Amy Clewell; amy@aibmr.com

Academic Editor: Steven J. Bursian

A 90-day repeated-dose oral toxicological evaluation was conducted according to GLP and OECD guidelines on the methylurate purine alkaloid theacrine, which is found naturally in certain plants. Four groups of Hsd.Brl.Han Wistar rats (ten/sex/group) were administered theacrine by gavage doses of 0 (vehicle only), 180, 300, and 375 mg/kg bw/day. Two females and one male in the 300 and 375 mg/kg bw/day groups, respectively, died during the study. Histological examination revealed centrilobular hepatocellular necrosis as the probable cause of death. In 375 mg/kg bw/day males, slight reductions in body weight development, food consumption, and feed efficiency, decreased weight of the testes and epididymides and decreased intensity of spermatogenesis in the testes, lack or decreased amount of mature spermatozoa in the epididymides, and decreased amount of prostatic secretions were detected at the end of the three months. At 300 mg/kg bw/day, slight decreases in the weights of the testes and epididymides, along with decreased intensity of spermatogenesis in the testes, and lack or decreased amount of mature spermatozoa in the epididymides were detected in male animals. The NOAEL was considered to be 180 mg/kg bw/day, as at this dose there were no toxicologically relevant treatment-related findings in male or female animals.

1. Introduction

Theacrine (1,3,7,9-tetramethyluric acid) is a methylurate, which is a class of purine alkaloids similar in structure to methylxanthines such as caffeine. Theacrine is often found as a methylated and oxidized metabolite of caffeine in methylxanthine-producing plants [1]. The two prominent theacrine-containing foods in the human diet are the fruits and seeds of *Theobroma grandiflorum* (cupuaçu) and kucha green tea from the leaves of *Camellia kucha* (*Camellia assamica* var. *kucha*) [2–8]. Kucha tea leaves have historically been consumed in certain regions of China as a tea and "healthy beverage" [9–11]. The theacrine content of expanding buds and young leaves of kucha has been reported as ~2.8% of dry weight and the content of mature leaves as ~1.3% [2, 3, 11]. As an estimate of possible exposure to theacrine from kucha tea, if one were to assume 2-3 grams of tea is used per cup at a theacrine content of 2.8%, a cup of tea

would contain approximately 56–84 mg of theacrine (equivalent to 0.8–1.2 mg/kg bw for a 70 kg person). Radiolabelled experiments show that theacrine is synthesized from caffeine in some plants including kucha [2, 4]. Levels of theacrine in cupuaçu plant parts are not well-characterized in the literature.

Only limited research, primarily in cell and animal lines, is available to highlight any potential impact theacrine may have when ingested by humans. Preliminary data from a seven-day oral repeated-dose study by Feduccia et al. [12] demonstrated that theacrine increased locomotor activity in rats while an older study showed a potential biphasic dose-response curve with regard to its effects on activity in mice [13]. Mechanistically, theacrine appears to have adenosine receptor antagonist activity [12]. Other reports have highlighted theacrine's potential to exert dopaminergic and other neurochemical activity suggesting dose-dependent anti-inflammatory, antifatigue, analgesic, and mood enhancing bioactivity, although studies in humans are lacking [14–16].

Theacrine exhibited hepatoprotective effects in a stress-induced liver damage mouse model as well as strong antioxidant capacity in vitro and in vivo [3, 17]. In opposition to effects typically seen with caffeine [18, 19], Feduccia et al. showed that intraperitoneal injections of up to 48 mg/kg theacrine did not induce sensitization or tolerance of its physiologic effect over the seven-day period of the study [12].

Few studies on the safety of theacrine were found in a comprehensive literature search. Brief results of an acute toxicity study in mice were published in which the authors calculated the LD_{50} of orally administered theacrine as 810.6 mg/kg bw (95% confidence interval 769.5–858.0 mg/kg bw) [14]. Similar to other purine alkaloids, theacrine was reported to induce chromosomal aberrations in onion root tips, in *Vicia faba* cells treated during the G2 stage of interphase and in Chinese hamster cells [20, 21]. However, no genotoxicity was found in an in vivo mouse micronucleus study at theacrine concentrations up to 325 mg/kg bw [22].

In contrast to results observed using *C. sinensis* (31 g/kg caffeine and 0 g/kg theacrine), intragastric administration of water extracts of theacrine-containing teas including *C. assamica* var. *kucha* (3 g/kg caffeine and 22 g/kg theacrine) did not lead to increases in blood pressure and heart rate in spontaneously hypertensive rats [10]. When rats were given 30 mg/kg caffeine, theobromine, or theacrine, only the caffeine treatment had a significant effect on cardiovascular parameters [10].

In a human study of 60 healthy men and women, theacrine was given daily (200 or 300 mg) for eight weeks [23, 24]. The two doses are equivalent to 2.6 and 3.8 mg/kg bw/day, respectively, for a 78 kg human (the average weight for male and female subjects in the study). Primary outcomes included fasting clinical safety markers (heart rate, blood pressure, lipid profiles, and hematologic and liver/kidney/immune function biomarkers), all of which fell within normal limits with no group × time interactions and no differences in side effect profiles as compared to controls. Theacrine was also given to 15 healthy subjects in a randomized double-blinded crossover study [25, 26]. A single 200 mg dose (or placebo) was administered, and side effect reports, hemodynamics, and biochemical markers of safety were collected over a 3-hour postdosing period, with no significant findings noted. Six subjects additionally participated in a separate 7-day open-label repeated-dose study comparing 100, 200, and 400 mg of theacrine, in which no side effects were noted [25, 26].

To investigate further the safety of oral consumption of theacrine, in the current work we report the results of a 90-day repeated-dose oral subchronic toxicity study in the Wistar rat.

2. Material and Methods

The 90-day study was conducted according to OECD GLP (ENV/MC/CHEM (98)17; OECD, Paris, 1998) and in compliance with OECD 408 (adopted 21st September 1998; 90-day study) [27] and *US FDA Redbook 2000*, IV.C.4.a (2003; 90-day study) guidelines [28]. Care and use of study animals were in compliance with the laboratory's Institutional Animal Care and Use Committee, the National Research Council Guide for Care and Use of Laboratory Animals [29], and the principles of the Hungarian Act 2011 CLVIII (modification of Hungarian Act 1998 XXVIII) regulating animal protection.

Synthetic 1,3,7,9-tetramethyluric acid (CAS number 2309-49-1; ≥98% pure as measured by high performance liquid chromatography (HPLC), proton nuclear magnetic resonance, and liquid chromatography-mass spectrometry methodologies) was supplied as the branded product TeaCrine® for use as the test article by its manufacturer (Compound Solutions, Inc., Carlsbad, CA). TeaCrine is a commercially available white crystalline powder. A 24-month stability study on this product was conducted at $25 \pm 2°C$ with $60 \pm 10\%$ relative humidity under conditions of commercial packaging and the compound remained stable throughout the testing period (data not shown). Batch number 48-KY20141102, which met all commercial specifications for the product (including ≥98% purity, ≤1% loss on drying, ≤0.5% residue on ignition, and commercial limits for heavy metals and microbial counts) was utilized for the study within the two-year shelf-life date. The specific purity level of this batch (per HPLC analysis) was 99.5%.

The dose levels of theacrine utilized in the study were 375, 300, and 180 mg/kg bw/day. These doses were chosen based on an unpublished 14-day repeated-dose oral toxicity study in Wistar rats that utilized ten animals per group (five rats/sex/group). The highest dose group of 500 mg/kg bw/day resulted in mortality of 5 of 5 males and 3 of 5 females and tremors in all animals; additionally one male animal died in the 400 mg/kg bw/day group. Remaining animals in the 400, 350, and 200 mg/kg bw/day groups survived without toxicological signs, and the NOAEL of the 14-day study was determined to be 350 mg/kg bw/day. Based on the results of this study and OECD 408 guidelines stating that the highest dose level should be chosen with the aim to induce toxicity but not death or severe suffering, the high dose for the 90-day study was selected as 375 mg/kg bw/day. The guidelines suggest a descending dose sequence aiming to demonstrate any dose-related responses and a NOAEL at the lowest dose level. While the guidelines state that twofold to fourfold intervals are frequently optimal for setting descending dose levels, in this case smaller intervals were utilized due to the narrow dose range in which adverse events appeared in the 14-day study and with an aim to detect the highest NOAEL possible (which a broader interval may have missed) to allow assessment of the margin of safety of doses used in human studies, such as the 200–300 mg per day dose (2.6–3.8 mg/kg bw/day for a 78 kg human) used in the study by Taylor et al. [24], which did not result in adverse events or findings in clinical safety markers.

The test article doses were prepared by suspending theacrine in 1% aqueous methylcellulose to achieve concentrations of 18, 30, and 37.5 mg/mL in order to provide a constant dosing volume of 10 mL/kg bw. Doses were prepared daily by careful weight measurement and administered within four hours. The control group received the same volume of 1% methylcellulose vehicle only.

Male and female SPF Hsd.Brl.Han Wistar rats (Toxi-Coop, Budapest, Hungary) were housed individually, with a 12-hour light-dark cycle at 19–25°C and 30–70% relative humidity, in type II polypropylene/polycarbonate cages with Lignocel® certified laboratory wood bedding. Cages were 22 cm (width) by 32 cm (length) by 19 cm (height), and cages and bedding were changed weekly. Animals received ssniff® SM R/M-Z+H complete diet for rats and mice and potable tap water ad libitum. The animals were acclimated for seven days prior to the start of dosing.

At the start of the experimental period, animals were approximately seven weeks old and weighed 206–233 g (males) and 131–151 g (females). Eighty male and female rats were stratified by body weight and randomly assigned to four dose groups containing 10 rats/sex/group. Theacrine was administered by gavage daily each morning at doses of 0 (vehicle-control), 180, 300, or 375 mg/kg bw/day.

Animals were observed twice daily for morbidity and mortality. General cage-side observations for clinical signs were made on two occasions during the acclimation period and once daily during the dosing period, at approximately the same time each day, after administration of the test article. Detailed clinical observations were conducted once weekly, and a functional observational battery (FOB) was performed during the final week to assess parameters such as general physical condition and behavior, response to handling, sensory reactions to various stimuli, grip strength, and motor activity [30]. Measurements of body weight were conducted twice during the acclimation period, on the first experimental day prior to treatment, twice weekly during weeks 1–4, once a week during weeks 5–13, and immediately prior to sacrifice. Food intake was determined and food efficiency calculated once weekly. Ophthalmological examination was carried out on all animals prior to the experimental period and prior to study termination in control and high-dose group animals.

After an overnight fast (approximately 16 hours) following final administration of the test article, three blood samples were collected from the retroorbital venous plexus under Isofluran CP® (CP-Pharma Handelsgesellschaft GmbH, Germany) anesthesia (0.25 mL in tripotassium ethylenediaminetetraacetic acid tubes for hematology measurements, 1.0 mL in sodium citrate tubes for blood coagulation measurements, and 2.5 mL in serum separator tubes for clinical chemistry measurements) after which the animals were euthanized by exsanguination from the abdominal aorta. Blood samples were analyzed for hematologic [hematocrit (HCT), hemoglobin (HGB), red blood cell (RBC), white blood cell (WBC), white blood cell differential (neutrophils (NEU), lymphocytes (LYM), monocytes (MONO), eosinophils (EOS) and basophils (BASO)), platelet (PLT), mean corpuscular volume (MCV), mean corpuscular hemoglobin (MCH), mean corpuscular hemoglobin concentration (MCHC), and reticulocyte (RET)], blood coagulation (activated partial thromboplastin time and prothrombin time) and clinical chemistry [sodium (Na$^+$), potassium (K$^+$), glucose (GLUC), cholesterol, urea concentration, creatinine

(CREA), total protein (TPROT), albumin (ALB), alanine aminotransferase (ALT), aspartate aminotransferase (AST), alkaline phosphatase (ALP), gamma glutamyl transferase (GGT), total bilirubin (TBIL), albumin/globulin ratio, bile acids, calcium (Ca^{++}), chloride (Cl$^-$), and inorganic phosphate (Pi)] parameters. Gross pathological examinations and determinations of selected absolute organ weights (liver, kidneys, adrenals, testes, epididymides, thymus, spleen, brain, heart, uterus with fallopian tubes, ovaries, and thyroid/parathyroid) were completed and relative organ weights (compared to body and brain weights) were calculated. Full histopathological examinations were conducted on the preserved organs and tissues (adrenals, aorta, bone marrow of the femur, brain (cerebrum, cerebellum, pons, and medulla oblongata), eyes, female mammary gland, gonads (testes with epididymides and ovaries), heart, kidney, large intestines, liver, lungs, submandibular and mesenteric lymph nodes, quadriceps muscle, esophagus, nasal turbinates, pancreas, pituitary, prostate, submandibular salivary glands, sciatic nerve, seminal vesicle, skin, small intestines, spinal cord at three levels, spleen, sternum, stomach, thymus, thyroid and parathyroid, trachea and urinary bladder, and uterus with vagina) of all animals of the control and high-dose groups. The adrenal glands, testes, and epididymides were also processed and examined histologically in all animals of the low- and mid-dose groups on the basis of the macroscopic observations at the necropsy (pale adrenal glands and smaller than normal testes and epididymides).

Statistical analyses were conducted using SPSS PC+ software (SPSS, Inc., Chicago, IL). Bartlett's homogeneity of variance test was used to assess heterogeneity of variance between groups and was followed by a one-way analysis of variance (ANOVA) if no significant heterogeneity was detected. Duncan's Multiple Range test was used to assess the significance of intergroup differences if a positive ANOVA result was obtained. Where significant heterogeneity was detected by Bartlett's test, the Kolmogorov-Smirnov test was performed to examine normally distributed data, and Kruskal-Wallis nonparametric one-way ANOVA, followed by the Mann-Whitney U test for intergroup comparisons of positive results, was used in the case of a nonnormal distribution. A p value of <0.05 was considered statistically significant, and statistically significant results were reported at $p < 0.05$ and $p < 0.01$ levels.

3. Results and Discussion

One male at 375 mg/kg bw/day and two females at 300 mg/kg bw/day were found dead on days 42, 33, and 67, respectively. There were no preceding clinical signs in the dead male and in one of the dead females. The other female exhibited a decrease in activity on the day before death. Necropsy observations of the dead animals revealed dark red liver (all) and lungs (male and one female), smaller than normal testes (male), clotted blood in the thoracic cavity near to the heart (male), cyanotic skin and subcutaneous connective tissue on the lower part of the abdomen (male), empty stomach (both females) and intestines (one female),

TABLE 1: Summary of necropsy findings.

| Organ | Observations* | Males (mg/kg bw/d) | | | | | Females (mg/kg bw/d) | | | | |
		Control	180	300	375 Died early	375 Survivors	Control	180	300 Died early	300 Survivors	375
	No macroscopic findings	10/10	9/10	6/10	0/1	0/9	9/10	6/10	0/2	6/8	3/10
Testes	Smaller than normal	0/10	0/10	4/10	1/1	9/9	/	/	/	/	/
Epididymides	Smaller than normal	0/10	0/10	4/10	0/1	9/9	/	/	/	/	/
Prostate	Smaller than normal	0/10	0/10	0/10	0/1	3/9	/	/	/	/	/
Adrenal glands	Pale	0/10	0/10	2/10	0/1	7/9	0/10	0/10	0/2	0/8	4/10
	Enlarged	0/10	0/10	0/10	0/1	0/9	0/10	0/10	1/2	0/8	0/10
Kidney (left side)	White compact formation on the surface	0/10	0/10	0/10	0/1	1/9	0/10	0/10	0/2	0/8	0/10
Skin	Alopecia	0/10	1/10	1/10	0/1	0/9	0/10	0/10	0/2	0/8	0/10
	Scar	0/10	0/10	1/10	0/1	2/9	0/10	0/10	0/2	0/8	0/10
	Cyanotic	0/10	0/10	0/10	1/1	0/9	0/10	0/10	0/2	0/8	0/10
Liver	Dark red	0/10	0/10	0/10	1/1	0/9	0/10	0/10	2/2	0/8	0/10
Lungs	Dark red	0/10	0/10	0/10	1/1	0/9	0/10	0/10	1/2	0/8	0/10
Thoracic cavity	Clotted blood near to the heart	0/10	0/10	0/10	1/1	0/9	0/10	0/10	0/2	0/8	0/10
Stomach	Empty	0/10	0/10	0/10	0/1	0/9	0/10	0/10	2/2	0/8	0/10
Intestines	Empty	0/10	0/10	0/10	0/1	0/9	0/10	0/10	1/2	0/8	0/10
Uterus	Hydrometra	/	/	/	/	/	1/10	4/10	1/2	2/8	4/10

*Number of animals with observations/number of animals examined.

/, not examined; mg/kg bw/day, milligrams per kilogram body weight per day.

hydrometra (one female), and enlarged adrenal glands (one female) (Table 1). During histopathological examination centrilobular hepatocellular necrosis was noted in all three animals (Figures 1 and 2). Chemically induced liver injury can lead to lipidosis, necrosis, fibrosis, and proliferation of organelles, hyperplasia of bile ducts or hepatocytes, and neoplasia [31]. Hepatocellular necrosis may be seen in aging and surviving untreated animals as well as those exposed to toxic chemicals. Necrosis may be coagulative in nature and characterized by homogenous eosinophilia and loss of cellular detail. Chemically induced necrosis is often zonal, most frequently centrilobular or periportal. Thus, the test article was considered to have most likely caused the centrilobular necrosis seen in these animals, and it was considered the probable cause of death.

Slight focal alveolar emphysema and congestion in the lungs and liver were also noted in the three dead animals and, along with the macroscopic changes in the lungs, liver, and heart and the cyanotic skin and subcutaneous connective tissue, were considered to have occurred due to circulatory disturbances developed during agony and/or death. Additionally, a decreased amount of spermatozoa in the epididymides and decreased intensity of spermatogenesis (defined by the proportion of tubuli containing mature spermatozoa) in the testes were observed in the male (Table 2).

In surviving animals, the daily cage-side and weekly detailed clinical observations and the FOB revealed no toxicologically relevant findings. A reduced body weight gain was detected in male and female animals in the 300 and 375 mg/kg bw/day groups and in male animals of the 180 mg/kg bw/day group between days 0 and 3 (Table 3). The reduced body weight gain of male animals in the 300 and 375 mg/kg bw/day groups resulted in lower mean body weight from day 3 to day 89 (Table 4) and lower mean total body weight gain with respect to controls. However, this reduced mean body weight gain on days 0 to 3 was fully compensated in male animals of the 180 mg/kg bw/day group and in both female groups (300 and 375 mg/kg bw/day) during the course of the treatment period resulting in no difference in the summarized mean body weight gain in these groups.

During week 1, food consumption was slightly decreased compared to controls in male and female treated animals in all dose groups and also occurred in male animals at 300 and 375 mg/kg bw/day on other weeks (Table 5). In accordance with the changes in body weight and food consumption, the mean feed efficiency was decreased in male animals at the 300 and 375 mg/kg bw/day dose levels during week 1 and transiently thereafter (Table 6).

No ophthalmologic abnormalities were observed in the control and 375 mg/kg bw/day groups prior to the start of

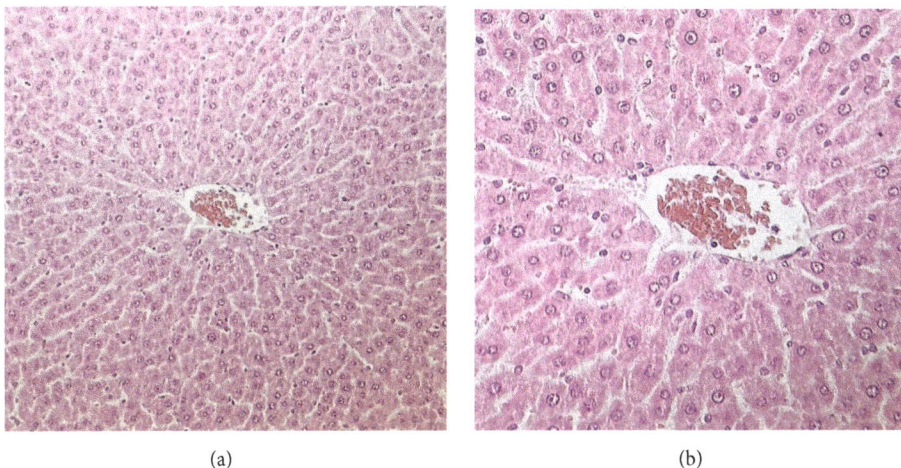

(a)

(b)

FIGURE 1: Intact (normal) hepatocytes around the central vein of a female rat at 375 mg/kg bw/day at terminal sacrifice. Haematoxylin and eosin staining; magnification 200x (a) and 400x (b).

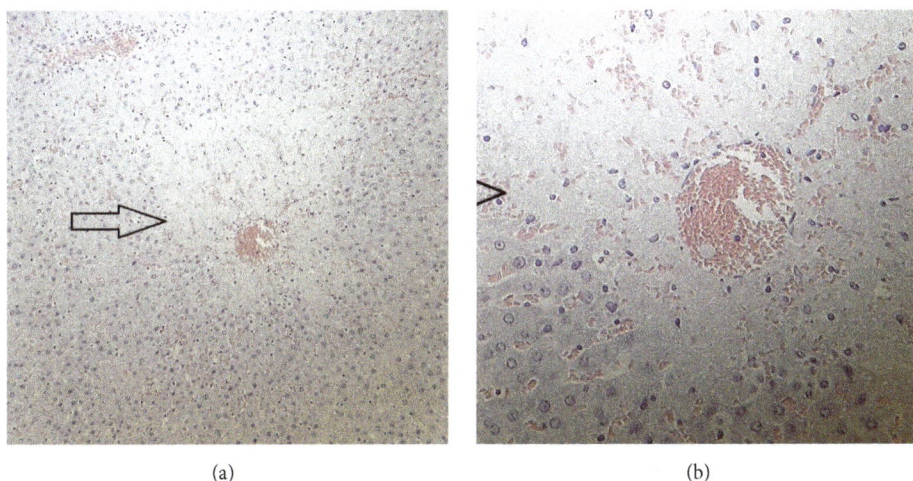

(a)

(b)

FIGURE 2: Centrilobular necrosis (arrows) in the liver of a female rat at 300 mg/kg bw/day found dead on day 33. Haematoxylin and eosin staining; magnification 200x (a) and 400x (b).

dosing or at the end of the treatment period (data not shown). Statistically significant differences between treatment and controls were noted in some hematological and clinical chemistry parameters in male and female animals and are shown in Tables 7 and 8, respectively. Statistically significant differences in MCHC and RET values as compared to controls in males and RBC values in both males and females were not clearly dose-dependent and fell well within historical control ranges and were thus not considered toxicologically relevant. EOS values appeared to decrease dose-dependently within historical ranges in both genders; however, decreases in this value are not generally considered biologically relevant. Significant differences in MCV and MCH levels were slight and values remained within historical control ranges in the 180 mg/kg bw/day group (and were within or marginal to historical control ranges in the mid- and high-dose groups). Related hematological parameters such as HGB and HCT were not different than controls, and no hematologically

related organ pathologies were noted. Thus the findings were not considered toxicologically adverse.

Slight but statistically significant increases were observed in liver ALT and AST enzyme activities in the 300 (ALT) and 375 (ALT and AST) mg/kg bw/day groups. Similarly, the mean CREA concentrations were slightly elevated in male treated animals. These slight, apparently dose-dependent changes may be indicative of a test article effect on hepatic and renal function; however, there were no related histopathological changes in the kidneys or livers of these animals to substantiate their relevance, and the values all remained well within historically normal ranges.

Interestingly, at lower doses in mice, theacrine (up to 30 mg/kg bw/day for seven days) was reported to protect against increases in ALT and AST levels induced by restraint stress [17]. Yet, in another recently published 90-day study, Crl: Sprague Dawley CD IGS rats given 150 mg/kg bw/day of the structurally similar compound, caffeine, also showed

TABLE 2: Summary of notable histopathology findings.

Organs	Observations*	Males Control	Males 180	Males 300	Males 375 Survivors	Males 375 Died early	Females Control	Females 180	Females 300 Survivors	Females 300 Died early	Females 375
Epididymides	Decreased amount of spermatozoa	0/10	0/10	1/10	1/9	1/1	/	/	/	/	/
	Lack of spermatozoa	0/10	0/10	2/10	8/9	0/1	/	/	/	/	/
Testes	Decreased intensity of spermatogenesis	0/10	0/10	5/10	9/9	1/1	/	/	/	/	/
Liver	Congestion	0/10	/	/	0/9	1/1	0/10	/	/	2/2	0/10
	Centrilobular necrosis	0/10	/	/	0/9	1/1	0/10	/	/	2/2	0/10
Lungs	Alveolar emphysema	2/10	/	/	1/9	1/1	2/10	/	/	2/2	2/10
	Hyperplasia of BALT	2/10	/	/	1/9	0/1	1/10	/	/	0/2	0/10
	Congestion	0/10	/	/	0/9	1/1	0/10	/	/	2/2	0/10
Prostate	Decreased amount of secretion	0/10	/	/	3/9	0/1	/	/	/	/	/
Skin	Exudative dermatitis	0/10	1/1	1/1	2/9	0/1	0/10	0/10	0/10	0/10	0/10
Uterus	Dilatation	/	/	/	/	/	1/10	/	/	0/2	4/9

*Number of animals with observations/number of animals examined.
/, not examined; BALT, bronchus associated lymphoid tissue; mg/kg bw/d, milligrams per kilogram body weight per day.

increases in AST, ALT, and CREA that fell within historical control ranges [32]. Significant differences in AST and ALT were reported in a National Toxicology Program study in Fischer 244 rats on caffeine at doses up to 287 mg/kg bw/day; however, no dose-related patterns were established [33]. Slight but significant increases in AST and ALT have also been reported in humans with consumption of coffee [34], although coffee/caffeine consumption has also been associated with protective effects against increases in liver enzymes (e.g., ALT) and liver protection in general [35–37]. Caffeine (and likely theacrine) is metabolized in the liver [33, 38] and thus high doses could theoretically have an effect on this organ due to high exposure chronically.

Other statistically significant differences in clinical chemistry values in various dose groups were slight and considered to be of little or no biological or toxicological relevance. For example, slight statistically significant differences in TBIL and K^+, as compared to controls, occurred only in one gender, were not dose-dependent, and remained well within the historical control ranges. GLUC and Na^+ values appeared to decrease statistically significantly and dose-dependently in both genders suggesting a possible test article effect, although all values remained well within historical control ranges. Differences in Cl^- and Pi did not show clear dose-response relationships.

Of note with regard to macroscopic findings (Table 1), smaller than normal testes (4/10 and 9/9) and epididymides (4/10 and 9/9) were observed in males of the 300 and 375 mg/kg bw/day groups, respectively. Three animals in the 375 mg/kg bw/day group also had smaller than normal prostates. Pale adrenal glands were observed in male animals at 300 mg/kg bw/day (2/10) and in male and female animals at 375 mg/kg bw/day (7/9 and 4/10, resp.). Other minor necropsy findings shown in Table 1 (e.g., white compact formation on the surface of the kidney, scarring, and alopecia in several groups) were considered to be individual findings in male animals as they are common observations in untreated experimental rats of this strain and age.

Decreased organ weights compared to controls were observed in male animals in the testes of the 300 (absolute and relative to brain weight) and 375 (absolute and relative to body and brain weights) mg/kg bw/day groups and epididymides of the 300 and 375 (absolute and relative to body and brain weights) mg/kg bw/day groups. Increased weights compared to controls were noted for adrenal glands in males at 375 (absolute and relative to body and brain weight) and 300 mg/kg bw/day (relative to body weight only). Decreases in thymus weight (absolute and relative to body and brain weight) were noted at 300 and 375 mg/kg bw/day in both male and female animals (Tables 9–11). Statistically significant

TABLE 3: Summary of mean body weight gain.

Group (mg/kg bw/d)		Body weight gain (g) between days																	Sum 0–89
		0–3	3–7	7–10	10–14	14–17	17–21	21–24	24–28	28–35	35–42	42–49	49–56	56–63	63–70	70–77	77–84	84–89	0–89
Males																			
Control	Mean	21.2	23.8	6.7	19.8	10.4	17.4	8.3	13.4	14.4	18.1	16.0	12.8	7.8	10.1	8.7	5.1	1.0	215.0
	SD	1.8	3.3	2.9	3.4	2.4	3.8	4.2	3.9	2.9	3.5	4.0	2.1	2.3	3.0	3.9	3.5	2.4	15.1
180	Mean	16.5	23.1	10.5	18.0	9.5	16.2	9.9	12.2	19.3	16.3	14.6	15.2	10.9	8.5	9.4	7.1	3.6	220.8
	SD	5.2	3.9	2.5	3.8	3.8	3.4	4.7	3.6	6.2	3.9	4.7	4.1	3.3	4.1	3.1	3.6	3.7	22.9
	SS	**																	
300	Mean	10.3	21.6	7.7	16.9	8.4	13.2	10.6	9.8	16.1	13.3	14.3	12.1	9.7	10.6	11.1	0.9	4.9	191.5
	SD	7.1	4.6	4.5	6.6	3.4	2.6	4.2	3.2	4.5	9.8	3.6	2.6	3.1	3.6	2.5	8.3	6.2	30.5
	SS	**					*											*	*
375	Mean	−1.7	22.7	10.0	15.9	10.5	15.3	9.3	9.4	11.9	12.1	12.3	10.9	7.0	9.8	10.8	5.2	7.9	181.9
	SD	12.5	3.6	5.2	6.0	3.8	3.1	4.2	8.0	6.2	5.7	6.9	6.2	5.5	4.2	5.3	6.1	2.0	27.7
	SS	**									*							**	**
	n	10	10	10	10	10	10	10	10	10	10	9	9	9	9	9	9	9	9
Females																			
Control	Mean	10.9	13.0	6.9	9.4	5.2	7.0	4.4	6.2	11.6	6.1	5.9	6.5	0.7	5.6	5.7	3.8	2.2	111.1
	SD	3.7	1.6	3.4	2.3	2.8	1.6	3.4	2.7	4.2	3.6	3.8	2.1	3.6	2.8	4.2	4.1	3.3	13.7
180	Mean	9.1	13.1	9.0	8.3	5.7	8.8	3.6	8.2	9.7	5.3	7.5	7.3	1.1	4.2	4.5	4.6	4.0	114.0
	SD	3.1	3.7	4.6	2.0	5.1	4.2	2.0	3.8	4.4	3.8	4.6	2.7	2.8	3.4	4.6	5.1	3.8	14.5
300	Mean	6.7	14.3	7.8	8.8	6.7	9.1	4.5	8.7	9.6	8.3	8.0	4.3	7.2	2.1	8.1	3.2	2.4	118.5
	SD	5.1	2.8	3.6	4.7	3.4	2.2	3.4	2.1	2.5	2.5	4.5	4.2	2.5	3.6	2.4	3.2	1.8	16.5
	n	10	10	10	10	10	10	10	10	9	9	9	9	9	8	8	8	8	8
	SS	*												**					
375	Mean	5.0	12.8	10.0	12.3	6.1	6.4	6.5	7.9	9.5	7.1	9.2	4.7	4.5	3.5	6.6	3.2	5.2	120.5
	SD	2.5	2.7	3.5	3.3	4.4	4.4	4.3	3.3	5.2	7.6	5.2	2.4	2.5	3.9	5.0	4.5	3.8	21.4
	SS	**												**					

mg/kg bw/d, milligrams per kilogram body weight per day; SD, standard deviation; g, grams; SS, statistical significance; n, number of animals.
* $p < 0.05$; ** $p < 0.01$. $n = 10$ unless otherwise stated.

TABLE 4: Summary of mean body weight.

Group (mg/kg bw/d)		Body weight (g) on days																	
		0	3	7	10	14	17	21	24	28	35	42	49	56	63	70	77	84	89
Males																			
Control	Mean	218.6	239.8	263.6	270.3	290.1	300.5	317.9	326.2	339.6	354.0	372.1	388.1	400.9	408.7	418.8	427.5	432.6	433.6
	SD	7.2	7.9	10.0	11.2	12.9	13.9	16.8	15.6	16.8	17.0	18.2	19.5	18.8	18.4	18.8	18.1	19.7	18.9
	n	10	10	10	10	10	10	10	10	10	10	10	10	10	10	10	10	10	10
180	Mean	218.3	234.8	257.9	268.4	286.4	295.9	312.1	322.0	334.2	353.5	369.8	384.4	399.6	410.5	419.0	428.4	435.5	439.1
	SD	7.2	10.9	12.0	12.2	15.5	17.5	15.7	16.0	15.9	18.4	19.4	21.7	21.5	22.1	23.8	24.0	26.1	26.2
	±%	0	-2	-2	-1	-1	-2	-2	-1	-2	0	-1	-1	0	0	0	0	1	1
	n	10	10	10	10	10	10	10	10	10	10	10	10	10	10	10	10	10	10
300	Mean	217.2	227.5	249.1	256.8	273.7	282.1	295.3	305.9	315.7	331.8	345.1	359.4	371.5	381.2	391.8	402.9	403.8	408.7
	SD	6.2	9.3	12.0	12.5	14.8	14.8	14.8	16.9	16.9	18.0	23.9	25.2	25.5	26.0	27.0	27.3	28.6	31.7
	±%	-1	-5	-6	-5	-6	-6	-7	-6	-7	-6	-7	-7	-7	-7	-6	-6	-7	-6
	SS		*	*	*	*	*	**	*	**	**	**	**	**	**	*	*	*	*
	n	10	10	10	10	10	10	10	10	10	10	10	10	10	10	10	10	10	10
375	Mean	217.1	215.4	238.1	248.1	264.0	274.5	289.8	299.1	308.5	320.4	332.5	348.2	359.1	366.1	375.9	386.7	391.9	399.8
	SD	5.5	13.4	12.0	11.0	13.3	14.3	14.8	15.9	17.1	16.4	18.3	16.7	20.0	22.9	23.7	25.1	28.2	28.4
	±%	-1	-10	-10	-8	-9	-9	-9	-8	-9	-9	-11	-10	-10	-10	-10	-10	-9	-8
	SS		**	**	**	**	**	**	**	**	**	**	**	**	**	**	**	**	*
	n	10	10	10	10	10	10	10	10	10	10	10	9	9	9	9	9	9	9
Females																			
Control	Mean	139.8	150.7	163.7	170.6	180.0	185.2	192.2	196.6	202.8	214.4	220.5	226.4	232.9	233.6	239.2	244.9	248.7	250.9
	SD	5.5	6.7	7.4	8.8	10.2	11.1	12.0	11.5	13.0	12.0	13.4	13.8	14.3	14.2	14.2	16.2	15.5	17.2
	n	10	10	10	10	10	10	10	10	10	10	10	10	10	10	10	10	10	10
180	Mean	140.1	149.2	162.3	171.3	179.6	185.3	194.1	197.7	205.9	215.6	220.9	228.4	235.7	236.8	241.0	245.5	250.1	254.1
	SD	5.9	6.1	4.5	5.0	4.8	6.3	8.2	8.4	9.7	11.4	11.9	13.3	14.0	13.9	14.0	14.0	15.6	15.8
	±%	0	-1	-1	0	0	0	1	1	2	1	0	1	1	1	1	0	1	1
	n	10	10	10	10	10	10	10	10	10	10	10	10	10	10	10	10	10	10
300	Mean	139.4	146.1	160.4	168.2	177.0	183.7	192.8	197.3	206.0	216.4	224.8	232.8	237.1	244.3	245.4	253.5	255.9	258.3
	SD	2.0	4.4	4.6	5.8	7.3	7.2	8.4	9.9	9.8	10.8	11.4	13.3	14.5	13.4	15.5	15.7	16.1	17.1
	±%	0	-3	-2	-1	-2	-1	0	0	2	1	2	3	2	5	3	4	3	3
	n	10	10	10	10	10	10	10	10	10	10	10	10	10	10	10	10	10	10
375	Mean	141.0	146.0	158.8	168.8	181.1	187.2	193.6	200.1	208.0	217.5	224.6	233.8	238.5	243.0	246.5	253.1	256.3	261.5
	SD	5.2	6.1	6.9	7.6	8.8	7.9	10.5	11.7	11.2	15.9	16.8	16.2	16.5	16.0	19.1	21.1	21.5	23.4
	±%	1	-3	-3	-1	1	1	1	2	3	1	2	3	2	4	3	3	3	4
	n	10	10	10	10	10	10	10	10	10	10	10	10	10	10	10	10	10	10

±%, percent deviation versus control; mg/kg bw/d, milligrams per kilogram body weight per day; SD, standard deviation; g, grams; SS, statistical significance; n, number of animals.
* $p < 0.05$; ** $p < 0.01$.

TABLE 5: Summary of food consumption.

Group (mg/kg bw/d)		Daily mean food consumption (g/animal/day) on weeks												
		1	2	3	4	5	6	7	8	9	10	11	12	13
Males														
Control	Mean	25.0	25.2	26.4	26.9	25.8	25.9	26.9	25.7	24.2	25.3	23.8	25.4	24.1
	SD	1.56	1.76	1.93	1.74	2.13	1.94	2.25	1.87	2.04	2.50	2.03	2.31	2.47
180	Mean	23.1	25.3	26.6	27.2	27.1	26.8	26.9	26.1	25.3	26.7	25.3	26.2	26.5
	SD	1.52	1.70	2.13	1.82	1.88	2.16	2.27	2.24	1.88	1.65	1.45	1.59	1.84
	±%	−7.7	0.4	0.9	1.1	5.1	3.3	0.1	1.7	4.8	5.9	6.3	3.2	10.2
	SS	*												*
300	Mean	21.0	23.6	23.6	24.9	24.5	24.4	24.9	23.9	23.7	24.8	23.7	24.1	24.1
	SD	1.72	1.43	2.52	1.22	1.16	1.40	1.69	1.47	1.40	1.23	1.47	1.93	2.21
	±%	−16	−6	−11	−7	−5	−6	−7	−7	−2	−2	0	−5	0
	SS	**		**	**			*	*					
375	Mean	18.2	22.8	24.4	24.7	23.2	23.2	24.4	23.2	22.6	23.8	23.2	24.6	24.7
	SD	2.76	2.48	1.62	1.43	1.86	1.71	1.54	1.94	1.86	2.04	2.15	2.76	2.21
	n	10	10	10	10	10	10	9	9	9	9	9	9	9
	±%	−27	−10	−8	−8	−10	−11	−9	−9	−7	−6	−2	−3	3
	SS	**	**	*	**	**	**	*	*					
Females														
Control	Mean	17.3	17.6	17.8	18.9	19.5	19.3	19.7	19.0	17.9	19.4	18.6	20.5	20.0
	SD	1.04	1.35	1.19	1.34	1.60	1.37	1.54	2.19	2.21	2.15	2.66	2.31	2.69
180	Mean	15.5	17.0	17.8	18.2	18.3	18.4	19.3	17.9	17.3	18.8	17.6	19.2	19.4
	SD	0.53	0.88	1.13	1.10	1.48	1.46	1.51	1.16	1.14	1.63	1.18	1.48	1.69
	±%	−10	−4	0	−4	−6	−5	−2	−6	−3	−3	−5	−6	−3
	SS	**												
		**												
300	Mean	14.6	16.5	17.8	18.4	18.4	18.7	19.5	18.1	17.8	18.8	18.9	20.5	19.6
	SD	1.81	1.13	1.41	1.12	1.39	0.98	1.61	1.46	1.03	0.68	2.83	3.47	1.18
	n	10	10	10	10	9	9	9	9	9	8	8	8	8
	±%	−15	−6	0	−3	−6	−3	−1	−5	0	−3	2	0	−2
	SS	**												
		**												
375	Mean	14.4	17.5	17.6	18.8	18.7	18.6	19.6	18.7	17.7	18.9	18.2	19.8	19.9
	SD	1.49	1.08	2.14	1.17	1.80	2.26	1.57	1.55	1.45	1.64	1.79	1.91	1.95
	±%	−16.9	−0.6	−1.0	−0.5	−4.2	−3.9	−0.3	−1.7	−1.2	−2.9	−2.1	−3.3	−0.2
	SS	**												

±%, percent deviation versus control; mg/kg bw/d, milligrams per kilogram body weight per day; SD, standard deviation; g, grams; SS, statistical significance; n, number of animals.
$^*p < 0.05$; $^{**}p < 0.01$. $n = 10$ unless otherwise stated.

differences in the weights of some organs in male animals (heart and kidneys) relative to body weight arose partially or fully from the body weight changes of these groups and were not seen in organ to brain weight ratios. Differences in some organ weights (absolute or relative) were observed only in the lower dose groups but not in the higher dose groups (liver, thyroid, and uterus) and, therefore, were not considered treatment-related.

In surviving animals, histological examination (Table 2) revealed decreased intensity of spermatogenesis in the seminiferous tubuli in all male animals at 375 mg/kg bw/day and in half of male animals at 300 mg/kg bw/day as compared to controls. In all animals with testicular findings, giant cells in the seminiferous tubuli were noted. Lack of mature spermatozoa in the ductuli of epididymides (2/10 at 300 mg/kg bw/day and 8/9 at 375 mg/kg bw/day to a moderate or severe degree) and decreased number of mature spermatozoa (1/10 at 300 mg/kg bw/day and 1/9 at 375 mg/kg bw/day in minimal or mild degree) were seen in male animals. The alterations in the testes and epididymides were not accompanied

TABLE 6: Summary of feed efficiency.

Group (mg/kg bw/d)		Feed efficiency (g bw/g food)													Sum
	Days	0–7	7–14	14–21	21–28	28–35	35–42	42–49	49–56	56–63	63–70	70–77	77–84	84–89	0–89
	Weeks	1	2	3	4	5	6	7	8	9	10	11	12	13	1–13
Males															
Control	Mean	0.26	0.15	0.15	0.12	0.08	0.10	0.09	0.07	0.05	0.06	0.05	0.03	0.02	0.10
	SD	0.02	0.02	0.02	0.02	0.01	0.02	0.02	0.02	0.01	0.01	0.02	0.02	0.02	0.01
180	Mean	0.24	0.16	0.14	0.12	0.10	0.09	0.08	0.08	0.06	0.04	0.05	0.04	0.04	0.09
	SD	0.03	0.01	0.02	0.03	0.03	0.02	0.02	0.02	0.02	0.02	0.02	0.02	0.01	0.01
	SS													*	
300	Mean	0.21	0.15	0.13	0.12	0.09	0.09	0.08	0.07	0.06	0.06	0.07	0.02	0.05	0.09
	SD	0.05	0.05	0.03	0.03	0.02	0.02	0.02	0.01	0.02	0.02	0.02	0.02	0.04	0.01
	SS	*												*	
375	Mean	0.15	0.14	0.14	0.11	0.08	0.07	0.07	0.07	0.05	0.06	0.07	0.04	0.06	0.09
	SD	0.08	0.07	0.05	0.05	0.03	0.03	0.04	0.04	0.03	0.02	0.03	0.02	0.02	0.01
	SS	**					*							**	
Females															
Control	Mean	0.20	0.13	0.10	0.08	0.08	0.05	0.05	0.05	0.02	0.05	0.05	0.03	0.04	0.07
	SD	0.02	0.02	0.02	0.03	0.03	0.02	0.02	0.02	0.02	0.01	0.03	0.02	0.02	0.01
180	Mean	0.20	0.15	0.11	0.09	0.07	0.04	0.05	0.06	0.02	0.04	0.05	0.05	0.06	0.07
	SD	0.04	0.04	0.04	0.03	0.03	0.03	0.05	0.02	0.01	0.02	0.02	0.03	0.03	0.01
	SS														
300	Mean	0.20	0.14	0.13	0.10	0.07	0.06	0.06	0.04	0.06	0.02	0.06	0.03	0.03	0.07
	SD	0.04	0.04	0.03	0.03	0.02	0.02	0.03	0.02	0.02	0.02	0.02	0.02	0.02	0.01
	SS									**	*				
375	Mean	0.18	0.18	0.10	0.11	0.08	0.07	0.07	0.04	0.04	0.04	0.06	0.04	0.07	0.07
	SD	0.02	0.04	0.04	0.03	0.03	0.02	0.04	0.02	0.02	0.01	0.03	0.02	0.03	0.01
	SS		**												*

±%, percent deviation versus control; mg/kg bw/d, milligrams per kilogram body weight per day; g bw/g food, grams body weight per grams of food; SD, standard deviation; g, grams; SS, statistical significance; n, number of animals.
$^*p < 0.05$; $^{**}p < 0.01$.

by inflammation, degeneration, or necrosis. The number and cytomorphology of interstitial testicular cells were the same as in control male animals. A decreased amount of secretion in the tubuli of the prostate was observed in three male animals at 375 mg/kg bw/day. In the remaining male animals of the 300 mg/kg bw/day group (5/10) and in all animals of the 180 mg/kg bw/day and control groups, the various spermatogenic cells (spermatogonia, spermatocytes, spermatids, and spermatozoa)—representing different phases in the development and differentiation of the spermatozoons—and the interstitial cells appeared normal. Similar effects have been reported in rats after consumption of high levels of the purine alkaloids theobromine and caffeine, namely, atrophy of the testes and epididymides and spermatogenic cell degeneration, although the mechanism by which this occurs is unknown [39, 40]. However in human studies, caffeine intake has not been associated with adverse effects related to semen quality, and fertility levels have, overall, not consistently been linked to caffeine intake [41].

There were no other treatment-related findings upon microscopic examination of the selected tissues. Findings that were not considered toxicologically relevant occurred in a few animals; for example, slight, focal alveolar emphysema was observed in the lungs of some male and female animals in control and high-dose groups with similar incidence. This finding is connected to hypoxia, dyspnea, and circulatory disturbance that occurs during exsanguination and was considered unrelated to test article administration [42]. Hyperplasia of bronchus-associated lymphoid tissue (BALT) was also observed in both the control and high-dose groups (with greater incidence in the control group). This is a physiological, immunomorphological phenomenon [43, 44] and is not considered toxicologically relevant. Dilatation of the uterine horns occurred in female animals of control and high-dose groups; this is considered a slight neurohormonal phenomenon connected to the estrus phase of the inner genital organs and not toxicologically relevant [45].

No histopathological findings were noted in the adrenal or thymus glands. Thus the pale adrenals and differences in organ weights of the adrenals and thymus were considered likely to be an indication of the adaptive process (the response of the organ to environmental variation in order to maintain

TABLE 7: Summary of statistically significant hematological findings.

| | Dose group (mg/kg bw/d) | | | | | | | | | |
| | Males | | | | | | Females | | | |
	Control n = 10	180 n = 10	300 n = 10	375 n = 9	Historical range	Control n = 10	180 n = 10	300 n = 8	375 n = 10	Historical range
WBC ($\times 10^9$/L)	7.91 ± 0.97	7.69 ± 1.49	6.69 ± 1.79	8.13 ± 1.65	4.60–13.86	6.20 ± 1.81	5.63 ± 1.02	*4.74 ± 0.98	6.57 ± 1.66	2.96–12.94
MONO (%)	2.82 ± 0.48	*3.70 ± 0.85	2.62 ± 1.17	2.67 ± 0.68	0.6–4.1	2.09 ± 0.64	2.26 ± 0.31	2.51 ± 0.45	1.81 ± 0.48	0.4–3.1
EOS (%)	1.41 ± 0.40	*1.04 ± 0.34	**0.78 ± 0.20	**0.69 ± 0.31	0.4–3.3	1.06 ± 0.43	0.78 ± 0.34	0.76 ± 0.32	**0.52 ± 0.20	0.5–2.0
RBC ($\times 10^{12}$/L)	9.51 ± 0.40	**8.43 ± 0.48	**8.31 ± 0.64	**8.34 ± 0.33	6.20–10.26	8.67 ± 0.28	**7.92 ± 0.40	**8.01 ± 0.52	*8.19 ± 0.67	7.61–9.31
HGB (g/L)	168.70 ± 5.93	162.00 ± 7.47	161.90 ± 10.84	163.67 ± 3.50	109–184	161.20 ± 3.77	*154.60 ± 6.82	158.88 ± 9.49	165.20 ± 6.99	145–169
MCV (fL)	48.04 ± 1.40	**52.96 ± 2.96	**53.94 ± 2.15	**54.17 ± 2.68	45.0–53.7	51.13 ± 2.09	**54.18 ± 2.71	**54.78 ± 2.15	**55.14 ± 1.65	47.0–55.0
MCH (pg)	17.75 ± 0.41	**19.24 ± 0.81	**19.51 ± 0.57	**19.66 ± 0.86	16.7–19.4	18.61 ± 0.62	*19.54 ± 0.89	**19.85 ± 0.56	**20.25 ± 1.29	17.3–19.7
MCHC (g/L)	369.70 ± 4.40	*363.70 ± 9.07	*361.80 ± 5.92	*362.89 ± 4.26	339–376	363.90 ± 5.90	360.60 ± 3.53	362.75 ± 5.50	367.20 ± 17.07	351–368
RET (%)	3.15 ± 0.30	**3.67 ± 0.32	**4.18 ± 1.72	**3.94 ± 0.56	2.51–4.65	3.93 ± 0.49	4.14 ± 0.79	3.91 ± 0.63	4.36 ± 1.22	3.17–6.16

Values are expressed as mean ± standard deviation. Historical Range based on data from 40 male and 38 female Hsd.Brl.Han Wistar control rats aged 19-20 weeks. mg/kg bw/d, milligrams per kilogram body weight per day; L, liter; fL, femtoliters; pg, picograms; n, number of animals; * p < 0.05 and ** p < 0.01.

TABLE 8: Summary of statistically significant clinical chemistry findings.

| | Dose group (mg/kg bw/d) | | | | | | | | | |
| | Males | | | | | Females | | | | |
	Control n = 10	180 n = 10	300 n = 10	375 n = 9	Historical range	Control n = 10	180 n = 10	300 n = 8	375 n = 10	Historical range
ALT (U/L)	54.97 ± 10.62	66.51 ± 7.29	*73.55 ± 18.09	***75.58 ± 18.09	38.5–98.0	58.26 ± 11.88	68.12 ± 12.14	*73.925 ± 17.23	**78.25 ± 14.91	31.4–84.1
AST (U/L)	94.64 ± 20.70	101.81 ± 12.75	98.25 ± 8.76	*112.53 ± 17.90	72.6–123.5	95.25 ± 16.82	89.75 ± 16.20	99.39 ± 17.46	*112.36 ± 20.00	75.0–116.6
ALP (U/L)	102.80 ± 20.47	**78.8 ± 10.89	*79.70 ± 12.28	89.44 ± 25.67	67–215	55.9 ± 17.25	72.90 ± 25.88	60.88 ± 35.45	73.40 ± 32.00	20–185
TBIL (µmol/L)	1.71 ± 0.23	1.69 ± 0.28	*2.07 ± 0.30	*2.09 ± 0.35	0.62–4.72	1.839 ± 0.45	1.44 ± 0.34	1.86 ± 0.38	1.85 ± 0.62	0.91–4.69
CREA (µmol/L)	28.70 ± 2.73	*32.76 ± 3.97	***34.35 ± 4.58	***35.97 ± 2.89	23.1–37.0	29.3 ± 2.32	29.51 ± 3.28	30.30 ± 3.55	31.15 ± 3.06	25.9–38.2
Urea (µmol/L)	7.48 ± 0.91	7.20 ± 0.88	7.64 ± 0.86	7.64 ± 0.82	4.14–9.62	6.947 ± 0.71	7.19 ± 1.04	6.83 ± 0.85	7.08 ± 0.82	4.79–9.71
GLUC (µmol/L)	6.04 ± 0.52	5.99 ± 0.53	5.62 ± 0.43	**5.35 ± 0.33	4.98–7.97	5.73 ± 0.49	5.71 ± 0.49	*5.10 ± 0.80	**4.53 ± 0.41	4.18–8.49
Pi (µmol/L)	1.90 ± 0.28	2.09 ± 0.25	2.09 ± 0.24	*2.39 ± 0.24	1.40–2.06	1.275 ± 0.16	*1.53 ± 0.16	**2.12 ± 0.20	**2.11 ± 0.39	1.3–2.1
Ca$^+$ (µmol/L)	2.67 ± 0.08	*2.58 ± 0.11	*2.56 ± 0.09	2.63 ± 0.07	2.39–2.75	2.617 ± 0.06	2.55 ± 0.10	2.57 ± 0.07	2.54 ± 0.10	2.4–2.8
Na$^+$ (µmol/L)	142.00 ± 1.05	**140.00 ± 1.49	**138.80 ± 1.14	**138.67 ± 0.87	137–147	140.6 ± 0.97	139.90 ± 1.79	139.25 ± 1.58	138.50 ± 2.51	137–147
K$^+$ (µmol/L)	4.41 ± 0.25	4.61 ± 0.39	4.23 ± 0.15	4.45 ± 0.26	3.62–5.31	3.921 ± 0.24	4.15 ± 0.21	4.28 ± 0.32	*4.24 ± 0.45	3.6–4.4
Cl$^-$ (µmol/L)	105.65 ± 0.98	**103.4 ± 1.70	**102.24 ± 0.98	**102.46 ± 1.34	101.0–106.6	104.66 ± 0.74	**103.56 ± 1.37	102.79 ± 1.15	102.79 ± 2.22	101.2–109.6
ALB (g/L)	34.21 ± 0.72	33.08 ± 0.88	32.03 ± 1.61	33.63 ± 1.19	31.5–36.7	35.77 ± 1.29	34.73 ± 1.10	34.76 ± 1.45	35.03 ± 2.04	32.9–41.1
TPROT (g/L)	62.59 ± 3.30	*59.7 ± 2.44	57.37 ± 2.30	61.22 ± 2.70	55.5–70.6	64.76 ± 3.53	62.09 ± 2.60	62.65 ± 2.66	64.29 ± 5.17	57.6–79.3

Values are expressed as mean ± standard deviation. Historical Range based on data from 40 male and 38 female (19 females for BUN and Pi) Hsd.Brl.Han Wistar control rats aged 19-20 weeks. mg/kg bw/d, milligrams per kilogram body weight per day; U/L, units per liter; µmol, micromol; g, gram; n, number of animals.
* $p < 0.05$; ** $p < 0.01$.

TABLE 9: Summary of organ weights.

Group (mg/kg bw/d)		Body weight	Brain	Liver	Kidneys	Heart	Thymus	Spleen	Testes or uterus	Epididymides or ovaries	Adrenals	Thyroids
									Organ weight (g)			
Males												
Control (n = 10)	Mean	422.0	2.16	10.00	2.28	1.14	0.44	0.71	3.49	1.62	0.077	0.028
	SD	17.52	0.16	0.96	0.20	0.09	0.12	0.10	0.34	0.09	0.01	0.01
180 (n = 10)	Mean	421.8	2.19	10.77	2.38	1.14	0.40	0.77	3.51	1.65	0.074	0.023
	SD	25.26	0.12	0.99	0.26	0.19	0.08	0.08	0.34	0.20	0.02	0.01
	±%	0.0	1	8	5	0	−8	9	1	2	−4	−19
	SS											*
300 (n = 10)	Mean	393.1	2.11	9.83	2.33	1.20	0.32	0.80	2.70	1.36	0.085	0.021
	SD	28.39	0.10	0.77	0.26	0.14	0.06	0.11	0.74	0.15	0.01	0.01
	±%	−7	−2	−2	3	5	−26	13	−23	−16	10	−26
	SS	*					**		**	**		**
375 (n = 9)	Mean	377.0	2.06	9.51	2.22	1.24	0.30	0.71	1.42	1.14	0.093	0.023
	SD	26.43	0.14	0.99	0.25	0.22	0.05	0.10	0.68	0.12	0.01	0.00
	±%	−11	−4	−5	−3	9	−31	1	−59	−30	20	−16
	SS	**					**		**	**	*	
Females												
Control (n = 10)	Mean	241.9	1.94	6.63	1.61	0.83	0.41	0.55	0.66	0.165	0.088	0.021
	SD	15.55	0.07	0.70	0.21	0.07	0.06	0.11	0.09	0.036	0.012	0.003
180 (n = 10)	Mean	242.5	2.01	7.41	1.59	0.77	0.38	0.63	0.88	0.154	0.085	0.022
	SD	14.74	0.11	0.62	0.14	0.05	0.05	0.10	0.28	0.027	0.018	0.006
	±%	0	4	12	−1	−7	−8	15	32	−7	−4	9
	SS					*			*			
300 (n = 8)	Mean	250.4	1.98	7.07	1.56	0.92	0.33	0.61	0.58	0.148	0.092	0.022
	SD	15.97	0.08	0.56	0.09	0.09	0.05	0.06	0.18	0.034	0.016	0.004
	±%	4	2	7	−3	11	−20	11	−12	−10	4	6
	SS					*	**					
375 (n = 10)	Mean	247.3	1.96	7.16	1.55	0.95	0.31	0.61	0.57	0.151	0.095	0.022
	SD	21.06	0.06	0.84	0.14	0.14	0.07	0.11	0.19	0.031	0.016	0.005
	±%	2.2	0.7	8.0	−3.5	14.7	−25.0	11.1	−13.2	−8.3	6.9	8.3
	SS											

±%, percent deviation versus control, mg/kg bw/d, milligrams per kilogram body weight per day; SD, standard deviation; g, grams; SS, statistical significance; n, number of animals.
* $p < 0.05$; ** $p < 0.01$.

TABLE 10: Summary of organ weights relative to body weight (%).

Group (mg/kg bw/d)		Organ weight relative to body weight (%)									
		Brain	Liver	Kidneys	Heart	Thymus	Spleen	Testes or uterus	Epididymides or ovaries	Adrenals	Thyroids
Males											
Control (n = 10)	Mean	0.512	2.371	0.538	0.271	0.104	0.167	0.825	0.384	0.018	0.007
	SD	0.031	0.206	0.032	0.017	0.027	0.019	0.051	0.024	0.003	0.001
180 (n = 10)	Mean	0.519	2.551	0.564	0.269	0.096	0.183	0.831	0.391	0.018	0.005
	SD	0.021	0.137	0.034	0.037	0.018	0.011	0.060	0.031	0.003	0.001
	±%	1	8	5	−1	−8	10	1	2	−5	−19
	SS		*				*				*
300 (n = 10)	Mean	0.540	2.502	0.593	0.305	0.082	0.203	0.692	0.347	0.022	0.005
	SD	0.054	0.099	0.045	0.031	0.011	0.021	0.201	0.046	0.003	0.001
	±%	5	6	10	13	−21	22	−16	−10	18	−20
	SS			**	*	*	**		*	*	*
375 (n = 9)	Mean	0.549	2.519	0.588	0.329	0.079	0.189	0.379	0.304	0.025	0.006
	SD	0.040	0.148	0.043	0.047	0.009	0.019	0.187	0.040	0.003	0.001
	±%	7	6	9	22	−23	13	−54	−21	35	−5
	SS			*	**	*	*	**	**	**	
Females											
Control (n = 10)	Mean	0.807	2.739	0.663	0.343	0.170	0.226	0.274	0.068	0.037	0.009
	SD	0.064	0.215	0.058	0.032	0.023	0.041	0.036	0.014	0.005	0.002
180 (n = 10)	Mean	0.831	3.051	0.656	0.316	0.155	0.260	0.359	0.064	0.035	0.009
	SD	0.040	0.110	0.049	0.023	0.017	0.034	0.107	0.013	0.007	0.002
	±%	3	11	−1	−8	−9	15	31	−6	−4	7
	SS		**					*			
300 (n = 8)	Mean	0.794	2.828	0.625	0.367	0.132	0.244	0.233	0.059	0.037	0.009
	SD	0.054	0.204	0.025	0.031	0.019	0.029	0.078	0.012	0.005	0.001
	±%	−2	3	−6	7	−23	8	−15	−13	0	2
	SS					**					
375 (n = 10)	Mean	0.796	2.892	0.628	0.384	0.125	0.245	0.231	0.061	0.038	0.009
	SD	0.071	0.200	0.039	0.048	0.023	0.026	0.068	0.013	0.006	0.002
	±%	−1	6	−5	12	−27	8	−15	−10	5	5
	SS				*	**					

±%, percent deviation versus control, mg/kg bw/d, milligrams per kilogram body weight per day; SD, standard deviation; SS, statistical significance; n, number of animals.
* $p < 0.05$; ** $p < 0.01$.

TABLE II: Summary of organ weight and body weight relative to brain weight (%).

Group (mg/kg bw/d)		Body weight	Organ weight and body weight relative to brain weight (%)								
			Liver	Kidneys	Heart	Thymus	Spleen	Testes or uterus	Epididymides or ovaries	Adrenals	Thyroids
Males											
Control (n = 10)	Mean	19608.6	465.49	105.54	52.99	19.90	32.71	161.64	75.55	3.58	1.29
	SD	1278.39	59.62	8.82	3.84	4.61	4.51	12.20	9.17	0.51	0.23
180 (n = 10)	Mean	19285.0	492.44	108.86	52.07	18.44	35.34	160.22	75.51	3.39	1.03
	SD	759.63	40.09	8.86	8.62	3.60	3.05	11.73	7.23	0.64	0.22
	±%	−1.7	6	3	−2	−7	8	−1	0	−5	−20
	SS										*
300 (n = 10)	Mean	18700.4	467.55	110.87	56.86	15.45	37.96	127.31	64.29	4.04	0.97
	SD	1910.29	48.08	13.13	7.56	3.34	6.61	32.03	6.09	0.64	0.23
	±%	−5	0	5	7	−22	16	−21	−15	13	−25
	SS					*			**		**
375 (n = 9)	Mean	18314.2	460.80	107.34	60.39	14.59	34.75	68.41	55.41	4.52	1.14
	SD	1352.12	35.16	7.32	10.94	2.47	5.35	31.26	5.53	0.45	0.18
	±%	−7	−1	2	14	−27	6	−58	−27	26	−12
	SS					**		**	**	**	
Females											
Control (n = 10)	Mean	12466.2	341.455	82.693	42.583	21.197	28.267	34.109	8.473	4.554	1.056
	SD	957.28	37.492	10.797	3.797	2.917	5.757	5.119	1.847	0.652	0.183
180 (n = 10)	Mean	12062.5	368.27	78.98	38.14	18.71	31.46	43.10	7.66	4.20	1.10
	SD	591.84	25.74	4.94	3.23	2.17	4.83	12.09	1.39	0.78	0.23
	±%	−3	8	−4	−10	−12	11	26	−10	−8	4
	SS				*			*			
300 (n = 8)	Mean	12642.0	356.58	78.94	46.31	16.71	30.83	29.21	7.48	4.63	1.10
	SD	863.82	20.88	4.51	4.30	2.80	3.60	8.44	1.66	0.77	0.23
	±%	1	4	−5	9	−21	9	−14	−12	2	4
	SS					**					
375 (n = 10)	Mean	12643.1	365.80	79.19	48.41	15.81	31.17	29.31	7.69	4.84	1.13
	SD	1076.51	40.84	6.37	6.57	3.62	5.39	9.33	1.45	0.85	0.25
	±%	1	7	−4	14	−25	10	−14	−9	6	7
	SS				*	**					

±%, percent deviation versus control, mg/kg bw/d, milligrams per kilogram body weight per day; SD, standard deviation; SS, statistical significance; n, number of animals.
*$p < 0.05$; **$p < 0.01$.

function/survival) or stress response, and the toxicological significance was considered equivocal as has also been seen with theobromine and caffeine consumption in rats [32, 39, 46, 47].

4. Conclusion

In summary, doses of up to 300 mg (3.8 mg/kg bw/day for a 78 kg human) given to healthy males and females in a previous clinical study did not result in any adverse effects or potential toxicological findings in numerous clinical safety markers [24]. In the present GLP and OECD 408 compliant toxicological study in Wistar rats, theacrine consumption was associated with mortality at 300 mg/kg bw/day in two of ten females and, at 375 mg/kg bw/day in one of ten males, with centrilobular hepatocellular necrosis considered the likely cause of death. Males in the 375 mg/kg bw/day group also had reductions in body weight gain, food consumption and feed efficiency, and decreased weight of the testes and epididymides, along with decreased intensity of spermatogenesis, amount of mature spermatozoa, and prostate secretions. Males of the 300 mg/kg bw/day similarly had decreased weight of testes and epididymides and decreased intensity of spermatogenesis and amount of mature spermatozoa. Based on observations made in this 90-day repeated-dose gavage toxicity study and the lack of toxicologically relevant findings in the low dose group, the NOAEL for theacrine is considered to be 180 mg/kg bw/day in male and female Wistar rats.

Competing Interests

The authors declare that they have no competing interests.

Acknowledgments

The authors would like to thank the following participating investigators for their contributions to the work: Viktória Balogh, Erzsébet Biczó, Ibolya Bogdán, Monika Csatári, Tímea Csörge, Ildikó Hermann, Isvánné Horváth, Zoltán Jakab, Klára Fritz Kovácsné, Viktória Matina, Ágota Jó Schüllerné, János Stáhl, Beatrix Szilágyi Sümeginé, Éva Szabó, Ferenc Szabó, Zsuzsanna Szabó, Edit Szám, Judit Szilák, Márta Tenk, Zsuzsanna Vuleta, and Levente Zoltán for the performance of experimental tasks and/or collection of data and Jared Brodin for copyediting and administrative support in preparation of the paper. The authors disclose that financial support for the research described herein was provided by Compound Solutions Inc. (Carlsbad, CA).

References

[1] J. B. Petermann and T. W. Baumann, "Metabolic relations between methylxanthines and methyluric acids in *Coffea* L.," *Plant Physiology*, vol. 73, no. 4, pp. 961–964, 1983.

[2] H. Ashihara, M. Kato, and A. Crozier, "Distribution, biosynthesis and catabolism of methylxanthines in plants," in *Methylxanthines*, B. B. Fredholm, Ed., vol. 200 of *Handbook of Experimental Pharmacology*, pp. 11–31, 2011.

[3] K. Li, X. Shi, X. Yang, Y. Wang, C. Ye, and Z. Yang, "Antioxidative activities and the chemical constituents of two Chinese teas, *Camellia kucha* and *C. ptilophylla*," *International Journal of Food Science and Technology*, vol. 47, no. 5, pp. 1063–1071, 2012.

[4] A. L. Anaya, R. Cruz-Ortega, and G. R. Waller, "Metabolism and ecology of purine alkaloids," *Frontiers in Bioscience*, vol. 11, no. 1, pp. 2354–2370, 2006.

[5] T. Lim, "*Theobroma grandiflorum*," in *Edible Medicinal and Non-Medicinal Plants: Volume 3, Fruits*, pp. 252–258, Springer, New York, NY, USA, 2012.

[6] M. Vasconcelos, M. da Silva, J. Maia, and O. Gottlieb, "Estudo químico de sementes do cupuaçu," *Acta Amazônica*, vol. 5, no. 3, pp. 293–295, 1975.

[7] T. Baumann and H. Wanner, "The 1,3,7,9-tetramethyluric acid content of cupu (*Theobroma grandiflorum* Schum.)," *Acta Amazônica*, vol. 10, no. 2, p. 425, 1980.

[8] F. Marx and J. G. S. Maia, "Purine alkaloids in seeds of Theobroma species from the Amazon," *Zeitschrift für Lebensmittel-Untersuchung und Forschung*, vol. 193, no. 5, pp. 460–461, 1991.

[9] G. Xie, R.-R. He, X. Feng et al., "The hypoglycemic effects of *Camellia assamica* var. *kucha* extract," *Bioscience, Biotechnology and Biochemistry*, vol. 74, no. 2, pp. 405–407, 2010.

[10] S.-B. Li, Y.-F. Li, Z.-F. Mao et al., "Differing chemical compositions of three teas may explain their different effects on acute blood pressure in spontaneously hypertensive rats," *Journal of the Science of Food and Agriculture*, vol. 95, no. 6, pp. 1236–1242, 2015.

[11] X.-Q. Zheng, C.-X. Ye, M. Kato, A. Crozier, and H. Ashihara, "Theacrine (1,3,7,9-tetramethyluric acid) synthesis in leaves of a Chinese tea, kucha (*Camellia assamica* var. *kucha*)," *Phytochemistry*, vol. 60, no. 2, pp. 129–134, 2002.

[12] A. A. Feduccia, Y. Wang, J. A. Simms et al., "Locomotor activation by theacrine, a purine alkaloid structurally similar to caffeine: involvement of adenosine and dopamine receptors," *Pharmacology Biochemistry and Behavior*, vol. 102, no. 2, pp. 241–248, 2012.

[13] J.-K. Xu, H. Kurihara, L. Zhao, and X.-S. Yao, "Theacrine, a special purine alkaloid with sedative and hypnotic properties from *Cammelia assamica* var. kucha in mice," *Journal of Asian Natural Products Research*, vol. 9, no. 7, pp. 665–672, 2007.

[14] Y. Wang, X. Yang, X. Zheng, J. Li, C. Ye, and X. Song, "Theacrine, a purine alkaloid with anti-inflammatory and analgesic activities," *Fitoterapia*, vol. 81, no. 6, pp. 627–631, 2010.

[15] G. Xie, M. Wu, Y. Huang et al., "Experimental study of the acrine on antidepressant effects," *Chinese Pharmacological Bulletin*, vol. 9, 2009.

[16] Y.-F. Li, M. Chen, C. Wang et al., "Theacrine, a purine alkaloid derived from *Camellia assamica* var. *kucha*, ameliorates impairments in learning and memory caused by restraint-induced central fatigue," *Journal of Functional Foods*, vol. 16, pp. 472–483, 2015.

[17] W.-X. Li, Y.-F. Li, Y.-J. Zhai, W.-M. Chen, H. Kurihara, and R.-R. He, "Theacrine, a purine alkaloid obtained from *Camellia assamica* var. *kucha*, attenuates restraint stress-provoked liver damage in mice," *Journal of Agricultural and Food Chemistry*, vol. 61, no. 26, pp. 6328–6335, 2013.

[18] O. Cauli, A. Pinna, V. Valentini, and M. Morelli, "Subchronic caffeine exposure induces sensitization to caffeine and cross-sensitization to amphetamine ipsilateral turning behavior independent from dopamine release," *Neuropsychopharmacology*, vol. 28, no. 10, pp. 1752–1759, 2003.

[19] P. Svenningsson, G. G. Nomikos, and B. B. Fredholm, "The stimulatory action and the development of tolerance to caffeine is associated with alterations in gene expression in specific brain regions," *The Journal of Neuroscience*, vol. 19, no. 10, pp. 4011–4022, 1999.

[20] B. A. Kihlman, "1,3,7,9-Tetramethyluric acid—a chromosome-damaging agent occurring as a natural metabolite in certain caffeine-producing plants," *Mutation Research/Reviews in Genetic Toxicology*, vol. 39, no. 3-4, pp. 297–315, 1977.

[21] B. A. Kihlman and G. Odmark, "Deoxyribonucleic acid synthesis and the production of chromosomal aberrations by streptonigrin, 8-ethoxycaffeine and 1,3,7,9-tetramethyluric acid," *Mutation Research—Fundamental and Molecular Mechanisms of Mutagenesis*, vol. 2, no. 6, pp. 494–505, 1965.

[22] J. Endres, N. Deshmukh, R. Glavitis et al., "A comprehensive toxicological assessment of the purine alkaloid theacrine," *The Toxicologist, Supplement to Toxicological Sciences*, vol. 150, no. 1, 2016, Abstract #1459.

[23] "Safety of Teacrine™, a non-habituating, naturally-occuring purine alkaloid over eight weeks of continuous use," in *Proceedings of the Annual Meeting of the International Society of Sport Nutrition*, S. Hayward, J. Mullins, S. Urbina et al., Eds., Austin, Tex, USA, 2015.

[24] L. Taylor, P. Mumford, M. Roberts et al., "Safety of TeaCrine®, a non-habituating, naturally-occurring purine alkaloid over eight weeks of continuous use," *Journal of the International Society of Sports Nutrition*, vol. 13, article 2, 2016.

[25] S. M. Habowski, J. E. Sandrock, A. W. Kedia, and T. N. Ziegenfuss, "The effects of Teacrine™, a nature-identical purine alkaloid, on subjective measures of cognitive function, psychometric and hemodynamic indices in healthy humans: a randomized, double-blinded crossover pilot trial," *Journal of the International Society of Sports Nutrition*, vol. 11, no. 1, article P49, 2014.

[26] T. N. Ziegenfuss, S. M. Habowski, J. E. Sandrock, A. W. Kedia, C. M. Kerksick, and H. L. Lopez, "A two-part approach to examine the effects of theacrine (TeaCrine®) supplementation on oxygen consumption, hemodynamic responses, and subjective measures of cognitive and psychometric parameters," *Journal of Dietary Supplements*, 2016.

[27] OECD, OECD 408. Guideline for the testing of chemicals: repeated dose 90-day oral toxicity study in rodents, Section 4, No. 408, adopted 21, pp. 1–10, September 1998.

[28] FDA and Redbook 2000, *Toxicological Principles for the Safety Assessment of Food Ingredients. IV.C.4.a. Subchronic Toxicity Studies with Rodents*, 2003.

[29] National Research Council, *Guide for the Care and Use of Laboratory Animals*, Committee for the Update of the Guide for the Care and Use of Laboratory Animals, Institute for Laboratory Animal Research, Division on Earth and Life Studies, National Research Council, Washington, DC, USA, 2011.

[30] S. Irwin, "Comprehensive observational assessment: Ia. A systematic, quantitative procedure for assessing the behavioral and physiologic state of the mouse," *Psychopharmacologia*, vol. 13, no. 3, pp. 222–257, 1968.

[31] S. Eustis, G. Boorman, T. Harada, and J. Popp, "Liver," in *Pathology of the Fischer Rat Reference and Atlas*, pp. 71–94, Academic Press, San Diego, Calif, USA, 1990.

[32] R. W. Kapp Jr., O. Mendes, S. Roy, R. S. McQuate, and R. Kraska, "General and genetic toxicology of guayusa concentrate (*Ilex guayusa*)," *International Journal of Toxicology*, vol. 35, no. 2, pp. 222–242, 2016.

[33] OECD SIDS, Cafeine, CAS: 58-08-2, UNEP Publications, Paris, France, 2002.

[34] A. J. Onuegbu, J. M. Olisekodiaka, O. E. Adebolu, A. Adesiyan, and O. E. Ayodele, "Coffee consumption could affect the activity of some liver enzymes and other biochemical parameters in healthy drinkers," *Medical Principles and Practice*, vol. 20, no. 6, pp. 514–518, 2011.

[35] A. A. Modi, J. J. Feld, Y. Park et al., "Increased caffeine consumption is associated with reduced hepatic fibrosis," *Hepatology*, vol. 51, no. 1, pp. 201–209, 2010.

[36] C. E. Ruhl and J. E. Everhart, "Coffee and caffeine consumption reduce the risk of elevated serum alanine aminotransferase activity in the United States," *Gastroenterology*, vol. 128, no. 1, pp. 24–32, 2005.

[37] C. E. Ruhl and J. E. Everhart, "Coffee and tea consumption are associated with a lower incidence of chronic liver disease in the United States," *Gastroenterology*, vol. 129, no. 6, pp. 1928–1936, 2005.

[38] EFSA, "Scientific opinion. Opinion on the safety of caffeine," *The EFSA Journal*, vol. 13, no. 5, 2015.

[39] J. H. Gans, "Comparative toxicities of dietary caffeine and theobromine in the rat," *Food and Chemical Toxicology*, vol. 22, no. 5, pp. 365–369, 1984.

[40] H. Funabashi, M. Fujioka, M. Kohchi, Y. Tateishi, and N. Matsuoka, "Collaborative work to evaluate toxicity on male reproductive organs by repeated dose studies in rats. 22) effects of 2- and 4-week administration of theobromine on the testis," *Journal of Toxicological Sciences*, vol. 25, pp. 211–221, 2000.

[41] J. D. Peck, A. Leviton, and L. D. Cowan, "A review of the epidemiologic evidence concerning the reproductive health effects of caffeine consumption: a 2000–2009 update," *Food and Chemical Toxicology*, vol. 48, no. 10, pp. 2549–2576, 2010.

[42] J. Vandenberghe, *Life-Span Data and Historical Data in Carcinogenicity Testing in Wistar Rats Crl:(WI) BR. Addendum 5.8*, Janssen Research Foundation, Department of Toxicology, Charles River Deutschland, Beerse, Belgium, 1990.

[43] G. Boorman and S. Eustis, "Lung," in *Pathology of the Fischer Rat: Reference and Atlas*, G. Boorman, S. Eustis, M. Elwell, and W. MacKenzie, Eds., pp. 339–367, Academic Press, San Diego, Calif, USA, 1990.

[44] W. Haschek, C. Rousseaux, and M. Wallig, "Respiratory system. Structure and cell biology. Physiology and functional considerations—lymphoid tissue," in *Fundamentals of Toxicologic Pathology*, p. 98, Elsevier, New York, NY, USA, 2009.

[45] J. Vidal, M. Mirsky, K. Colman, K. Whitney, and D. Creasy, "Reproductive system and mammary gland," in *Toxicologic Pathology Nonclinical Safety Assessment*, chapter 18, pp. 717–830, CRC Press, Boca Raton, Fla, USA, 2013.

[46] M. Hamlin and D. Banas, "Adrenal gland," in *Pathology of the Fischer rat Reference and Atlas*, pp. 501–518, Academic Press, San Diego, Calif, USA, 1990.

[47] N. E. Everds, P. W. Snyder, K. L. Bailey et al., "Interpreting stress responses during routine toxicity studies: a review of the biology, impact, and assessment," *Toxicologic Pathology*, vol. 41, no. 4, pp. 560–614, 2013.

9

Evaluating the Effects of Tetrachloro-1,4-benzoquinone, an Active Metabolite of Pentachlorophenol, on the Growth of Human Breast Cancer Cells

Binbing Ling, Bosong Gao, and Jian Yang

Drug Discovery and Development Research Group, College of Pharmacy and Nutrition, University of Saskatchewan, 107 Wiggins Road, Saskatoon, SK, Canada S7N 5E5

Correspondence should be addressed to Jian Yang; jian.yang@usask.ca

Academic Editor: Brad Upham

Tetrachloro-1,4-benzoquinone (TCBQ), an active metabolite of pentachlorophenol (PCP), is genotoxic and potentially carcinogenic. As an electrophilic and oxidative molecule, TCBQ can conjugate with deoxyguanosine in DNA molecules and/or impose oxidative stress in cells. In the current study, we investigated the effects of TCBQ on intracellular ROS production, apoptosis, and cytotoxicity against three different subtypes of human breast cancer cells. Luminal A subtype MCF7 (ER$^+$, PR$^+$, HER2$^-$) cells maintained the highest intracellular ROS level and were subjected to TCBQ-induced ROS reduction, apoptosis, and cytotoxicity. HER2 subtype Sk-Br-3 (ER$^-$, PR$^-$, HER2$^+$) cells possessed the lowest intracellular ROS level. TCBQ promoted ROS production, inhibited apoptosis, and elevated cytotoxicity (due to necrosis) against Sk-Br-3 cells. Triple-negative/basal-like subtype MDA-MB-231 cells were less sensitive towards TCBQ treatment. Therefore, the effect of prolonged exposure to PCP and its active metabolites on cancer growth is highly cancer-cell-type specific.

1. Introduction

Pentachlorophenol (PCP), a potent uncoupler of oxidative phosphorylation, was widely used as a low-cost and effective farm pesticide in agriculture and wood preservative in timber industry in the last century [1–5]. Because of its high toxicity to fish, farm animals, and human, PCP was banned from agricultural usage in the 1980s [3, 5–8]. PCP is highly resistant to biodegradation due to the introduction of high and obstructive halogenation, making it one of the most persistent pollutants in the environment [9, 10]. Furthermore, PCP is reasonably soluble (10–20 mg/L) and can be spread to unpolluted areas *via* rain or human activities, making it a continuous source of contamination to fruits, vegetables, and grains [3, 11, 12].

The daily net intake of PCP is about 0.05 μg/kg and 16 μg/kg of body weight for Canadians and Americans, respectively [12, 13]. However, it could reach as high as 24,000 μg for people occupationally exposed to PCP (i.e., 282 μg/kg for a man with the Canadian national average body weight of 85 kg and 343 μg/kg for a woman with the Canadian national average body weight of 70 kg) [14]. Because of its high lipophilicity, PCP can easily cross skin, respiratory tract, and gastrointestinal tract and be distributed in different tissues [3]. The half-life ($t_{1/2}$) of PCP ranges from 33 hours to 16 days in human bodies [14]. Liver and kidney contain the highest levels after PCP exposures [14]. Extended exposure to PCP may cause serious diseases such as neurological disorders, immune disorders, and cancers [15–17]. PCP was also found in breast milk and could be passed to infants by breastfeeding [18, 19]. PCP exposure has been implied as a causal factor for women's repeated miscarriages, endocrine disorders, and even breast cancer [20–22]. The toxicity of PCP is most likely due to the formation of a highly reactive metabolite, tetrachloro-1,4-benzoquinone (TCBQ) [23, 24]. As an electrophilic molecule, TCBQ forms adducts with deoxyguanosine in DNA molecules, causing genotoxic effects to cells [23–25]. Furthermore, TCBQ is susceptible to quick reduction to generate tetrachlorosemiquinone (TCSQ) radicals and imposes oxidative stress in cells. It has been shown that TCBQ increased the intracellular ROS level by about 10-fold in human hepatoma HepG2 cells after 24 h of exposure [23, 24]. These studies implicate that TCBQ is genotoxic and potentially carcinogenic to both human and animals.

In contrast to the vast studies on genotoxic and cytotoxic effects of PCP and its reactive metabolite TCBQ to normal human cells, little is known on how continued exposure to PCP or TCBQ could affect the growth of cancer cells. As a genotoxic and oxidative compound, TCBQ may be a double-edged sword. On the one hand, it may initiate carcinogenesis in normal cells and/or promote cancer cell growth by elevating the intracellular ROS level. On the other hand, TCBQ may cause cell death *via* forming adducts with cancer cell DNA molecules and/or induce cell apoptosis through increasing the intracellular ROS level above the apoptotic threshold in cancer cells. To gain an insight into how extended PCP exposure could affect tumor growth for women with breast cancer, we undertook an *in vitro* study to elucidate the effects of TCBQ on oxidative stress, apoptosis, and cytotoxicity against human breast cancer cells. In spite of big differences in morphology, growth, survival, migration, invasiveness, and metastasis, breast cancer cells are commonly divided into 4 subtypes, luminal A (ER^+ and/or PR^+, $HER2^-$), luminal B (ER^+ and/or PR^+, $HER2^+$), HER2 (ER^-, PR^-, $HER2^+$), and triple-negative/basal-like (ER^-, PR^-, $HER2^-$), based on expression of three cell surface receptors, estrogen receptor (ER), progesterone receptor (PR), and HER2/neu receptor (HER2). The weakly invasive luminal A subtype MCF7 (ER^+, PR^+, $HER2^-$) cell line, weakly invasive HER2 subtype Sk-Br-3 (ER^-, PR^-, $HER2^+$), and highly invasive triple-negative MDA-MB-231 (ER^-, PR^-, $HER2^-$) were selected for this study.

2. Materials and Methods

2.1. Materials. TCBQ and $2',7'$-dichlorofluorescein diacetate (DCFH-DA) were purchased from Sigma-Aldrich Canada (Oakville, ON, Canada). Human breast cancer cell lines MCF7 (ER^+, PR^+, $HER2^-$), Sk-Br-3 (ER^-, PR^-, $HER2^+$), and MDA-MB-231 (ER^-, PR^-, $HER2^-$) were purchased from the American Type Culture Collection (ATCC) (Manassas, VA, USA). ATCC-recommended cell culture media for each cell line were purchased from Cedarlane Canada (Burlington, ON, Canada). Cell apoptosis assay kit, Caspase-Glo® 3/7 Assay, and cytotoxicity assay kit, CytoTox96® Nonradioactive Cytotoxicity Assay, were purchased from Promega Corporation (Madison, WI, USA).

2.2. Cell Culture. Human breast cancer cell lines MCF7, Sk-Br-3, and MDA-MB-231 were cultured in T-75 culture flasks under ATCC-recommended cell culture conditions at 37°C in a Forma™ Series II Water-Jacketed CO_2 Incubator from ThermoFisher Scientific Inc. (Waltham, MA, USA). Cell lines MCF7 and Sk-Br-3 were cultured with 5% CO_2, whereas cell line MDA-MB-231 was cultured with 0% CO_2. Culture media were changed every 2-3 days for each cell line.

2.3. Intracellular ROS Measurement. All experiments in the current study were carried out in triplicate. Intracellular ROS level was measured using probe DCFH-DA in the MCF7, Sk-Br-3, and MDA-MB-231 cells with and without TCBQ treatment under normoxic condition. DCFH-DA was prepared in stock solution of 10 mM in dimethyl sulfoxide (DMSO). Working solution of DCFH-DA was prepared by diluting the stock solution with the respective cell culture media with a final concentration of 0.1 mM. Cells of each cell line were plated on a black flat-bottom 96-well plate at 10,000 cells per well and incubated at 37°C for 18 h. Working solution (5 μL) was added to each well and allowed to react with the cells for 30 min before being aspirated out. The cells were then washed with 200 μL 1x PBS (phosphate buffered saline) buffer twice. Finally, 100 μL 1x PBS buffer was added to each well and fluorescence was read at extinction of 485 nm and emission of 528 nm using an Agilent 8453E UV-visible Spectroscopy System (Agilent Technologies Canada, Mississauga, ON, Canada).

2.4. Apoptosis and Cytotoxicity Assays. The cultured breast cancer MCF7, Sk-Br-3, or MDA-MB-231 cells were plated in 96-well plates (10,000 cells/well) and grown to 70–80% confluence before being treated with TCBQ (final concentrations: 0.16 μM, 0.31 μM, 0.63 μM, 1.25 μM, 2.5 μM, 5 μM, and 10 μM) for 18 h. The optimal exposure time was determined by a pilot study. Treatment with DMSO, in which TCBQ stock solution was prepared, was used as negative control. Apoptosis (caspase 3/7 level) and cytotoxicity (lactate dehydrogenase level) were measured using the Caspase-Glo 3/7 Assay and the CytoTox96 Nonradioactive Cytotoxicity Assay, respectively.

2.5. Statistical Analyses. The experimental data were processed using Microsoft Excel 2010 and presented as mean ± standard deviation. One-way ANOVA with Dunnett's comparison as posthoc analysis was performed with GraphPad Prism 6 (GraphPad Software, Inc., La Jolla, CA, USA). A P value of less than 0.05 was considered to be statistically significant.

3. Results and Discussion

3.1. Intracellular ROS Level under Normoxia. Reactive oxygen species (ROS), which are short-lived and normally generated as byproducts of mitochondrial energy metabolism, play important roles in cell growth, cell signaling, and homeostasis in normal cells [26–28]. Persistently elevated ROS level is a characteristic phenomenon for tumorigenesis, tumor growth, and cancer metastasis [26, 29]. However, measuring and comparing the intracellular ROS across different types of cancer cells or tissues is a challenging task as the ROS level is significantly influenced by the cancer microenvironment, intracellular signaling regulation, and the type and degree of hypoxia. In the current study, we measured the intracellular ROS level in human breast cancer MCF7, Sk-Br-3, and MDA-MB-231 cells under normoxic condition. Although our measurement may not necessarily represent the pathophysiological situation, it allowed us to cross-compare the intracellular ROS of different types of breast cancer cells on the same scale and make reasonable prediction

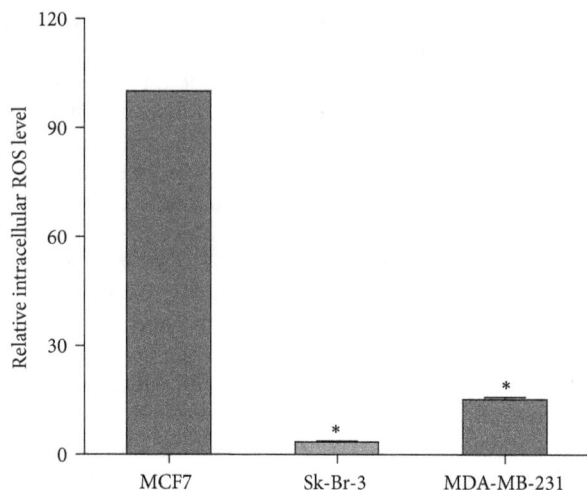

FIGURE 1: Relative intracellular ROS level in human breast cancer MCF7, Sk-Br-3, and MDA-MB-231 cells under normoxic condition. The highest intracellular ROS level was observed in MCF7 cells and set as 100.

on the effects of exogenously administered agents such as oxidative compounds and chemotherapy drugs on ROS production. As shown in Figure 1, the weakly invasive luminal A subtype MCF7 cells maintained the highest intracellular ROS level among all three cancer cell lines. The respective intracellular ROS level in the weakly invasive HER2 subtype Sk-Br-3 cells and highly invasive triple-negative MDA-MB-231 cells was only about $3.5 \pm 0.3\%$ ($P < 0.01$) and $15.3 \pm 0.6\%$ ($P < 0.01$) of that in the MCF7 cells. Our study results were consistent with observation that Sk-Br-3 and MDA-MB-231 cells exhibited a much lower basal oxygen consumption level, relied more on glycolysis rather than oxidative phosphorylation for energy production, and had much higher uptake of F^{18}-fluorodeoxyglucose (FDG) than MCF7 cells [30–32]. Lower oxidative phosphorylation would lead to less ROS in Sk-Br-3 and MDA-MB-231 cells. Furthermore, MCF7 cells are likely more tolerable to ROS and may have a much higher apoptotic threshold than Sk-Br-3 and MDA-MB-231 cells.

3.2. Effects of TCBQ on the Intracellular ROS Level. As an oxidative compound, TCBQ was shown to increase the intracellular ROS level by almost 10-fold in human hepatoma HepG2 cells at $5 \mu M$ concentration after 24 h of exposure [23]. Higher concentration of TCBQ did not further enhance ROS generation, implicating that TCBQ has already reached a plateau for its function on ROS production in HepG2 cells. Therefore, we examined the effect of TCBQ on ROS production in MCF7, SK-Br-3, and MDA-MB-231 cells with its concentration ranging from $0.16 \mu M$ to $10 \mu M$ (~39 $\mu g/kg$ to 2459 $\mu g/kg$, covering the range of previously reported PCP exposure levels and assuming all PCP could be metabolized to TCBQ quickly). Interestingly, TCBQ inhibited instead of promoting ROS production in MCF7 and MDA-MB-231 cells (Figures 2(a) and 2(c)). MCF7 cells gave a bell-shaped response towards TCBQ with the maximum inhibition of ROS production (57% decrease compared to the control,

statistically significant) at $0.63 \mu M$, whereas MDA-MB-231 showed a U-shaped response towards TCBQ treatment with approximately 36% and 42% reduction of ROS compared to the control (statistically significant) at $0.16 \mu M$ and $10 \mu M$, respectively. As for Sk-Br-3 cells, TCBQ increased the intracellular ROS production in a concentration-dependent manner with ROS production dwindled along with elevated TCBQ concentration (Figure 2(b)). The intracellular ROS level was increased by 66% compared to the control at $0.16 \mu M$ of TCBQ; and TCBQ lost its function on ROS production when its concentration surpassed $2 \mu M$. However, the change in ROS level compared to control was statistically insignificant at all TCBQ concentrations. Recently, it was reported that quinone compounds were able to regulate ROS production both positively and negatively in human HEK293 cells [33]. Our current results reinforced and complemented to this study that the effect of quinones on ROS production is highly compound-type specific and cell-type specific. However, it is unknown how TCBQ decreased ROS production in the MCF7 and MDA-MB-231 cells and increased ROS production in the Sk-Br-3 cells even though the ROS increase was statistically insignificant. It has been reported in previous studies that the expression level of glutathione peroxidase (GPx) was much higher in Sk-Br-3 and MDA-MB-231 cells than MCF7 cells and the expression of GPx-1 was increased upon PCP treatment in murine melanoma B16F10 cells [34, 35]. Therefore, we speculated that the different effects of TCBQ on ROS production might be related to its capability of altering intracellular glutathione (GSH) level, which, in turn, is determined by the expression level of GSH-related enzymes such as GPx, glutathione reductase (GR), and glutathione S-transferase (GST). We will undertake further studies to confirm whether the TCBQ effect on ROS production is indeed via changing the expression of GSH-related enzymes.

3.3. Apoptotic Effects. A very recent study showed that 1,4-benzoquinone (BQ) induced cell apoptosis in a concentration-dependent manner in mouse bone marrow cells [36]. However, another study reported that TCBQ induced oxidative stress but not apoptosis in male Kunming mice [37]. Low level of oxidative stress could trigger protein kinase D1- (PKD1-) mediated cell survival while high level of oxidative stress could initiate apoptosis via activating c-Jun N-terminal kinases (JNKs) to downregulate various antiapoptotic proteins [38–41]. Taking into consideration our current observed effects of TCBQ on ROS production, it is rational to hypothesize that the apoptotic effect of TCBQ is also likely to be cell-type specific. To examine our hypothesis, we measured the apoptotic effect (caspase 3/7 level) of TCBQ against the three breast cancer cell lines. As illustrated in Figure 3, cell apoptosis was increased in MCF7 cells (statistically significant) but decreased in Sk-Br-3 and MDA-MB-231 cells (statistically insignificant) throughout the TCBQ concentration range.

In general, MCF7 cells gave a concentration-dependent response towards TCBQ (Figure 3(a)). Apoptosis was increased by more than 59% compared to the control at TCBQ concentration of $0.31 \mu M$ and reached a plateau of 108% as TCBQ concentration reached $5 \mu M$. We speculated that

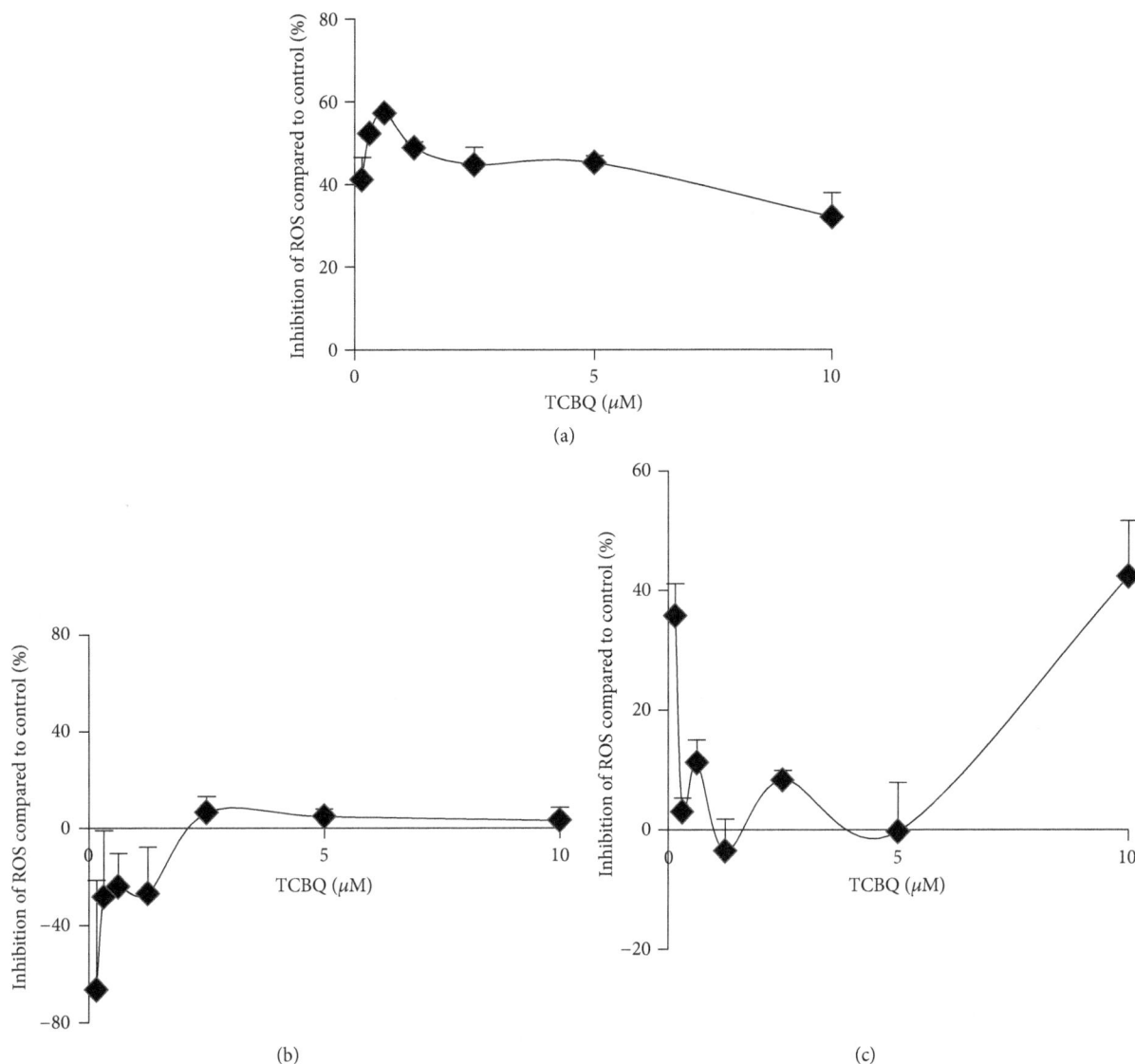

FIGURE 2: Effects of TCBQ on intracellular ROS production in human breast cancer MCF7 (a), Sk-Br-3 (b), and MDA-MB-231 (c) cells under normoxic condition. The concentration of TCBQ was $0.16\,\mu M$, $0.31\,\mu M$, $0.63\,\mu M$, $1.25\,\mu M$, $2.5\,\mu M$, $5\,\mu M$, and $10\,\mu M$, respectively. Treatment with DMSO was used as negative control. The inhibition of ROS production (%) compared to control was statistically significant at all TCBQ concentrations towards the MCF7 cells, statistically insignificant at all TCBQ concentrations towards the Sk-Br-3 cells, and statistically significant at TCBQ concentration of $0.16\,\mu M$ and $10\,\mu M$ towards the MDA-MB-231 cells. Statistical analysis was performed by one-way ANOVA with Dunnett's comparison as posthoc analysis.

decreased ROS production in the MCF7 cells might alleviate PKD1 activation, which, in turn, elevated cell apoptosis *via* downregulating the expression of antiapoptotic proteins. As for Sk-Br-3 and MDA-MB-231 cells, apoptosis was reduced upon TCBQ treatment. Sk-Br-3 cells showed a reverse bell-shaped response towards TCBQ treatment with the maximum inhibition of apoptosis (~30%) at concentrations around $1\,\mu M$ (Figure 3(b)). It is possible that increase in intracellular ROS level upon TCBQ treatment triggered PKD1-mediated cell survival. MDA-MB-231 cells were insensitive to TCBQ treatment and maintained relatively flat inhibition of apoptosis of less than 15% (Figure 3(c)). It is highly doubtful that TCBQ adopted the same mechanism to elicit

its antiapoptotic functions in Sk-Br-3 and MDA-MB-231 cells as it caused opposite effects on intracellular ROS production in these two types of cancer cells even though the antiapoptotic functions were not statistically significant. Further studies are required to confirm whether TCBQ possesses any antiapoptotic effects against the Sk-Br-3 and MDA-MB-231 cells under different culture conditions such as hypoxia and identify the underlying mechanism on how TCBQ prompts its proapoptotic or antiapoptotic functions towards different human breast cancer cells.

3.4. Cytotoxic Effects. As an active electrophilic molecule, TCBQ conjugates with $2'$-deoxyguanosine of DNA molecules

(a)

(b)

(c)

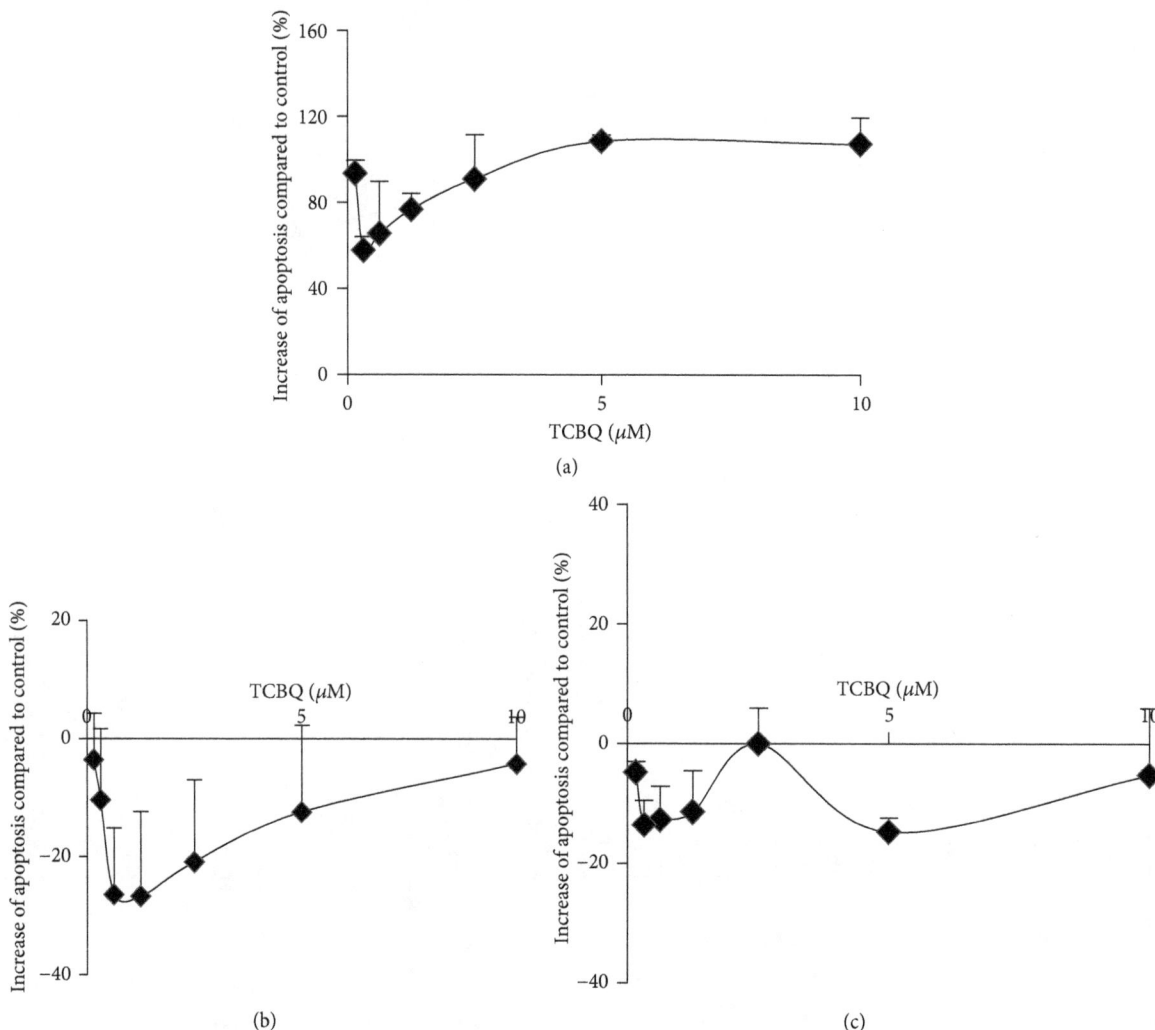

FIGURE 3: Apoptotic (caspase 3/7 level) effect of TCBQ towards human breast cancer MCF7 (a), Sk-Br-3 (b), and MDA-MB-231 (c) cells. The concentration of TCBQ was 0.16 μM, 0.31 μM, 0.63 μM, 1.25 μM, 2.5 μM, 5 μM, and 10 μM, respectively. Treatment with DMSO was used as negative control. Apoptosis was increased upon TCBQ treatment towards the MCF7 cells. The increase of apoptosis (%) compared to control was statistically significant at all TCBQ concentrations. However, apoptosis was decreased upon TCBQ treatment against the Sk-Br-3 and MDA-MB-231 cells. The decrease of apoptosis (%) compared to control was statistically insignificant at all TCBQ concentrations towards both cell lines. Statistical analysis was performed by one-way ANOVA with Dunnett's comparison as posthoc analysis.

to form dichlorobenzoquinone-1,N^2-etheno-2$'$-deoxyguanosine [25]. This conjugation reaction could initiate two opposite responses inside human body. Firstly, it may cause gene mutations, which could subsequently lead to carcinogenesis. However, it is still debatable whether chlorinated pesticides as well as their metabolites such as TCBQ could initiate carcinogenesis, as PCP was shown to promote rather than induce hepatocarcinogenesis in B6C3F$_1$ mice [42]. Secondly, the conjugation between TCBQ and 2$'$-deoxyguanosine may provoke apoptosis and/or necrosis, a common mechanism adopted by alkylating chemotherapy drugs like carboplatin to kill cancer cells. Herein, we examined whether TCBQ could impose cytotoxic effect (necrosis + apoptosis) against the breast cancer cells. As shown in Figure 4, TCBQ was cytotoxic only to MCF7 (TCBQ concentration > 0.3 μM) and Sk-Br-3 cells. MCF7 cells gave a log-shaped response

towards TCBQ treatment with a maximum of 31% increase in cytotoxicity compared to the control at concentration higher than 2.5 μM (Figure 4(a)). However, TCBQ exhibited cell-protective effect when its concentration was reduced to 0.16 μM. It was unknown what factors contributed to the cell-protective (proliferation or survival) effects. The observed lower cytotoxic effects (less than 31% increase compared to control) than apoptotic effects (59–109% increase compared to control) were due to the different mechanism of the assay kits. The apoptosis assay kit, Caspase-Glo 3/7 Assay, measures the caspase 3/7 activity, whereas the cytotoxicity assay kit, CytoTox96 Nonradioactive Cytotoxicity Assay, measures lactate dehydrogenase (LDH) release upon cell lysis. Thus, at the end of 18 h of TCBQ treatment, some of the MCF7 cells that underwent apoptosis might be still alive with intact cell membranes, resulting in lower observed

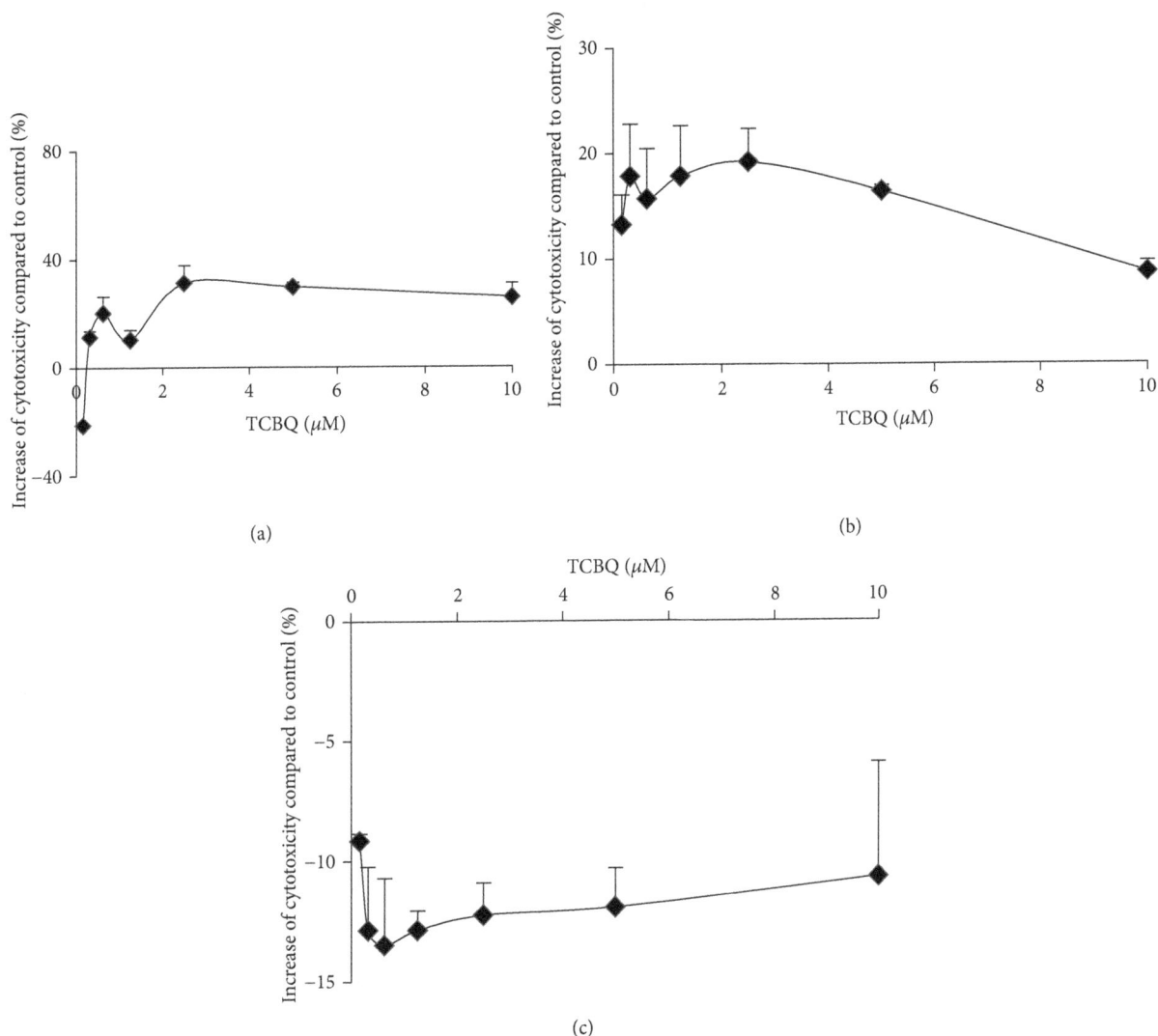

FIGURE 4: Cytotoxic effect of TCBQ towards human breast cancer MCF7 (a), Sk-Br-3 (b), and MDA-MB-231 (c) cells. The concentration of TCBQ was 0.16 μM, 0.31 μM, 0.63 μM, 1.25 μM, 2.5 μM, 5 μM, and 10 μM, respectively. Treatment with DMSO was used as negative control. Cytotoxicity was increased upon TCBQ treatment against both MCF7 and Sk-Br-3 cells. The increase of cytotoxicity (%) compared to control was statistically significant at TCBQ concentration of 0.16 μM, 0.63 μM, 1.25 μM, 2.5 μM, and 5 μM towards the MCF7 cells and at TCBQ concentration of 0.16 μM, 0.31 μM, 0.63 μM, 1.25 μM, 2.5 μM, and 5 μM towards the Sk-Br-3 cells, respectively. However, cytotoxicity was decreased upon TCBQ treatment towards the MDA-MB-231 cells. The decrease of cytotoxicity (%) compared to control was statistically significant at TCBQ concentration of 0.31 μM, 0.63 μM, 1.25 μM, 2.5 μM, 5 μM, and 10 μM. Statistical analysis was performed by one-way ANOVA with Dunnett's comparison as posthoc analysis.

cytotoxicity. Sk-Br-3 cells showed a very shallow bell-shaped response towards TCBQ with a maximum of 19% increase in cytotoxicity at concentration of 2.5 μM (Figure 4(b)). MDA-MB-231 cells were less sensitive to TCBQ treatment and maintained a stable marginal cell-protective effect (~12% decrease in cytotoxicity compared to the control, statistically significant except at 0.16 μM) throughout the whole TCBQ concentration range (Figure 4(c)). Thus, the cytotoxic effect of TCBQ was as well cell-type specific against human breast cancer cells.

4. Conclusion

In the current study, we showed that effects of TCBQ, an active metabolite of PCP, on intracellular ROS production,

apoptosis, and cytotoxicity were cell-type specific against human breast cancer. Triple-negative MDA-MB-231 cells were less sensitive to TCBQ treatment. Our results implicated that cell type was the decisive factor in determining whether continued exposure to PCP as well as its active metabolites such as TCBQ would promote or inhibit tumor growth. Of course, the exposure level of PCP also plays an important role in tumor growth. To our knowledge, this was the first study to examine how continued exposure of PCP could affect breast cancer cell growth *via* its highly reactive metabolite TCBQ and demonstrated that breast cancer cell type was a decisive factor for the PCP or TCBQ effects. Further cell line and mouse xenograft studies are warranted to establish a relationship between effect of continued PCP and TCBQ exposure and the four common breast cancer molecular subtypes (luminal A, luminal B, HER2, and triple-negative/basal-like). The underlying mechanisms for the effects of PCP and TCBQ on proliferation, apoptosis, and cytotoxicity, as well as metabolic profile of PCP in normal and breast cancer cells, will also be investigated.

Abbreviations

ROS: Reactive oxygen species
ER: Estrogen receptor
PR: Progesterone receptor
HER2: HER2/neu receptor.

Conflict of Interests

The authors have declared that no conflict of interests exists.

Acknowledgments

This work was supported in part by a research grant from the Canadian Breast Cancer Foundation and an internal grant from the College of Pharmacy and Nutrition, University of Saskatchewan.

References

[1] D. G. Crosby, "Environmental chemistry of pentachlorophenol," *Pure and Applied Chemistry*, vol. 53, pp. 1051–1080, 1981.

[2] R. E. Cline, R. H. Hill Jr., D. L. Phillips, and L. L. Needham, "Pentachlorophenol measurements in body fluids of people in log homes and workplaces," *Archives of Environmental Contamination and Toxicology*, vol. 18, no. 4, pp. 475–481, 1989.

[3] P. G. Jorens and P. J. C. Schepens, "Human pentachlorophenol poisoning," *Human and Experimental Toxicology*, vol. 12, no. 6, pp. 479–495, 1993.

[4] C. Colosio, M. Maroni, W. Barcellini et al., "Toxicological and immune findings in workers exposed to pentachlorophenol (PCP)," *Archives of Environmental Health*, vol. 48, no. 2, pp. 81–88, 1993.

[5] K. A. McAllister, H. Lee, and J. T. Trevors, "Microbial degradation of pentachlorophenol," *Biodegradation*, vol. 7, no. 1, pp. 1–40, 1996.

[6] M. M. Hanumante and S. S. Kulkarni, "Acute toxicity of two molluscicides, mercuric chloride and pentachlorophenol to a freshwater fish (*Channa gachua*)," *Bulletin of Environmental Contamination and Toxicology*, vol. 23, no. 6, pp. 725–727, 1979.

[7] R. Frank, H. E. Braun, K. I. Stonefield, J. Rasper, and H. Luyken, "Organochlorine and organophosphorus residues in the fat of domestic farm animal species, Ontario, Canada 1986–1988," *Food Additives and Contaminants*, vol. 7, no. 5, pp. 629–636, 1990.

[8] D. L. McCarthy, A. A. Claude, and S. D. Copley, "In vivo levels of chlorinated hydroquinones in a pentachlorophenol-degrading bacterium," *Applied and Environmental Microbiology*, vol. 63, no. 5, pp. 1883–1888, 1997.

[9] P. Valenti, M. Recanatini, P. Da Re, L. Cima, and P. Giusti, "Halogenated dimefline-type derivatives," *Archiv der Pharmazie*, vol. 316, no. 5, pp. 421–426, 1983.

[10] J. R. Dimmock, "Problem solving learning: applications in medicinal chemistry," *The American Journal of Pharmaceutical Education*, vol. 64, no. 1, pp. 44–49, 2000.

[11] A. Bevenue, J. N. Ogata, and J. W. Hylin, "Organochlorine pesticides in rainwater, Oahu, Hawaii, 1971-1972," *Bulletin of Environmental Contamination and Toxicology*, vol. 8, no. 4, pp. 238–241, 1972.

[12] H. A. Hattemer-Frey and C. C. Travis, "Pentachlorophenol: environmental partitioning and human exposure," *Archives of Environmental Contamination and Toxicology*, vol. 18, no. 4, pp. 482–489, 1989.

[13] S. Coad and R. C. Newhook, "PCP exposure for the Canadian general population: a multimedia analysis," *Journal of Exposure Analysis and Environmental Epidemiology*, vol. 2, no. 4, pp. 391–413, 1992.

[14] B. G. Reigner, F. Y. Bois, and T. N. Tozer, "Assessment of pentachlorophenol exposure in humans using the clearance concept," *Human and Experimental Toxicology*, vol. 11, no. 1, pp. 17–26, 1992.

[15] J. Dahlgren, R. Warshaw, J. Thornton, C. P. Anderson-Mahoney, and H. Takhar, "Health effects on nearby residents of a wood treatment plant," *Environmental Research*, vol. 92, no. 2, pp. 92–98, 2003.

[16] H.-M. Chen, Y.-H. Lee, R.-J. Chen, H.-W. Chiu, B.-J. Wang, and Y.-J. Wang, "The immunotoxic effects of dual exposure to PCP and TCDD," *Chemico-Biological Interactions*, vol. 206, no. 2, pp. 166–174, 2013.

[17] P. A. Demers, H. W. Davies, M. C. Friesen et al., "Cancer and occupational exposure to pentachlorophenol and tetrachlorophenol (Canada)," *Cancer Causes and Control*, vol. 17, no. 6, pp. 749–758, 2006.

[18] H. C. Hong, H. Y. Zhou, T. G. Luan, and C. Y. Lan, "Residue of pentachlorophenol in freshwater sediments and human breast milk collected from the Pearl River Delta, China," *Environment International*, vol. 31, no. 5, pp. 643–649, 2005.

[19] D. M. Guvenius, A. Aronsson, G. Ekman-Ordeberg, Å. Bergman, and K. Norén, "Human prenatal and postnatal exposure to polybrominated diphenyl ethers, polychlorinated biphenyls, polychlorobiphenylols, and pentachlorophenol," *Environmental Health Perspectives*, vol. 111, no. 9, pp. 1235–1241, 2003.

[20] J. de Maeyer, P. J. C. Schepens, P. G. Jorens, and R. Verstraete, "Exposure to pentachlorophenol as a possible cause of miscarriages," *British Journal of Obstetrics and Gynaecology*, vol. 102, no. 12, pp. 1010–1011, 1995.

[21] I. Gerhard, A. Frick, B. Monga, and B. Runnebaum, "Pentachlorophenol exposure in women with gynecological and endocrine dysfunction," *Environmental Research*, vol. 80, no. 4, pp. 383–388, 1999.

[22] R. Patel and R. J. Rosengren, "The oestrogenicity of pentachlorophenol and paracetamol," *Australasian Journal of Ecotoxicology*, vol. 6, pp. 81–84, 2000.

[23] I. E. Schroeder, J. J. van Tonder, and V. Steenkamp, "Comparative toxicity of pentachlorophenol with its metabolites tetrachloro-1,2-hydroquinone and tetrachloro-1,4-benzoquinone in HepG2 cells," *Open Toxicology Journal*, vol. 5, no. 1, pp. 11–20, 2012.

[24] H. Dong, D. Xu, L. Hu, L. Li, E. Song, and Y. Song, "Evaluation of N-acetyl-cysteine against tetrachlorobenzoquinone-induced genotoxicity and oxidative stress in HepG2 cells," *Food and Chemical Toxicology*, vol. 64, pp. 291–297, 2014.

[25] T. N. T. Nguyen, A. D. Bertagnolli, P. W. Villalta, P. Bühlmann, and S. J. Sturla, "Characterization of a deoxyguanosine

adduct of tetrachlorobenzoquinone: dichlorobenzoquinone-1,N^2-etheno-2'-deoxyguanosine," *Chemical Research in Toxicology*, vol. 18, no. 11, pp. 1770–1776, 2005.

[26] W. D. Landry and T. G. Cotter, "ROS signalling, NADPH oxidases and cancer," *Biochemical Society Transactions*, vol. 42, no. 4, pp. 934–938, 2014.

[27] M. Schieber and N. S. Chandel, "ROS function in redox signaling and oxidative stress," *Current Biology*, vol. 24, no. 10, pp. R453–R462, 2014.

[28] E. D. Yoboue, A. Mougeolle, L. Kaiser, N. Averet, M. Rigoulet, and A. Devin, "The role of mitochondrial biogenesis and ROS in the control of energy supply in proliferating cells," *Biochimica et Biophysica Acta*, vol. 1837, no. 7, pp. 1093–1098, 2014.

[29] E. I. Chen, "Mitochondrial dysfunction and cancer metastasis," *Journal of Bioenergetics and Biomembranes*, vol. 44, no. 6, pp. 619–622, 2012.

[30] A. Aliaga, J. A. Rousseau, R. Ouellette et al., "Breast cancer models to study the expression of estrogen receptors with small animal PET imaging," *Nuclear Medicine and Biology*, vol. 31, no. 6, pp. 761–770, 2004.

[31] D. S. Harischandra and D. Hockenbery, "Bioenergetic differences in breast cancer cell lines," in *Proceedings of the AACR Metabolism and Cancer Conference*, La Jolla, Calif, USA, 2009.

[32] H. Pelicano, W. Zhang, J. Liu et al., "Mitochondrial dysfunction in some triple-negative breast cancer cell lines: role of mTOR pathway and therapeutic potential," *Breast Cancer Research*, vol. 16, no. 5, article 434, 2014.

[33] M. V. C. Nguyen, B. Lardy, F. Rousset et al., "Quinone compounds regulate the level of ROS production by the NADPH oxidase Nox4," *Biochemical Pharmacology*, vol. 85, no. 11, pp. 1644–1654, 2013.

[34] R. S. Esworthy, M. A. Baker, and F.-F. Chu, "Expression of selenium-dependent glutathione peroxidase in human breast tumor cell lines," *Cancer Research*, vol. 55, no. 4, pp. 957–962, 1995.

[35] S. J. Kang, B. R. Choi, E. K. Lee et al., "Inhibitory effect of dried pomegranate concentration powder on melanogenesis in B16F10 melanoma cells; involvement of p38 and PKA signaling pathways," *International Journal of Molecular Sciences*, vol. 16, no. 10, pp. 24219–24242, 2015.

[36] P. W. Chow, Z. Abdul Hamid, K. M. Chan, S. H. Inayat-Hussain, and N. F. Rajab, "Lineage-related cytotoxicity and clonogenic profile of 1,4-benzoquinone-exposed hematopoietic stem and progenitor cells," *Toxicology and Applied Pharmacology*, vol. 284, no. 1, pp. 8–15, 2015.

[37] D. Xu, L. Hu, C. Su et al., "Tetrachloro-p-benzoquinone induces hepatic oxidative damage and inflammatory response, but not apoptosis in mouse: the prevention of curcumin," *Toxicology and Applied Pharmacology*, vol. 280, no. 2, pp. 305–313, 2014.

[38] Z.-W. Xu, H. Friess, M. W. Büchler, and M. Solioz, "Overexpression of Bax sensitizes human pancreatic cancer cells to apoptosis induced by chemotherapeutic agents," *Cancer Chemotherapy and Pharmacology*, vol. 49, no. 6, pp. 504–510, 2002.

[39] E. Cadenas, "Mitochondrial free radical production and cell signaling," *Molecular Aspects of Medicine*, vol. 25, no. 1-2, pp. 17–26, 2004.

[40] P. Storz, H. Döppler, C. Ferran, S. T. Grey, and A. Toker, "Functional dichotomy of A20 in apoptotic and necrotic cell death," *Biochemical Journal*, vol. 387, no. 1, pp. 47–55, 2005.

[41] G.-Y. Liou and P. Storz, "Reactive oxygen species in cancer," *Free Radical Research*, vol. 44, no. 5, pp. 479–496, 2010.

[42] T. Umemura, S. Kai, R. Hasegawa, K. Sai, Y. Kurokawa, and G. M. Williams, "Pentachlorophenol (PCP) produces liver oxidative stress and promotes but does not initiate hepatocarcinogenesis in B6C3F$_1$ mice," *Carcinogenesis*, vol. 20, no. 6, pp. 1115–1120, 1999.

10

Macro- and Microelemental Composition and Toxicity of Unsweetened Natural Cocoa Powder in Sprague-Dawley Rats

Isaac Julius Asiedu-Gyekye,[1] **Samuel Frimpong-Manso,**[2] **Benoit Banga N'guessan,**[1] **Mahmood Abdulai Seidu,**[3] **Paul Osei-Prempeh,**[1] **and Daniel Kwaku Boamah**[4]

[1]*Department of Pharmacology and Toxicology, University of Ghana School of Pharmacy, College of Health Sciences, Legon, Ghana*
[2]*Department of Pharmaceutical Chemistry, University of Ghana School of Pharmacy, College of Health Sciences, Legon, Ghana*
[3]*Department of Medical Laboratory Sciences (Pathology), School of Biomedical and Allied Health Sciences,*
 University of Ghana, Legon, Ghana
[4]*Geological Survey Department, Accra, Ghana*

Correspondence should be addressed to Isaac Julius Asiedu-Gyekye; ijasiedu-gyekye@ug.edu.gh

Academic Editor: Syed Ali

Unsweetened natural cocoa powder (UNCP) is a pulverized high-grade powder of compressed solid blocks which remains after extraction. Little scientific data is available concerning its safety despite the presence of potential toxic elements. Elemental composition in UNCP was analyzed with ED-XRF spectroscopy. Single oral high dose toxicity study was conducted on adult male Sprague-Dawley rats (150 g) by the limit test method. One group received water and the test group 2000 mg/kg UNCP. All animals were observed for 14 days and then euthanized for haematological, biochemical, and histopathological examinations. Thirty-eight (38) elements were found in UNCP. There was an increase in HDL cholesterol ($p < 0.05$), reduction in LDL cholesterol ($p > 0.05$), alkaline phosphatase ($p < 0.05$), and creatinine levels, and slight increase in urea levels ($p > 0.05$). Haematological changes were not significant. Histopathological analysis showed no toxic effect on the heart, liver, kidney, lungs, testis, and spleen. Intestinal erosion was observed in the test group. UNCP appears to be relatively safe when taken as a single oral high dose of 2000 mg/kg b.w.t. in rats. Caution should however be exercised at high doses due to the high elemental content of copper and high possibility of intestinal lining erosion.

1. Introduction

Natural products (secondary metabolites) including cocoa have been the most successful source of potential drug leads [1, 2]. Extensive research is being carried out on plant materials gathered from the rain forests and other places for their potential medicinal value and potential toxic effects [3]. As such, the demand for herbal remedies has been increasingly rising in industrialized countries as it is in developing countries [4].

The medicinal and pharmacological importance of *Theobroma Cacao* and its powder, unsweetened natural cocoa powder (UNCP) as nutraceutical and as traditional medicine, has been well investigated. In Ghana and other parts of Africa, UNCP is used as remedy for managing bronchial asthma, as an aphrodisiac, antidiabetic, anti-inflammatory, cardioprotective, antihypertensive, and antimalarial agent [5–11]. In Ghana and West Africa, UNCP is a common beverage [1].

Cocoa powder is prepared after removal of the cocoa butter from powdered cocoa beans via fermentation, drying and bagging, winnowing, roasting, grinding, and pressing. The solid blocks of compressed cocoa remaining after extraction (press cake) are pulverised into a fine powder to produce a high-grade cocoa powder.

The chemical composition of cocoa has been well investigated using various methods [12–15]. UNCP contains about 1.9% theobromine and 0.21% caffeine [16]. Proanthocyanidin being a constituent of unsweetened natural cocoa powder has been found to be capable of destroying the mucosal lining of the gastrointestinal tract [17]. Besides, micro- and macroelements present in plants may interfere with the availability of secondary metabolites in UNCP which may easily modulate their pharmacological activity [18]. The presence of toxic heavy metals in medicinal plants can also pose as a threat to the health of consumers [19]. For the safety of consumers, the World Health Organization states maximum permissible levels in raw plant materials for only cadmium ($0.3\,mg\,kg^{-1}$), arsenic ($1\,mg\,kg^{-1}$), and lead ($10\,mg\,kg^{-1}$) [20].

Toxicity studies on this nutraceutical are rare. Cocoa per se has not attracted much interest to the scientific world probably because of its long term usage with very little reported adverse effects. There have been reports on the potential carcinogenicity and teratogenicity, that is, bilateral testicular atrophy and aspermatogenesis of cocoa [21, 22]. Besides, Sertoli cells have been identified as the main target for theobromine toxicity accompanying cocoa administration [23].

It is against this background that this study is being conducted to determine the elemental composition and safety of this important nutraceutical.

2. Materials and Methods

2.1. Energy Dispersive X-Ray (ED-XRF) Measurements.
Generally, the X-ray fluorescence (XRF) is a fast, accurate, and nondestructive analytical technique used for the elemental and chemical analysis of powdered, solid, and liquid samples [19, 24–26].

Sample of processed cocoa powder was purchased (Batch number BT620IT; FDA/DK06-070) from a supermarket. The sample was sieved using sieve of 180 microns. Three samples were prepared and sieved with a mesh size (aperture) of $180\,\mu m$ into a fine powder and kept in a dry well-labelled container. Before pelletation, the sample was kept in an oven at $60^{\circ}C$ overnight. Due to their morphology and the loose nature, triplicate weighed samples—4000 mg/sample—were added separately to 900 mg Fluxana H Elektronic BM-0002-1 (Licowax C micropowder PM-Hoechstwax) as binder; the mixture was homogenized using the RETSCH Mixer Mill (MM301) for 3 min and pressed manually with SPECAC hydraulic press for 2 min with a maximum pressure limit of 15 tons (15000 kg) into pellets of 32 mm in diameter and 3 mm thickness for subsequent XRF measurements. Time between pelletation and measurement was kept short to avoid deformation of the flat surfaces of the pellets. SPECTRO X-Lab 2000 spectrometer (Geological Survey Department, Accra, Ghana) enhanced with three-axial geometry to reduce background noise due to radiation polarization and its monochromatic radiations emitted from the X-ray tube to excite the atoms of the samples were used for simultaneous analysis and measurement of the elemental content of the samples. This spectrometer is equipped with Rh anode and 400 W Pd X-ray tube, a 0.5 mm Be end window tube, a Si (Li) detector (resolution of 148 eV – 1000 cps Mn Kα), available targets (Al$_2$O$_3$ and B4C used as a BARKLA polarizer), HOPG (High Oriented Pyrolitic Graphite) as a BRAGG polarizer, Al, Mo, and Co as secondary target, and 0.5 mm Be side window. It has a carousel (circular rotating sample changer) inside a sample chamber with a capacity of 20 sample holder disc (32 mm) for sequential sample analyses. The radiation chamber was cooled using liquid nitrogen. Its computer-based multichannel analyzer-SPECTRO X-Lab Pro Software package (Turbiquant) controlled and computed spectral analysis and collected, evaluated, and stored data. Combination of these different targets gave a typical detection limit for light elements (Si, Al, Mg, and Na) in the range of 25–50 ppm. For heavy metals, 1–5 ppm was the limit of detection. This spectrometer was factory calibrated using a number of international rock standards.

2.2. Preparation of UNCP.
Calculated amount (9.6 g) of Brown Gold Natural Cocoa Powder from Hords Company Ltd., (Batch number BT620IT) registered with the Ghana Food and Drugs Authority (FDA/DK06-070) was dissolved in warm distilled water (40 mL) with stirring making a concentration of 240 mg/mL (of the UNCP). The preparation was then administered to the animals via oral gavage based on their individual body weights.

2.3. Animal Experimentation.
Twenty (20) adult male Sprague-Dawley rats of average weight 150 g were purchased from the Animal House Department of the Korle-Bu Teaching Hospital, Korle-Bu, Accra. The rats were acclimatized to laboratory environment ($20–24^{\circ}C$), $60 \pm 1\%$ humidity with a 12 h light-darkness cycle for 7 days prior to experimentation. The rats had access to standard laboratory diet and water ad libitum. The experimental procedures were approved by the departmental ethical and protocol review committee and the Noguchi Memorial Institute for Medical Research Institutional Animal Care and Use Committee with protocol number 2013-01-3E and also conducted in accordance with international ethical guidelines.

2.4. Experimental Design.
The Sprague-Dawley rats were randomly assigned to the experimental group and the control group for 7 days before the start of the experiment. Both groups contained ten (10) rats each. All rats had access to water and food except for a 12 hour fasting period before the administration of the unsweetened natural cocoa powder. The experimental group of rats received the unsweetened natural cocoa powder at the dose of 2000 mg/kg while the control group received an equal volume of distilled water. This was based on the fact that the initial testing of 300 mg/kg and 1200 mg/kg to single rats each did not result in any death.

2.5. Effect of UNCP on Body and Relative Organ Weights.
Selected organs like the liver, kidney, heart, lungs, testis, spleen, and intestines were excised quickly and placed in ice-cold saline to wash off blood, trimmed of fat and connective tissues, blot dried, and finally weighed on a balance. The organ-to-body weight index (OBI) was calculated as the ratio of organ weight and the body weight of the animal before sacrifice ×100. Body weight of rats were also taken dosing, a week after dosing on Day 7 and before sacrificing them on Day 14.

2.6. Effect of UNCP on Haematological Parameters. Two millilitres (2 mL) of blood from euthanized SD rats was drawn out by cardiac puncture and then transferred into EDTA test tubes. An automated haematology analyzer was used to estimate the counts of the various parameters considered in this study. Peripheral blood smear was also done to examine the nature of blood cells.

2.7. Effect of UNCP on Serum Biochemistry. 1 mL of the blood of sacrificed rats was collected by means of cardiac puncture. The blood sample was allowed to stand and then centrifuged at 4000 rpm for 15 minutes using a Wiperfuge centrifuge with the serum collected separately into Eppendoff tubes for the measurement of the biochemical parameters.

2.8. Histopathology Examination. The liver, kidney, heart, lungs, spleen, testis, and small intestinal organs were immediately fixed in 10% buffered formaldehyde solution for 24 h. Samples of the tissues were then paraffin embedded and sectioned at 5 μm thickness. Sectioned tissues were mounted on slides and stained with haematoxylin and eosin (H&E). The sections were evaluated microscopically for histological changes under a light microscope (Olympus BX 51TF).

2.9. Statistical Analysis and Data Evaluation. Statistical analysis of the data was done using GraphPad Prism Software version 5.0. Results were expressed as mean ± standard error of mean, $n = 5$. Significant difference between dosed groups and control was evaluated by performing student's one-tailed t-test. p values less than 0.05 were considered statistically significant.

3. Results

3.1. Energy Dispersive X-Ray (ED-XRF) Measurements. A total of thirty-eight (38) macro-12 elements (sodium (Na), magnesium (Mg), aluminium (Al), silicon (Si), phosphorus (P), sulphur (S), chlorine (Cl), potassium (K), calcium (Ca), titanium (Ti), manganese (Mn), and iron (Fe)) and micro-26 elements (vanadium (V), chromium (Cr), cobalt (Co), nickel (Ni), copper (Cu), zinc (Zn), gallium (Ga), arsenic (As), rubidium (Rb), strontium (Sr), yttrium (Y), zirconium (Zr), niobium (Nb), molybdenum (Mo), antimony (Sb), iodine (I), cesium (Cs), barium (Ba), lanthanum (La), cerium (Ce), hafnium (Hf), tantalum (Ta), lead (Pb), bismuth (Bi), thorium (Th), uranium (U)) (Table 1) were identified and evaluated.

3.2. Microelements. These elements either in % w/w or in ppm were converted to their respective amounts in milligrams. For example, an average of triplicate measurements of elements such as magnesium (Mg) in percentage was converted as (0.837+0.83+0.809/3 = 0.8253/100 * 4000 mg = 33.0133 mg 4000 mg^{-1}) and lead (Pb) in parts per million (ppm) was calculated as an average of triplicate measurement:

$$0.9 + 0.9 + \frac{0.9}{3} = \frac{0.9}{1000000} * 4000 \tag{1}$$

$$= 0.0036 \text{ mg } 4000 \text{ mg}^{-1}.$$

TABLE 1: Mean and standard deviation (SD) of measured elements (mg/4000 mg).

	Element	Mean/SD mg/4000 mg
Macroelements	Na	2.4666 ± 0.00
	Mg	33.0133 ± 0.02
	Al	14.0093 ± 0.01
	Si	15.3880 ± 0.02
	P	64.3866 ± 0.00
	S	30.9120 ± 0.00
	Cl	2.3616 ± 0.00
	K	149.0667 ± 0.03
	Ca	11.0146 ± 0.00
	Ti	0.0232 ± 0.00
	Mn	0.4093 ± 0.00
	Fe	1.0309 ± 0.00
Microelements	V	0.2320 ± 1.73
	Cr	0.4200 ± 17.44
	Co	0.0108 ± 0.10
	Ni	0.0638 ± 1.16
	Cu	0.2984 ± 1.71
	Zn	0.4086 ± 0.74
	Ga	0.0024 ± 0.00
	As	0.0020 ± 0.00
	Rb	0.1698 ± 0.49
	Sr	0.1064 ± 0.20
	Y	0.0016 ± 0.00
	Zr	0.0125 ± 0.42
	Nb	0.0070 ± 0.29
	Mo	0.0044 ± 0.00
	Sb	0.0043 ± 0.06
	I	0.0133 ± 0.15
	Cs	0.0232 ± 0.10
	Ba	0.0620 ± 5.81
	La	0.0480 ± 0.00
	Ce	0.0849 ± 4.97
	Hf	0.0148 ± 0.17
	Ta	0.0213 ± 0.06
	Pb	0.0036 ± 0.00
	Bi	0.0024 ± 0.00
	Th	0.0020 ± 0.00
	U	0.0112 ± 0.10

Simple statistics (mean and standard) of the results were calculated to gain a better understanding of the results (Table 1).

3.3. Effects of Treatment on Food, Water Intake, and Body Weight. Food and water intake of the treated animals that received 2000 mg/kg body weight and control group remained relatively the same. There was generally no increase

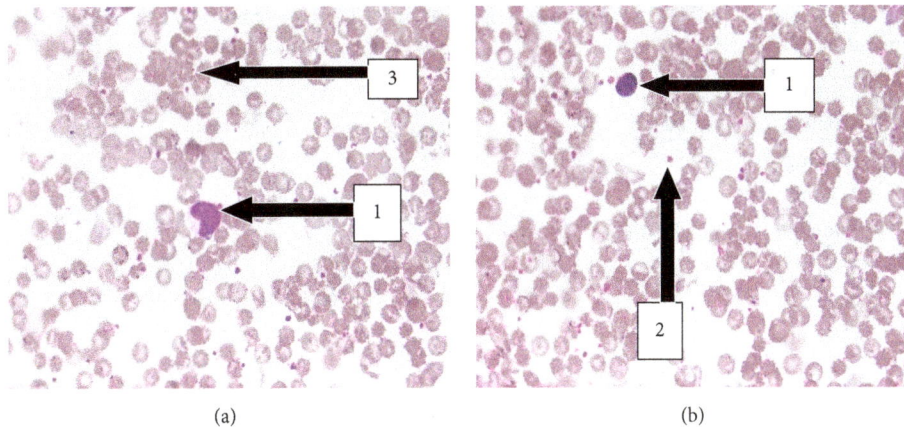

FIGURE 1: Leishman stained peripheral blood smear plate (20x). (a) Peripheral blood smear plate of control male SD rats showing normal distribution of blood cells. Note the white blood cell (1), platelet (2), and red blood cell (3). (b) Peripheral blood smear plate of treated animals of dose 2000 mg/kg showing normal distribution of WBCs, RBCs, and platelets. Note the normocytic and normochromic nature of the RBCs.

in the intake of food and water by both the control and experimental SD rats. General physical observations such as abnormality of the eyes, skin and fur, coma, convulsion, tremors, diarrhea, lethargy, sleep, morbidity, and then mortality were all not observed to have happened.

From Day 1 to Day 14, there were no significant changes in the body weight of the SD rats that survived at the end of the experiment as in Table 3. However, there was a slight decrease in the weight of the treatment group from Day 1 to Day 14.

3.4. Clinical Signs and Mortality Patterns.
At the dose level tested, no untoward clinical signs were observed in all the rats used. There were no changes in the nature of the stool, urine, and an eye colour of all the rats. No mortality was observed in the treatment or control rat groups.

3.5. Effects on Relative Organ Weight.
There were no significant changes in the relative weights of the liver, kidney, heart, lungs, spleen, and testis of the treated rats in relation to the control groups. However, the treated rats consistently showed slightly reduced organ weight values as compared to the control group rats. This is as shown in Table 3.

3.6. Effects on Haematological Parameters.
There were generally no significant changes in the various haematological parameters of the treatment group in comparison with the control group as shown in Table 3. There was an increased value for the percentage eosinophil and monocyte of the treated group as compared to the control group. This increase was however not statistically significant. Similarly there was a marginal increase for the eosinophil and basophil numbers of the treatment group in comparison with the control group. The platelet number for the treatment groups however reduced in comparison with that of the control group.

The peripheral blood smear also showed no significant changes in the size, colour, and nature of the red blood cells and white blood cells when the treatment group was compared with the control group.

3.7. Effects on Serum Biochemistry.
Biochemical profile which includes liver function indices, kidney function indices, and lipid profile of the treated rats and that of the control rats are presented in Table 4.

The acute oral administration of UNCP at the limit dose of 2000 mg/kg body weight did not cause any statistically significant change in the serum proteins and bilirubin as well as some electrolytes (slight decrease in sodium and slight increase in potassium). Blood urea nitrogen increased ($p > 0.05$) while creatinine levels reduced ($p > 0.05$) compared to the control. The levels of the liver marker enzymes (aspartate transaminase, gamma glutamyl transferase, and alanine transferase) of treated animals were not significantly different from that of the control. There was however a reduction in ALP levels ($p < 0.05$). Changes in serum biochemistry in male SD rats receiving 2000 mg/kg b.w.t. of UNCP are shown in Table 5 and changes in haematological indices in male SD rats receiving 2000 mg/kg b.w.t. of UNCP are shown in Table 6.

3.8. Histopathological Changes

3.8.1. Effects of UNCP Treatment on Histology of the Liver, Kidney, Heart, Lungs, Testis, Spleen, and Small Intestines.
The results of histopathology changes in the liver, kidney, heart, lungs, testis, spleen, and small intestines are summarized in Figures 1–7. The various organs from the control group had a normal histology and appearance. Generally, there were no observable changes in the architecture of the various organs of the treatment rats in comparison with the control.

The histology of the liver and the kidney was consistent with the normal liver and kidney function indices obtained in the serum biochemical analysis. The lipid profile was also consistent with the normal nature of the heart and the liver since both organs had no fatty tissues on observation.

However, the histology of the small intestines of animals that received UNCP showed mild changes as compared to that of the control rats. There were mild erosion of the lining of the small intestines. As such there was only a mild inflammatory response with less cellular infiltration.

TABLE 2: Recommended daily allowance: mg (RDA, lit values) and percentage RDA of elements in UNCP.

Element	RDA (men)	RDA (women)	% RDA (men)	% RDA (women)
Na	1500 mg	1500 mg	0.51	0.51
Mg	420 mg	320 mg	24.60	32.30
P	700 mg	700 mg	28.70	28.70
Cl	2300 mg	2300 mg	0.32	0.32
K	4700 mg	4700 mg	10.00	10.00
Ca	1000 mg	1000 mg	3.40	3.40
Mn	2.3 mg	1.8 mg	56.50	72.20
Fe	8 mg	18 mg	40.25	17.90
Cr	35 μg	25 μg	3750.00	5250.00
Cu	900 μg	900 μg	103.60	103.60
Zn	11 mg	8 mg	11.60	16.00
Mo	45 μg	45 μg	30.60	30.60
I	150 μg	150 μg	27.78	27.78

4. Discussion

Most people believe that herbal medicines have no side effects or any potential risks due to their natural origins and are often considered as healthy food supplements and not drugs. Most herbs used for medicinal purposes are usually prescribed by the consumers and there is a lack of control and review concerning the dose, frequency, and route of administration. Active components found in these medicinal herbs have the potential of causing toxicity in humans.

This study focused on the acute toxicity effect of UNCP in male SD rats. The increased use of this natural product has called for concerns over both the efficacy and safety of the product.

UNCP contains phytochemicals such as tannins, saponins, cardiac glycosides, terpenoids, and flavonoids [27] which are normally responsible for both therapeutic and toxic effects of various plant and herbal extracts or products [28].

Evaluating UNCP as nutraceutical, the assumption was that the average African weighs 60.70 kg. UNCP will provide the following nutritional values per every 4000 mg of UNCP and its corresponding % RDA as represented in Tables 1 and 2. Magnesium contributes about 25% of the minimum amount of magnesium the human body requires per day (Table 2). Evaluating UNCP's medicinal value, for example, elements believed to be involved in the pathophysiology of hypertension and dysrhythmias and other cardiovascular diseases [29–31], sodium 0.51% (both men and women), magnesium 25% (men) and 32% (women), potassium 10%, and calcium 3%, were considered. High copper 104% (both men and women) and chromium (3750% in men/5250% in women) both implicated in pathophysiology of diabetes further justify cocoa's traditional usage as traditional medicine.

WHO's permissible limits of lead and arsenic are 0.00016 mg/kg and 0.0010 mg/kg, respectively [32]. Heavy metals determined in UNCP were Pb – 0.0036 mg and As –

TABLE 3: Changes of body weight of adult male SD rats treated with 2000 mg/kg body weight of solution of UNCP.

DAY	CTRL	UNCP	p value
Day 1	112.5 ± 12.50	142 ± 8.000	0.0526
Day 7	115.0 ± 10.00	142.0 ± 7.176	0.3618
Day 14	112.5 ± 7.500	135.0 ± 7.000	0.0522

TABLE 4: Changes in relative organ weight of male SD rats dosed with 2000 mg/kg body weight of UNCP solution.

ORGANS	CTRL	UNCP	p value
Liver	8.605 ± 4.225	7.454 ± 1.263	0.3260
Kidney	0.6000 ± 0.05000	0.5500 ± 0.02739	0.3618
Heart	8.605 ± 4.225	7.454 ± 1.263	0.3534
Lungs	0.8500 ± 0.05000	0.7600 ± 0.02915	0.3618
Spleen		7.454 ± 1.263	0.0829
Testis		1.224 ± 0.02502	0.3618

TABLE 5: Changes in serum biochemistry in male SD rats receiving 2000 mg/kg b.w.t. of UNCP.

Parameter	UNITS	CTRL	UNCP	p value
Creatinine	μmol/L	43.25 ± 2.925	40.61 ± 1.158	0.3618
Urea UV	mmol/L	8.605 ± 4.225	8.854 ± 1.263	0.2880
Bilirubin total	μmol/L	0.795 ± 0.0144	0.625 ± 0.165	0.3960
ALT	U/L	125 ± 0.722	120 ± 5.01	0.1999
Albumin	g/L	40.5 ± 0.442	39.0 ± 0.692	0.2046
AST	U/L	2.49 ± 0.358	2.52 ± 0.541	0.3263
Total protein	g/L	73.1 ± 1.02	70.6 ± 3.09	0.6061
Triglycerides	mmol/L	1.28 ± 0.160	0.943 ± 0.116	0.1185
Bilirubin direct	μmol/L	0.555 ± 0.0240	1.38 ± 0.489	0.1791
ALP	U/L	707 ± 7.86	535 ± 40.7	0.0103
GGT	U/L	1.20 ± 0.200	2.40 ± 1.44	0.4316
HDL cholesterol	mmol/L	0.560 ± 0.0372	0.755 ± 0.0349	0.0060
Cholesterol	mmol/L	2.08 ± 0.0854	2.15 ± 0.129	0.6616
LDL cholesterol	mmol/L	1.27 ± 0.0740	0.934 ± 0.124	0.0810
Na$^+$	mmol/L	137 ± 0.479	133 ± 0.477	0.0002
K$^+$	mmol/L	5.75 ± 0.132	6.44 ± 0.293	0.1098
Ca^{2+}	mmol/L	0.845 ± 0.0132	0.858 ± 0.0180	0.5200

0.002 mg corresponding to 0.0002 mg/kg and 0.0001 mg/kg, respectively, with the assumption that the average African weighs 60.7 kg. These values are far below WHO guidelines (Table 2). The high content of Cu^{2+} (0.2984 mg per 4 g UNCP) should be of concern especially at high doses since copper has been shown to play a role in the pathogenesis of Wilson's syndrome and liver damage [33, 34] while the high content of chromium could have beneficial effect in the management of diabetes mellitus and cardiovascular disorders [17, 29, 35]. The relationship between these elements, nutrition, and

TABLE 6: Changes in haematological indices in male SD rats receiving 2000 mg/kg b.w.t. of UNCP.

Parameter	Ctrl	UNCP	p value
WBC	8.605 ± 4.225	7.454 ± 1.263	0.3618
Neut. number	2.020 ± 0.4400	1.858 ± 0.3836	0.4109
Lymph number	5.985 ± 3.435	4.864 ± 1.111	0.3422
Mono. number	0.3700 ± 0.220	0.3740 ± 0.1225	0.4936
Eosin. number	0.2250 ± 0.125	0.3520 ± 0.07439	0.2045
Baso. number	0.0050 ± 0.005	0.0060 ± 0.002449	0.4228
Neut.%	27.65 ± 8.450	25.38 ± 4.450	0.4021
Lymph.%	65.80 ± 7.600	63.90 ± 6.119	0.4348
Mono.%	4.000 ± 0.6000	5.700 ± 1.642	0.2828
Eosin.%	2.500 ± 0.2000	4.940 ± 0.9553	0.0941
RBC	7.360 ± 1.060	7.156 ± 0.5533	0.4290
HGB	12.20 ± 1.500	12.38 ± 1.048	0.4646
HCT	36.05 ± 4.050	37.82 ± 3.269	0.3877
MCV	49.20 ± 1.600	52.76 ± 0.9405	0.0515
MCH	16.65 ± 0.3500	17.28 ± 0.2354	0.1037
MCHC	33.80 ± 0.4000	32.76 ± 0.3696	0.0862
RDW-CV	17.05 ± 3.150	15.74 ± 1.105	0.3106
RDW-SD	27.00 ± 2.000	27.70 ± 1.064	0.3746
PLT	696.5 ± 324.5	498.4 ± 166.3	0.2855

medicine observed suggests that micro- and macroelements of herbal products should not be envisage always as contaminants.

There are concerns however with regard to the copper content in UNCP; with inference from dose translation from animal to human studies according to Reagan-Shaw et al. [36] which takes into account the body surface area of the animal species and man, then K_m (i.e., body weight/surface area) for human adult and rat could be estimated as 37 and 6, respectively [36]. The human equivalent dose (HED) of 2000 mg/kg UNCP in rats corresponds to approximately 324.32 mg/kg HED. This is equivalent to 19,686.224 mg UNCP (approx. 8 teaspoonful if a teaspoonful of UNCP = 2.5 g) for a normal human weight of 60.70 kg. The amount of copper contained in 19,686.224 mg UNCP is 1.469 mg. This may imply that an individual weighing 60.70 kg could have detrimental consequences if 8 teaspoonfuls of UNCP are ingested especially equivalent amounts on a daily basis.

Body weight changes between the control group and the experimental group that were taken on Day 1, Day 7, and Day 14 with respect to dosing were found not to be statistically significant ($p > 0.05$). The increase in the body weight for both groups for the first week after dosing was about 10 grams (8.3%), which was consistent with other observations [37]. This could be attributed to the increase in the food consumption of the animals within the first week after dosing. There was however a decrease in weight of the SD rats on the 2nd week after dosing by 8.3% and 22.2% ($p < 0.05$) for the control and test group, respectively. The decrease in body weight with the control animals is consistent with the corresponding decrease in their food and water intake while that for the test animals might be explained by the

reduction in the food and water intake as well as the ability of UNCP to react with nutrients in the body including stored fat, carbohydrate, and protein [6].

Generally there was a 10.90% ($p > 0.05$) reduction of the organ weight in the test group as compared to the control group. The relative organ weight of the control and experimental group of SD rats was however very similar and thus no significant changes in organ weight were observed.

Hepatic assessment revealed a significant decrease in ALP ($p < 0.05$) and a slight reduction in bilirubin levels ($p > 0.05$) of the UNCP treated group in comparison with the controls. AST and ALT levels were not much affected ($p > 0.05$) by the administration of UNCP solution (Figure 5) as have been observed by other researchers [38, 39]. The plasma protein levels remained relatively unchanged compared with the controls ($p > 0.05$) which may indicate that UNCP has not got any adverse effect on the liver, a situation that is consistent with the histopathological results. It is most likely that the liver being an organ capable of regenerating damaged tissue may not be impaired early following an insult from a toxicant [40].

There was an increase in HDL cholesterol ($p < 0.05$), a decrease in the level of triglycerides, and LDL cholesterol of the UNCP group ($p > 0.05$) in comparison with that of the control while cholesterol levels remained relatively unchanged (Figure 5). This is consistent with the findings of Hammerstone et al. [41] that flavonoids and procyanidins [17] in UNCP possess lipid lowering abilities. The first human clinical study performed showed that 35 g of delipidated cocoa decreased LDL oxidation between 2 h and 4 h after ingestion [17]. An increase in HDL cholesterol ($p < 0.05$) and reduction in LDL cholesterol of the treated group in comparison with the control group were however recorded which agrees with the work of Galleano et al. [35]. This might possibly explain the antihyperlipidaemic and antihypertensive effect of UNCP observed in other studies [7, 10, 11]. The slight reduction in Na levels supports the diuretic effect of UNCP beneficial in blood pressure control. However, this urine output was not monitored neither did the test animals show significant increase in water consumption. It is highly possible that a much prolonged administration of UNCP could have had significant and pronounced effects on these parameters.

There was a slight increase in the level of urea and K^+ ($p > 0.05$) while creatinine levels reduced in the UNCP group as compared to the control group ($p > 0.05$) (Figure 6). Histopathology evaluation of the liver, kidney, heart, lungs, spleen, and the testis of the animals that received UNCP showed no toxic effect as compared to that of the control group. It is obvious that both hepatic and renal effects which showed normal morphology in the treated male SD rats and control are consistent with the results for the kidney and liver function tests. UNCP solution therefore is not likely to have toxic effect on the kidney when administered in a single oral high dose of 2000 mg/kg.

Haematological results showed a decrease (28.44%, $p > 0.05$) in the level of platelet in the UNCP group in comparison with the controls. Polyphenols in cocoa have been found to reduce platelet count. Neutrophil and lymphocyte polymorph

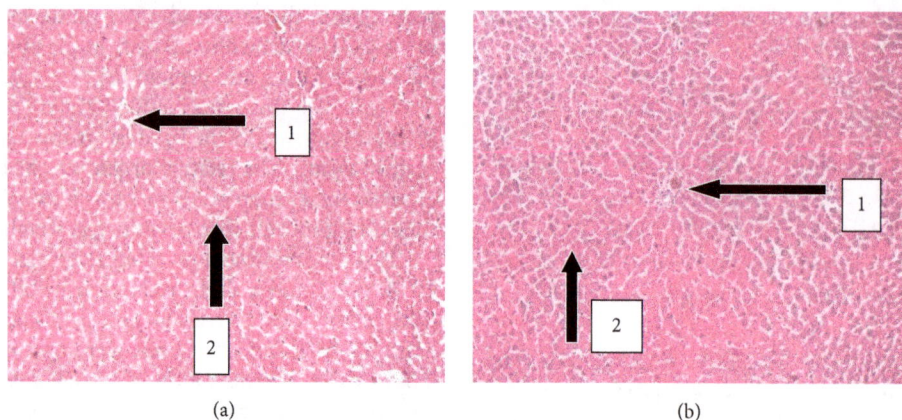

(a)   (b)

FIGURE 2: H&E stained section of livers at 20x magnification. (a) Liver sections of control rat showing normal histology. Note the presence of the central vein with no congestion and cellular infiltration (1) and sinusoids with no dilatation (2). (b) Liver sections of treated male SD rats (2000 mg/kg) with normal central vein, sinusoids, and hepatocytes.

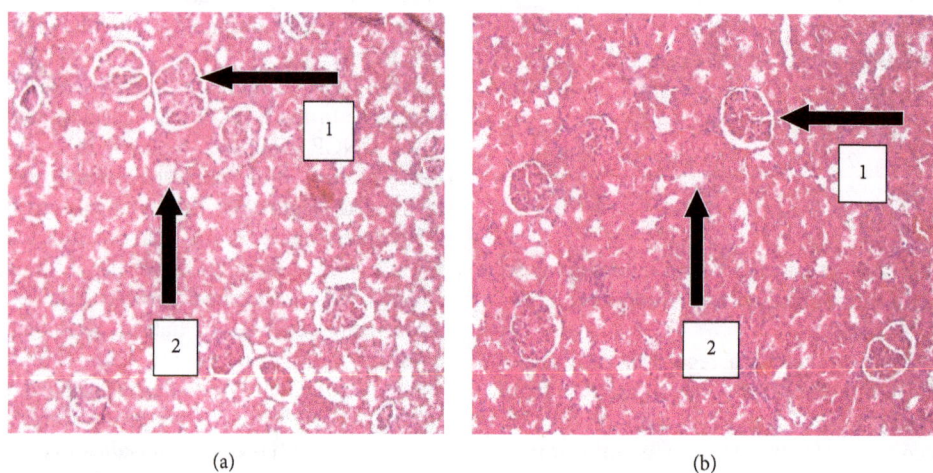

(a)   (b)

FIGURE 3: H&E stained sections of kidneys at 20x magnification. (a) Kidney sections of control male SD rats showing normal histology. Note the presence of the glomerular capsule with no necrosis, degeneration, and congestion (1) and normal convoluted tubules with no tubular casts (2). (b) Kidney section of treated animals (2000 mg/kg) with normal glomerulus and renal tubules with no congestion and cellular infiltration.

of white blood cells showed a slight decrease of 8.02% and 18.73%, respectively ($p > 0.05$) (Figure 6). Negligible difference between the experimental and control group was observed in the case of haemoglobin (1.48%) and red blood cells (2.77%, $p > 0.05$). These results are contrary to other studies where a forty-eight day administration of an aqueous Venaco cocoa powder was found to increase platelet and white blood cell levels while liver enzymes, HCT, and HGB levels remained relatively unchanged [42]. However, there have been other studies with unexplainable contradictory results where platelets and leucocytes have increased during natural cocoa administration [43, 44]. There remains much investigation into these scientific observations. Besides, there was no significant difference between the actual measurement of the width of the erythrocyte distribution curve and the mean erythrocyte size (RDW-CV and RDW-SD) when compared to the control ($p > 0.05$). This is confirmed by the peripheral blood smear which showed normal red blood cells

with respect to their shape, size, and colour (Figure 1). They were therefore normocytic and normochromic. Thus UNCP is likely not to have produced any toxic effect on the red blood cell, white blood cell, and platelet according to the peripheral blood smear.

One notable effect of UNCP was on the small intestines in the form of erosions of the mucosal lining of the villi, an effect which was not observed in the animals that received equivalent volumes of the vehicle (distilled water) (Figure 8). This could be caused by the high concentration of proanthocyanidins contained in the 2000 mg/kg dose of UNCP (approx. 2.5 g in man). This proanthocyanidins have been found to instigate the destruction of the mucosal lining of the gastrointestinal tract, haemorrhagic gastroenteritis in rabbits, striking lesions in the digestive tract of sheep, and congestion of the intestinal wall in rats [17]. Though considered safe, proanthocyanidin-rich products at high concentrations could result in intestinal erosions. Since the UNCP used in

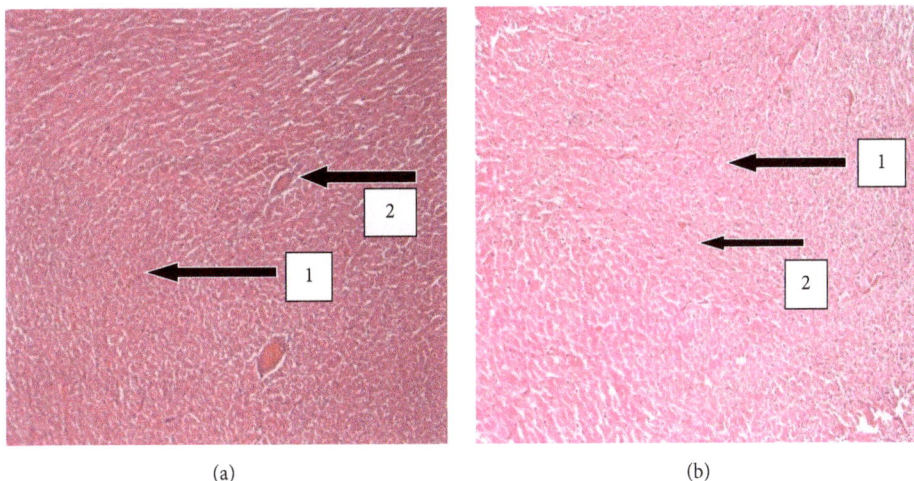

(a)　　　　　　　　(b)

FIGURE 4: H&E stained sections of hearts at 20x magnification. (a) Heart sections of control SD rats showing normal myocardium. Note the presence of the myocardial fibres with no necrosis (1) and coronary vessels carrying blood normally to the heart (2). (b) Heart sections of treated animals (2000 mg/kg) showing normal histology and branched myofibrils.

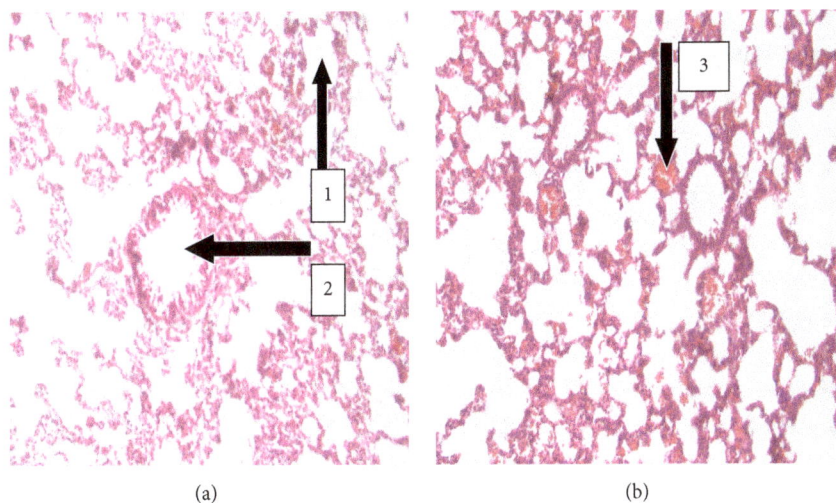

(a)　　　　　　　　(b)

FIGURE 5: H&E stained sections of lungs at 20x magnification. (a) Lung sections of control rats showing normal histology. Note the presence of the alveoli with its surrounding interalveolar septa (1), bronchus (2), and pulmonary vessels with normal blood flow (3). (b) Lung sections of treated animal (2000 mg/kg) showing normal structure of the bronchi and alveoli.

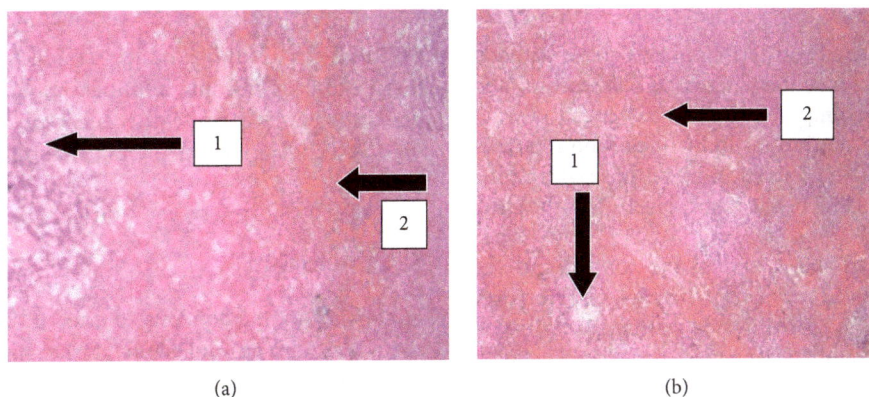

(a)　　　　　　　　(b)

FIGURE 6: H&E stained sections of the spleen at 20x magnification. (a) Spleen sections of control SD rats showing normal histology. Note the presence of the white pulp (1) and the red pulp (2). (b) Spleen sections of treated male SD rats (2000 mg/kg) of UNCP showing intact splenic pulps.

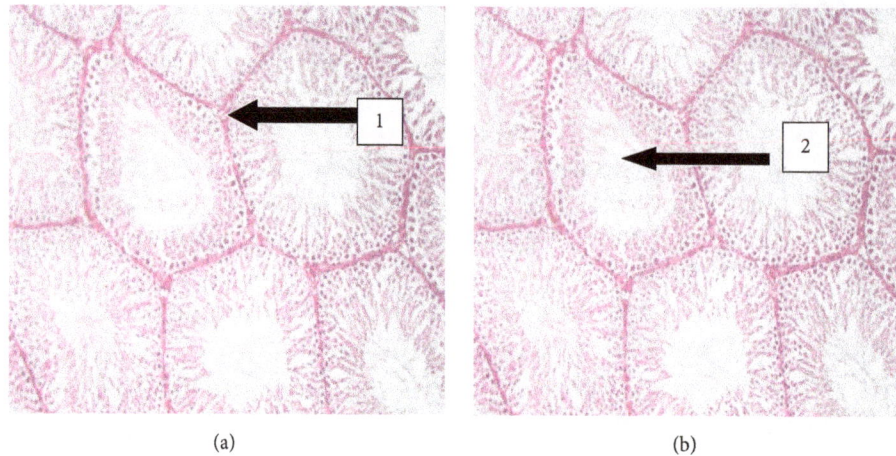

(a)   (b)

FIGURE 7: H&E stained sections of the testis at the magnification of 20x. (a) Testis sections of control SD rats showing normal histology. Note the presence of the intact seminiferous tubules (1) and the Sertoli cells which produces spermatozoa (2). (b) Testis sections of treated animals (2000 mg/kg) showing normal seminiferous tubules with intact spermatogenesis.

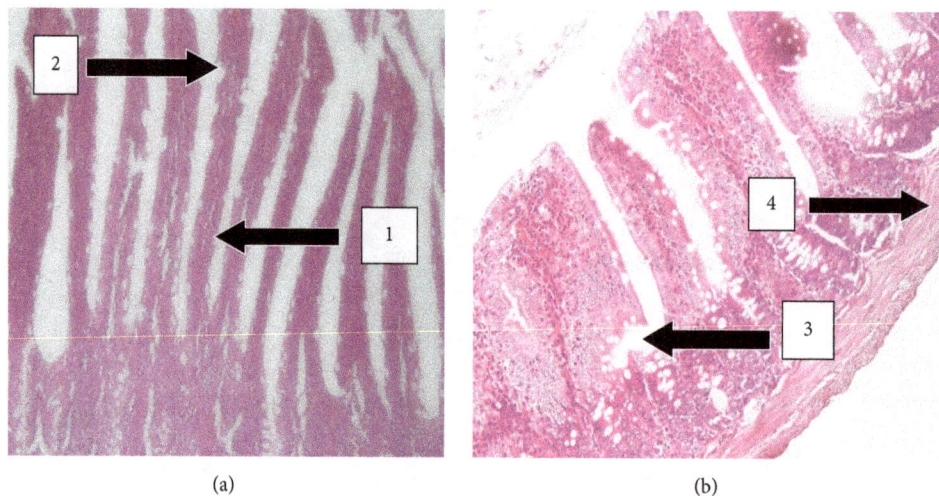

(a)   (b)

FIGURE 8: H&E stained sections of the small intestines at 20x magnification. (a) Small intestine sections of control male SD rats showing normal histology. Note the presence of the villi (1), goblet cells which produces mucus (2), and basement membrane with no proliferation (4). (b) Small intestine section of the UNCP treated male SD rats (2000 mg/kg) showing moderate changes and erosion of the mucosal lining of the villi (3).

this study is a nonalkalized powder, it is likely to have a greater percentage of total polyphenols, increased epicatechin, and proanthocyanidins as compared to alkalized cocoa powder [45]. This should be a caution for individuals who regularly take high quantities of UNCP as beverage or those with peptic ulcer diseases, since UNCP has some level of cumulative properties.

The morphology of the spleen in the control and the UNCP group also showed normalcy with no tissue necrosis, hyperplasia, or depopulation and thus was concurrent with the results of the haematological analysis.

The lungs, testis, and heart also showed no signs of toxicity in the experimental animals and thus unsweetened natural cocoa powder could be considered to have no toxic effect on these organs at the dose administered in SD rats. In another study, Tarka et al. (1982; 1991) have shown the potential of cocoa to produce teratogenic and reproductive toxicity during chronic administration [21, 22]. This study has attempted to relate the effect of high dose nonalkalized UNCP and its elemental composition in laboratory animals.

5. Conclusion

In conclusion, the aqueous solution of unsweetened natural cocoa powder administered at the single oral high dose of 2000 mg/kg appears to be relatively safe in male SD rats. Caution should however be taken when using UNCP especially in high quantities or amounts since it is capable of causing considerable damage to the mucosal lining of the small intestines.

Abbreviations

ED-XRF:　Energy dispersive X-ray
RDA:　Recommended daily allowance
UNCP:　Unsweetened natural cocoa powder
ALT:　Alanine aminotransferase
AST:　Aspartate aminotransferase
CK:　Creatinine kinase
ALB:　Albumin
ALP:　Alkaline phosphatase
HDL:　High density lipoprotein
LDL:　Low density lipoprotein
VLDL:　Very low density lipoproteins
ANOVA:　Analysis of variance
GAFCO:　Ghana Agriculture Food Company
LD_{50}:　Lethal dose
SD:　Sprague-Dawley
SDR:　Sprague-Dawley Rats
HCT:　Haematocrit
HD:　High dose
HGB:　Haemoglobin
LD:　Low dose
LYM%:　Lymphocytes percentage
LYM#:　Lymphocyte count
MCH:　Mean corpuscular haemoglobin
MCHC:　Mean corpuscular haemoglobin concentration
MCV:　Mean corpuscular volume
MPV:　Mean platelet volume
PDW:　Platelet distribution width
P-LCR:　Platelet larger cell ratio
PLT:　Platelet
RBC:　Red blood cells
RDW-CV:　Coefficient of variation in red cell distribution width
RDW-SD:　Standard deviation in red cell distribution width
TP:　Total protein
WBC:　White blood cells
Lympho.:　Lymphocytes
Eosin.:　Eosinophils
Baso.:　Basophils
RDW-SD:　Standard deviation in red cell distribution width
RDW-CV:　Coefficient of variation in red cell distribution width
PDW:　Platelet distribution width
MPV:　Mean platelet volume.

Ethical Approval

The study protocol was approved by the departmental ethical and protocol review committee and the Noguchi Memorial Institute for Medical Research Institutional Animal Care and Use Committee with protocol approval number 2013-01-3E.

Competing Interests

The authors hereby declare there are no competing interests in the above research conducted and publication of the paper.

Acknowledgments

The authors acknowledge the valuable effort of Abraham Terkpertey for the various roles he played as participating investigators in executing this experiment.

References

[1] F. K. Addai, "Natural cocoa as diet-mediated antimalarial prophylaxis," *Medical Hypotheses*, vol. 74, no. 5, pp. 825–830, 2010.

[2] B. B. Mishra and V. K. Tiwari, "Natural products: an evolving role in future drug discovery," *European Journal of Medicinal Chemistry*, vol. 46, no. 10, pp. 4769–4807, 2011.

[3] G. Kumar, G. S. Banu, P. V. Pappa, M. Sundararajan, and M. R. Pandian, "Hepatoprotective activity of *Trianthema portulacastrum* L. against paracetamol and thioacetamide intoxication in albino rats," *Journal of Ethnopharmacology*, vol. 92, no. 1, pp. 37–40, 2004.

[4] T. A. Abere, P. E. Okoto, and F. O. Agoreyo, "Antidiarrhoea and toxicological evaluation of the leaf extract of *Dissotis rotundifolia triana* (Melastomataceae)," *BMC Complementary and Alternative Medicine*, vol. 10, article 71, 2010.

[5] T. L. Dillinger, P. Barriga, S. Escárcega, M. Jimenez, D. S. Lowe, and L. E. Grivetti, "Food of the gods: cure for humanity? A cultural history of the medicinal and ritual use of chocolate," *Journal of Nutrition*, vol. 130, no. 8, pp. 2057–2072, 2000.

[6] L. Alemanno, T. Ramos, A. Gargadenec, C. Andary, and N. Ferriere, "Localization and identification of phenolic compounds in *Theobroma cacao* L. somatic embryogenesis," *Annals of Botany*, vol. 92, no. 4, pp. 613–623, 2003.

[7] E. L. Ding, S. M. Hutfless, X. Ding, and S. Girotra, "Chocolate and prevention of cardiovascular disease: a systematic review," *Nutrition & Metabolism*, vol. 3, article 2, 2006.

[8] D. Taubert, R. Berkels, W. Klaus, and R. Roesen, "Nitric oxide formation and corresponding relaxation of porcine coronary arteries induced by plant phenols: essential structural features," *Journal of Cardiovascular Pharmacology*, vol. 40, no. 5, pp. 701–713, 2002.

[9] K. B. Miller, W. J. Hurst, M. J. Payne et al., "Impact of alkalization on the antioxidant and flavanol content of commercial cocoa powders," *Journal of Agricultural and Food Chemistry*, vol. 56, no. 18, pp. 8527–8533, 2008.

[10] I. Andújar, M. C. Recio, R. M. Giner, and J. L. Ríos, "Cocoa polyphenols and their potential benefits for human health," *Oxidative Medicine and Cellular Longevity*, vol. 2012, Article ID 906252, 23 pages, 2012.

[11] S. Arranz, P. Valderas-Martinez, G. Chiva-Blanch et al., "Cardioprotective effects of cocoa: clinical evidence from randomized clinical intervention trials in humans," *Molecular Nutrition & Food Research*, vol. 57, no. 6, pp. 936–947, 2013.

[12] C. Andres-Lacueva, M. Monagas, N. Khan et al., "Flavanol and flavonol contents of cocoa powder products: influence of the manufacturing process," *Journal of Agricultural and Food Chemistry*, vol. 56, no. 9, pp. 3111–3117, 2008.

[13] A. Caligiani, D. Acquotti, M. Cirlini, and G. Palla, "1H NMR study of fermented cocoa (*Theobroma cacao* L.) beans," *Journal of Agricultural and Food Chemistry*, vol. 58, no. 23, pp. 12105–12111, 2010.

[14] M. Del Rosario Brunetto, L. Gutiérrez, Y. Delgado et al., "Determination of theobromine, theophylline and caffeine in

cocoa samples by a high-performance liquid chromatographic method with on-line sample cleanup in a switching-column system," *Food Chemistry*, vol. 100, no. 2, pp. 459–467, 2007.

[15] J. Wollgast and E. Anklam, "Review on polyphenols in *Theobroma cacao*: changes in composition during the manufacture of chocolate and methodology for identification and quantification," *Food Research International*, vol. 33, no. 6, pp. 423–447, 2000.

[16] C. Awortwe, I. J. Asiedu-Gyekye, E. Nkansah, and S. Adjei, "Unsweetened natural cocoa has anti-asthmatic potential," *International Journal of Immunopathology and Pharmacology*, vol. 27, no. 2, pp. 203–212, 2014.

[17] M. Rusconi and A. Conti, "*Theobroma cacao* L., the food of the gods: a scientific approach beyond myths and claims," *Pharmacological Research*, vol. 61, no. 1, pp. 5–13, 2010.

[18] R. Eyal, "Micro-elements in agriculture," *Practical Hydroponics and Greenhouses*, pp. 39–48, 2007.

[19] World Health Organization, *Quality Control Methods for Medicinal Plant Materials*, WHO Offset Publication, WHO, Geneva, Switzerland, 1998.

[20] J. M. Carvelho, L. G. Ferrerira, P. Amorim, M. L. M. Marques, and M. T. Ramos, "Heavy metals in macrophyte algae using Xray fluorescence," *Environmental Toxicology Chemistry*, vol. 16, no. 4, pp. 807–812, 1997.

[21] S. M. Tarka and H. H. Cornish, "The toxicology of cocoa and methylxanthines: a review of the literature," *CRC Critical Reviews in Toxicology*, vol. 9, no. 4, pp. 275–312, 1982.

[22] S. M. Tarka Jr., R. B. Morrissey, J. L. Apgar, K. A. Hostetler, and C. A. Shively, "Chronic toxicity/carcinogenicity studies of cocoa powder in rats," *Food and Chemical Toxicology*, vol. 29, no. 1, pp. 7–19, 1991.

[23] W. Ying and D. P. Waller, "Theobromine toxicity on Sertoli cells and comparison with cocoa extract in male rats," *Toxicology Letters*, vol. 70, no. 2, pp. 155–164, 1994.

[24] M. J. Anjos, R. T. Lopes, E. F. O. Jesus, S. M. Simabuco, and R. Cesareo, "Quantitative determination of metals in radish using x-ray fluorescence spectrometry," *X-Ray Spectrometry*, vol. 31, no. 2, pp. 120–123, 2002.

[25] C. Vázquez, N. Bárbara, and S. López, "XRF analysis of micronutrients in endive grown on soils with sewage sludge," *X-Ray Spectrometry*, vol. 32, no. 1, pp. 57–59, 2003.

[26] R. E. López De Ruiz, R. A. Olsina, and A. N. Masi, "Different analytical methodologies for the preconcentration and determination of trace chromium by XRF in medicinal herbs with effects on metabolism," *X-Ray Spectrometry*, vol. 31, no. 2, pp. 150–153, 2002.

[27] R. Subhashini, U. S. Mahadeva Rao, P. Sumathi, and G. Gunalan, "A comparative phytochemical analysis of cocoa and green tea," *Indian Journal of Science and Technology*, vol. 3, no. 2, pp. 188–192, 2010.

[28] H. O. Mbagwu, R. A. Anene, and O. O. Adeyemi, "Analgesic, antipyretic and anti-inflammatory properties of *Mezoneuron benthamianum Baill* (Caesalpiniaceae)," *Nigerian Quarterly Journal of Hospital Medicine*, vol. 17, no. 1, pp. 35–41, 2007.

[29] H. Nguyen, O. A. Odelola, J. Rangaswami, and A. Amanullah, "A review of nutritional factors in hypertension management," *International Journal of Hypertension*, vol. 2013, Article ID 698940, 12 pages, 2013.

[30] M. Houston, "The role of magnesium in hypertension and cardiovascular disease," *The Journal of Clinical Hypertension*, vol. 13, no. 11, pp. 843–847, 2011.

[31] B. Sontia and R. M. Touyz, "Role of magnesium in hypertension," *Archives of Biochemistry and Biophysics*, vol. 458, no. 1, pp. 33–39, 2007.

[32] R. Masironi, *Trace Elements in Relation to cArdiovascular Diseases: Status of the Joint WHO/IAEA Research Programme*, WHO Offset Publication, WHO, Geneva, Switzerland, 1973.

[33] O. Bandmann, K. H. Weiss, and S. G. Kaler, "Wilson's disease and other neurological copper disorders," *The Lancet Neurology*, vol. 14, no. 1, pp. 103–113, 2015.

[34] P. Dusek, P. M. Roos, T. Litwin, S. A. Schneider, T. P. Flaten, and J. Aaseth, "The neurotoxicity of iron, copper and manganese in Parkinson's and Wilson's diseases," *Journal of Trace Elements in Medicine and Biology*, vol. 31, pp. 193–203, 2015.

[35] M. Galleano, P. I. Oteiza, and C. G. Fraga, "Cocoa, chocolate, and cardiovascular disease," *Journal of Cardiovascular Pharmacology*, vol. 54, no. 6, pp. 483–490, 2009.

[36] S. Reagan-Shaw, M. Nihal, and N. Ahmad, "Dose translation from animal to human studies revisited," *The FASEB Journal*, vol. 22, no. 3, pp. 659–661, 2008.

[37] Taconic Technical Library, *Hematological Clinical Chemistry values Sprague-Dawley Rats*, 2003.

[38] C. A. Pieme, V. N. Penlap, B. Nkegoum et al., "Evaluation of acute and subacute toxicities of aqueous ethanolic extract of leaves of *Senna alata* (L.) Roxb. (Ceasalpiniaceae)," *African Journal of Biotechnology*, vol. 5, no. 3, pp. 283–289, 2006.

[39] S. K. Ramaiah, "A toxicologist guide to the diagnostic interpretation of hepatic biochemical parameters," *Food and Chemical Toxicology*, vol. 45, no. 9, pp. 1551–1557, 2007.

[40] O. A. Salawu, B. A. Chindo, A. Y. Tijani, I. C. Obidike, and T. A. Salawu, "Acute and sub-acute Toxicological evaluation of the methanolic stem bark extract of *Crossopteryx febrifuga* in rats," *African Journal of Pharmacy and Pharmacology*, vol. 3, pp. 621–626, 2009.

[41] J. F. Hammerstone, S. A. Lazarus, A. E. Mitchell, R. Rucker, and H. H. Schmitz, "Identification of procyanidins in cocoa (*Theobroma cacao*) and chocolate using high-performance liquid chromatography/mass spectrometry," *Journal of Agricultural and Food Chemistry*, vol. 47, no. 2, pp. 490–496, 1999.

[42] S. Heptinstall, J. May, S. Fox, C. Kwik-Uribe, and L. Zhao, "Cocoa flavanols and platelet and leukocyte function: recent *in vitro* and *ex vivo* studies in healthy adults," *Journal of Cardiovascular Pharmacology*, vol. 47, no. 2, pp. S197–S205, 2006.

[43] F. K. Abrokwah, K. A. Asamoah, and P. K. A. Esubonteng, "Effects of the intake of natural cocoa powder on some biochemical and haematological indices in the rat," *Ghana Medical Journal*, vol. 43, no. 4, p. 164, 2009.

[44] C. O. Ibegbulem, P. C. Chikezie, and E. C. Dike, "Growth rate, haematologic and atherogenic indicators of rats fed with cocoa beverages," *Journal of Molecular Pathophysiology*, vol. 4, no. 2, p. 77, 2015.

[45] T. H. Stanley, A. T. Smithson, A. P. Neilson, R. C. Anantheswaran, and J. D. Lambert, "Analysis of cocoa proanthocyanidins using reversed phase high-performance liquid chromatography and electrochemical detection: application to studies on the effect of alkaline processing," *Journal of Agricultural and Food Chemistry*, vol. 63, no. 25, pp. 5970–5975, 2015.

11

Cisplatin-Associated Ototoxicity: A Review for the Health Professional

Jessica Paken,[1] Cyril D. Govender,[1] Mershen Pillay,[1] and Vikash Sewram[1,2,3]

[1]Discipline of Audiology, School of Health Sciences, University of KwaZulu-Natal, Private Bag X54001, Durban 4000, South Africa
[2]African Cancer Institute, Faculty of Medicine and Health Sciences, Stellenbosch University, P.O. Box 241,
 Cape Town 8000, South Africa
[3]Division of Community Health, Faculty of Medicine and Health Sciences, Stellenbosch University, P.O. Box 241,
 Cape Town 8000, South Africa

Correspondence should be addressed to Vikash Sewram; vsewram@sun.ac.za

Academic Editor: Brad Upham

Cisplatin is an effective drug used in the treatment of many cancers, yet its ototoxic potential places cancer patients, exposed to this drug, at risk of hearing loss, thus negatively impacting further on a patient's quality of life. It is paramount for health care practitioners managing such patients to be aware of cisplatin's ototoxic properties and the clinical signs to identify patients at risk of developing hearing loss. English peer-reviewed articles from January 1975 to July 2015 were assessed from PubMed, Science Direct, and Ebscohost. Seventy-nine articles and two books were identified for this review, using MeSH terms and keywords such as "ototoxicity", "cisplatin", "hearing loss", and "ototoxicity monitoring". This review provides an up-to-date overview of cisplatin-associated ototoxicity, namely, its clinical features, incidence rates, and molecular and cellular mechanisms and risk factors, to health care practitioners managing the patient with cancer, and highlights the need for a team-based approach to complement an audiological monitoring programme to mitigate any further loss in the quality of life of affected patients, as there is currently no otoprotective agent recommended routinely for the prevention of cisplatin-associated ototoxicity. It also sets the platform for effective dialogue towards policy formulation and strengthening of health systems in developing countries.

1. Introduction

Cancer places a huge burden on society and has been identified as the leading cause of death in both more and less economically developed countries [1]. Projections based on the GLOBOCAN 2012 estimates predict a substantive increase to 19.3 million new cancer cases per year by 2025, due to growth and ageing of the global population. South Africa, like other developing countries, is also experiencing an increase in the overall burden of disease attributable to cancer, with the number of new cancer cases predicted to increase by 46% by 2030 [2]. This is likely to result in an increase in the use of cancer chemotherapy agents, which assist in preventing the proliferation, invasion, and metastases of the cancer cells [3].

The basis for chemotherapy is anticancer drugs containing platinum, that is, cisplatin (cis-diamminedichloroplatinum II) and carboplatin (cis-diammine 1,1-cyclobutane dicarboxylatoplatinum II) [4]. Other chemotherapy drugs include nitrogen mustard, amino-nicotinamide, dichloromethotrexate, bleomycin, and 5-fluorouracil [5, 6]. The first of these drugs, that is, cisplatin, consists of a divalent Pt (II) central atom and four ligands of cis-positioned pairs of chlorine atoms or amine groups [3].

Since its discovery in the 1970s [7], cisplatin continues to be hailed as one of the most potent cancer chemotherapeutics in children and adults, as it is unique and unmatched in its effectiveness against many cancers [4], namely, osteogenic sarcoma, medulloblastoma, testicular, cervical, and ovarian cancers [8]. Similarly, its toxicity profile is expansive, involving the gastrointestinal, hematologic, renal, and auditory systems [8]. While the use of saline hydration and mannitol diuresis may prevent nephrotoxicity, neurotoxicity is still not curable or preventable [9].

Ototoxicity refers to the hearing disorder that results from the temporary or permanent inner ear dysfunction after treatment with an ototoxic drug [10]. Other drug classes known to have ototoxic properties include aminoglycosides, loop diuretics, quinine, nonsteroidal anti-inflammatory drugs [11], and antiretroviral therapy (ART) [12]. This is of concern in South Africa, as it is estimated that 12.2% of the population (6.4 million persons) were HIV positive in 2012, which is 1.2 million more people living with HIV than in 2008 (10.6%, or 5.2 million) [13]. Resultantly, ART exposure had almost doubled from 16.6% in 2008 to 31.2% in 2012 [13]. Not only will many infected people be at risk for ototoxicity due to ARTs, but a large number will also be susceptible to HIV-related cancers, such as Kaposi's sarcoma, Non-Hodgkin's lymphoma, and cervical cancer, as well as infectious diseases such as tuberculosis, conditions that often require pharmacological therapy with the adverse side effect of ototoxicity. It is possible that their treatments could consist of simultaneous use of more than one ototoxic drug, increasing the likelihood of ototoxicity. All health care professionals managing patients with cancer should therefore be knowledgeable about the ototoxic properties of cisplatin.

However, Malhotra [7] indicated that most oncologists in India do not make referrals for audiological evaluations of patients receiving cisplatin, while a study in South Africa revealed that the effects of ototoxicity, the role of audiologists, and need for their expertise were not fully realized by the oncologists sampled [14]. This is further supported by evidence from the South African study of Khoza-Shangase and Jina [15] which indicated that most general practitioners sampled also do not appear to carry out ototoxicity monitoring strategies, despite being aware of their own role within an ototoxicity monitoring programme. This review therefore aims to serve as resource for health professionals to enhance their understanding of ototoxicity as well as their roles within an ototoxicity monitoring programme by providing an overview and description of this condition in patients diagnosed with cancer and receiving cisplatin chemotherapy.

2. Method

The review identified peer-reviewed articles available from January 1975 to July 2015 on the topic of cisplatin-associated ototoxicity and ototoxicity monitoring and included English articles only. The same researcher conducted the literature search and reviewed the abstracts and articles for inclusion in the study. Studies were identified using keyword and MeSH term searches of electronic databases depicted in Table 1. A manual search of relevant authors and journals was also completed. The references cited by each publication, review, or book chapter were reviewed in order to locate additional potential publications.

In order to be selected, the article had to present data on either cisplatin ototoxicity and/or ototoxicity monitoring in human participants, and no research designs were excluded. Running these searches yielded a total of 2106 records, of which 1581 were excluded based on the title and/or abstract as well as duplication. Eighty-five relevant articles, comprising six national and 79 international articles, were selected. Information was also obtained from four internationally published books. A perusal of narrative reviews of other auditory

TABLE 1: Search and MeSH terms used in the literature search.

Electronic database	Search term	MeSH term
PubMed (Medline)	Ototoxicity [All Fields] AND monitoring [All Fields]	(("cisplatin" [MeSH Terms] OR "cisplatin" [All Fields]) AND ototoxicity [All Fields]) OR (("cisplatin" [MeSH Terms] OR "cisplatin" [All Fields]) AND ("hearing loss" [MeSH Terms] OR ("hearing" [All Fields] AND "loss" [All Fields]) OR "hearing loss" [All Fields]))
Science Direct		"cisplatin ototoxicity" or "cisplatin hearing loss" "ototoxicity monitoring"
Ebscohost	Cisplatin ototoxicity or cisplatin hearing loss Ototoxicity monitoring	

pathologies was conducted in an attempt to determine areas of significance for an overview of cisplatin ototoxicity. This resulted in the following eight areas being included: the mechanisms of cisplatin ototoxicity, clinical presentation, risk factors, incidence rates in adults and children, the effect on quality of life, ototoxicity monitoring, otoprotective strategies, and management of an ototoxic hearing loss.

2.1. The Mechanisms of Cisplatin Ototoxicity. Cisplatin ototoxicity is produced by several distinct mechanisms [16] as depicted in Figure 1. One such mechanism, the antioxidant model, involves the formation of reactive oxygen species (ROS) within the cochlea and consequent reduction in antioxidant enzymes following exposure to cisplatin chemotherapy [16–20]. Another mechanism of cisplatin ototoxicity involves the significant contribution of nicotinamide adenine dinucleotide phosphate oxidase 3 isoform (NOX3) to the generation of reactive oxygen species within the cochlea, when activated by cisplatin [17, 21], while a third mechanism relates to the activation of transient receptor potential vanilloid 1 channel (TRPV1) [22–24].

The molecular mechanisms of cisplatin ototoxicity therefore include the following:

(i) "Creation of reactive oxygen species,

(ii) Depletion of antioxidant glutathione and its regenerating enzymes,

(iii) Increased rate of lipid peroxidation,

(iv) Oxidative modifications of proteins,

(v) Nucleic acids damage by caspase system activation and

(vi) S-Nitrosylation of cochlear proteins" [25].

With the cellular mechanisms of cisplatin-associated ototoxicity including damage to the outer hair cells, supporting cells,

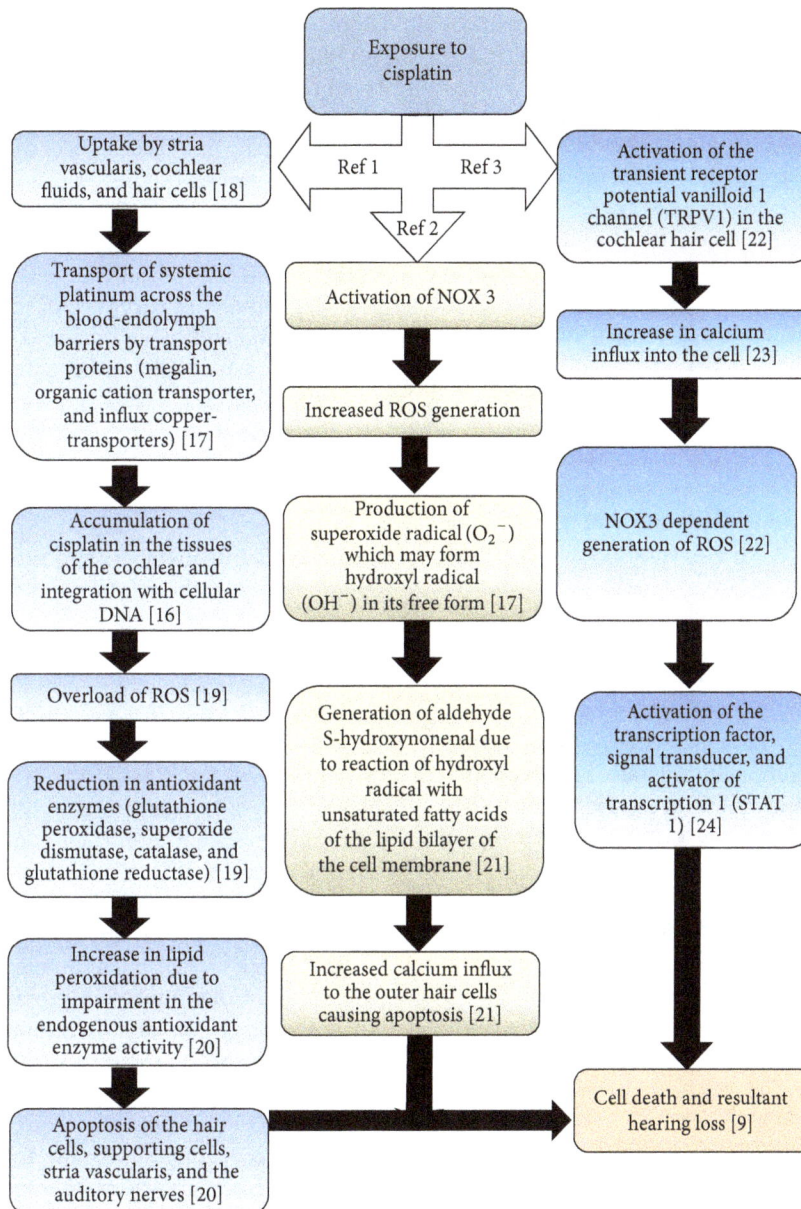

FIGURE 1: Mechanisms of cisplatin ototoxicity REF 1 [16–20], REF 2 [17, 21], and REF 3 [22–24].

marginal cells of the stria vascularis, spiral ligament, and the spiral ganglion cells [25], it is evident that the structures of the inner ear are most susceptible to damage by cisplatin chemotherapy, with apoptotic degeneration of the hair cell in the organ of Corti being most prominent [26]. The outer hair cells in the basal turn of the cochlea are most affected [27, 28]. This leads to an initial elevation of high frequency audiometric thresholds, followed by a progressive loss into the lower frequencies with continued therapy [27, 28]. Knowledge of the different mechanisms of cisplatin ototoxicity is important for health care professionals as it will create an awareness of its complexity and the resulting clinical presentation.

2.2. Clinical Presentation and Risk Factors. Cisplatin-associated ototoxicity usually manifests as irreversible, progressive

[8], bilateral, high frequency sensorineural hearing loss [29] with tinnitus [30]. The latter may occur with or without a hearing loss [29] and may be permanent or transient, sometimes disappearing a few hours after treatment [31] or alternatively persisting a week after treatment [32]. While most of the hearing loss is permanent, there is sometimes sporadic and partial recovery [31]. In addition, rare cases of unilateral hearing loss have been reported, which are usually explained by tumour location and surgical or therapeutic intervention on the affected side [33]. Moreover, the hearing loss is not always symmetrical [33, 34], with Jenkins et al. [34] finding that 75% of women on cisplatin chemotherapy displayed an asymmetry of hearing thresholds of at least 10 dB between ears posttreatment. Schmidt et al. [33], in their investigation of 55 children on cisplatin chemotherapy, found that the high

frequency hearing thresholds were slightly elevated in the left ear and that males had a greater degree of hearing loss than the females.

The degree of hearing loss is often variable and is related to the dose; that is, the higher the cumulative dose, the greater the ototoxic effect [35, 36]. The duration, number of cycles administered [37], and method of administration [38] also influence cisplatin-associated ototoxicity. Additional factors that may increase ototoxicity include exposure to concomitant noise [39], chemicals, and other ototoxic medications [35]. Furthermore, evidence also shows that melanin content is related to an increased risk of cisplatin-associated ototoxicity [40]. Individuals with dark eyes and therefore a higher melanin content in the cochlear are at greater risk of ototoxic damage, as the melanin causes retention of the platinum within the cochlear and subsequently increases the risk of damage [41, 42]. Individuals presenting with renal insufficiency, that is, high levels of serum creatinine, are at a greater risk for cisplatin-associated ototoxicity [35]. Genetic risk factors, such as megalin and glutathione S-transferases gene polymorphism, have also been reported to influence cisplatin ototoxicity [43], as do physiological factors such as age, with younger children [44] and older adults (older than 46 years) [45] presenting with a greater severity of hearing damage. Preexposure hearing ability may also impact on incidence rates [35, 46]. Awareness of these risk factors may assist health care professionals with informational counselling of the patient receiving cisplatin chemotherapy.

2.3. Cisplatin-Associated Hearing Loss in Adults and Children.
The incidence of cisplatin ototoxicity is variable in adults (Table 2) and children (Table 3). The variations may be due to a number of factors, such as differences in the dose, both within a cycle and the total amount administered over multiple cycles, time interval between courses, method of administration, and treatment duration, as well as differences in patient population. Further exploration in this regard is therefore necessary.

2.4. Quality of Life.
Ototoxicity poses a major problem to the cancer patient, as the quality of life after receiving cisplatin chemotherapy may be negatively affected due to hearing loss, resulting in social, emotional, and vocational difficulties, as effective communication is often hindered. Tasks that normal hearing persons take for granted may become challenging and frustrating [58]. In addition, an individual's safety may be compromised due to the hearing loss, as appropriate response to alarms and warning signals may be delayed. Furthermore, a hearing loss may also result in psychosocial and physical health problems, as well as depression and social isolation [59]. Hence, hearing loss, often referred to as the "invisible condition," has serious visible ramifications on the quality of life of a hearing impaired individual [58]. This is particularly relevant if the individual has already experienced the hearing world, as the hearing function is never restored to normal, even though patients may benefit from the use of assistive listening devices, such as hearing aids and cochlear implants [10].

The impact of an ototoxic hearing loss may be more profound for infants and young children who are at a critical stage of their speech and language development [60]. Furthermore, the high frequency nature of an ototoxic hearing loss may result in speech recognition and comprehension being compromised [61], resulting in possible neurocognitive and psychosocial delays [62]. There is also an elevated risk for academic learning problems and psychosocial difficulties in school-aged children and adolescents [63]. Literature indicated that childhood survivors of neuroblastoma had twice the rate of difficulties, as indicated by parent reports, with reading and math skills, and/or attention and a higher risk of a general learning disability than those without a hearing loss. There was also poorer self-reported quality of life scores in these children with regard to school functioning [63]. Hence, cisplatin-associated ototoxicity further complicates the morbidity of cancer patients [8], as it would also isolate them from family members and significant others at a time when they require the greatest support.

2.5. Ototoxicity Monitoring.
Advancements in medical knowledge and technology, such as screening and early detection of several cancers, have resulted in notable improvements in relative five-year survival rates for cancer [64, 65]. Therefore, improving the quality of life after cisplatin-based chemotherapy becomes increasingly important, and resulting comorbidities such as ototoxicity can be managed appropriately and immediately [14] if adequate monitoring is in place.

The nature of ototoxicity is such that it often goes undetected until speech intelligibility is affected [66] and is usually detected when a communication problem becomes evident [67]. Communication problems, such as constantly asking for repetition or not responding when spoken to, signify that the hearing loss has progressed to the frequencies important for understanding speech [67]. In this case, an audiological monitoring programme can avert, to a large extent, the reduced quality of life as a result of hearing loss, as patients on cisplatin chemotherapy can be identified early, counselled, monitored, and managed appropriately through interventions in a logical, systematic, and coherent manner.

Audiological monitoring should aim to identify the hearing loss early and reduce its impact on the individual's life by means of proper medical and hearing intervention [68]. Prospective audiological evaluations remain the only reliable method for detecting ototoxicity before it becomes symptomatic [69]. An ototoxicity monitoring programme should involve a health care team comprising of an oncology nurse, oncologists, audiologist, and pharmacist to ensure effective sustainability of such a programme, if implemented, with the patient being the central focus. The audiologist is involved in identifying an ototoxic hearing loss, informing the oncologist of such a development, counselling the patient and their family, and prescribing amplification devices, such as hearing aids and cochlear implants [70]. Early identification of an ototoxic hearing loss provides oncologists with an opportunity to adjust the chemotherapy regimen in order to reduce or prevent further deterioration of hearing [70]. The oncologist

TABLE 2: Studies reflecting cisplatin-associated hearing loss in adults.

Study	Country	Type of study	Audiological tests conducted	Patient population	Number of patients who developed ototoxicity
Malgonde et al. [47]	India	Prospective	Pure tone audiometry (frequencies not specified) and short increment sensitivity index test	34 patients with head and neck cancers receiving cisplatin containing chemotherapy and concomitant radiation therapy	34 (100%)
Whitehorn et al. [48]	South Africa	Retrospective cross-sectional	Air (0.25–8 kHz) and bone conduction pure tone audiometry	107 patients receiving cisplatin containing chemotherapy, irrespective of the type of the cancer	59 (55.1%)
Nitz et al. [49]	Germany	Prospective longitudinal trinational population-based	Air (0.125–8 kHz) and bone conduction pure tone audiometry	1 patient with soft-tissue sarcoma and 16 with osteosarcoma, receiving cisplatin and/or carboplatin containing chemotherapy	6 (35.3%)
Arora et al. [8]	India	Prospective, randomized, observational	Pure tone air (0.25–16 kHz) and bone conduction audiometry Results are reflective of frequencies 4 to 16 kHz.	57 patients receiving cisplatin containing chemotherapy: 10 patients (low dose group, carcinoma of the larynx) 35 patients (middle dose group, head and neck cancers, carcinoma of the cervix) 12 patients (high dose group, carcinoma of the lung and carcinoma of the testis)	— 6 (60%) 35 (100%) 12 (100%)
Dell'Aringa et al. [50]	Brazil	Case series	Tympanometry, acoustic reflex threshold testing, distortion product otoacoustic emissions (DPOAEs), air (0.25–8 kHz) and bone conduction pure tone audiometry, speech audiometry	17 patients with extracranial head and neck cancers receiving cisplatin containing chemotherapy and concomitant radiation therapy	12 (70.5%), left ears; 11 (64.7%), right ears
Schultz et al. [51]	Brazil	Prospective	Full audiometric evaluations, with only air (0.25–8 kHz) and bone conduction pure tone audiometry thresholds computed	31 patients receiving cisplatin containing chemotherapy, irrespective of the type of cancer	12 (38%), NCI criteria; 19 (65%), Brock et al.'s criteria; 17 (54%), ASHA criteria; 9 (29%), David and Silverman's criteria
Zuur et al. [52]	The Netherlands	Prospective	Air (0.125–16 kHz) and bone conduction pure tone audiometry	60 patients with locally advanced head and neck cancer, receiving cisplatin containing chemotherapy and concomitant radiation therapy	19 (31%), up to 8 kHz; 28 (47%), up to 16 kHz

TABLE 2: Continued.

Study	Country	Type of study	Audiological tests conducted	Patient population	Number of patients who developed ototoxicity
Dutta et al. [36]	India	Prospective	Pure tone audiometry (frequencies not specified)	60 patients receiving cisplatin containing chemotherapy, type of cancer not indicated	9 (15%)
				51, low dose group	6 (12%)
				9, high dose group	3 (33%)
Strumberg et al. [53]	Germany	Retrospective	Pure tone air (0.125–12 kHz) and bone conduction audiometry, transient evoked otoacoustic emissions test (TEOAE)	32 patients with testicular cancer receiving cisplatin containing chemotherapy	21 (70%)
Nagy et al. [54]	USA	Retrospective	Tympanometry, air (0.25–8 KHz) conduction pure tone audiometry	53 patients with oesophageal, lung, or head and neck cancer receiving cisplatin containing chemotherapy and concomitant radiation therapy (only for head and neck cancer)	19 (36%)
Bokemeyer et al. [35]	Germany	Retrospective	Pure tone air (0.5–8 kHz) and bone audiometry	86 patients with testicular cancer receiving cisplatin containing chemotherapy	57 (66%)
Waters et al. [32]	Canada	Retrospective	Pure tone air (0.25–8 kHz) and bone conduction audiometry, immittance audiometry, and speech audiometry	60 patients with advanced ovarian carcinomas receiving cisplatin containing chemotherapy	
				39, low dose, short treatment (25 from LDE group and 14 new cases after treatment modification)	6 (15%)
				8, low dose, blocks	0 (0%)
				25, low dose, extended treatment	9 (36%)
				13, high dose, short treatment	12 (92%)

and nurses should also counsel patients on the side effects of cisplatin, including ototoxicity, in an attempt to prepare them for treatment outcomes and help them set realistic expectations [71]. Pharmacists who have access to a patient's medication list may also alert the oncologists and audiologists to those who are on other ototoxic medication and therefore at a greater risk for cisplatin-induced ototoxicity. Effective management of such patients using evidence-based practices may improve management of those with cancer [72], ensuring that they and their families are counselled and appropriate interventions are timeously implemented. The principles of early identification and early intervention are a part of

ototoxicity monitoring, and the audiologist can manage such a programme [56].

In countries without ototoxicity management guidelines, the "Guidelines for the Audiological Management of Individuals receiving Cochleotoxic Drug Therapy" developed by the American Association of Speech-Language-Hearing Association [69] may, consequently, guide the audiologist in the implementation of an ototoxicity monitoring programme within a local, regional, or national setting. For widespread acceptance and use, ototoxicity monitoring programmes need to incorporate efficient and cost-effective ototoxicity identification techniques [67], while considering the health

TABLE 3: Studies reflecting cisplatin-associated hearing loss in children.

Study	Country	Type of study	Audiological tests conducted	Patient population	Number of patients who developed ototoxicity
Nitz et al. [49]	Germany	Prospective longitudinal trinational population-based	Air (0.125–8 kHz) conduction pure tone audiometry	93 patients with osteosarcoma and 19 with soft-tissue sarcoma receiving cisplatin and/or carboplatin containing chemotherapy	55 (49.1%)
Knight et al. [55]	USA	Prospective	Otoscopy, tympanometry, pure tone audiometry (0.5–8 kHz), DPOAEs, and ABR	32 children with different types of cancers treated with cisplatin and/or carboplatin containing chemotherapy	20 (62.5%)
			Otoscopy, tympanometry, extended pure tone audiometry (0.5–16 kHz), and DPOAEs	17 children with different types of cancers treated with cisplatin and/or carboplatin containing chemotherapy	16 (94.1%)
Coradini et al. [44]	Brazil	Retrospective	Tympanometry, pure tone audiometry (0.25–8 kHz), TEAOEs, and DPOAEs	23 children with malignant hepatic tumour, osteosarcoma, and germ cell tumours receiving cisplatin containing chemotherapy	12 (52%), pure tone; 5 (22%), TEOAEs; 16 (71%), DPOAEs
Bertolini et al. [56]	France	Prospective	Otoscopy, immittance audiometry, speech audiometry, play audiometry or free-field audiometry, conventional pure tone audiometry (frequencies not specified), or ABR (depending on the age of the participant)	102 children with either neuroblastoma, hepatoblastoma, germ cell tumour, or osteosarcoma	—
				96 received cisplatin and/or carboplatin containing chemotherapy	39 (41%)
				52 received cisplatin only	19 (37%)
Stavroulaki et al. [57]	Greece	Prospective	Otoscopy, immittance audiometry, pure tone audiometry (0.25–8 kHz), TEOAEs, and DPOAEs	12 children with either neuroblastoma, osteosarcoma, medulloblastoma, rhabdomyosarcoma, or primitive neuroectodermal tumour receiving cisplatin containing chemotherapy	6 (50%)

care system and demographics of the patient population being managed. For any population receiving ototoxic medication, the following should be considered: "(1) the patient's level of alertness or ability to respond reliably; (2) the most appropriate times during the treatment protocol for test administration, and; (3) the test should comprise the baseline, monitoring and post-treatment evaluations" [73]. Appropriate time intervals for audiological assessments may differ depending on the type of cancer as well as the frequency and dose of cisplatin (Figure 2) [69].

The audiological assessments should incorporate a detailed case history, otoscopic examination, immittance audiometry, speech audiometry, DPOAEs, and conventional and extended high frequency audiometry (i.e., up to 20 000 Hz) (HFA) [69, 73]. These procedures are all conducted for the baseline assessment and the six-month follow-up evaluation

TABLE 4: Clinical significance and limitations of HFA and OAEs.

HFA (>8kHz)	OAEs
Clinical significance for ototoxicity	
(i) HFA is considered to be the most sensitive test to identify ototoxic hearing loss [8, 55, 75].	(i) OAES is considered a noninvasive objective measure of cochlear outer hair cell function [76].
(ii) HFA is not as affected by middle ear pathologies as OAEs [11].	(ii) DPOAEs can be regarded as a more sensitive measure for the early detection of hearing loss than conventional pure tone audiometry [44].
(iii) The criteria of change for ototoxicity is established [11].	(iii) OAEs is time efficient [11].
	(iv) DPOAEs provide frequency specific information [67].
Limitations	
(i) HFA is not standardised [11].	(i) OAEs are significantly affected by middle ear pathology [37].
(ii) HFA is not commonly used, due to the need for additional equipment such as circum-aural headphones [77].	(ii) There is no universal value for the criteria of change indicating ototoxicity [76].
(iii) HFA may not always be applicable, as patients with hearing loss in the conventional frequency range may not have measurable hearing in the extended high frequency range [78].	(iii) OAEs are absent in patients with moderate degrees of hearing loss [67].
(iv) Test efficiency may be affected due to HFA being time consuming [70].	(iv) OAEs have a limited frequency range (generally up to 8000 Hz) [67].

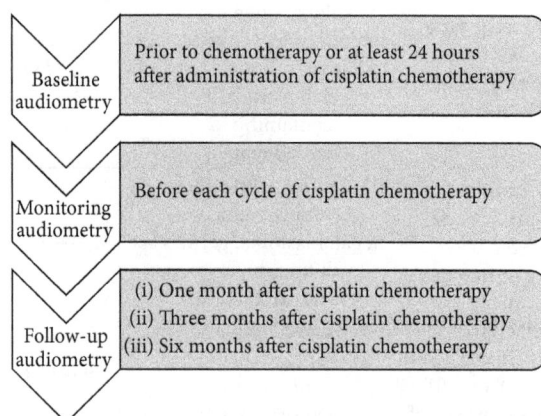

FIGURE 2: Timelines for audiological assessments [69].

[69, 73]. While auditory brainstem response may be used, it is not considered a standard procedure for monitoring ototoxicity [73].

Monitoring audiological evaluations during treatment and the one- and three-month follow-up evaluations include case interview, otoscopy, and immittance audiometry as well as air conduction pure tone and objective testing [73]. However, full-frequency threshold testing is impractical for many patients on cisplatin chemotherapy, as these individuals are often extremely ill and easily fatigued. The use of abbreviated threshold monitoring procedures that are clinically practical for these patients is therefore recommended. One such method involves the use of the sensitive range for ototoxicity (SRO). This is "the highest frequency with a threshold at or below 100 dB SPL followed by the next six lower adjacent frequencies in 1/6-octave steps or the one octave range near the highest audible frequency" [73]. SRO is usually determined during the baseline evaluation and is dependent on each

patient's hearing threshold configuration. During monitoring evaluations, air conduction thresholds should be determined within the patient's defined SRO. However, full-frequency testing should be conducted within the same session if an ASHA significant hearing change is noted within the SRO [69].

If a patient on cisplatin chemotherapy is still responsive and alert, the protocol presented above would be suitable. However, a patient who has limited responsiveness may be required to undergo the same audiological evaluations, except speech audiometry. Patients who are responsive as well as those who have limited responses can undergo both behavioural and objective testing. However, those patients who are too ill or too young to respond should undergo only objective testing, such as otoscopy, tympanometry, acoustic reflexes, and DPOAEs or ABRs [73].

While pure tone audiometry in the conventional frequency range is suitable for evaluating hearing in the range responsible for speech understanding, as well as for differential diagnosis, it is less sensitive to detecting early ototoxic change [11, 70]. The two tests identified as being the most important for the early detection of cisplatin ototoxicity are HFAs and OAEs, each also having limitations (see Table 4) [70]. Therefore, using each test in isolation may not be as effective as utilizing a test battery approach, as it increases the chances of obtaining reliable audiologic monitoring data over time. In addition, these two tests could be used to complement one another in every cycle of chemotherapy to ensure the earliest detection of ototoxicity [74].

The otoxicity monitoring protocol proposed by ASHA [69] represents an aggressive and ideal approach for monitoring ototoxicity and is dependent on a country's infrastructure and resource constraints. The ASHA [69] guidelines may therefore not be generalized to a country without considering the contextual factors that may influence its applicability to that country. However, it does provide guidance towards creating a roadmap that countries, such as South Africa, may aspire towards in implementing an ototoxicity monitoring programme. Similar to India [79], no programmes have been formally implemented to identify and monitor ototoxicity in patients on cancer chemotherapy in South Africa. As a result, there is no contextually relevant research to steer the implementation of an accountable and effective ototoxicity monitoring program in the country. This is probably one of the main reasons for ototoxicity monitoring programmes not being commonplace in local hospitals and clinics. In addition, the health of South Africans is characterized by a quadruple burden of disease, encompassing the occurrence of infectious diseases, the rise of noncommunicable diseases, and perinatal and maternal disorders, as well as injuries and violence [80], which may result in cancer receiving low priority for health care services. However, the creation of an audiological monitoring programme allows for better control of cancer related comorbidities.

2.6. Otoprotective Strategies. Over the years, a number of studies have investigated the use of otoprotectants with cisplatin, their purpose being to protect the inner ear from any injury while not interfering with the antitumor effects of cisplatin [61]. Otoprotective strategies include reducing the formation of free radicals by maintaining glutathione levels and antioxidant activity [27]. Three mechanisms may provide protection against cisplatin, these being endogenous molecules, exogenous agents, or a combination of exogenous agents that trigger endogenous protective mechanisms. However, endogenous agents are not effective against cisplatin when the dose exceeds a certain threshold [17, 81].

Nearly all of the otoprotective agents are sulfur- or sulfhydryl-containing compounds (thio compounds), known as antioxidants, and potent heavy metal chelators [82]. The numerous otoprotective agents utilized in clinical and animal studies include Amifostine, D-or L-Methionine, methylthiobenzoic acid, lipoic acid, tiopronin, glutathione ester, sodium thiosulfate [83], Melatonin [84], Vitamin E [85], N-acetylcysteine [86], Dexamethasone [87], and Resveratrol [88]. However, none of these agents have been found to be unequivocally beneficial in preventing cisplatin ototoxicity and no agent is currently recommended for routine use [7]. Further research is therefore needed to find new methods and optimize old ones to prevent and/or treat hearing loss during cisplatin therapy. In addition, intratympanic administration of medication together with gene therapy needs to be further explored [25]. Intratympanic administration involves the diffusion of the otoprotective agent across the round window into the inner ear, where its therapeutic effect is exerted. An advantage of this method of administration is that there are higher concentrations of the otoprotective agent in the inner ear, this being in comparison to the use of oral or parenteral administration, without potentially reducing the efficacy of the cisplatin treatment [89, 90]. The disadvantage of this procedure, however, is that each ear would have to be treated with a moderately invasive procedure [91]. Alternatively, gene therapy may prove to be beneficial in protecting an individual against cisplatin-induced hearing loss as several genes,

namely, megalin, glutathione-S-transferases, Thiopurine S-methyltransferase, and catechol-O-methyl transferase, may be responsible for susceptibility to hearing loss [9].

2.7. Management of an Ototoxic Hearing Loss. If a cisplatin-associated hearing loss results in communication difficulties, it is the audiologist's ethical responsibility to begin or recommend aural rehabilitation [69]. However, this intervention should not only occur once hearing loss has been detected but before the patient begins the cisplatin chemotherapy. Aural rehabilitation techniques such as speech reading and counselling on compensatory communication strategies should be conducted. The counselling should include spouses and significant other, as hearing loss may not only impact the person with cancer but also frequent communication partners [92]. Patients with sensorineural hearing loss due to the use of cisplatin may also benefit from the use of assistive listening devices such as hearing aids or cochlear implants [10]. Children with ototoxic hearing loss may also require the use of personal frequency modulated systems in the classroom.

Furthermore, with the recent developments in hearing aid technology, a patient with an ototoxic hearing loss is more likely to receive the desired amplification benefit. These developments in technology include

(i) "Extended bandwidth" hearing aids. These hearing aids are able to amplify sounds at and above 8000 Hz. However, there is limited data indicating significant improvements in speech recognition with the use of this technology [93].

(ii) Hearing aids with frequency lowering technology achieved by linear frequency transposition, nonlinear frequency compression, or spectral envelope warping. Frequency lowering is used to overcome the limits of either the bandwidth of the device or the functional bandwidth of the ear, by lowering high frequency energy to a region that is more likely to provide and/or benefit from audible sound [94]. While there are no published studies suggesting one approach to be superior to another, frequency lowering technology has been found to improve audibility and speech understanding of high frequency sounds [93]. Commercially available types of frequency lowering signal processing include frequency transposition (Widex), nonlinear frequency compression (Phonak), and frequency translation (Starkey). These processors are commercially labelled as Audibility Extender, SoundRecover, and Spectral IQ, respectively [94].

3. Conclusion

This review has highlighted that cisplatin ototoxicity is a frequent adverse event of cisplatin chemotherapy that may negatively affect the quality of life of patients with cancer. The different molecular and cellular mechanisms involved in cisplatin-associated ototoxicity highlight the complexity of this condition and the consequent difficulty in identifying an effective otoprotective agent. The varying incidence rates reported in both adults and paediatrics may be due to the different audiological tests employed in the monitoring of the cancer patient's hearing status and therefore highlight the importance of the use of extended high frequency audiometry and DPOAEs in ototoxicity monitoring. An audiological monitoring programme comprising a team of health care professionals, knowledgeable about cisplatin ototoxicity, may therefore serve to improve evidence-based service delivery to these patients.

Disclosure

This manuscript has been presented at the ENT/SAAA/SASLHA Congress 2015 in South Africa, Audiology Australia National Conference 2016, and the World Congress of Audiology 2016.

Competing Interests

The authors declare that they have no competing interests.

Authors' Contributions

Jessica Paken collected the data and wrote the first draft of the manuscript. Cyril D. Govender, Mershen Pillay, and Vikash Sewram critically reviewed and provided input of intellectual content. All authors read and approved the final manuscript.

Acknowledgments

The study is supported by the Medical Research Council of South Africa in terms of the National Health Scholarship Programme provided for this purpose by the National Department of Health. The study also received financial support from Oticon Foundation.

References

[1] L. A. Torre, F. Bray, R. L. Siegel, J. Ferlay, J. Lortet-Tieulent, and A. Jemal, "Global cancer statistics, 2012," *CA Cancer Journal for Clinicians*, vol. 65, no. 2, pp. 87–108, 2015.

[2] J. Ferlay, I. Soerjomataram, M. Ervik et al., *GLOBOCAN 2012 v1.0, Cancer Incidence and Mortality Worldwide: IARC CancerBase No. 11 [Internet]*, International Agency for Research on Cancer, Lyon, France, 2013.

[3] L. P. Rybak, "Cancer and Ototoxicity of chemotherapeutics," in *Pharmacology and Ototoxicity for Audiologists*, K. C. M. Campbell, Ed., pp. 138–162, Thomson Delmar Learning: United States, 2007.

[4] K. M. Reavis, G. McMillan, D. Austin et al., "Distortion-product otoacoustic emission test performance for ototoxicity monitoring," *Ear and Hearing*, vol. 32, no. 1, pp. 61–74, 2011.

[5] L. Luxon, J. M. Furman, A. Martini, and S. D. G. Stephens, *Textbook of Audiological Medicine: Clinical Aspects of Hearing and Balance*, Taylor & Francis, London, UK, 2003.

[6] R. J. Roeser, M. Valente, and H. Hosford-Dunn, *Audiology Diagnosis*, Thieme, New York, NY, USA, 2000.

[7] H. Malhotra, "Cisplatin ototoxicity," *Indian Journal of Cancer*, vol. 46, no. 4, pp. 262–263, 2009.

[8] R. Arora, J. S. Thakur, R. K. Azad, N. K. Mohindroo, D. R. Sharma, and R. K. Seam, "Cisplatin-based chemotherapy: add high-frequency audiometry in the regimen," *Indian Journal of Cancer*, vol. 46, no. 4, pp. 311–317, 2009.

[9] D. Mukherjea and L. P. Rybak, "Pharmacogenomics of cisplatin-induced ototoxicity," *Pharmacogenomics*, vol. 12, no. 7, pp. 1039–1050, 2011.

[10] J. G. Yorgason, J. N. Fayad, and F. Kalinec, "Understanding drug ototoxicity: molecular insights for prevention and clinical management," *Expert Opinion on Drug Safety*, vol. 5, no. 3, pp. 383–399, 2006.

[11] N. Schellack and A. Naude, "An overview of pharmacotherapy-induced ototoxicity," *South African Family Practice*, vol. 55, no. 4, pp. 357–365, 2013.

[12] N. Stearn and D. W. Swanepoel, "Sensory and neural auditory disorders associated with HIV/AIDS," in *HIV/AIDS Related Communication, Hearing and Swallowing Disorders*, D. W. Swanepoel and B. Louw, Eds., pp. 243–288, Plural Publishing, San Diego, Calif, USA, 2010.

[13] O. Shisana, T. Rehle, L. C. Simbayi et al., *South African National HIV Prevalence, Incidence and Behaviour Survey, 2012*, Human Sciences Research Council, Pretoria, South Africa, 2014.

[14] V. De Andrade, K. Khoza-Shangase, and F. Hajat, "Perceptions of oncologists at two state hospitals in Gauteng regarding the ototoxic effects of cancer chemotherapy: a pilot study," *African Journal of Pharmacy and Pharmacology*, vol. 3, no. 6, pp. 307–318, 2009.

[15] K. Khoza-Shangase and K. Jina, "Ototoxicity monitoring in general medical practice: exploring perceptions and practices of general practitioners about drug-induced auditory symptoms," *Innovations in Pharmaceuticals and Pharmacotherapy*, vol. 1, no. 3, pp. 250–259, 2013.

[16] M. S. Gonçalves, A. F. Silveira, A. R. Teixeira, and M. A. Hyppolito, "Mechanisms of cisplatin ototoxicity: theoretical review," *Journal of Laryngology & Otology*, vol. 127, no. 6, pp. 536–541, 2013.

[17] L. P. Rybak, "Mechanisms of cisplatin ototoxicity and progress in otoprotection," *Current Opinion in Otolaryngology & Head and Neck Surgery*, vol. 15, no. 5, pp. 364–369, 2007.

[18] Y. Olgun, "Cisplatin ototoxicity: where we are?" *Journal of International Advanced Otology*, vol. 9, no. 3, pp. 403–416, 2013.

[19] L. P. Rybak, K. Husain, C. Morris, C. Whitworth, and S. Somani, "Effect of protective agents against cisplatin ototoxicity," *American Journal of Otology*, vol. 21, no. 4, pp. 513–520, 2000.

[20] K. C. M. Campbell, J. Kalkanis, and F. R. Glatz, "Ototoxicity: mechanisms, protective agents, and monitoring," *Current Opinion in Otolaryngology and Head and Neck Surgery*, vol. 8, no. 5, pp. 436–440, 2000.

[21] K. Ikeda, H. Sunose, and T. Takasaka, "Effects of free radicals on the intracellular calcium concentration in the isolated outer hair cell of the guinea pig cochlea," *Acta Oto-Laryngologica*, vol. 113, no. 1-2, pp. 137–141, 1993.

[22] D. Mukherjea, S. Jajoo, C. Whitworth et al., "Short interfering RNA against transient receptor potential vanilloid 1 attenuates cisplatin-induced hearing loss in the rat," *Journal of Neuroscience*, vol. 28, no. 49, pp. 13056–13065, 2008.

[23] T. Karasawa and P. S. Steyger, "An integrated view of cisplatin-induced nephrotoxicity and ototoxicity," *Toxicology Letters*, vol. 237, no. 3, pp. 219–227, 2015.

[24] N. C. Schmitt, E. W. Rubel, and N. M. Nathanson, "Cisplatin-induced hair cell death requires STAT1 and is attenuated by

epigallocatechin gallate," *Journal of Neuroscience*, vol. 29, no. 12, pp. 3843–3851, 2009.

[25] F. Chirtes and S. Albu, "Prevention and restoration of hearing loss associated with the use of cisplatin," *BioMed Research International*, vol. 2014, Article ID 925485, 2014.

[26] A. Callejo, L. Sedó-Cabezón, I. Juan, and J. Llorens, "Cisplatin-induced ototoxicity: effects, mechanisms and protection strategies," *Toxics*, vol. 3, no. 3, pp. 268–293, 2015.

[27] L. P. Rybak and V. Ramkumar, "Ototoxicity," *Kidney International*, vol. 72, no. 8, pp. 931–935, 2007.

[28] J. Schacht, A. E. Talaska, and L. P. Rybak, "Cisplatin and aminoglycoside antibiotics: hearing loss and its prevention," *The Anatomical Record: Advances in Integrative Anatomy and Evolutionary Biology*, vol. 295, no. 11, pp. 1837–1850, 2012.

[29] M. Sakamoto, K. Kaga, and T. Kamio, "Extended high-frequency ototoxicity induced by the first administration of cisplatin," *Otolaryngology—Head and Neck Surgery*, vol. 122, no. 6, pp. 828–833, 2000.

[30] R. R. Reddel, R. F. Kefford, J. M. Grant, A. S. Coates, R. M. Fox, and M. H. Tattersall, "Ototoxicity in patients receiving cisplatin: importance of dose and method of drug administration," *Cancer Treatment Reports*, vol. 66, no. 1, pp. 19–23, 1982.

[31] M. J. Moroso and R. L. Blair, "A review of cis-platinum ototoxicity," *Journal of Otolaryngology*, vol. 12, no. 6, pp. 365–369, 1983.

[32] G. S. Waters, M. Ahmad, A. Katsarkas, G. Stanimir, and J. McKay, "Ototoxicity Due to Cis-diamminedichloro-platinum in the treatment of ovarian cancer: influence of dosage and schedule of administration," *Ear and Hearing*, vol. 12, no. 2, pp. 91–102, 1991.

[33] C.-M. Schmidt, A. Knief, A. K. Lagosch, D. Deuster, and A. Am Zehnhoff-Dinnesen, "Left-right asymmetry in hearing loss following cisplatin therapy in children—the left ear is slightly but significantly more affected," *Ear and Hearing*, vol. 29, no. 6, pp. 830–837, 2008.

[34] V. Jenkins, R. Low, and S. Mitra, "Hearing sensitivity in women following chemotherapy treatment for breast cancer: results from a pilot study," *Breast*, vol. 18, no. 5, pp. 279–283, 2009.

[35] C. Bokemeyer, C. C. Berger, J. T. Hartmann et al., "Analysis of risk factors for cisplatin-induced ototoxicity in patients with testicular cancer," *British Journal of Cancer*, vol. 77, no. 8, pp. 1355–1362, 1998.

[36] A. Dutta, M. D. Venkatesh, and R. C. Kashyap, "Study of the effects of chemotherapy on auditory function," *Indian Journal of Otolaryngology and Head and Neck Surgery*, vol. 57, no. 3, pp. 226–228, 2005.

[37] G. C. Allen, C. Tiu, K. Koike, A. K. Ritchey, M. Kurs-Lasky, and M. K. Wax, "Transient-evoked otoacoustic emissions in children after cisplatin chemotherapy," *Otolaryngology—Head and Neck Surgery*, vol. 118, no. 5, pp. 584–588, 1998.

[38] J. Kopelman, A. S. Budnick, R. B. Sessions, M. B. Kramer, and G. Y. Wong, "Ototoxicity of high-dose cisplatin by bolus administration in patients with advanced cancers and normal hearing," *Laryngoscope*, vol. 98, no. 8, pp. 858–864, 1988.

[39] M. A. Gratton, R. J. Salvi, B. A. Kamen, and S. S. Saunders, "Interaction of cisplatin and noise on the peripheral auditory system," *Hearing Research*, vol. 50, no. 1-2, pp. 211–223, 1990.

[40] R. M. Barr-Hamilton, L. M. Matheson, and D. G. Keay, "Ototoxicity of cis-platinum and its relationship to eye colour," *Journal of Laryngology and Otology*, vol. 105, no. 1, pp. 7–11, 1991.

[41] M. A. Mujica-Mota, J. Schermbrucker, and S. J. Daniel, "Eye color as a risk factor for acquired sensorineural hearing loss: a review," *Hearing Research*, vol. 320, pp. 1–10, 2015.

[42] B. S. Larsson, "Interaction between chemicals and melanin," *Pigment Cell Research*, vol. 6, no. 3, pp. 127–133, 1993.

[43] G. Kirkim, Y. Olgun, S. Aktas et al., "Is there a gender-related susceptibility for cisplatin ototoxicity?" *European Archives of Oto-Rhino-Laryngology*, vol. 272, no. 10, pp. 2755–2763, 2015.

[44] P. P. Coradini, L. Cigana, S. G. A. Selistre, L. S. Rosito, and A. L. Brunetto, "Ototoxicity from cisplatin therapy in childhood cancer," *Journal of Pediatric Hematology/Oncology*, vol. 29, no. 6, pp. 355–360, 2007.

[45] L. Helson, E. Okonkwo, L. Anton, and E. Cvitkovic, "Cis-platinum ototoxicity," *Clinical Toxicology*, vol. 13, no. 4, pp. 469–478, 1978.

[46] L. B. Melamed, M. A. Selim, and D. Schuchman, "Cisplatin ototoxicity in gynecologic cancer patients. A preliminary report," *Cancer*, vol. 55, no. 1, pp. 41–43, 1985.

[47] M. S. Malgonde, P. Nagpure, and M. Kumar, "Audiometric patterns in ototoxicity after radiotherapy and chemotherapy in patients of head and neck cancers," *Indian Journal of Palliative Care*, vol. 21, no. 2, pp. 164–167, 2015.

[48] H. Whitehorn, M. Sibanda, M. Lacerda et al., "High prevalence of cisplatin-induced ototoxicity in Cape Town, South Africa," *South African Medical Journal*, vol. 104, no. 4, pp. 288–291, 2014.

[49] A. Nitz, E. Kontopantelis, S. Bielack et al., "Prospective evaluation of cisplatin- and carboplatin-mediated ototoxicity in paediatric and adult soft tissue and osteosarcoma patients," *Oncology Letters*, vol. 5, no. 1, pp. 311–315, 2013.

[50] A. H. B. Dell'Aringa, M. L. Isaac, G. V. Arruda et al., "Audiological findings in patients treated with radio- and concomitant chemotherapy for head and neck tumors," *Radiation Oncology*, vol. 4, no. 1, article 53, 2009.

[51] C. Schultz, M. V. S. Goffi-Gomez, P. H. P. Liberman, and A. L. Carvalho, "Report on hearing loss in oncology," *Brazilian Journal of Otorhinolaryngology*, vol. 75, no. 5, pp. 634–641, 2009.

[52] C. L. Zuur, Y. J. W. Simis, R. S. Verkaik et al., "Hearing loss due to concurrent daily low-dose cisplatin chemoradiation for locally advanced head and neck cancer," *Radiotherapy and Oncology*, vol. 89, no. 1, pp. 38–43, 2008.

[53] D. Strumberg, S. Brügge, M. W. Korn et al., "Evaluation of long-term toxicity in patients after cisplatin-based chemotherapy for non-seminomatous testicular cancer," *Annals of Oncology*, vol. 13, no. 2, pp. 229–236, 2002.

[54] J. L. Nagy, D. J. Adelstein, C. W. Newman, L. A. Rybicki, T. W. Rice, and P. Lavertu, "Cisplatin ototoxicity. The importance of baseline audiometry," *American Journal of Clinical Oncology: Cancer Clinical Trials*, vol. 22, no. 3, pp. 305–308, 1999.

[55] K. R. Knight, D. P. Kraemer, C. Winter, and E. A. Neuwelt, "Early changes in auditory function as a result of platinum chemotherapy: use of extended high-frequency audiometry and evoked distortion product otoacoustic emissions," *Journal of Clinical Oncology*, vol. 25, no. 10, pp. 1190–1195, 2007.

[56] P. Bertolini, M. Lassalle, G. Mercier et al., "Platinum compound-related ototoxicity in children: long-term follow-up reveals continuous worsening of hearing loss," *Journal of Pediatric Hematology/Oncology*, vol. 26, no. 10, pp. 649–655, 2004.

[57] P. Stavroulaki, N. Apostolopoulos, J. Segas, M. Tsakanikos, and G. Adamopoulos, "Evoked otoacoustic emissions—an approach for monitoring cisplatin induced ototoxicity in children," *International Journal of Pediatric Otorhinolaryngology*, vol. 59, no. 1, pp. 47–57, 2001.

[58] N. Tye-Murray, *Foundations of Aural Rehabilitation: Children, Adults, and Their Family Members*, Cengage Learning, Boston, Mass, USA, 2014.

[59] K. G. Herbst and C. Humphrey, "Hearing impairment and mental state in the elderly living at home," *British Medical Journal*, vol. 281, no. 6245, pp. 903–905, 1980.

[60] E. A. Neuwelt and P. Brock, "Critical need for international consensus on ototoxicity assessment criteria," *Journal of Clinical Oncology*, vol. 28, no. 10, pp. 1630–1632, 2010.

[61] T. Langer, A. am Zehnhoff-Dinnesen, S. Radtke, J. Meitert, and O. Zolk, "Understanding platinum-induced ototoxicity," *Trends in Pharmacological Sciences*, vol. 34, no. 8, pp. 458–469, 2013.

[62] A. Yancey, M. S. Harris, A. Egbelakin, J. Gilbert, D. B. Pisoni, and J. Renbarger, "Risk factors for cisplatin-associated ototoxicity in pediatric oncology patients," *Pediatric Blood & Cancer*, vol. 59, no. 1, pp. 144–148, 2012.

[63] J. G. Gurney, J. M. Tersak, K. K. Ness, W. Landier, K. K. Matthay, and M. L. Schmidt, "Hearing loss, quality of life, and academic problems in long-term neuroblastoma survivors: a report from the Children's Oncology Group," *Pediatrics*, vol. 120, no. 5, pp. e1229–e1236, 2007.

[64] A. Jemal, R. Siegel, J. Xu, and E. Ward, "Cancer statistics, 2010," *CA Cancer Journal for Clinicians*, vol. 60, no. 5, pp. 277–300, 2010.

[65] R. L. Siegel, K. D. Miller, and A. Jemal, "Cancer statistics, 2015," *CA Cancer Journal for Clinicians*, vol. 65, no. 1, pp. 5–29, 2015.

[66] D. Konrad-Martin, W. J. Helt, K. M. Reavis et al., "Ototoxicity: early detection and monitoring," *The ASHA Leader*, vol. 10, pp. 1–14, 2005.

[67] S. A. Fausti, D. J. Wilmington, P. V. Helt, W. J. Helt, and D. Konrad-Martin, "Hearing health and care: the need for improved hearing loss prevention and hearing conservation practices," *Journal of Rehabilitation Research and Development*, vol. 42, no. 4, supplement 2, pp. 45–61, 2005.

[68] L. C. B. Jacob, F. P. Aguiar, A. A. Tomiasi, S. N. Tschoeke, and R. F. De Bitencourt, "Auditory monitoring in ototoxicity," *Brazilian Journal of Otorhinolaryngology*, vol. 72, no. 6, pp. 836–844, 2006.

[69] American Speech-Langauge-Hearing Association, "Audiologic management of individuals receiving cochleotoxic drug therapy," *ASHA*, vol. 36, supplement 12, pp. 11–19, 1994.

[70] American Academy of Audiology, Position statement and clinical practice guidelines: ototoxicity monitoring, 2009, http://audiology-web.s3.amazonaws.com/migrated/OtoMonGuidelines.pdf_539974c40999c1.58842217.pdf.

[71] T. Dabrowski and F. Hussain-Said, "The audiologists role in ototoxicity monitoring," *Advance for Audiologists*, vol. 10, no. 3, p. 54, 2010.

[72] N. Schellack, A. M. Wium, K. Ehlert, Y. Van Aswegen, and A. Gous, "Establishing a pharmacotherapy induced ototoxicity programme within a service-learning approach," *The South African Journal of Communication Disorders*, vol. 62, no. 1, pp. 1–7, 2015.

[73] S. A. Fausti, W. J. Helt, and J. S. Gordon, "Audiologic monitoring for ototoxicity and patients management," in *Pharmacology and Ototoxicity for Audiologists*, C. K. M. Campbell, Ed., pp. 230–251, Thomson Delmar Learning: United States, 2007.

[74] K. K. Yu, C. H. Choi, Y.-H. An et al., "Comparison of the effectiveness of monitoring cisplatin-induced ototoxicity with extended high-frequency pure-tone audiometry or distortion-product otoacoustic emission," *Korean Journal of Audiology*, vol. 18, no. 2, pp. 58–68, 2014.

[75] S. A. Fausti, V. D. Larson, D. Noffsinger, R. H. Wilson, D. S. Phillips, and C. G. Fowler, "High-frequency audiometric monitoring strategies for early detection of ototoxicity," *Ear and Hearing*, vol. 15, no. 3, pp. 232–239, 1994.

[76] K. C. M. Campbell, "Detection of ototoxicity," *Seminars in Hearing*, vol. 32, no. 2, pp. 196–202, 2011.

[77] T. Frank, "High-frequency (8 to 16 kHz) reference thresholds and intrasubject threshold variability relative to ototoxicity criteria using a Sennheiser HDA 200 earphone," *Ear and Hearing*, vol. 22, no. 2, pp. 161–168, 2001.

[78] D. Osterhammel, "High frequency audiometry. Clinical aspects," *Scandinavian Audiology*, vol. 9, no. 4, pp. 249–256, 1980.

[79] R. S. Chauhan, R. K. Saxena, and S. Varshey, "The role of ultrahigh-frequency audiometry in the early detection of systemic drug-induced hearing loss," *Ear, Nose & Throat Journal*, vol. 90, no. 5, pp. 218–222, 2011.

[80] B. M. Mayosi, A. J. Flisher, U. G. Lalloo, F. Sitas, S. M. Tollman, and D. Bradshaw, "The burden of non-communicable diseases in South Africa," *The Lancet*, vol. 374, no. 9693, pp. 934–947, 2009.

[81] L. P. Rybak, C. A. Whitworth, D. Mukherjea, and V. Ramkumar, "Mechanisms of cisplatin-induced ototoxicity and prevention," *Hearing Research*, vol. 226, no. 1-2, pp. 157–167, 2007.

[82] M. Y. Huang and J. Schacht, "Drug-induced ototoxicity: pathogenesis and prevention," *Medical Toxicology and Adverse Drug Experience*, vol. 4, no. 6, pp. 452–467, 1989.

[83] L. P. Rybak and C. A. Whitworth, "Ototoxicity: therapeutic opportunities," *Drug Discovery Today*, vol. 10, no. 19, pp. 1313–1321, 2005.

[84] R. J. Reiter, D.-X. Tan, A. Korkmaz, and L. Fuentes-Broto, "Drug-mediated ototoxicity and tinnitus: alleviation with melatonin," *Journal of Physiology and Pharmacology*, vol. 62, no. 2, pp. 151–157, 2011.

[85] J. G. Kalkanis, C. Whitworth, and L. P. Rybak, "Vitamin E reduces cisplatin ototoxicity," *Laryngoscope*, vol. 114, no. 3, pp. 538–542, 2004.

[86] W.-T. Choe, N. Chinosornvatana, and K. W. Chang, "Prevention of cisplatin ototoxicity using transtympanic N-acetylcysteine and lactate," *Otology & Neurotology*, vol. 25, no. 6, pp. 910–915, 2004.

[87] A. L. Hughes, N. Hussain, R. Pafford, and K. Parham, "Dexamethasone otoprotection in a multidose cisplatin ototoxicity mouse model," *Otolaryngology—Head and Neck Surgery (United States)*, vol. 150, no. 1, pp. 115–120, 2014.

[88] Y. Olgun, G. Kýrkím, E. Kolatan et al., "Friend or foe? Effect of oral resveratrol on cisplatin ototoxicity," *Laryngoscope*, vol. 124, no. 3, pp. 760–766, 2014.

[89] T. Marshak, M. Steiner, M. Kaminer, L. Levy, and A. Shupak, "Prevention of cisplatin-induced hearing loss by intratympanic dexamethasone: a randomized controlled study," *Otolaryngology—Head and Neck Surgery*, vol. 150, no. 6, pp. 983–990, 2014.

[90] A. A. McCall, E. E. L. Swan, J. T. Borenstein, W. F. Sewell, S. G. Kujawa, and M. J. McKenna, "Drug delivery for treatment of inner ear disease: current state of knowledge," *Ear & hearing*, vol. 31, no. 2, pp. 156–165, 2010.

[91] L. P. Rybak, D. Mukherjea, S. Jajoo, and V. Ramkumar, "Cisplatin ototoxicity and protection: clinical and experimental studies," *The Tohoku Journal of Experimental Medicine*, vol. 219, no. 3, pp. 177–186, 2009.

[92] N. G. Govender, N. Maistry, N. Soomar, and J. Paken, "Hearing loss within a marriage: perceptions of the spouse with normal hearing," *South African Family Practice*, vol. 56, no. 1, pp. 50–56, 2014.

[93] S. Neumann and J. Wolfe, "What's new and notable in hearing aids: a friendly guide for parents and hearing aid wearers," *Volta Voices*, vol. 20, no. 3, pp. 24–29, 2013.

[94] V. Parsa, S. Scollie, D. Glista, and A. Seelisch, "Nonlinear frequency compression: effects on sound quality ratings of speech and music," *Trends in Amplification*, vol. 17, no. 1, pp. 54–68, 2013.

12

Neurotoxic Effect of Benzo[a]pyrene and Its Possible Association with 6-Hydroxydopamine Induced Neurobehavioral Changes during Early Adolescence Period in Rats

Saroj Kumar Das,[1,2] Bhupesh Patel,[1] and Manorama Patri[1]

[1]Department of Zoology, School of Life Sciences, Ravenshaw University, Cuttack, Odisha 753003, India
[2]Department of High Altitude Physiology, Defence Institute of High Altitude Research, Leh 901205, India

Correspondence should be addressed to Manorama Patri; mpatri@ravenshawuniversity.ac.in

Academic Editor: Maria Teresa Colomina

Exposure to persistent genotoxicants like benzo[a]pyrene (B[a]P) during postnatal days causes neurobehavioral changes in animal models. However, neurotoxic potential of B[a]P and its association with 6-hydroxydopamine (6-OHDA) induced neurobehavioral changes are yet to be explored. The growth of rat brain peaks at the first week of birth and continues up to one month with the attainment of adolescence. Hence, the present study was conducted on male Wistar rats at postnatal day 5 (PND 5) following single intracisternal administration of B[a]P to compare with neurobehavioral and neurotransmitter changes induced by 6-OHDA at PND 30. Spontaneous motor activity was significantly increased by 6-OHDA showing similar trend following B[a]P administration. Total distance travelled in novel open field arena and elevated plus maze was significantly increased following B[a]P and 6-OHDA administration. Neurotransmitter estimation showed significant alleviation of dopamine in striatum following B[a]P and 6-OHDA administration. Histopathological studies of striatum by hematoxylin and eosin (H&E) staining revealed the neurodegenerative potential of B[a]P and 6-OHDA. Our results indicate that B[a]P-induced spontaneous motor hyperactivity in rats showed symptomatic similarities with 6-OHDA. In conclusion, early postnatal exposure to B[a]P in rats causing neurobehavioral changes may lead to serious neurodegenerative consequences during adolescence.

1. Introduction

Exposure to environmental contaminants poses a significant threat to normal growth and differentiation of the developing brain [1]. It has also been reported that nervous system is susceptible to toxic chemicals and subsequent developmental perturbation may lead to long-term irreversible consequences that affect nervous system function in adult animals [2]. Benzo[a]pyrene (B[a]P), a polycyclic aromatic hydrocarbon (PAH), is known for its neurotoxic potential causing neurobehavioral alterations in animal models [3]. Reports also suggest that exposure to B[a]P through early postnatal development leads to impairment in locomotor activity in adolescence [4]. A recent report revealed that subchronic oral administration of B[a]P in rats leads to spontaneous locomotor hyperactivity [5]. Behavioral and motor dysfunction following exposure to environmental toxicants like B[a]P is well documented but the neurodegenerative potential of these compounds cannot be ignored.

Exposure to B[a]P produces neuromuscular, physiological, autonomic abnormalities and also shows decreased responsiveness to sensory stimuli [6, 7]. Earlier reports suggest that microinjection of diesel exhaust fraction containing PAH into rat hippocampus and striatum leads to neuronal lesions [8]. Epidemiological study also revealed that parental occupational exposure to PAH was associated with an increased risk of neuroectodermal tumors in children [9]. Maternal exposure to airborne PAHs during pregnancy was associated with a reduction in head circumference, lower IQ, and reduced cognitive functioning in children [10].

Investigation into pathophysiological manifestations following exposure to persistent anthropogenic neurotoxicants like benzo[a]pyrene might address new insight into their neurodegenerative potential. Studies have also addressed the effect of highly specific neurotoxin 6-hydroxydopamine (6-OHDA) on catecholaminergic neurons with an extensive and irreversible loss of dopaminergic neurons in the mesencephalon which is associated with behavioral deficits [11–13]. Investigation of potential environmental neurotoxicants like B[a]P in animal model provides a new insight into serious human neurodegenerative diseases.

The purpose of the present study was to investigate the neurotoxic potential of B[a]P following intracisternal administration during early phase of postnatal development and its consequences in early adolescent period of rats. We also investigated the neurotoxic effect of benzo[a]pyrene and its possible association with 6-hydroxydopamine induced neurobehavioral changes during early adolescence period.

2. Materials and Methods

2.1. Chemicals and Reagents. The chemicals used in this experimentation were procured from Sigma-Aldrich Chemicals (St. Louis, MO, USA), unless otherwise mentioned such as benzo[a]pyrene (B[a]P, catalogue number B1760), corn oil (catalogue number C8267), 6-hydroxydomine hydrochloride (6-OHDA, catalogue number H4381), and paraformaldehyde.

2.2. Experimental Animals. Pregnant Wistar rats (*Rattus norvegicus*) were maintained in home cages in standard laboratory conditions and fed laboratory chow and filtered water ad libitum. The animals were subjected to 12 hr light and 12 hr dark cycle in standard laboratory environment. Temperature and humidity were maintained at 25–28°C and 60–65%, respectively.

2.3. Experimental Design and Toxicant Administration. Five-day-old male Wistar pups were arbitrarily consigned to lactating dams and intracisternal administration of B[a]P and 6-OHDA was carried out at postnatal day 5 [14]. The B[a]P solution was freshly prepared by dissolving $2 \mu g/kg$ BW of B[a]P into $10 \mu L$ of corn oil and was subsequently used for intracisternal administration while the control rats received only corn oil ($10 \mu L$). Rats of 6-OHDA group were injected with $25 g/kg$, desipramine in $100 \mu L$ (i.p.), 30 minutes before 6-OHDA injection. Then $150 \mu g/kg$ BW of 6-OHDA dissolved in $10 \mu L$ of saline (containing 0.2% ascorbic acid as antioxidant) was injected into rats of 6-OHDA group while rats of control group received $10 \mu L$ saline solution, respectively [15]. Five-day-old male Wistar pups were designated into four groups (12 male pups/group), namely, control A (corn oil); B[a]P (B[a]P dissolved in corn oil); control B (saline); and 6-OHDA (6-OHDA dissolved in saline). We aimed to study the neurodegenerative potential of B[a]P and its symptomatic similarities with 6-OHDA induced neurobehavioral alteration, rather than address the

confounding effect as a result of coadministration of these neurotoxicants.

2.4. Evaluation of Spontaneous Motor Activity (SMA). The standard experimental paradigm was followed for evaluation of SMA with slight modification [5]. SMA of rats at PND 30 was individually measured in a home cage with a Supermex system (Muromachi Kikai, Ikeda, Japan). The sensor monitored the motion and movement of the animal. Rats were maintained on a 12 h light: dark cycle during the recording and total distance covered for a period of 24 hr was recorded and the data was represented in 2 hr intervals as absolute time. Food and water were supplied at the beginning of recordings and rats were never disturbed in anyway.

2.5. Open Field Test. Open field test was conducted to assess the explorative behavior of rats [16]. Open field activity was monitored in a circular arena (75 m diameter and 1.5 cm height) wall with grey color paint. The animals were placed individually in a specific side of the wall of the arena and the time spent in the central zone and total distance travelled were automatically monitored for 5 min using ANY Maze software (Stoelting Co., USA). The apparatus was cleaned with 70% ethanol solution after testing each subject.

2.6. Elevated Plus Maze Test. Briefly, elevated plus maze consisted of two opposite open arms (50 cm long × 10 cm wide) and two enclosed arms (50 × 10 × 40 cm) that extended from a common central platform (10 × 10 cm), elevated 75 cm above the floor. Time spent in open arm and total distance travelled were recorded and considered as an indicator of general locomotor activity independent of anxiety [17]. The video-tracking system (ANY Maze software, Stoelting Co., USA) was set for 5 min of recording. The apparatus was cleaned with 70% ethanol and dried with paper towels before testing with another rodent.

2.7. Sample Preparation and Analysis. After completion of behavioral recording, rats of all the experimental groups were sacrificed after being deeply anesthetized with sodium pentobarbital and subsequently perfused intracardially with ice-cold 0.1 M phosphate buffer saline (PBS) followed by 4% paraformaldehyde [18]. Brain samples were cryoprotected in 30% sucrose in PBS for 48 hr and then serial cryosectioning was carried out for histopathological studies. For biochemical and molecular study, rats were sacrificed by cervical dislocation and the requisite brain region was immediately dissected out at 4°C in ice-cold 0.1 M PBS and then snap frozen in liquid nitrogen. The samples were then stored at −80°C until further analysis.

2.8. Quantitative Estimation of Dopamine by HPLC-ECD. Quantification of striatal dopamine level was carried out by high performance liquid chromatography-electrochemical detector (HPLC-ECD) with minor modification [19]. Briefly, 100 mg wet brain tissue (striatum) was homogenized by sonication in 0.5 mL of 0.2 M $HClO_4$ (perchloric acid) containing isoproterenol as an internal standard substance. The homogenized tissue was then kept in ice bath for 30 min.

and then subjected to centrifugation for 2 min. at 20,000 ×g and then the supernatant was added with 1 M sodium acetate to adjust the pH 3.0. After that 10 μL of sample solution was injected into a separation column (Eicompak SC-5ODS, ID 3.0 × 100 mm) in a HPLC-ECD system for measurement of dopamine and the result was expressed as ng/mg of protein.

2.9. Histopathological Study by Hematoxylin and Eosin Staining. Brains were postfixed in 4% paraformaldehyde for 24 hr and then washed for 24 h under running tap water and dehydrated in graded series of ethanol concentrations (50%, 70%, 90%, and 100%) [20]. Then they were cleared in xylene, embedded in paraffin wax, serially sectioned at 7 mm thickness, and stained with hematoxylin and eosin (H&E). The slides were observed under microscope and images of striatal region were taken with requisite magnification with the help of a digital camera (Olympus, BX43F, Japan). The area and perimeter of the neurons were measured with the help of ocular micrometer.

2.10. Statistical Analysis. The mean and standard error of mean of each set, that is, control A, B[a]P, control B, and 6-OHDA, were calculated. The post hoc analysis was done by the Newman-Keuls test in all experimental groups by using one-way ANOVA. Difference below the probability level 0.05 was considered statistically significant. Bonferroni posttest was conducted to study the effect of B[a]P and 6-OHDA on SMA by using two-way ANOVA and difference below the probability level $p < 0.001$ was considered statistically significant.

3. Results

3.1. Assessment of Spontaneous Motor Activity. B[a]P administration to rat neonates at PND 5 led to significant increase in spontaneous motor activity during 24 hr of recording ($F_{(3,528)}$ = 380.8, $p < 0.001$) when compared to rats of control A group (Figure 1). Similarly, intracisternal administration of 6-OHDA to rats pups significantly increased the spontaneous motor activity ($F_{(3,528)}$ = 380.8, $p < 0.001$) with respect to control B and B[a]P treated rats (Figure 1).

3.2. Open Field Test (OFT). Open field test showed significant increase in the stay time at center in B[a]P group as compared to control A ($F_{(3,44)}$ = 11.71, $p < 0.05$) (Figure 2(a)). However the total distance travelled in OFT was significantly augmented following 6-OHDA administration ($F_{(3,44)}$ = 14.69, $p < 0.05$) as compared to control B group (Figure 2(b)). Similarly, there was a significant increase in total distance travelled in B[a]P treated group when compared to control A ($F_{(3,44)}$ = 14.69, $p < 0.05$). The results showed significant increase in total distance travelled in OFT following 6-OHDA administration ($F_{(3,44)}$ = 14.69, $p < 0.05$) which showed similar effects following B[a]P administration.

3.3. Elevated Plus Maze Test (EPM). The analysis of the stay time in open arm following B[a]P administration showed significant increase when compared to the control A group

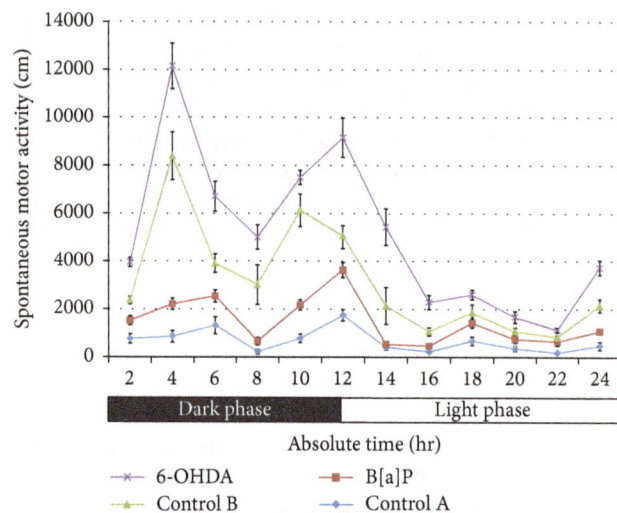

FIGURE 1: Spontaneous motor activity (SMA). Graph showing significant increase ($p < 0.001$) in SMA after 24 hrs of recording following B[a]P and 6-OHDA administration. The data were represented as mean ± SEM ($n = 12$/group).

($F_{(3,44)}$ = 84.96, $p < 0.05$) whereas no significant difference was observed between 6-OHDA and control B groups (Figure 3(a)). The B[a]P and 6-OHDA administration also showed significant increase in total distance travelled in EPM ($F_{(3,44)}$ = 28.23, $p < 0.05$) as compared to control A and control B, respectively (Figure 3(b)).

3.4. Measurement of Dopamine (DA) in Striatum. Dopamine (DA) level in striatum significantly ($F_{(3,20)}$ = 14.79, $p < 0.05$) declined in B[a]P treated group as compared to control A (Figure 4). Comparable depletion of DA was detected in striatum following intracisternal administration of B[a]P as compared to 6-OHDA group ($F_{(3,20)}$ = 14.79, $p < 0.05$) (Figure 4).

3.5. Histopathological Assessment of Striatum by Hematoxylin and Eosin (H&E) Staining. The histopathological examination of striatal region following H&E staining showed significant increase in abnormal striatal neuron morphology in B[a]P and 6-OHDA treated groups (Figure 5(a)). The mean area ($F_{(3,20)}$ = 7.985, $p < 0.05$) and perimeter ($F_{(3,20)}$ = 8.603, $p < 0.05$) of striatal neurons were significantly decreased in B[a]P treated group as compared to control A and similar alleviation of mean area ($F_{(3,20)}$ = 7.985, $p < 0.05$) and perimeter ($F_{(3,20)}$ = 8.603, $p < 0.05$) of striatal neurons was also observed in 6-OHDA group as compared to control B (Figures 5(b) and 5(c)). However, there was a significant increase in pyknotic cell counts in 6-OHDA group when compared with B[a]P.

4. Discussion

Polycyclic aromatic hydrocarbons (PAHs) are predominantly anthropogenic in source and are liberated as a consequence of partial combustion carbon containing organic compounds

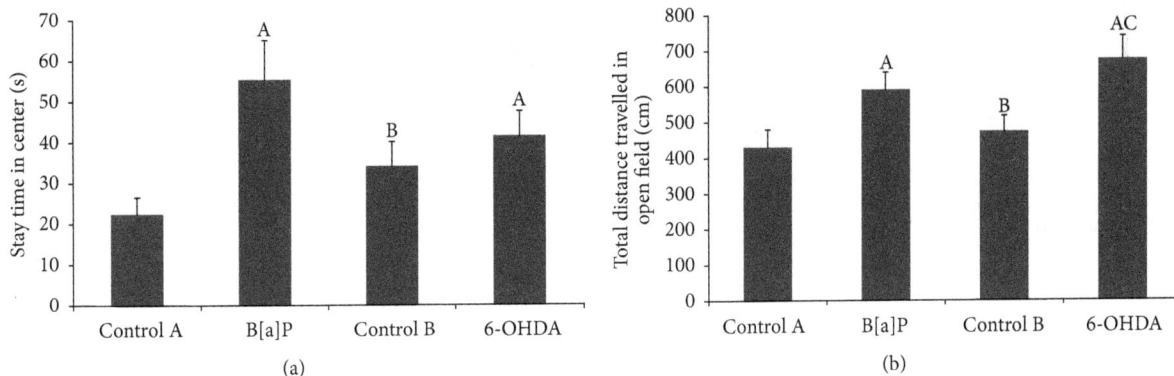

FIGURE 2: Open field test. Graphs showing alterations in time spent in central zone and total distance travelled in open field arena ((a) and (b)). Values are expressed as mean ± SEM (n = 12/group). "A" denotes $p < 0.05$ when compared to control A group, "B" denotes $p < 0.05$ when compared to B[a]P group, and "C" denotes $p < 0.05$ when compared to control B group.

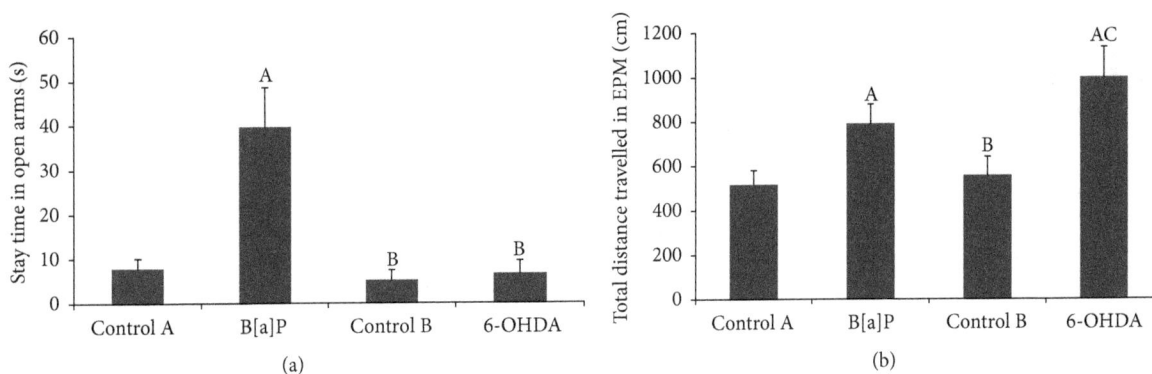

FIGURE 3: Elevated plus maze test. Graphs showing alterations in (a) time spent in open arm and (b) total distance travelled in elevated plus maze. Values are expressed as mean ± SEM (n = 12/group). "A" denotes $p < 0.05$ when compared to control A group, "B" denotes $p < 0.05$ when compared to B[a]P group, and "C" denotes $p < 0.05$ when compared to control B group.

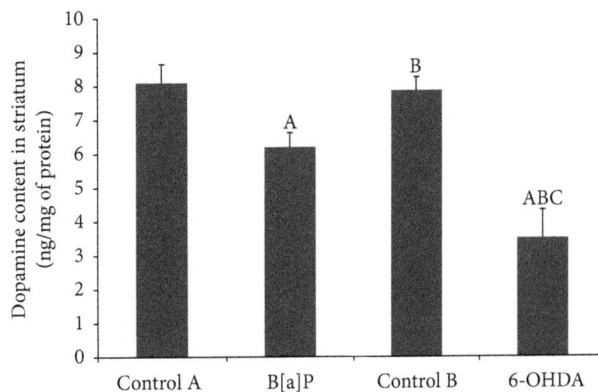

FIGURE 4: Quantification of dopamine level in striatum by HPLC-ECD. The graph showed significant alteration in striatal dopamine level following B[a]P and 6-OHDA administration when compared to their respective control groups. Values are expressed as mean ± SEM (n = 6/group). "A" denotes $p < 0.05$ when compared to control A group, "B" denotes $p < 0.05$ when compared to B[a]P group, and "C" denotes $p < 0.05$ when compared to control B group.

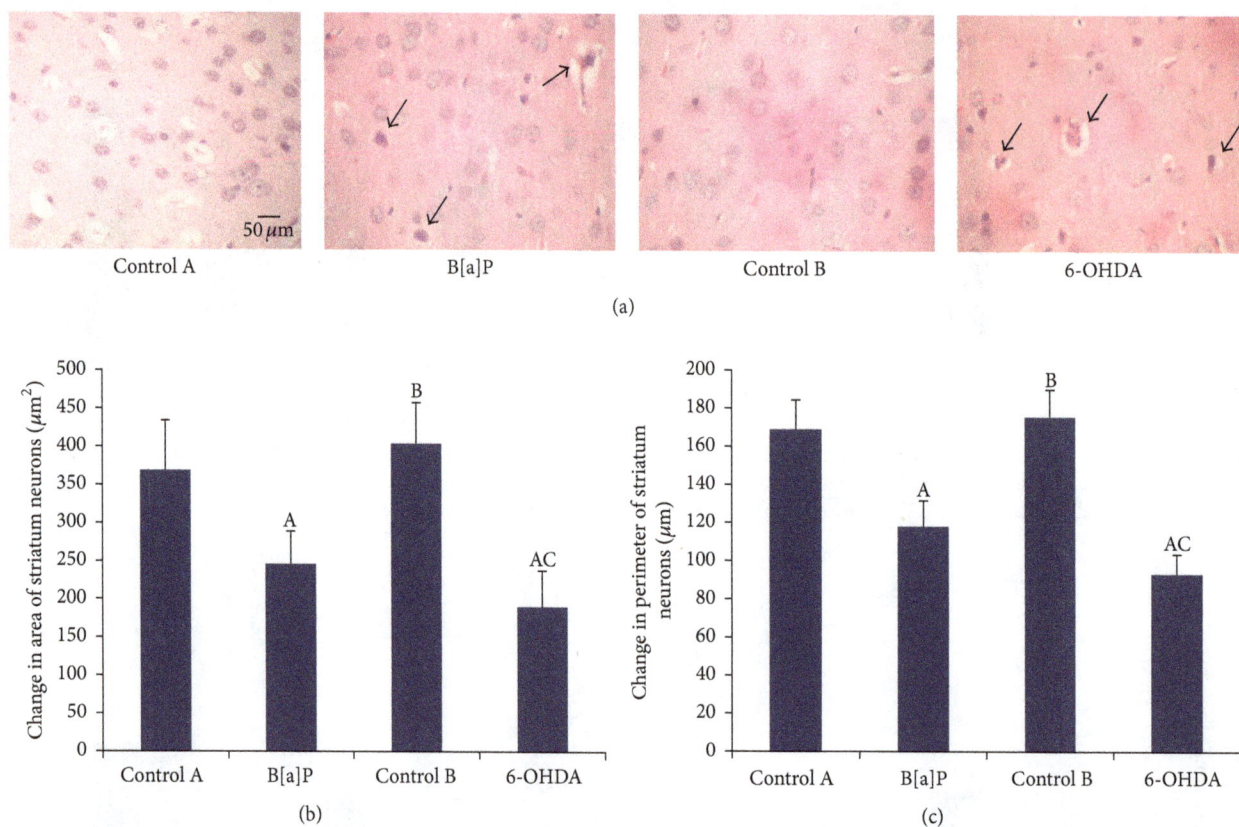

FIGURE 5: Histopathological study by hematoxylin and eosin staining. Representative microscopic images of hematoxylin and eosin staining of striatal neurons (a). Magnification at 10x (scale bar = 50 μm). Arrow head depicts degenerative neurons. Histogram represents striatal neuronal area and perimeter ((b) and (c)). Values are expressed as mean ± SEM (n = 6/group). "A" denotes $p < 0.05$ when compared to control A group, "B" denotes $p < 0.05$ when compared to B[a]P group, and "C" denotes $p < 0.05$ when compared to control B group.

[21, 22]. Benzo[a]pyrene (B[a]P) is extensively used as a prototype of PAH which demonstrates significant genotoxicity. Further, humans and rodents differ with respect to their sensitivity to varying doses of B[a]P and previous findings suggested that humans were 10–100 times more sensitive to toxic effects of B[a]P than rodents [23]. Additionally, infants and children are exceptionally susceptible to environmental neurotoxicants at levels far below those known to harm adults [24]. As the early phase of postnatal life is involved with rapid phase of growth and development, it becomes a target of exposure to environment neurotoxicants, the rapid growth period in rat neonates straddling the first (1-2) weeks of life to acquire numerous novel motor and sensory skills during the early stage of development [25].

B[a]P induced motor dysfunction leading to spontaneous motor hyperactivity in rodents addresses possible consequences of serious neurological problems [5]. Several studies have been conducted to show spontaneous motor dysfunction and its association with neurodegenerative symptoms following administration of potent neurotoxicants [26, 27]. Substantial evidence suggests that early postnatal exposure to B[a]P drastically alters the motor functions [28]. This neurodegenerative predisposition is potentially related to alleviated dopamine level at striatum [29]. During early stage

of postnatal development striatal dopaminergic neurons regulate the storage and release of dopamine. As the blood-brain barrier is not fully developed in rat neonates, 6-OHDA, a potent neurotoxicant, might adversely affect the brain development during early adolescence period.

Hence, the present study was conducted at PND 5 in male Wistar pups following single intracisternal administration of B[a]P that showed significant increase in spontaneous motor activity at PND 30. The above findings are in agreement with the earlier studies [5]. Further investigation showed that neonatal 6-OHDA administration leads to spontaneous motor hyperactivity in adolescent rats and the findings are in agreement with previous reports [30]. Novel open field exploration study was also considered to address the spontaneous locomotor activity [31]. Our results demonstrated that 6-OHDA administration leads to significant increase in total distance travelled in both OFT and EPM and similar behavioral change was also found after B[a]P administration. The motor dysfunction following B[a]P administration was found to be positively associated with the neurobehavioral manifestation induced by potent neurotoxicant, that is, 6-OHDA, and the above findings are in agreement with previous reports [32, 33]. The behavioral observations as stay time in OFT and EPM significantly increased in the group to which B[a]P was administered as compared to control. However, no significant difference was observed after 6-OHDA administration, from which it can be inferred that intracisternal B[a]P administration has anxiolytic potential and the findings are in agreement with the previous report [4].

We extended our findings to ascertain the possible relationship of neurobehavioral manifestation induced by intracisternal administration of B[a]P with that of dopamine level in striatum of adolescent rats. Our results showed significant alleviation of striatal dopamine level following B[a]P administration and the result finds support from previous report [20]. Similarly, 6-OHDA administration leads to significant decrease in dopamine level as compared to B[a]P and the above findings are in agreement with previous report [34, 35]. The possible effect of neonatal B[a]P administration on striatal dopamine level during adolescence was found to be linked with the effect of 6-OHDA. The findings of striatal dopamine alleviation by B[a]P administration were significantly associated with altered histopathological observation. Our results demonstrated a significant decrease in area and perimeter of striatal neurons following B[a]P administration. The above findings are comparable with the neurodegenerative symptoms exhibited by 6-OHDA and our results are supported by previous report [15]. The possible neurodegenerative consequences following B[a]P administration at PND 5 and its neurobehavioral manifestation in adolescent rats may be associated with reduced striatal dopamine level. The basic findings of the present study indicate that 6-OHDA produces alterations in behavior that are similar to those produced by B[a]P.

5. Conclusion

In conclusion, the findings suggest that early postnatal life is highly susceptible to environmental neurotoxicants leading to neurobehavioral perturbation in adolescence. Early exposure to potent environmental neurotoxicants like B[a]P may lead to reduction in dopamine neurotransmitter level that can cause striatal neurodegeneration. We addressed a pioneer effect of B[a]P exposure during early postnatal life leading to neurodegenerative processes and its symptomatic similarities with progressive neurodegenerative diseases.

Ethical Approval

All protocols followed in the experiments were ratified by the ethics board of the institute (SOA University, Odisha, India) according to the guidelines of the "Committee for the Purpose of Control and Supervision of Experiments on Animals" of the Govt. of India. Utmost care was taken to decrease suffering of animals throughout the sampling and drug administration.

Conflict of Interests

The authors declare no competing interests.

Acknowledgments

Research funding from the Department of Science and Technology, WOS A Fellowship (No. SR/WOS-A/LS-22/2009) to Manorama Patri are acknowledged. The authors acknowledge the contribution of Mr. Ritendra Mishra, DIHAR, DRDO, who helped in copyediting and proofreading of the paper.

References

[1] J. L. Jacobson and S. W. Jacobson, "Intellectual impairment in children exposed to polychlorinated biphenyls in utero," *The New England Journal of Medicine*, vol. 335, no. 11, pp. 783–789, 1996.

[2] S. J. Barone, K. P. Das, T. L. Lassiter, and L. D. White, "Vulnerable processes of nervous system development: a review of markers and methods," *NeuroToxicology*, vol. 21, no. 1-2, pp. 15–36, 2000.

[3] C. R. Saunders, S. K. Das, A. Ramesh, D. C. Shockley, and S. Mukherjee, "Benzo(a)pyrene-induced acute neurotoxicity in the F-344 rat: role of oxidative stress," *Journal of Applied Toxicology*, vol. 26, no. 5, pp. 427–438, 2006.

[4] C. Chen, Y. Tang, X. Jiang et al., "Early postnatal benzo(a)pyrene exposure in sprague-dawley rats causes persistent neurobehavioral impairments that emerge postnatally and continue into adolescence and adulthood," *Toxicological Sciences*, vol. 125, no. 1, Article ID kfr265, pp. 248–261, 2012.

[5] É. S. Maciel, R. Biasibetti, A. P. Costa et al., "Subchronic oral administration of Benzo[a]pyrene impairs motor and cognitive behavior and modulates S100B levels and MAPKs in rats," *Neurochemical Research*, vol. 39, no. 4, pp. 731–740, 2014.

[6] C. R. Saunders, D. C. Shockley, and M. E. Knuckles, "Behavioral effects induced by acute exposure to benzo(a) pyrene in F-344 rats," *Neurotoxicity Research*, vol. 3, no. 6, pp. 557–579, 2001.

[7] C. R. Saunders, A. Ramesh, and D. C. Shockley, "Modulation of neurotoxic behavior in F-344 rats by temporal disposition of benzo(a)pyrene," *Toxicology Letters*, vol. 129, no. 1-2, pp. 33–45, 2002.

[8] H. Andersson, E. Lindqvist, R. Westerholm, K. Grägg, J. Almén, and L. Olson, "Neurotoxic effects of fractionated diesel exhausts following microinjections in rat hippocampus and striatum," *Environmental Research*, vol. 76, no. 1, pp. 41–51, 1998.

[9] S. Cordier, B. Lefeuvre, G. Filippini et al., "Parental occupation, occupational exposure to solvents and polycyclic aromatic hydrocarbons and risk of childhood brain tumors (Italy, France, Spain)," *Cancer Causes and Control*, vol. 8, no. 5, pp. 688–697, 1997.

[10] F. P. Perera, V. Rauh, W.-Y. Tsai et al., "Effects of transplacental exposure to environmental pollutants on birth outcomes in a multiethnic population," *Environmental Health Perspectives*, vol. 111, no. 2, pp. 201–205, 2003.

[11] M. J. Zigmond and E. M. Stricker, "Animal models of parkinsonism using selective neurotoxins: clinical and basic implications," *International Review of Neurobiology*, vol. 31, pp. 1–79, 1989.

[12] M. Gerlach and P. Riederer, "Animal models of Parkinson's disease: an empirical comparison with the phenomenology of the disease in man," *Journal of Neural Transmission*, vol. 103, no. 8-9, pp. 987–1041, 1996.

[13] R. Iancu, P. Mohapel, P. Brundin, and G. Paul, "Behavioral characterization of a unilateral 6-OHDA-lesion model of Parkinson's disease in mice," *Behavioural Brain Research*, vol. 162, no. 1, pp. 1–10, 2005.

[14] B. A. Shaywitz, R. D. Yager, and J. H. Klopper, "Selective brain dopamine depletion in developing rats: an experimental model of minimal brain dysfunction," *Science*, vol. 191, no. 4224, pp. 305–308, 1976.

[15] O. T. Korkmaz, H. Ay, E. Ulupinar, and N. Tunçel, "Vasoactive intestinal peptide enhances striatal plasticity and prevents dopaminergic cell loss in Parkinsonian rats," *Journal of Molecular Neuroscience*, vol. 48, no. 3, pp. 565–573, 2012.

[16] S. K. Das, I. Baitharu, K. Barhwal, S. K. Hota, and S. B. Singh, "Early mood behavioral changes following exposure to monotonous environment during isolation stress is associated with altered hippocampal synaptic plasticity in male rats," *Neuroscience Letters*, vol. 612, pp. 231–237, 2016.

[17] H. Khoshbouei, M. Cecchi, and D. A. Morilak, "Amplication of the noradrenergic response to stress elicits galanin-mediated anxiolytic effects in central amygdala," *Pharmacology, Biochemistry & Behavior*, vol. 71, no. 3, pp. 407–417, 2002.

[18] S. K. Das, K. Barhwal, S. K. Hota, M. K. Thakur, and R. B. Srivastava, "Disrupting monotony during social isolation stress prevents early development of anxiety and depression like traits in male rats," *BMC Neuroscience*, vol. 16, article 2, 2015.

[19] P. Stephanou, M. Konstandi, P. Pappas, and M. Marselos, "Alterations in central monoaminergic neurotrasmission induced by polycyclic aromatic hydrocarbons in rats," *European Journal of Drug Metabolism and Pharmacokinetics*, vol. 23, no. 4, pp. 475–481, 1998.

[20] D. Davenport, G. Camougis, and J. F. Hickok, "Analyses of the behaviour of commensals in host-factor. 1. A hesioned polychaete and a pinnotherid crab," *Animal Behaviour*, vol. 8, no. 3-4, pp. 209–218, 1960.

[21] A. Motelay-Massei, D. Ollivon, B. Garban, K. Tiphagne-Larcher, I. Zimmerlin, and M. Chevreuil, "PAHs in the bulk atmospheric deposition of the Seine river basin: source identification and apportionment by ratios, multivariate statistical techniques and scanning electron microscopy," *Chemosphere*, vol. 67, no. 2, pp. 312–321, 2007.

[22] M. Patri, A. Singh, and B. N. Mallick, "Protective role of noradrenaline in benzo[a]pyrene-induced learning impairment in developing rat," *Journal of Neuroscience Research*, vol. 91, no. 11, pp. 1450–1462, 2013.

[23] D. R. Davila, D. L. Romero, and S. W. Burchiel, "Human T cells are highly sensitive to suppression of mitogenesis by polycyclic aromatic hydrocarbons and this effect is differentially reversed by α-naphthoflavone," *Toxicology and Applied Pharmacology*, vol. 139, no. 2, pp. 333–341, 1996.

[24] B. Weiss, "Vulnerability of children and the developing brain to neurotoxic hazards," *Environmental Health Perspectives*, vol. 108, no. 3, pp. 375–381, 2000.

[25] B. Kolb and I. Q. Whishaw, "Plasticity in the neocortex: mechanisms underlying recovery from early brain damage," *Progress in Neurobiology*, vol. 32, no. 4, pp. 235–276, 1989.

[26] L.-G. Chia, D.-R. Ni, L.-J. Cheng, J.-S. Kuo, F.-C. Cheng, and G. Dryhurst, "Effects of 1-methyl-4-phenyl-1,2,3,6-tetrahydropyridine and 5,7-dihydroxytryptamine on the locomotor activity and striatal amines in C57BL/6 mice," *Neuroscience Letters*, vol. 218, no. 1, pp. 67–71, 1996.

[27] E. Rousselet, C. Joubert, J. Callebert et al., "Behavioral changes are not directly related to striatal monoamine levels, number of nigral neurons, or dose of Parkinsonian toxin MPTP in mice," *Neurobiology of Disease*, vol. 14, no. 2, pp. 218–228, 2003.

[28] J. Bouayed, F. Desor, H. Rammal et al., "Effects of lactational exposure to benzo[α]pyrene (B[α]P) on postnatal neurodevelopment, neuronal receptor gene expression and behaviour in mice," *Toxicology*, vol. 259, no. 3, pp. 97–106, 2009.

[29] D. Blum, S. Torch, N. Lambeng et al., "Molecular pathways involved in the neurotoxicity of 6-OHDA, dopamine and MPTP: contribution to the apoptotic theory in Parkinson's disease," *Progress in Neurobiology*, vol. 65, no. 2, pp. 135–172, 2001.

[30] Y. Masuo, M. Ishido, M. Morita, S. Oka, and E. Niki, "Motor activity and gene expression in rats with neonatal 6-hydroxydopamine lesions," *Journal of Neurochemistry*, vol. 91, no. 1, pp. 9–19, 2004.

[31] A. B. Richards, T. A. Scheel, K. Wang, M. Henkemeyer, and L. F. Kromer, "EphB1 null mice exhibit neuronal loss in substantia nigra pars reticulata and spontaneous locomotor hyperactivity," *European Journal of Neuroscience*, vol. 25, no. 9, pp. 2619–2628, 2007.

[32] S. Grealish, L. Xie, M. Kelly, and E. Dowd, "Unilateral axonal or terminal injection of 6-hydroxydopamine causes rapid-onset nigrostriatal degeneration and contralateral motor impairments in the rat," *Brain Research Bulletin*, vol. 77, no. 5, pp. 312–319, 2008.

[33] V. Gaur, S. L. Bodhankar, V. Mohan, and P. A. Thakurdesai, "Neurobehavioral assessment of hydroalcoholic extract of *Trigonella foenum-graecum* seeds in rodent models of Parkinson's disease," *Pharmaceutical Biology*, vol. 51, no. 5, pp. 550–557, 2013.

[34] S. Zhang, X.-H. Gui, L.-P. Huang et al., "Neuroprotective effects of β-asarone against 6-hydroxy dopamine-induced parkinsonism via JNK/Bcl-2/beclin-1 pathway," *Molecular Neurobiology*, vol. 53, no. 1, pp. 83–94, 2016.

[35] M. V. Mabandla, M. Nyoka, and W. M. Daniels, "Early use of oleanolic acid provides protection against 6-hydroxydopamine induced dopamine neurodegeneration," *Brain Research*, vol. 1622, pp. 64–71, 2015.

13

Impact of Exposure to Fenitrothion on Vital Organs in Rats

Rasha Abdel-Ghany,[1] **Ebaa Mohammed,**[1] **Shimaa Anis,**[1] **and Waleed Barakat**[1,2]

[1]*Department of Pharmacology & Toxicology, Faculty of Pharmacy, Zagazig University, Zagazig, Egypt*
[2]*Department of Pharmacology & Toxicology, Faculty of Pharmacy, Tabuk University, Tabuk, Saudi Arabia*

Correspondence should be addressed to Waleed Barakat; waled055@yahoo.com

Academic Editor: Steven J. Bursian

This study was designed to investigate the impact of oral administration of fenitrothion (10 mg/kg) on liver, kidney, brain, and lung function in rats. The effect was studied on days 7, 14, 21, 28, and 42. Our results have shown deterioration in liver function as evidenced by the elevation in serum ALT, AST, ALP, and bilirubin and reduction in albumin and hepatic glycogen. This was associated with a state of hyperglycemia and hyperlipidemia and increased prothrombin time, while hemoglobin content was reduced. In addition, the kidney function was reduced as indicated by the elevation in serum creatinine, uric acid, and BUN, while the serum levels of magnesium, potassium, and sodium were reduced. This study also showed an impairment in brain neurotransmitter (elevated 5-HT, glutamate, GABA, and reduced dopamine and norepinephrine level). This was associated with a reduction in the barrier capacity in brain and lung. Fenitrothion also caused a decrease in cholinesterase activity in serum, lung, and brain activity associated with a state of oxidative stress in all tested organs and hyperammonemia. These results support the hazards of pesticide use and shows the importance of minimizing pesticide use or discovering new safe pesticides.

1. Introduction

Organophosphorus pesticides (OPs) are among the most widely used insecticides globally and they are readily available commercially for domestic and industrial purposes [1]. The widespread use of OPs by public health and agricultural programs has led to severe environmental pollution [2, 3] that constitutes a significant potential health hazard because of the possibility of the acute or chronic poisoning of humans and animals [4].

Fenitrothion is one of the most widely used organophosphorus pesticides mainly used in agriculture for controlling chewing and sucking insects. It is also used for the control of flies, mosquitos, and cockroaches in public health programs and/or indoor use [5].

Organophosphates affect many vital organs; chronic toxicity with organophosphorus pesticides may cause extreme injury in liver cells [6]. Liver enzymes, endogenous antioxidant status, and essential trace elements were found to be adversely affected after chronic OPs intoxication to rats [7]. In addition, hematological parameters such as hemoglobin,

leucocyte count, and coagulation of blood have been considered as bioindicators of toxicities following chronic exposure to malathion [8] and pyrethroids [9, 10].

Neuronal necrosis has been observed in multiple cortical and subcortical regions in experimental rats exposed to OPs [6] as soman [11, 12], fenthion [13], and methamidophos [14]. In addition, symptoms of chronic OPs toxicity vary between headache, sweating, Parkinson's, alterations in memory, and psychiatric or neuropsychological dysfunction [15, 16]. In addition, the key findings of OPs toxicity in respiratory system include shortness of breath and rapidly progressive bradypnea leading to apnea due to loss of central inspiratory drive causing central failure of breathing [17]. Chronic exposure to organophosphorus pesticides leads to kidney failure [18]. It has also been reported that pesticides exposure was associated with kidney cancer [1].

The present study was designed to evaluate the consequences of oral fenitrothion administration for 42 consecutive days on liver function and its possible deleterious action on brain, lung, and kidney in albino rats.

2. Materials and Methods

Fenitrothion (Sumithion 50®, 500 mg/mL) was purchased from Kafr Elzayat Co. for Insecticide Ind., (Kafr Elzayat, Egypt). Fenitrothion emulsion was freshly diluted in distilled water to 10 mg/mL and orally administered at a dose of 1 mL/kg rat body weight which corresponds to 10 mg/kg. The difference in administered volume among animals was not more than 12% based on body weight differences. The dose of fenitrothion was selected based on a previous study that used fenitrothion at 10 and 20 mg/kg [19].

2.1. Animals. Male albino rats weighing 160 ± 10 g were obtained from National Research Center (Cairo, Egypt) and were housed in plastic cages and allowed free access to a standard diet and tap water. The rats were housed at 23 ± 2°C 12 hr dark/light cycle. All experimental procedures were approved by the Ethical Committee for Animal Handling at Zagazig University (ECAHZU) (number P7-3-2013 and number P8-3-2013).

Animals were randomly allocated into 6 groups (n = 10) treated daily with the following: C (control group treated with oral distilled water, 1 mL/kg for 42 days), F1 (oral fenitrothion, 1 mL/kg for 7 days), F2 (oral fenitrothion, 1 mL/kg for 14 days), F3 (oral fenitrothion, 1 mL/kg for 21 days), F4 (oral fenitrothion, 1 mL/kg for 28 days), and F6 (oral fenitrothion, 1 mL/kg for 42 days).

At the end of the experiment, after overnight fasting, blood was collected from the retroorbital plexus and centrifuged at 3500 rpm for 15 minutes with or without heparin and serum/plasma was collected and stored at −20°C. Animals were sacrificed by decapitation and liver, brain cortex, lung, and kidney were excised for preparation of tissue homogenates. The cortex was chosen because the control centers of consciousness and memory are located mainly in cerebral cortex [20].

2.2. Methods. AChE activity in brain cortex and lung tissue was determined colorimetrically using acetylthiocholine iodide and 5,5′-dithiobis (nitrobenzoate) (DTNB) at 412 nm [21]; amino acids content was determined fluorometrically using ninhydrin at excitation of 377 nm and emission of 451 nm for both glutamate and GABA [22, 23], while content of monoamines was determined fluorometrically using n-heptane at excitation at 320 nm and emission at 480 nm for DA, excitation at 380 nm and emission at 480 nm for NE, and excitation at 355 nm and emission at 470 nm for 5-HT [23]. Water content in brain and lung tissue was determined using wet and dry weight method [24]. Evans blue extravasation in brain and lung tissue was determined colorimetrically using Evans blue dye at 610 nm [24, 25].

Liver glycogen content was determined by the gravimetric method using KoH, trichloroacetic acid, and absolute ethanol [26] and catalase (CAT) activity in tissue (liver, brain, lung, and kidney) was determined colorimetrically using potassium dichromate at 570 nm, reduced glutathione (GSH) content in tissue (liver, brain, lung, and kidney) was determined colorimetrically using 5,5′-dithiobis (nitrobenzoate) (DTNB) at 412 nm, and malondialdehyde (MDA)

content in tissue (liver, brain, lung, and kidney) was determined colorimetrically using thiobarbituric acid (TBA) and trichloroacetic acid at 535 nm [27–29].

The following parameters were assayed in serum using kits supplied by Biodiagnostic Co. (Cairo, Egypt): ALT and AST [30], ALP [31], butyrylcholinesterase activity [32], total bilirubin [33], albumin [34], sodium [35], potassium [36], magnesium [37], cholesterol [38], HDL-cholesterol [39], LDL-cholesterol [40], blood urea nitrogen (BUN) [41], creatinine, and uric acid contents [42].

Hemoglobin content [43], glucose level [44], and prothrombin time [45] were determined in blood using kits supplied by Biodiagnostic Co. (Cairo, Egypt).

Liver, serum, brain, lung, and kidney total protein content were determined by colorimetric method using a kit supplied by Biodiagnostic Co. (Cairo, Egypt) [46].

Liver, serum, and brain ammonia content were determined by colorimetric method using a kit supplied by Biodiagnostic Co. (Cairo, Egypt) [47].

2.3. Statistical Analysis. Data are expressed as means ± SD. The statistical significance of the data was determined using one-way analysis of variance (ANOVA) followed by Tukey's post hoc test using SPSS software package version 10. The level of significance was taken as $p < 0.05$.

3. Results

3.1. Effect on Some Liver Functions. Administration of fenitrothion for 7, 14, 21, 28, and 42 days (F1, F2, F3, F4, and F6, resp.) caused a significant gradual increase in serum ALT activity compared with control group (48, 49.6, 52.1, 56.3, and 58.1 versus 41.3 u/l), AST activity compared with control group (96.2, 114.8, 126.9, 143.9, and 151.9 versus 62.5 u/l), ALP activity compared with control group (137.8, 161.8, 199.4, 251.3, and 250.3 versus 112.1 u/l) (Figure 1(a)), and serum total bilirubin level compared with control group (0.56, 0.9, and 0.93 versus 0.32 mg/dL) (Figure 1(b)).

On the other hand, administration of fenitrothion for 7, 14, 21, 28, and 42 days (F1, F2, F3, F4, and F6, resp.) caused a significant gradual decrease in serum albumin compared with control group (4.11, 3.73, 3.59, 3.17, and 3.1 versus 4.89 g/dL) (Figure 1(c)) and liver glycogen content compared with control group (3.06, 2.64, 2.16, and 2.1 versus 3.9 g/100 g liver) (Figure 1(d)).

3.2. Effects on Liver Histopathology. Administration of fenitrothion for 7, 14, 21, 28, and 42 days (F1, F2, F3, F4, and F6, resp.) caused significant gradual deterioration in liver tissue starting by disorganized lobular patterns in hepatic parenchyma, followed by congested hepatic tissue and programmed cell death (apoptosis) and focal necrosis and widening of the hepatic sinusoids beside cell swelling in the remaining hepatic parenchyma, and ending with interstitial lymphocytic aggregations and interlobular thickened edematous fibrous tissue (Figure 2).

3.3. Effect on Some Hematologic Parameters. Administration of fenitrothion for 14, 21, 28, and 42 days (F2, F3, F4, and F6,

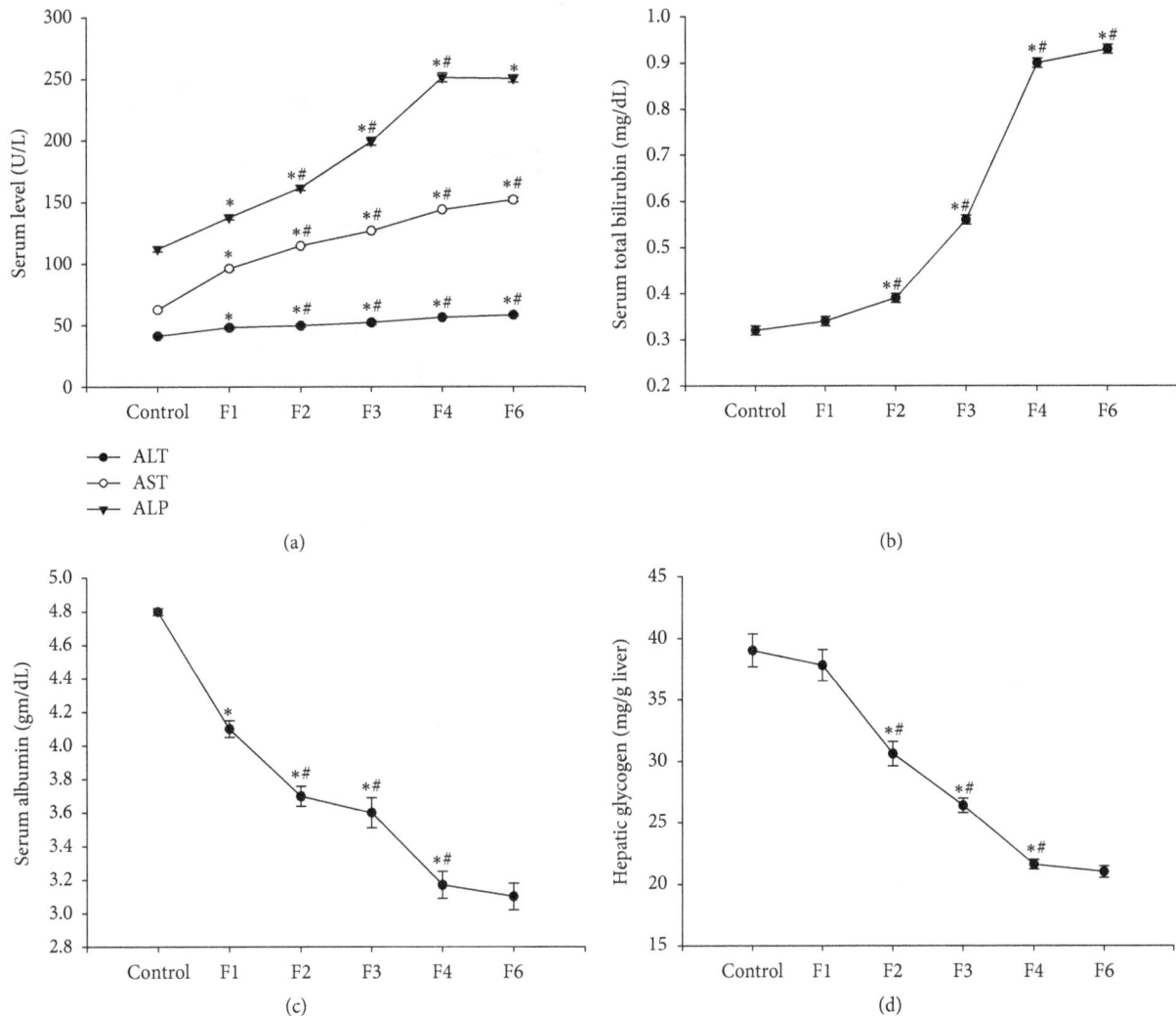

FIGURE 1: Effects of fenitrothion (10 mg/kg) for 1, 2, 3, 4, and 6 weeks (F1, F2, F3, F4, and F6, resp.) on some liver functions in rats. Data are expressed as mean ± SD. $N = 10$. *Significantly different from control group; #significantly different from fenitrothion at the previous time point at $p < 0.05$ using ANOVA followed by LSD and Tukey's post hoc test.

resp.) showed a significant gradual increase in blood glucose level compared with control group (104.43, 137.41, 153.63, and 168.66 versus 88.96 mg/dL) (Figure 3(a)) and prothrombin time compared with control group (16.88, 17.12, 18.22, and 18.56 versus 16.12 sec.) (Figure 3(b)).

This was accompanied by a significant decrease in blood hemoglobin content (by 12, 19, and 24%, resp.) compared with control group starting from week 3 of fenitrothion administration (F3) that continued throughout the experiment (F4 and F6) (Figure 3(c)).

Administration of fenitrothion for 14, 21, 28, and 42 days (F2, F3, F4, and F6, resp.) showed a state of hyperlipidemia as evidenced by the significant gradual elevation in serum cholesterol compared with control group (59.33, 72.49, 90.96, and 94.76 versus 51.35 mg/dL) and LDL content compared with control group (16.9, 22.8, 29.7, 31.51, and 35.67 versus 13.61 mg/dL) and the reduction in serum HDL compared with

control group (32.7, 24.6, 17.2, and 14.7 versus 40.6 mg/dL) compared with control group (Figure 3(d)).

3.4. Effect on Kidney Function. Administration of fenitrothion for 14, 21, 28, and 42 days (F2, F3, F4, and F6, resp.) caused a significant gradual increase in serum creatinine content compared with control group (0.88, 0.93, 1.01, 1.32, and 1.39 versus 0.87 mg/dL) (Figure 4(a)) and uric acid (Figure 4(b)), while serum blood urea nitrogen (BUN) content compared with control group (24, 25, 35, 40, and 44 versus 24 mg/dL) was increased starting from F3 (Figure 4(c)).

3.5. Effects on Kidney Histopathology. Administration of fenitrothion for 7, 14, 21, 28, and 42 days (F1, F2, F3, F4, and F6, resp.) caused a gradual significant histopathological changes in kidney tissue starting from minor changes in renal tubules as well as glomeruli at the cortical portion and ending with

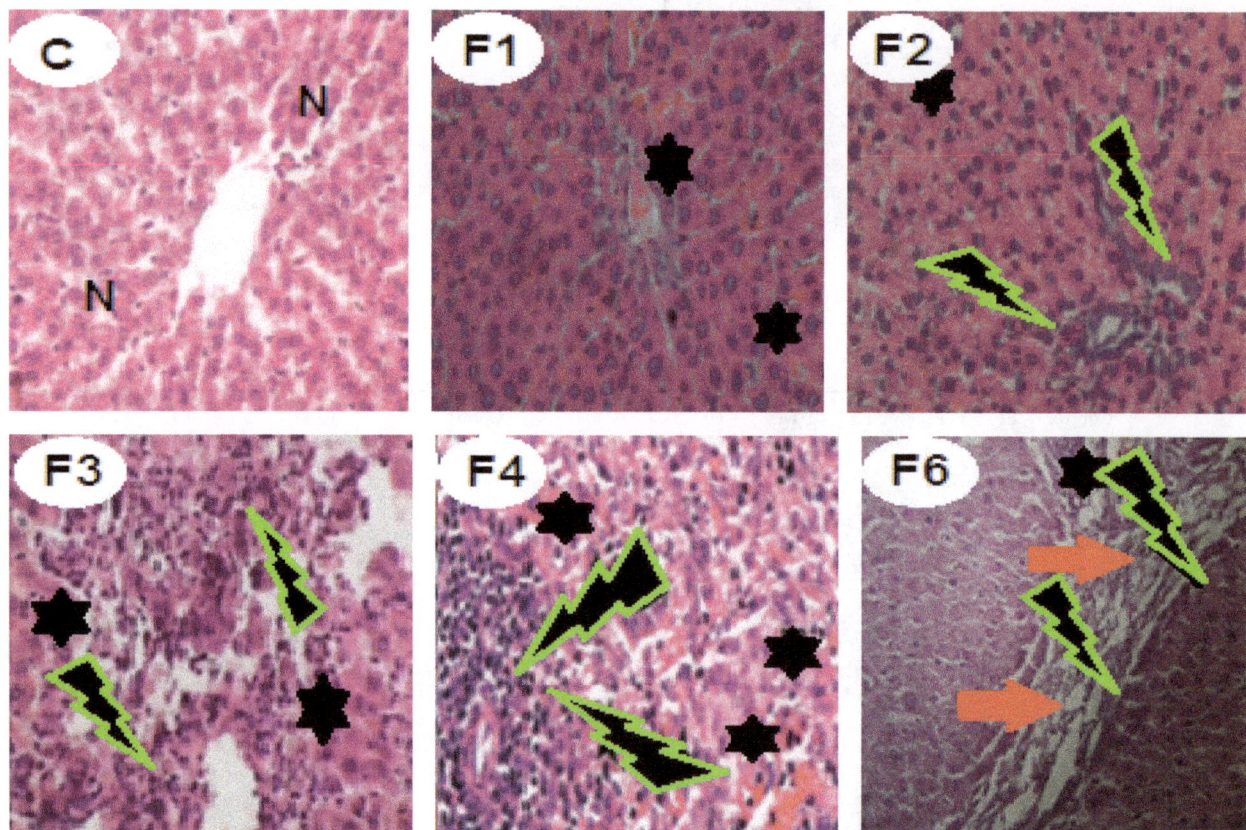

FIGURE 2: Effects of fenitrothion on liver histopathology in rats using H & E staining (×400). C: normal hepatic parenchyma, F1: mild congested, disorganized hepatic lobules and slight cell swelling, F2: moderate cell swelling associated with apoptosis and focal necrosis, F3: moderate degenerated and ballooned necrotic hepatocytes with lymphocytic aggregation and cell infiltration, F4: severe disappearance of hepatocytes and large areas of congestion, lymphocytic aggregation, and inflammation, and F6: thickened interlobular tissue by edematous fibrous tissue and congested blood vessels. N: normal liver cells. Black star: congested cells with cytoplasmic vacuolation. Green lightning: lymphocytic aggregation. Red arrow: edematous fibrous tissue.

severe degenerative changes in kidney tissue compared with control group (Figure 5).

3.6. Effect on Electrolyte. Administration of fenitrothion for 7, 14, 21, 28, and 42 days (F1, F2, F3, F4, and F6, resp.) induced a significant gradual reduction in serum magnesium content compared with control group (0.93, 0.83, 0.7, 0.64, and 0.45 versus 1.1 mmol/l), potassium content compared with control group (2.17, 1.78, 1.08, and 0.61 versus 2.62 mmol/l), and sodium content compared with control group (105.4, 90.6, 69.9, 58.2, and 47.6 versus 118.2 mmol/l) (Figures 6(a), 6(b), and 6(c)).

3.7. Effect on Brain Neurotransmitters. Administration. of fenitrothion for 14, 21, 28, and 42 days (F2, F3, F4 and F6, resp.) showed a significant gradual increase in brain 5-HT content compared with control group (427.88, 527.89, 627.38, and 752.46 versus 359.21 μg/g protein), glutamate content compared with control group (23.37, 32.9, 45.09, and 46.46 versus 20.24 μmol/g protein), and GABA content in cortex compared with control group (20.18, 23.84, 30.5, and 35.35 versus 18.34 μmol/g protein) (Figures 7(a), 7(b), and 7(c)).

On the other hand, administration of fenitrothion for 14, 21, 28, and 42 days (F2, F3, F4, and F6, resp.) was associated with a significant gradual reduction in brain DA content compared with control group (69.99, 59.71, 50.09, and 47.27 versus 91.72 μg/g protein) and NE content in brain cortex compared with control group (16, 12.42, 8.53, and 4.41 versus 18.34 μg/g protein) (Figures 7(d) and 7(e), resp.).

3.8. Effect on Brain and Lung Barrier Integrity. Administration of fenitrothion for 7, 14, 21, 28, and 42 days (F1, F2, F3, F4, and F6, resp.), revealed a significant gradual decrease in blood brain barrier integrity as evidenced by the increase in Evans blue extravasation in brain compared with control group (13.7, 15.14, 17.1, 19.06, and 21.42 versus 12.91 μg/g protein) (Figure 8(a)). This was accompanied by a significant increase in brain water content compared with control group (0.84, 0.87, 0.88, and 0.91 versus 0.79 g) starting from F2 (Figure 8(b)).

Similarly, administration of fenitrothion for 14, 21, 28, and 42 days (F2, F3, F4, and F6, resp.) revealed a significant gradual decrease in lung barrier integrity as evidenced by the increase in Evans blue extravasation in lung compared

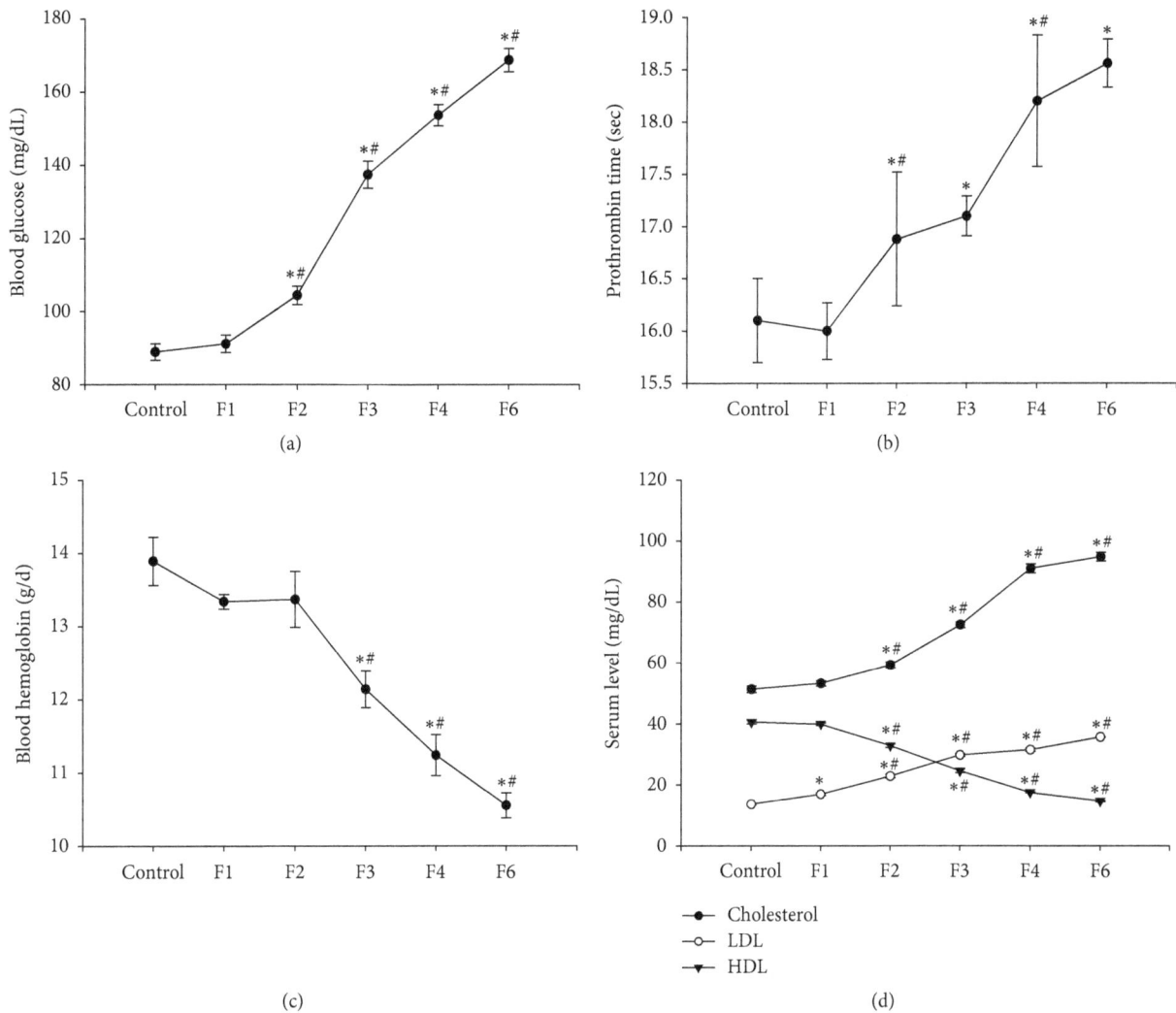

FIGURE 3: Effects of fenitrothion (10 mg/kg) for 1, 2, 3, 4, and 6 weeks (F1, F2, F3, F4, and F6, resp.) on some blood parameters in rats. Data are expressed as mean ± SD. $N = 10$. *Significantly different from control group; #significantly different from fenitrothion at the previous time point at $p < 0.05$ using ANOVA followed by Tukey's post hoc test.

with control group (18.31, 19.63, and 21.44 versus 17.19 μg/g protein) (Figure 8(c)) which was also accompanied by a significant increase in lung water content compared with control group (0.86, 0.9, and 0.91 versus 0.8 g) starting from F2 (Figure 8(d)).

3.9. Effects on Brain Histopathology. Administration of fenitrothion for 7, 14, 21, 28, and 42 days (F1, F2, F3, F4, and F6, resp.) caused significant gradual deterioration in brain tissue starting by focal scattered hemorrhagic areas. Later on, intense haemorrhage and narrow spaces with early encephalomalacia became visible in both lateral ventricles. This was followed by demyelination of nerve axon in the white matter, encephalomalacia, cytotoxic edema, neuronal degeneration, and intense microgliosis (Figure 9).

3.10. Effects on Lung Histopathology. Administration of fenitrothion for 7, 14, 21, 28, and 42 days (F1, F2, F3, F4,

and F6, resp.), caused significant gradual deterioration in the histopathology of lung tissue starting by focal hypertrophied smooth muscles of the pulmonary blood vessels and thickened intra-alveolar septa and ending with prevalent hypertrophied smooth muscles, interstitial hemorrhages with narrow alveolar spaces, and intense thickened septa with perivascular leukocytic aggregation compared to control group (Figure 10).

3.11. Effects on Cholinesterase Activity and Ammonia Content. Administration of fenitrothion for 7, 14, 21, 28, and 42 days (F1, F2, F3, F4, and F6, resp.) caused a significant gradual decrease in serum butyrylcholinesterase activity compared with control group (9696.3, 8557.64, 7879.32, 7544.74, and 6963.54 versus 16380 u/l), lung acetylcholinesterase activity compared with control group (272.41, 228.03, 170.32, 104.28, and 76.16 versus 302.49 μmol/min/mg protein), and brain acetylcholinesterase compared with control group (439.68,

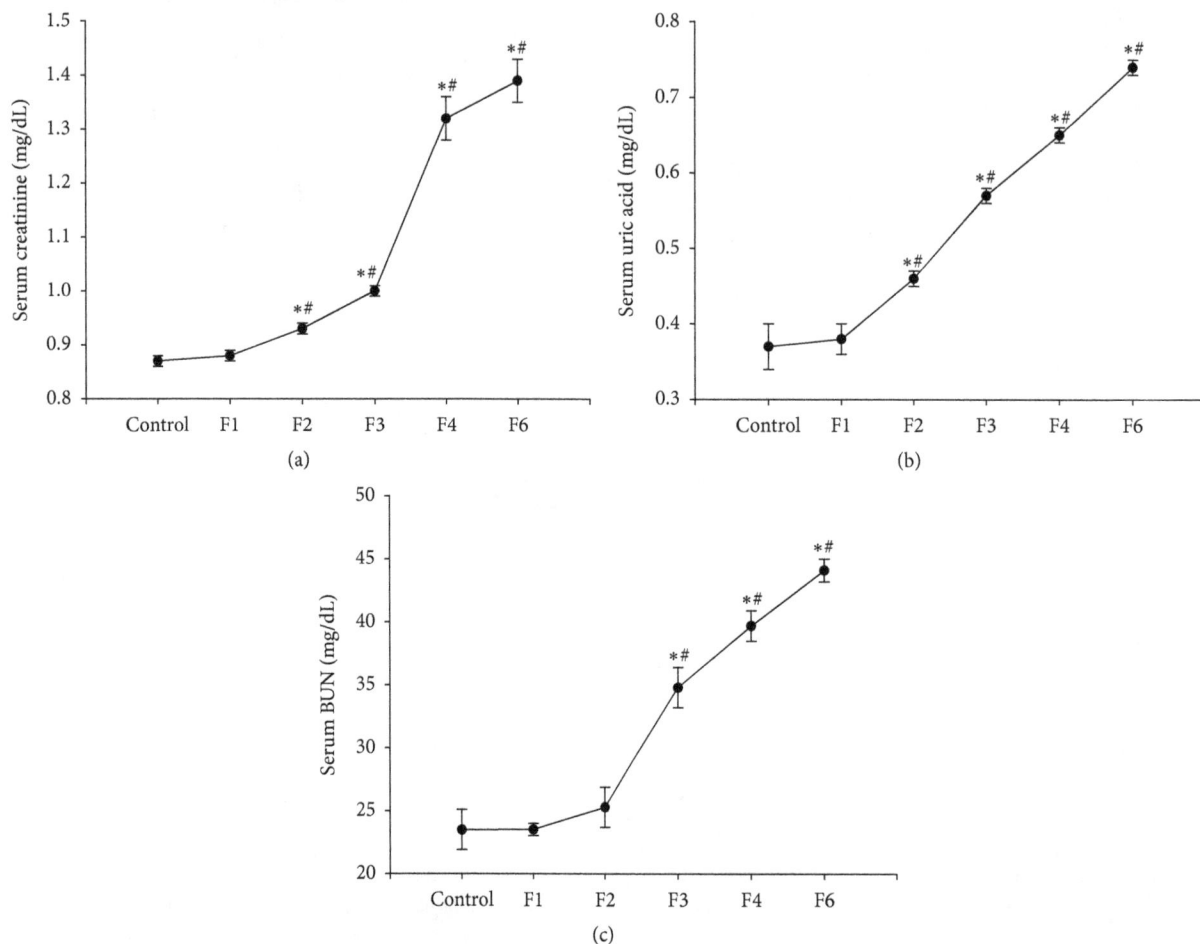

FIGURE 4: Effects of fenitrothion (10 mg/kg) for 1, 2, 3, 4, and 6 weeks (F1, F2, F3, F4, and F6, resp.) on some kidney functions in rats. Data are expressed as mean ± SD. N = 10. *Significantly different from control group; #significantly different from fenitrothion at the previous time point at $p < 0.05$ using ANOVA followed by Tukey's post hoc test.

399.16, 324.57, 207.26, and 155.76 versus 464.93 μmol/min/mg protein) (Figures 11(a), 11(b) and 11(c)).

On the other hand, fenitrothion caused a significant increase in liver ammonia content compared with control group (0.073, 0.1, 0.133, 0.183, and 0.202 versus 0.058 μmol/g protein) starting from the first week of administration (F1) and continuing throughout the experiment (F2, F3, F4, and F6). In addition, fenitrothion caused a significant increase in ammonia content in serum compared with control group (0.025, 0.036, 0.047, and 0.065 versus 0.022 μmol/l) and brain ammonia content compared with control group (0.083, 0.093, 0.11, and 0.124 versus 0.072 μmol/g protein) starting from week 2 of fenitrothion administration (F2) and continuing throughout the experiment (F3, F4, and F6) as shown in Figure 11(d).

3.12. Effect on Oxidative Stress Biomarkers. Administration of fenitrothion caused a significant initial increase in catalase (CAT) activity after 7 days (F1) in liver, brain, kidney, and lung compared with control group (0.085 versus 0.069, 0.37 versus 0.34, 0.06 versus 0.053, and 0.18 versus 0.14 μmole/min/mg,

resp.). However, continued administration of fenitrothion caused a gradual significant decrease in CAT activity in liver, brain, kidney, and lung after 21, 28, and 42 days (F3, F4, and F6, resp.) compared with control group (0.06, 0.048, and 0.041 versus 0.069 in liver, 0.3, 0.24, and 0.22 versus 0.34 in brain, 0.048, 0.041, and 0.034 versus 0.053 in kidney, and 0.11, 0.08, and 0.06 versus 0.14 μmole/min/mg in lung) (Figure 12(a)).

Similarly, fenitrothion caused a significant initial increase in glutathione content (GSH) after 7 days (F1) in liver, brain, kidney, and lung compared with control group (3.2 versus 2.8, 1.57 versus 1.34, 2.02 versus 1.7, and 6.8 versus 5.9 mg/g, resp.). This was followed by a gradual significant decrease in GSH content in liver, brain, kidney, and lung after 21, 28, and 42 days (F3, F4, and F6, resp.) compared with control group (2.7, 2.4, and 1.98 versus 2.8 in liver, 1.14, 1.05, and 1.01 versus 1.34 in brain, 1.4, 1.3, and 1.02 versus 1.7 in kidney, and 4.84, 3.85, and 3.05 versus 5.92 mg/g in lung) (Figure 12(b)).

On the other hand, administration of fenitrothion for 7 days (F1) caused a significant decrease in malondialdehyde (MDA) content in liver, brain, lung, and kidney compared

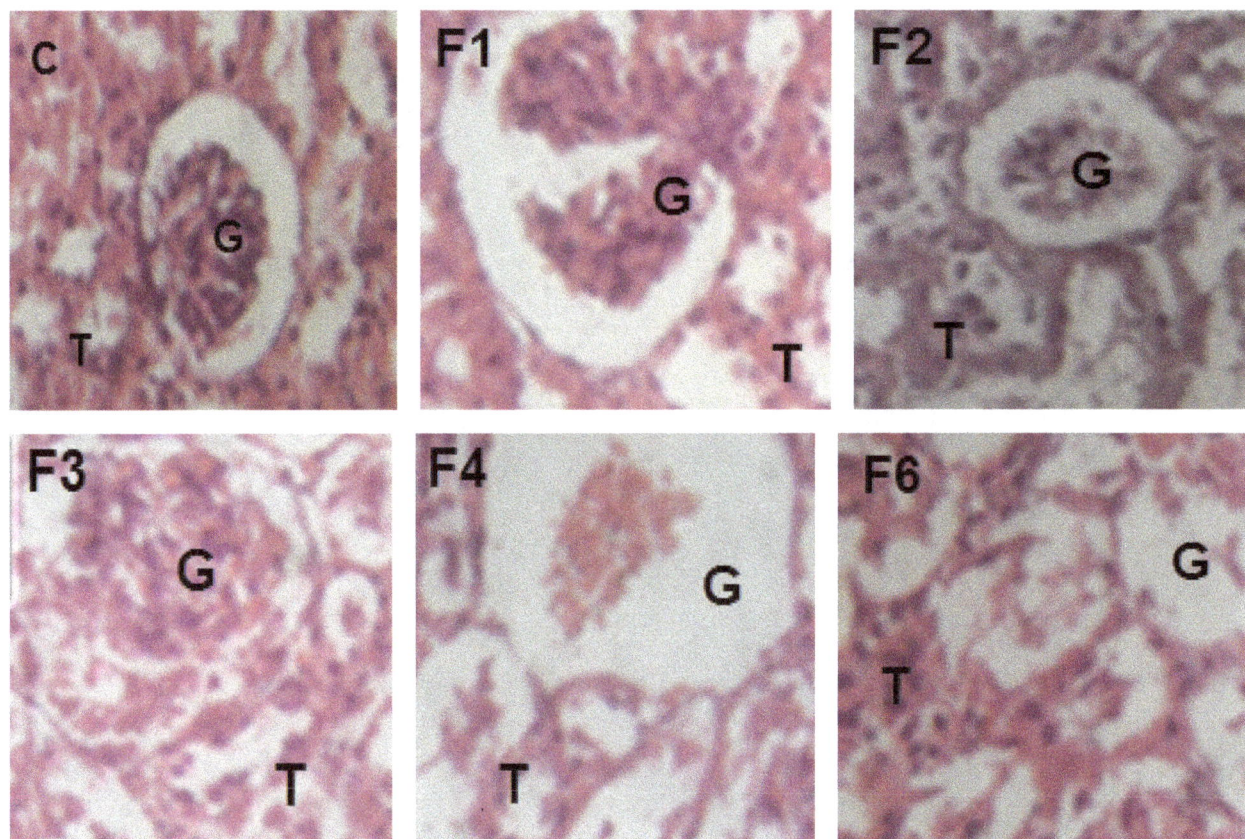

FIGURE 5: Effects of fenitrothion on kidney histopathology in rats using H & E staining (×400). C: normal segments of nephrons, interstitium, and blood vessels, F1: degenerative changes in glomeruli and tubules, F2: partial necrosis of glomerular tafts and some renal tubular epithelium in renal cortex, F3: focal intense degenerative changes in renal tubules and few shrunken glomeruli, F4: diffuse necrotic changes in renal tubules and glomeruli, and F6: marked necrosis of tubular cells, atrophy of the glomeruli, and areas of interstitial infiltration of round cells. G: renal glomeruli and T: renal tubule.

with control group (4.1 versus 5.2, 2.5 versus 2.7, 5.4 versus 5.7, and 8.57 versus 10.96 μmole/g, resp.). Continued administration of fenitrothion caused a gradual significant decrease in MDA content in liver, brain, kidney, and lung after 14, 21, 28, and 42 days (F2, F3, F4, and F6, resp.) compared with control group (6.8, 10, 13.6, and 14 versus 5.2 in liver, 4.1, 5.1, 5.7, and 6.34 versus 2.7 in brain, 7.04, 8.8, 11.3, and 11.93 versus 5.7 in kidney, and 13.05, 17.99, 21.8, and 21.65 versus 10.96 μmole/g in lung) (Figure 12(c)).

4. Discussion

This study was designed to investigate the effect of the organophosphorus pesticide: fenitrothion (10 mg/kg/day, p.o. for 6 weeks) on vital organs (liver, blood, kidney, brain, and lung) in albino rats.

Concerning the effect of fenitrothion on hepatocellular integrity, this study showed significant gradual increase in ALT and AST activity compared to control group starting from the first week. These results coincide with previous studies that showed a significant increase in liver enzymes in rats exposed to organophosphorus insecticides as fenitrothion [48].

The alteration in these enzymes might be attributed to hepatocellular damage and alteration in permeability of cell membrane leading to leakage of these enzymes into blood stream [49].

In the present study, fenitrothion administration gradually increased ALP activity as compared to control group. This result is in agreement with Kalender at al. [1], who reported that malathion treated rats had significantly higher ALP activity than the control group. This change may be in response to enhanced dephosphorylation of ALP for further metabolism of fenitrothion to be excreted with bile or due to defect in ALP excretion in bile by hepatocytes [50].

In the present study, fenitrothion treated rats showed significant gradual increase in the level of bilirubin which is a normal metabolic product of hemoglobin in red blood cells [51] as previously shown by Jayusman et al. [5] who reported that ingestion of pesticides caused a significant increase in bilirubin level.

Additionally, hyperbilirubinemia is toxic to the central nervous system and may lead to a sequence of neurological symptoms and signs termed bilirubin encephalopathy [52].

The present study showed a gradual decrease in albumin content which coincides with [53] who showed reduction in

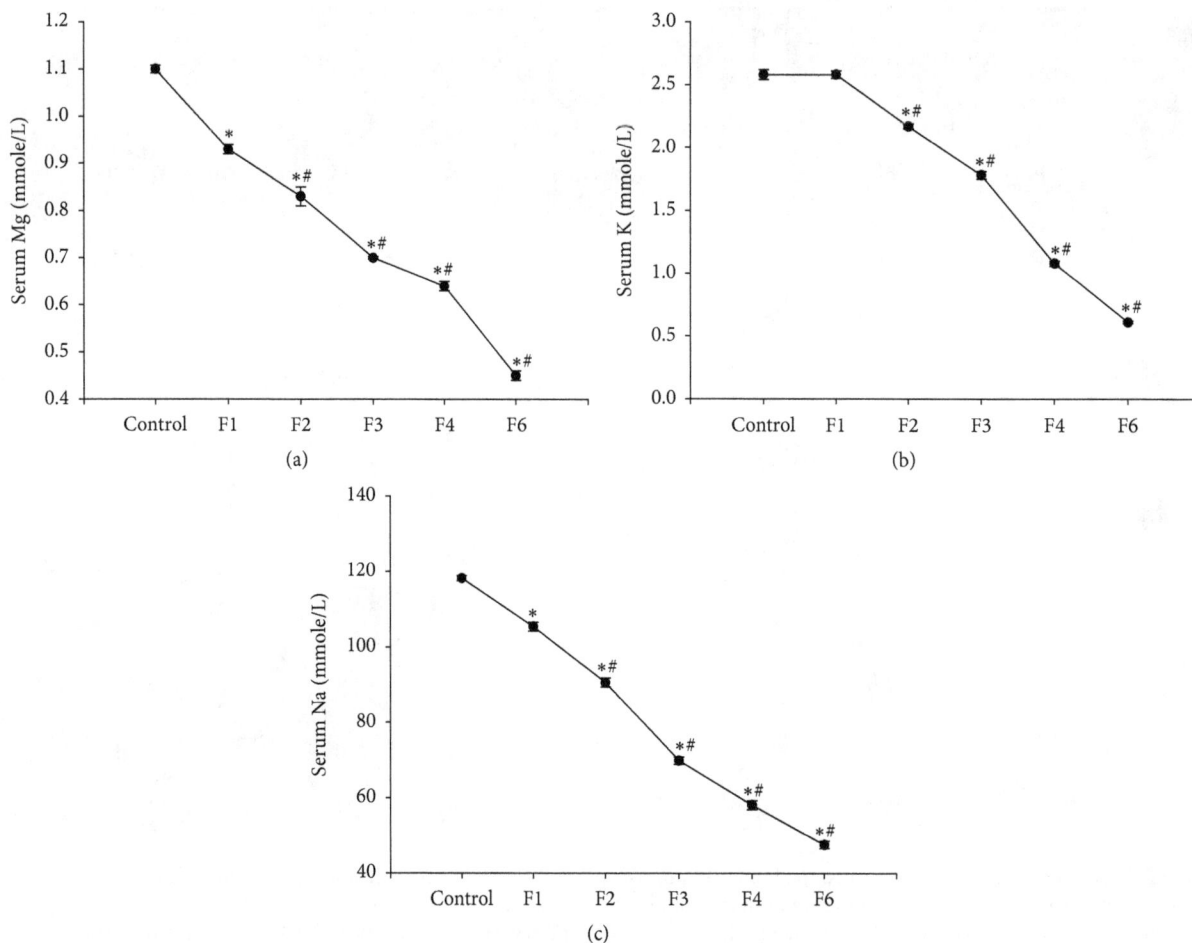

FIGURE 6: Effects of fenitrothion (10 mg/kg) for 1, 2, 3, 4, and 6 weeks (F1, F2, F3, F4, and F6, resp.) on serum electrolytes in rats. Data are expressed as mean ± SD. $N = 10$. *Significantly different from control group; #significantly different from fenitrothion at the previous time point at $p < 0.05$ using ANOVA followed by Tukey's post hoc test.

albumin content after OPs exposure confirming the failure in liver functions [54]. The reduction in albumin content may reflect increased albumin metabolism [55] or decreased hepatic capacity to synthesize proteins due to increased number of injured hepatocytes [56].

The present study showed that fenitrothion administration caused deterioration in glucose homeostasis as evidenced by significant gradual increase in blood glucose level and a drop in hepatic glycogen content; a previous study have reported that chronic exposure to OPs participates in hyperglycemia and depletion of glycogen content in liver and muscle [57, 58].

This might be attributed to disturbed glucose transport and glycogen metabolism [59]. Additionally, increased blood glucose level may result from an imbalance between hepatic output of glucose and its peripheral uptake [60] or as a consequence of abruptly increased catabolism to meet higher OP induced energy demands [61].

In addition, fenitrothion caused a significant gradual increase in prothrombin time starting from week 2. Reference [53] showed alteration in coagulation after OPs exposure

confirming the failure in liver functions and decreased hepatic capacity to synthesize coagulation factors [56].

The current study showed that exposure to fenitrothion was accompanied by a significant gradual decrease in the level of hemoglobin from the first week which might explain the state of hyperbilirubinemia since bilirubin is a normal metabolic product of hemoglobin in red blood cells [51]. These results are in accordance with those obtained by [62], who reported that OPs exposure altered hematological parameters in rats.

The reduction in hemoglobin level might be attributed to impairment of biosynthesis of heme in bone marrow [63] or binding of OPs on iron, followed by a lack of incorporation of iron in hemoglobin [64].

The current study has shown a gradual increase in serum cholesterol and LDL and gradual decrease in HDL after administration of fenitrothion. These results are in accordance with those obtained by Kalender at al. [1]. Liver is involved in lipid synthesis, metabolism, and transportation and changes in plasma lipid level could serve as a simple marker for assessing liver disorders [65]. These alterations in

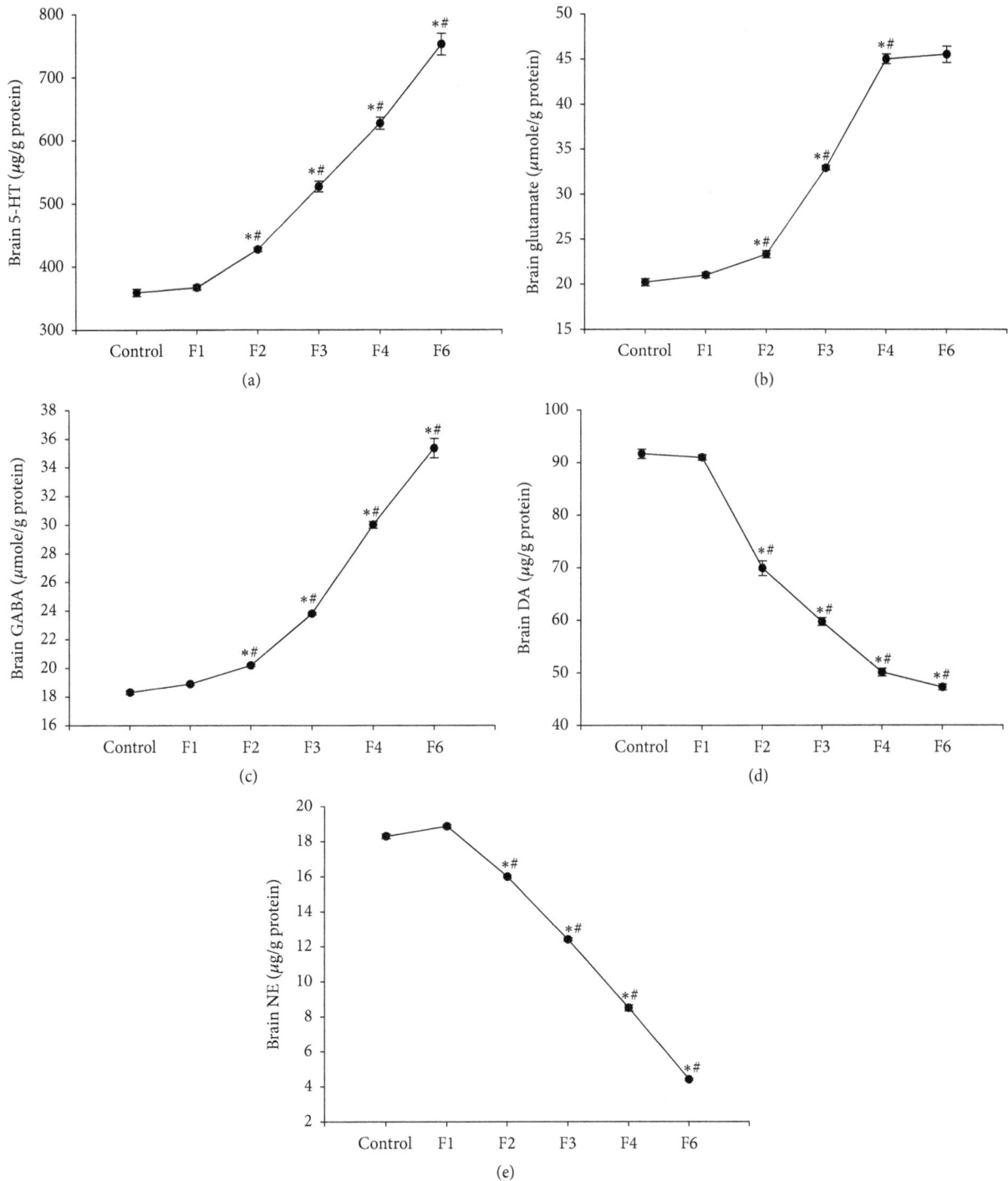

FIGURE 7: Effects of fenitrothion (10 mg/kg) for 1, 2, 3, 4, and 6 weeks (F1, F2, F3, F4, and F6, resp.) on some brain neurotransmitters in rats. Data are expressed as mean ± SD. $N = 10$. *Significantly different from control group; #significantly different from fenitrothion at the previous time point at $p < 0.05$ using ANOVA followed by Tukey's post hoc test.

lipid profile might be attributed to the effect of fenitrothion on the permeability of hepatocyte cell membrane or blockage of the bile duct which reduces or stops cholesterol secretion into the duodenum [1]. Also, this could be attributed to increased hepatic synthesis and/or diminished hepatic degradation of lipids due to reduced lipoprotein lipase activity [66].

This study showed that fenitrothion caused a gradual elevation in BUN, serum creatinine, and serum uric acid starting from third week indicating functional damage of the kidney. These results coincide with previous studies which demonstrated that the kidney is one of the target organs of OPs [67, 68].

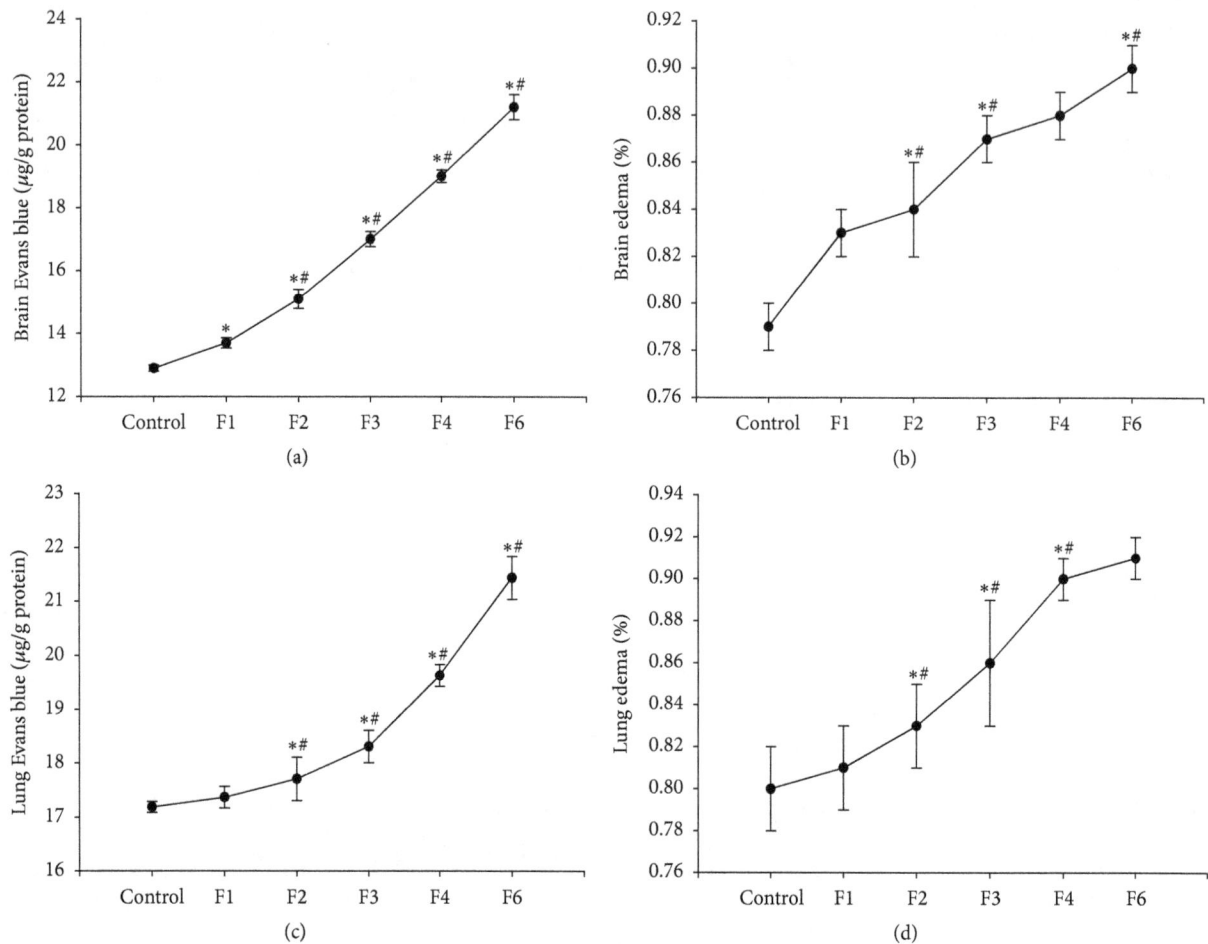

FIGURE 8: Effects of fenitrothion (10 mg/kg) for 1, 2, 3, 4, and 6 weeks (F1, F2, F3, F4, and F6, resp.) on barrier integrity in rats. Data are expressed as mean ± SD. $N = 10$. *Significantly different from control group; #significantly different from fenitrothion at the previous time point at $p < 0.05$ using ANOVA followed by Tukey's post hoc test.

In this study, fenitrothion caused a gradual decrease in serum Mg^{++}, K^+, and Na^+ content. The present findings are consistent with [69] that reported that exposure to pesticides caused decrease in serum Mg, K, and Na level. The importance of serum electrolytes is correlated with their involvement in many vital activities including muscle contraction, maintenance of acid-base balance, and nerve impulse conduction [70].

Gumz et al. [71] correlated these changes with alteration of the membrane configuration accompanied by cell membrane damage and disorders in membrane permeability leading to alteration in electrolyte balance.

Additionally, Mossalam et al. [72] showed that lipid peroxidation products generated by pesticides can cause DNA damage and directly inhibit protein synthesis including Na^+/K^+ ATPase.

Hypokalemia can exacerbate hepatic encephalopathy by increasing renal ammoniagenesis and hence increasing systemic ammonia level [73]. Furthermore, Giuliani and Peri [74] reported that, during hyponatremia, excess water enters the brain and the cells get swollen producing hyponatremic encephalopathy.

In the present study, fenitrothion caused a gradual increase in brain glutamate, GABA, and serotonin (5-HT) content, while the contents of norepinephrine and dopamine were gradually decreased. Rivera-Espinosa et al. [75] have previously reported similar changes of brain neurotransmitters after liver injury. Additionally, Ahmed et al. [76] have previously reported similar changes of brain neurotransmitters after OPs exposure. Additionally, exposures to pesticides have been reported to cause permanent alterations in GABAergic, serotonergic [77], and dopaminergic systems [78].

The changes observed in GABAergic tone might be due to modulation of central and peripheral benzodiazepine receptors [79], while changes in glutamatergic, dopaminergic, and cholinergic system were attributed to disturbances in the synthesis and degradation of amino acids by the liver [80] and amino acid efflux from and/or reuptake by astrocytes [81].

In the present study, a gradual increase in Evans blue extravasation in brain tissue and brain water content was observed following fenitrothion administration. Like other OPs, fenitrothion can alter and cross the BBB, leading to neurological damage [82]. With the alteration in BBB permeability, brain water and sodium content are increased

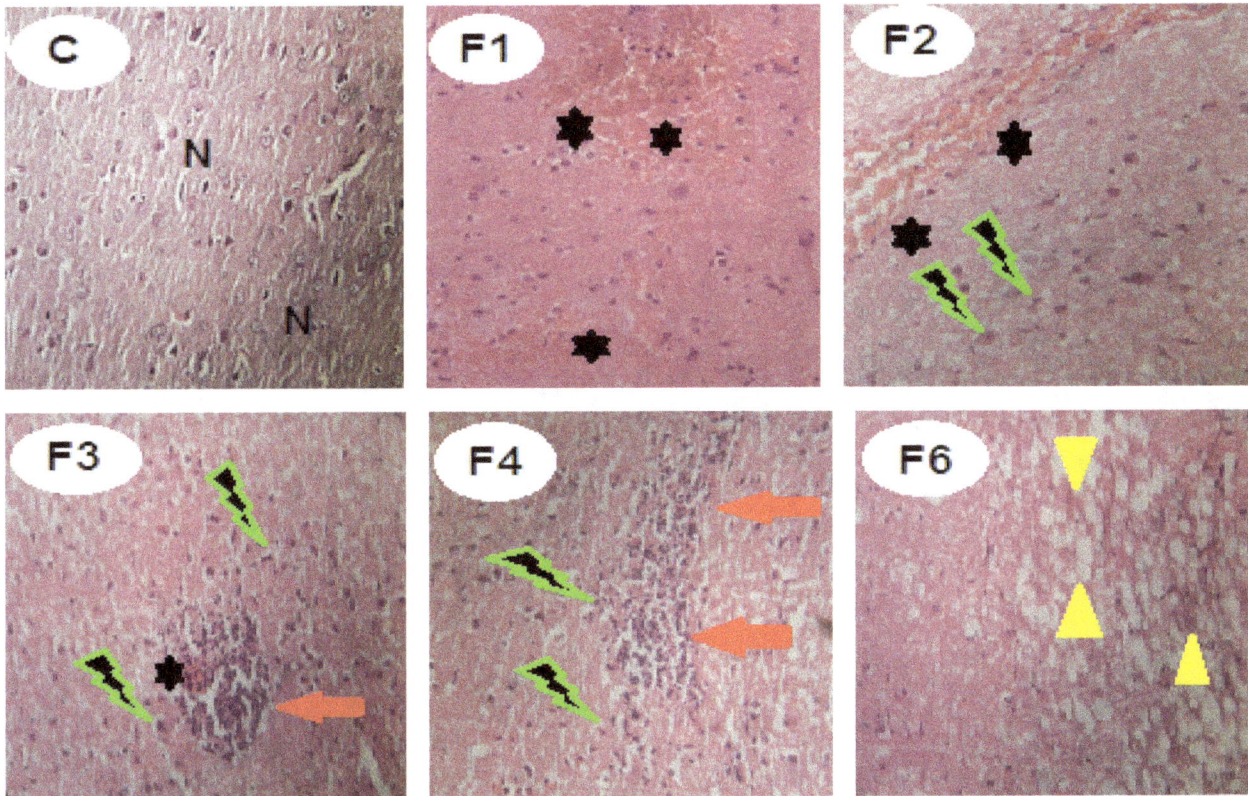

FIGURE 9: Effects of fenitrothion on brain histopathology in rats using H & E staining (×400). C: normal brain tissue, F1: focal hemorrhagic areas in the cortex, F2: scattered hemorrhage in brain ventricles and cytotoxic edema, F3: focal hemorrhagic areas, cytotoxic edema, degenerated neurons, and focal microgliosis, F4: cytotoxic edema and intense microgliosis, and F6: degenerated neurons, demyelination of the white matter axons, and encephalomalacia. N: normal brain cells. Black star: hemorrhagic area. Green lightning: cytotoxic edema. Red arrow: degenerated neurons and focal microgliosis. Yellow head arrow: demyelination of the white matter axons and encephalomalacia.

causing brain edema as previously reported [82]. In addition, metabolism of ammonia in astrocytes leads to glutamine accumulation that may contribute to astrocyte swelling, cytotoxic brain edema impaired astrocyte/neuronal communication, and synaptic plasticity [83].

In a similar manner, a gradual increase in EBE in lung tissue and lung water content was observed after fenitrothion administration. OPs can alter and cross the pleural membrane and cause lung injury through different mechanisms including ROS generation leading to pulmonary dysfunction. With the increase in pleural permeability of pulmonary microvessels, lung water content was increased profoundly causing lung edema [84].

Additionally, fluid accumulation causing brain and lung edema may also be due to the decreased production of albumin by the liver. As albumin production diminishes, fluid begins to leak from vessels causing edema that can lead to alteration of mental status and increasing in breathing rate and effort [85].

Organophosphorus pesticides have been reported to induce toxicity in mammals by inhibiting butyrylcholinesterase activity (BuChE) [86] and acetylcholinesterase (AChE), which leads to the accumulation of acetylcholine and the subsequent activation of cholinergic muscarinic and nicotinic receptors [87], leading to neuronal excitation and

then paralysis of cholinergic transmission [88]. Therefore, acetylcholinesterase (AChE) and butyrylcholinesterase (BuChE) inhibition are a well-accepted index of organophosphorus insecticides intoxication [89].

The present study has demonstrated a gradual decline in serum BuChE and brain and lung AChE activity starting from first week of fenitrothion administration. Cholinesterases inhibition may be due to direct effect of fenitrothion [90] or indirect effect of hyperammonemia and/or decreased synthetic function of the liver as a result to hepatopathy [91].

Ammonia is normally converted to urea in the liver by a series of enzymatic reactions [92]. One important finding of this study was the gradual elevation in liver ammonia starting from the first week of fenitrothion administration while a significant gradual increase in plasma and brain ammonia started from the second week.

These results coincide with those reported by Scott et al. [93], who showed a significant increase in plasma ammonia following liver injury in rats, and Penchalamma and Jacop [94] who reported the elevation in ammonia level in liver, blood, and kidney after OPs exposure.

The elevated serum ammonia content can cross the blood brain barrier (BBB) [95] causing hepatic encephalopathy through several mechanisms, including impaired brain energy metabolism and autoregulation of blood flow [79],

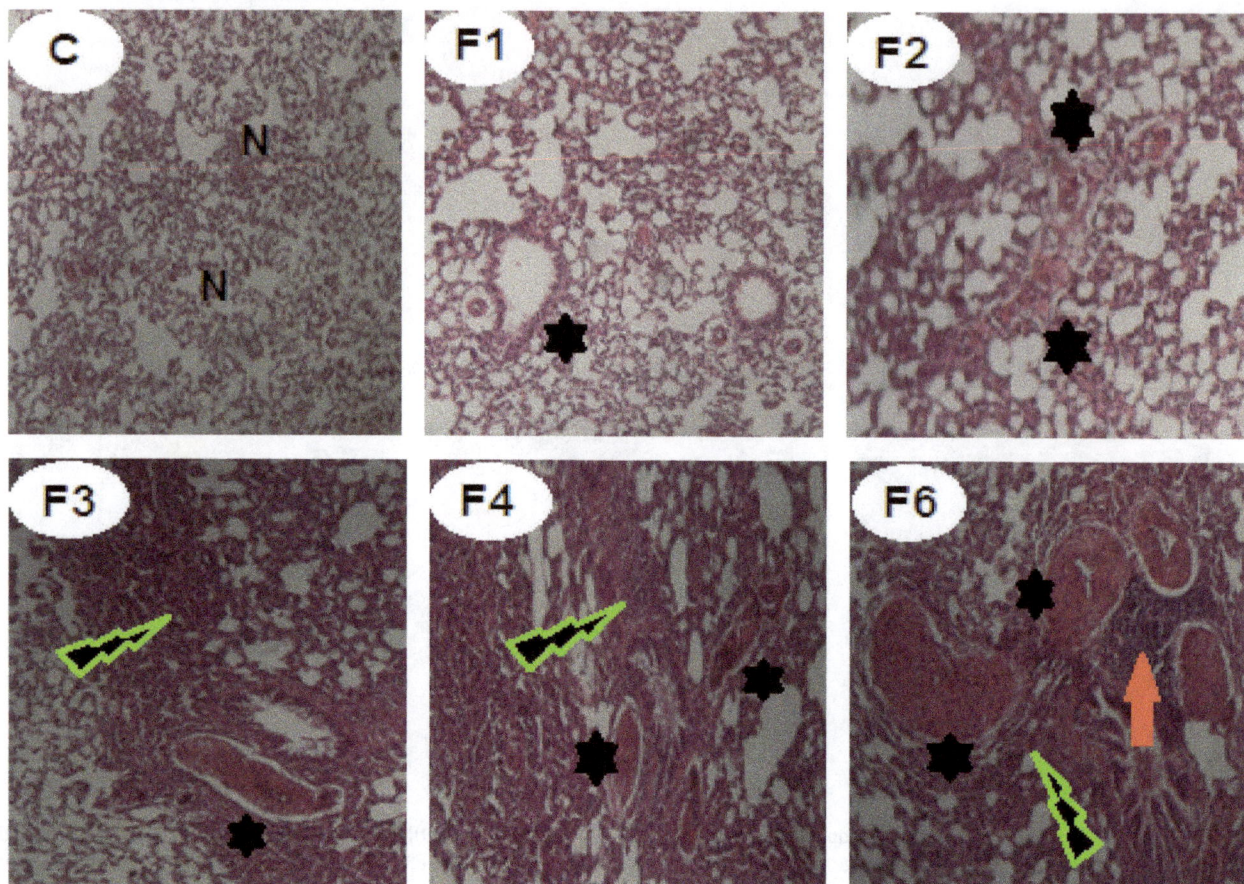

FIGURE 10: Effects of fenitrothion on lung histopathology in rats using H & E staining (×400). C: normal lung tissue, F1: slight hypertrophied vascular smooth muscles, F2: mild hypertrophied vascular smooth muscles, F3: moderate hypertrophied vascular smooth muscles and thickened intra-alveolar septa, F4: severe hypertrophied vascular smooth muscles and thickened intra-alveolar septa, and F6: severe hypertrophied vascular smooth muscles, interstitial hemorrhages with narrow alveolar spaces, and intense thickened septa with perivascular leukocytic aggregation. N: normal lung cells. Black star: hypertrophied vascular smooth muscles. Green lightning: thickening in the alveolar septa. Red arrow: perivascular leukocytic aggregation.

free radical production, changes in lipid composition in brain due to alteration in lipid profile, increased BBB permeability, and brain edema [93].

In normal subjects, intestinal ammonia, produced from nitrogen products, is taken up by the liver and metabolized to urea. Liver disease, whether acute or chronic, is usually accompanied by diminished hepatic urea synthesis, depriving the body of its main route of ammonia detoxification [96].

Ammonia was shown to cause imbalance between excitatory and inhibitory neurotransmitters [79]. Therefore, ammonia content is widely used in the diagnosis of hepatic encephalopathy in cirrhotic patients with altered mental status [97].

The current study has shown that administration of fenitrothion resulted in an initial increase in antioxidant defense mechanisms as evidenced by initial increase in catalase activity and glutathione content and an initial decrease in malondialdehyde content in the first week which was reversed with continued administration of fenitrothion culminating in a state of oxidative stress in the liver, brain, lung, and kidney.

This indicates an initial attempt of the body to combat the oxidative stress state induced by fenitrothion which failed and resulted in an evident state of oxidative stress in liver, brain, and lung. Organophosphorus pesticides have been reported to cause oxidative stress and changes in antioxidant status system [98, 99]. Similar effects of OPs were previously reported by [1] in liver, [100] in brain, [101] in lung, and [67] in kidney.

Organophosphorus pesticide may induce oxidative stress through their "redox-cycling" activity, where they generate superoxide anions and hydrogen peroxide, or through ROS generation via changes in normal antioxidant homeostasis that results in depletion of antioxidants [102].

Organophosphorus pesticides have been shown to induce inflammation and cell infiltration [103].

In the present study the altered histopathological features of liver, brain, and lung were consistent with the biochemical changes and authenticated the injury caused by fenitrothion. Fenitrothion administration caused liver cell injury and congestion of some hepatic cells (in 1st week), apoptosis, focal necrosis and hepatic cell swelling (in 2nd week),

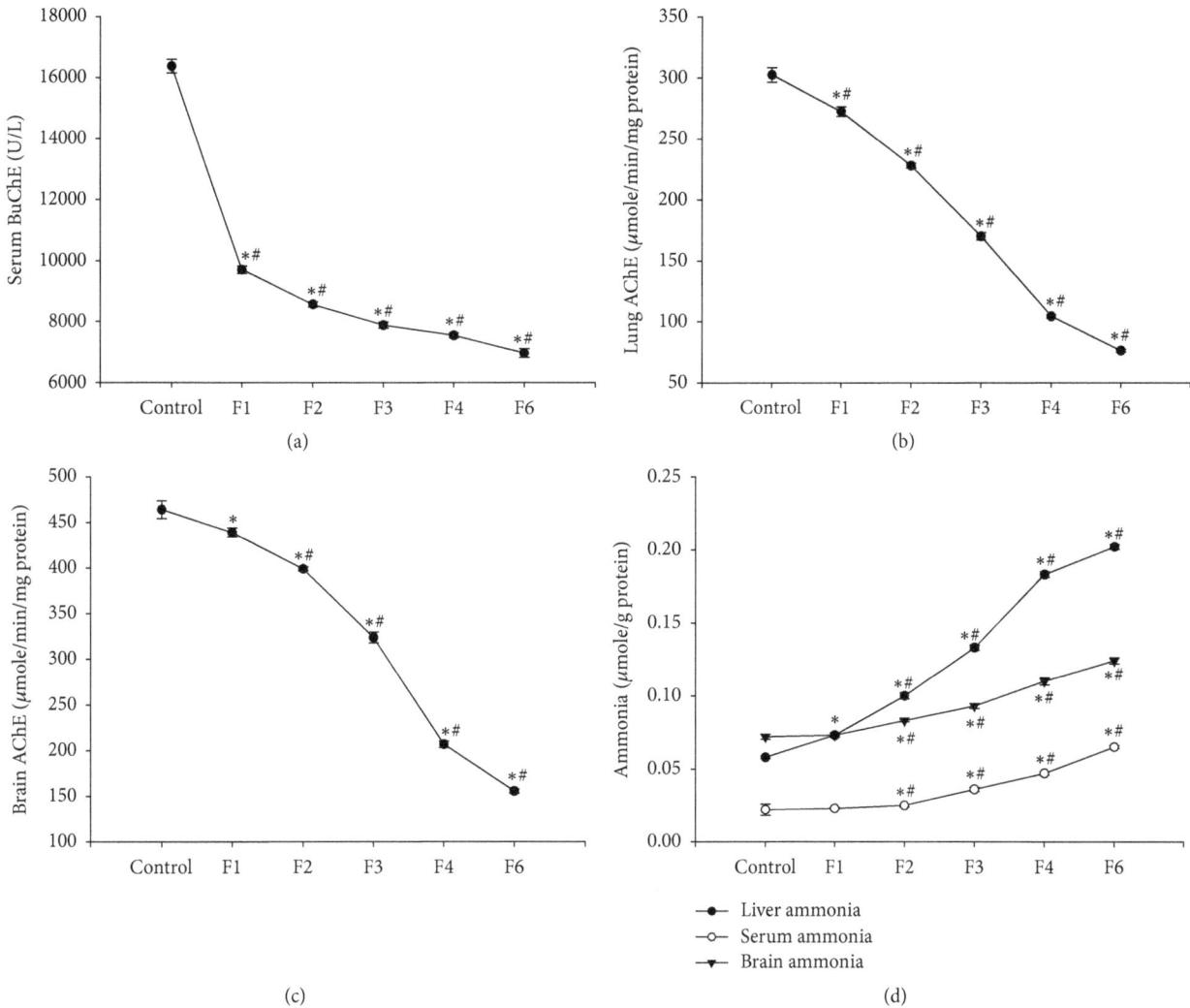

FIGURE 11: Effects of fenitrothion (10 mg/kg) for 1, 2, 3, 4, and 6 weeks (F1, F2, F3, F4, and F6, resp.) on cholinesterase activity and ammonia level in rats. Data are expressed as mean ± SD. $N = 10$. *Significantly different from control group; #significantly different from fenitrothion at the previous time point at $p < 0.05$ using ANOVA followed by Tukey's post hoc test.

ballooned necrotic hepatocytes with lymphocytic aggregation and cell infiltration (in 3rd week), large areas of congestion, lymphocytic aggregation and inflammation (in 4th week), interlobular tissue thickened by edematous fibrous tissue, and congested blood vessels (in 6th week). These changes are in line with data recorded by [104, 105].

Additionally, marked histopathological alterations in brain tissue were observed following fenitrothion administration including focal scattered hemorrhagic areas in cortex (in 1st week), ischemic changes in brain neurons and cytotoxic edema (in 2nd week), cytotoxic edema, degenerated neurons, and focal microgliosis (in 3rd week), cytotoxic edema and intense microgliosis (in 4th week), and finally degenerated neurons, demyelination of the white matter axons and encephalomalacia (in 6th week). Similar alterations were previously reported in chlorpyrifos (OPs) intoxicated animals [106].

Furthermore, marked histopathological alterations were observed in the lung of fenitrothion treated groups including slight hypertrophied vascular smooth muscles (in 1st week), mild hypertrophied vascular smooth muscles (in 2nd week), moderate hypertrophied vascular smooth muscles and thickened intra-alveolar septa (in 3rd week), severe hypertrophied vascular smooth muscles and thickened intra-alveolar septa (in 4th week), and severe hypertrophied vascular smooth muscles, interstitial hemorrhages with narrow alveolar spaces and intense thickened septa with perivascular leukocytic aggregation (in 6th week). These findings are supported by previous studies [84, 107].

5. Conclusion

In conclusion, these results demonstrated that intoxication with fenitrothion induced significant damage of the liver,

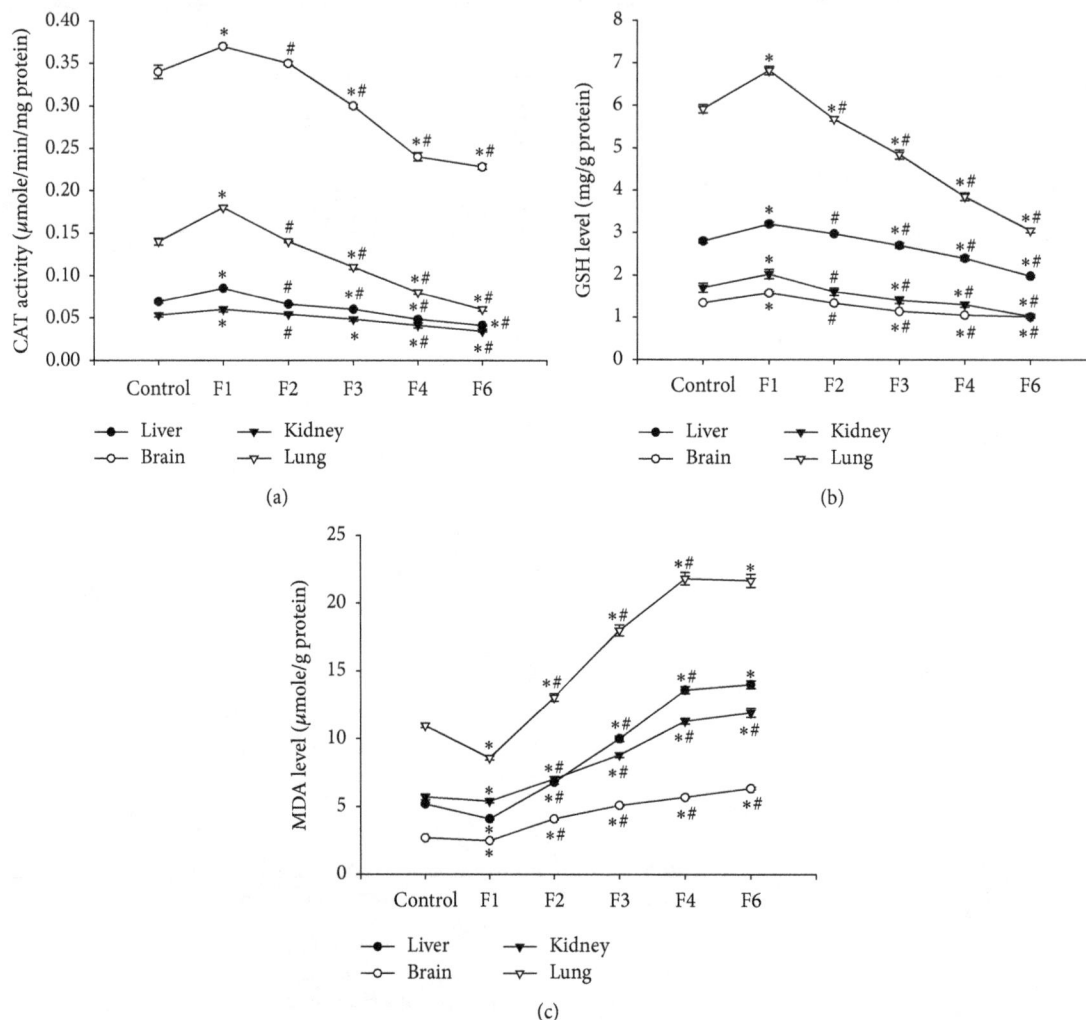

FIGURE 12: Effects of fenitrothion (10 mg/kg) for 1, 2, 3, 4, and 6 weeks (F1, F2, F3, F4, and F6, resp.) on antioxidant state in rats. Data are expressed as mean ± SD. $N = 10$. *Significantly different from control group. #Significantly different from fenitrothion at the previous time point at $p < 0.05$ using ANOVA followed by Tukey's post hoc test.

brain, lung, and kidney leading to imbalance in liver, brain, lung, and kidney functions. Interestingly, the liver was the first to be affected by fenitrothion administration which might imply a delayed effect of fenitrothion on the kidney, brain, and lung due to pharmacokinetic influences or that the damaged liver has affected other organs through elevated ammonia, bilirubin, or defects in hepatic synthesis of vital proteins as albumin and clotting factors.

These results support the hazards of pesticide use and shows the importance of minimizing pesticide use or discovering new safe pesticides.

Competing Interests

The authors declare that they have no conflict of interests.

Authors' Contributions

Ebaa Mohammed and Shimaa Anis equally contributed to this work.

Acknowledgments

This work was funded by the Academy for Scientific Research and Technology, Egypt (R11/2013-25/05/2014). All experiments were performed at the Department of Pharmacology, Faculty of Pharmacy, Zagazig University, Egypt.

References

[1] S. Kalender, F. G. Uzun, D. Durak, F. Demir, and Y. Kalender, "Malathion-induced hepatotoxicity in rats: the effects of vitamins C and E," *Food and Chemical Toxicology*, vol. 48, no. 2, pp. 633–638, 2010.

[2] M. M. Lasram, A. B. Annabi, N. E. Elj et al., "Metabolic disorders of acute exposure to malathion in adult Wistar rats," *Journal of Hazardous Materials*, vol. 163, no. 2-3, pp. 1052–1055, 2009.

[3] R. Rekha, S. Raina, and S. Hamid, "Histopathological effects of pesticide-cholopyrifos on kidney in albino rats," *International Journal of Research in Medical Sciences*, vol. 1, no. 4, p. 465, 2013.

[4] A. F. Hernández, T. Parrón, A. M. Tsatsakis, M. Requena, R. Alarcón, and O. López-Guarnido, "Toxic effects of pesticide mixtures at a molecular level: their relevance to human health," *Toxicology*, vol. 307, pp. 136–145, 2013.

[5] P. A. Jayusman, S. B. Budin, A. R. Ghazali, I. S. Taib, and S. R. Louis, "Effects of palm oil tocotrienol-rich fraction on biochemical and morphological alterations of liver in fenitrothion-treated rats," *Pakistan Journal of Pharmaceutical Sciences*, vol. 27, no. 6, pp. 1873–1880, 2014.

[6] S. V. Kumar, M. Fareedullah, Y. Sudhakar, B. Venkateswarlu, and E. A. Kumar, "Current review on organophosphorus poisoning," *Archives of Applied Science Research*, vol. 2, no. 4, pp. 199–215, 2010.

[7] S. H. Orabi, B. E. Elbialy, and S. M. Shawky, "Ameliorating and hypoglycemic effects of zinc against acute hepatotoxic effect of chlorpyrifos," *Global Veterinaria*, vol. 10, no. 4, pp. 439–446, 2013.

[8] D. Durak, F. G. Uzun, S. Kalender, A. Ogutcu, M. Uzunhisarcikli, and Y. Kalender, "Malathion-induced oxidative stress in human erythrocytes and the protective effect of vitamins C and E in vitro," *Environmental Toxicology*, vol. 24, no. 3, pp. 235–242, 2009.

[9] T. Vani, N. Saharan, S. D. Roy et al., "Alteration in haematological and biochemical parameters of *Catla catla* exposed to sub-lethal concentration of cypermethrin," *Fish Physiology and Biochemistry*, vol. 38, no. 6, pp. 1577–1584, 2012.

[10] M. A. Al-Damegh, "Toxicological impact of inhaled electric mosquito-repellent liquid on the rat: a hematological, cytokine indications, oxidative stress and tumor markers," *Inhalation Toxicology*, vol. 25, no. 5, pp. 292–297, 2013.

[11] J. M. Petras, "Soman neurotoxicity," *Fundamental and Applied Toxicology*, vol. 1, no. 2, p. 242, 1981.

[12] T. Kadar, G. Cohen, R. Sahar, D. Alkalai, and S. Shapira, "Long-term study of brain lesions following soman, in comparison to DFP and metrazol poisoning," *Human and Experimental Toxicology*, vol. 11, no. 6, pp. 517–523, 1992.

[13] B. Veronesi, K. Jones, and C. Pope, "The neurotoxicity of subchronic acetylcholinesterase (AChE) inhibition in rat hippocampus," *Toxicology and Applied Pharmacology*, vol. 104, no. 3, pp. 440–456, 1990.

[14] J. R. Pelegrino, E. E. Calore, P. H. N. Saldiva, V. F. Almeida, N. M. Peres, and L. Vilela-de-Almeida, "Morphometric studies of specific brain regions of rats chronically intoxicated with the organophosphate methamidophos," *Ecotoxicology and Environmental Safety*, vol. 64, no. 2, pp. 251–255, 2006.

[15] T. Dassanayake, V. Weerasinghe, U. Dangahadeniya et al., "Long-term event-related potential changes following organophosphorus insecticide poisoning," *Clinical Neurophysiology*, vol. 119, no. 1, pp. 144–150, 2008.

[16] H. E. Speed, C. A. Blaiss, A. Kim et al., "Delayed reduction of hippocampal synaptic transmission and spines following exposure to repeated subclinical doses of organophosphorus pesticide in adult mice," *Toxicological Sciences*, vol. 125, no. 1, pp. 196–208, 2012.

[17] J. L. Carey, C. Dunn, and R. J. Gaspari, "Central respiratory failure during acute organophosphate poisoning," *Respiratory Physiology and Neurobiology*, vol. 189, no. 2, pp. 403–410, 2013.

[18] A. M. Attia and H. Nasr, "Dimethoate-induced changes in biochemical parameters of experimental rat serum and its neutralization by black seed (Nigella sativa L.) oil," *Slovak Journal of Animal Science*, vol. 2, pp. 87–94, 2009.

[19] M. E. A. Elhalwagy, N. S. Darwish, and E. M. Zaher, "Prophylactic effect of green tea polyphenols against liver and kidney injury induced by fenitrothion insecticide," *Pesticide Biochemistry and Physiology*, vol. 91, no. 2, pp. 81–89, 2008.

[20] B. J. Baars, S. Franklin, and T. Z. Ramsøy, "Global workspace dynamics: cortical 'binding and propagation' enables conscious contents," *Frontiers in Psychology*, vol. 4, article 200, 2013.

[21] G. L. Ellman, K. D. Courtney, V. Andres Jr., and R. M. Featherstone, "A new and rapid colorimetric determination of acetylcholinesterase activity," *Biochemical Pharmacology*, vol. 7, no. 2, pp. 88–95, 1961.

[22] I. P. Lowe, E. Robins, and G. S. Eyerman, "The fluorometric measurement of glutamic decarboxylase and its distribution in brain," *Journal of Neurochemistry*, vol. 3, no. 1, pp. 8–18, 1958.

[23] M. J. G. Harrison, C. D. Marsden, and P. Jenner, "Effect of experimental ischemia on neurotransmitter amines in the gerbil brain," *Stroke*, vol. 10, no. 2, pp. 165–168, 1979.

[24] X. Zhang, H. Li, S. Hu et al., "Brain edema after intracerebral hemorrhage in rats: the role of inflammation," *Neurology India*, vol. 54, no. 4, pp. 402–407, 2006.

[25] M. Kaya, R. Kalayci, M. Küçük et al., "Effect of losartan on the blood-brain barrier permeability in diabetic hypertensive rats," *Life Sciences*, vol. 73, no. 25, pp. 3235–3244, 2003.

[26] C. A. Good, H. M. Kramer, and M. Somogyi, "The determination of glycogen," *The Journal of Biological Chemistry*, vol. 100, pp. 485–491, 1933.

[27] E. Beutler, O. Duron, and B. M. Kelly, "Improved method for the determination of blood glutathione," *The Journal of Laboratory and Clinical Medicine*, vol. 61, pp. 882–888, 1963.

[28] A. K. Sinha, "Colorimetric assay of catalase," *Analytical Biochemistry*, vol. 47, no. 2, pp. 389–394, 1972.

[29] T. Yoshioka, K. Kawada, T. Shimada, and M. Mori, "Lipid peroxidation in maternal and cord blood and protective mechanism against activated-oxygen toxicity in the blood," *American Journal of Obstetrics & Gynecology*, vol. 135, no. 3, pp. 372–376, 1979.

[30] S. Reitman and S. Frankel, "A colorimetric method for the determination of serum glutamic oxalacetic and glutamic pyruvic transaminases," *American Journal of Clinical Pathology*, vol. 28, no. 1, pp. 56–63, 1957.

[31] A. Belfield and D. M. Goldberg, "Revised assay for serum phenyl phosphatase activity using 4-amino-antipyrine," *Enzyme*, vol. 12, no. 5, pp. 561–573, 1971.

[32] M. Knedel and R. Böttger, "A kinetic method for determination of the activity of pseudocholinesterase (acylcholine acylhydrolase 3.1. 1.8.)," *Klinische Wochenschrift*, vol. 45, no. 6, pp. 325–327, 1967.

[33] M. I. Walters and H. W. Gerarde, "An ultramicromethod for the determination of conjugated and total bilirubin in serum or plasma," *Microchemical Journal*, vol. 15, no. 2, pp. 231–243, 1970.

[34] B. T. Doumas, W. A. Watson, and H. G. Biggs, "Albumin standards and the measurement of serum albumin with bromcresol green," *Clinica Chimica Acta*, vol. 258, no. 1, pp. 21–30, 1997.

[35] P. Trinder, "A rapid method for the determination of sodium in serum," *The Analyst*, vol. 76, no. 907, pp. 596–599, 1951.

[36] F. W. Sunderman Jr. and F. W. Sunderman, "Studies in serum electrolytes. XXII. A rapid, reliable method for serum potassium using tetraphenylboron," *American Journal of Clinical Pathology*, vol. 29, no. 2, pp. 95–103, 1958.

[37] E. Gindler and D. Heth, *Colorimetric Determination with Bound Calmagite of Magnesium in Human Blood Serum*, Clinical Chemistry, American Association for Clinical Chemistry, Washington, DC, USA, 1971.

[38] W. Richmond, "Preparation and properties of a cholesterol oxidase from Nocardia sp. and its application to the enzymatic assay of total cholesterol in serum," *Clinical Chemistry*, vol. 19, no. 12, pp. 1350–1356, 1973.

[39] M. Burstein, H. R. Scholnick, and R. Morfin, "Rapid method for the isolation of lipoproteins from human serum by precipitation with polyanions," *Journal of Lipid Research*, vol. 11, no. 6, pp. 583–595, 1970.

[40] H. Wieland and D. Seidel, "A simple specific method for precipitation of low density lipoproteins," *Journal of Lipid Research*, vol. 24, no. 7, pp. 904–909, 1983.

[41] J. K. Fawcett and J. E. Scott, "A rapid and precise method for the determination of urea," *Journal of Clinical Pathology*, vol. 13, no. 2, pp. 156–159, 1960.

[42] D. Barham and P. Trinder, "An improved colour reagent for the determination of blood glucose by the oxidase system," *Analyst*, vol. 97, no. 1151, pp. 142–145, 1972.

[43] D. L. Drabkin and J. H. Austin, "Spectrophotometric studies I. Spectrophotometric constants for common hemoglobin derivatives in human, dog, and rabbit blood," *The Journal of Biological Chemistry*, vol. 98, no. 2, pp. 719–733, 1932.

[44] P. Trinder, "Determination of blood glucose using an oxidase-peroxidase system with a non-carcinogenic chromogen," *Journal of Clinical Pathology*, vol. 22, no. 2, pp. 158–161, 1969.

[45] R. Hull, J. Hirsh, R. Jay et al., "Different intensities of oral anticoagulant therapy in the treatment of proximal-vein thrombosis," *The New England Journal of Medicine*, vol. 307, no. 27, pp. 1676–1681, 1982.

[46] R. Henry, D. Cannon, and J. Winkelman, *Clinical Chemistry: Principles and Technics*, Harper & Row, Hagerstown, Md, USA, 1974.

[47] K. Konitzer and S. Voigt, "Direct determination of ammonium in blood and tissue extracts by means of the phenol by chlorite reaction," *Clinica Chimica Acta; International Journal of Clinical Chemistry*, vol. 8, article 5, 1963.

[48] J. A. Patil, A. J. Patil, and S. P. Govindwar, "Biochemical effects of various pesticides on sprayers of grape gardens," *Indian Journal of Clinical Biochemistry*, vol. 18, no. 2, pp. 16–22, 2003.

[49] B. Kavitha, S. Shruthi, S. P. Rai, and Y. Ramachandra, "Phytochemical analysis and hepatoprotective properties of *Tinospora cordifolia* against carbon tetrachloride-induced hepatic damage in rats," *Journal of Basic and Clinical Pharmacy*, vol. 2, no. 3, pp. 139–142, 2011.

[50] N. K. Jain and A. K. Singhai, "Protective effects of *Phyllanthus acidus* (L.) Skeels leaf extracts on acetaminophen and thioacetamide induced hepatic injuries in Wistar rats," *Asian Pacific Journal of Tropical Medicine*, vol. 4, no. 6, pp. 470–474, 2011.

[51] S. W. Oh, E. S. Lee, S. Kim et al., "Bilirubin attenuates the renal tubular injury by inhibition of oxidative stress and apoptosis," *BMC Nephrology*, vol. 14, article 105, 2013.

[52] G. Bortolussi, E. Codarin, G. Antoniali et al., "Impairment of enzymatic antioxidant defenses is associated with bilirubin-induced neuronal cell death in the cerebellum of Ugt1 KO mice," *Cell Death & Disease*, vol. 6, no. 5, Article ID e1739, 2015.

[53] A.-T. H. Mossa, A. A. Refaie, and A. Ramadan, "Effect of exposure to mixture of four organophosphate insecticides at no observed adverse effect level dose on rat liver: the protective role

of vitamin C," *Research Journal of Environmental Toxicology*, vol. 5, no. 6, pp. 323–335, 2011.

[54] C. Heneghan, A. Ward, R. Perera et al., "Self-monitoring of oral anticoagulation: systematic review and meta-analysis of individual patient data," *The Lancet*, vol. 379, no. 9813, pp. 322–334, 2012.

[55] K. A. Amin and K. S. Hashem, "Deltamethrin-induced oxidative stress and biochemical changes in tissues and blood of catfish (Clarias gariepinus): antioxidant defense and role of alpha-tocopherol," *BMC Veterinary Research*, vol. 8, article 45, 2012.

[56] M. Anusha, M. Venkateswarlu, V. Prabhakaran, S. S. Taj, B. P. Kumari, and D. Ranganayakulu, "Hepatoprotective activity of aqueous extract of *Portulaca oleracea* in combination with lycopene in rats," *Indian Journal of Pharmacology*, vol. 43, no. 5, pp. 563–567, 2011.

[57] C. I. Acker and C. W. Nogueira, "Chlorpyrifos acute exposure induces hyperglycemia and hyperlipidemia in rats," *Chemosphere*, vol. 89, no. 5, pp. 602–608, 2012.

[58] R. Nagaraju, A. K. R. Joshi, and P. S. Rajini, "Organophosphorus insecticide, monocrotophos, possesses the propensity to induce insulin resistance in rats on chronic exposure," *Journal of Diabetes*, vol. 7, no. 1, pp. 47–59, 2015.

[59] A. D. Southam, A. Lange, A. Hines et al., "Metabolomics reveals target and off-target toxicities of a model organophosphate pesticide to roach (*Rutilus rutilus*): implications for biomonitoring," *Environmental Science & Technology*, vol. 45, no. 8, pp. 3759–3767, 2011.

[60] M. Pakzad, S. Fouladdel, A. Nili-Ahmadabadi et al., "Sublethal exposures of diazinon alters glucose homostasis in Wistar rats: biochemical and molecular evidences of oxidative stress in adipose tissues," *Pesticide Biochemistry and Physiology*, vol. 105, no. 1, pp. 57–61, 2013.

[61] A. A. Malekirad, M. Faghih, M. Mirabdollahi, M. Kiani, A. Fathi, and M. Abdollahi, "Neurocognitive, mental health, and glucose disorders in farmers exposed to organophosphorus pesticides," *Archives of Industrial Hygiene and Toxicology*, vol. 64, no. 1, pp. 1–8, 2013.

[62] S. M. Ismail, "Protective effects of vitamin C against biochemical toxicity induced by malathion pesticides in male albino rat," *Journal of Evolutionary Biology Research*, vol. 5, no. 1, pp. 1–5, 2013.

[63] B. Mehra, P. Sharma, U. Kaushik, and S. Joshi, "Effect of fytolan on haematology and serum parameters of male albino rats," *World Journal of Pharmaceutical Sciences*, vol. 3, pp. 817–829, 2014.

[64] I. A. Hundekari, A. N. Suryakar, and D. B. Rathi, "Acute organophosphorus pesticide poisoning in North Karnataka, India: oxidative damage, haemoglobin level and total leukocyte," *African Health Sciences*, vol. 13, no. 1, pp. 129–136, 2013.

[65] M. Muthulingam, P. Mohandoss, N. Indra, and S. Sethupathy, "Antihepatotoxic efficacy of Indigofera tinctoria (Linn.) on paracetamol induced liver damage in rats," *International Journal of Pharmaceutical and Biomedical Research*, vol. 1, no. 1, pp. 13–18, 2010.

[66] H. A. Hassan and M. I. Yousef, "Ameliorating effect of chicory (*Cichorium intybus* L.)-supplemented diet against nitrosamine precursors-induced liver injury and oxidative stress in male rats," *Food and Chemical Toxicology*, vol. 48, no. 8-9, pp. 2163–2169, 2010.

[67] S. A. Mansour and A.-T. H. Mossa, "Oxidative damage, biochemical and histopathological alterations in rats exposed

to chlorpyrifos and the antioxidant role of zinc," *Pesticide Biochemistry and Physiology*, vol. 96, no. 1, pp. 14–23, 2010.

[68] R. R. Elzoghby, A. F. Hamoda, A. Abed-Ftah, and M. Farouk, "Protective role of vitamin C and green tea extract on malathion-induced hepatotoxicity and nephrotoxicity in rats," *American Journal of Pharmacology and Toxicology*, vol. 9, no. 3, pp. 177–188, 2014.

[69] V. Sundaram, V. Manne, and A. M. S. Al-Osaimi, "Ascites and spontaneous bacterial peritonitis: recommendations from two United States centers," *Saudi Journal of Gastroenterology*, vol. 20, no. 5, pp. 279–287, 2014.

[70] H. R. Pohl, J. S. Wheeler, and H. E. Murray, "Sodium and potassium in health and disease," in *Interrelations between Essential Metal Ions and Human Diseases*, pp. 29–47, Springer, Berlin, Germany, 2013.

[71] M. L. Gumz, L. Rabinowitz, and C. S. Wingo, "An integrated view of potassium homeostasis," *The New England Journal of Medicine*, vol. 373, no. 1, pp. 60–72, 2015.

[72] H. H. Mossalam, O. A. Abd-El Aty, E. N. Morgan, S. Youssaf, and A. M. H. Mackawy, "Biochemical and ultra structure studies of the antioxidant effect of aqueous extract of hibiscus sabdariffa on the nephrotoxicity induced by organophosphorous pesticide (malathion) on the adult albino rats," *Journal of American Science*, vol. 7, no. 12, pp. 561–572, 2011.

[73] I. D. Weiner, W. E. Mitch, and J. M. Sands, "Urea and ammonia metabolism and the control of renal nitrogen excretion," *Clinical Journal of the American Society of Nephrology*, vol. 10, no. 8, pp. 1444–1458, 2015.

[74] C. Giuliani and A. Peri, "Effects of Hyponatremia on the Brain," *Journal of Clinical Medicine*, vol. 3, no. 4, pp. 1163–1177, 2014.

[75] L. Rivera-Espinosa, E. Floriano-Sánchez, J. Pedraza-Chaverrí et al., "Contributions of microdialysis to new alternative therapeutics for hepatic encephalopathy," *International Journal of Molecular Sciences*, vol. 14, no. 8, pp. 16184–16206, 2013.

[76] M. A. E. Ahmed, H. I. Ahmed, and E. M. El-Morsy, "Melatonin protects against diazinon-induced neurobehavioral changes in rats," *Neurochemical Research*, vol. 38, no. 10, pp. 2227–2236, 2013.

[77] D. C. Jones and G. W. Miller, "The effects of environmental neurotoxicants on the dopaminergic system: a possible role in drug addiction," *Biochemical Pharmacology*, vol. 76, no. 5, pp. 569–581, 2008.

[78] J. Zhang, H. Dai, Y. Deng et al., "Neonatal chlorpyrifos exposure induces loss of dopaminergic neurons in young adult rats," *Toxicology*, vol. 336, pp. 17–25, 2015.

[79] H. Cichoż-Lach and A. Michalak, "Current pathogenetic aspects of hepatic encephalopathy and noncirrhotic hyperammonemic encephalopathy," *World Journal of Gastroenterology*, vol. 19, no. 1, pp. 26–34, 2013.

[80] B. Moghaddam and D. Javitt, "From revolution to evolution: the glutamate hypothesis of schizophrenia and its implication for treatment," *Neuropsychopharmacology*, vol. 37, no. 1, pp. 4–15, 2012.

[81] M. Sidoryk-Wegrzynowicz and M. Aschner, "Manganese toxicity in the central nervous system: the glutamine/glutamate-γ-aminobutyric acid cycle," *Journal of Internal Medicine*, vol. 273, no. 5, pp. 466–477, 2013.

[82] Y. Avraham, N. C. Grigoriadis, T. Poutahidis et al., "Cannabidiol improves brain and liver function in a fulminant hepatic failure-induced model of hepatic encephalopathy in mice," *British Journal of Pharmacology*, vol. 162, no. 7, pp. 1650–1658, 2011.

[83] D. Häussinger and B. Görg, "Interaction of oxidative stress, astrocyte swelling and cerebral ammonia toxicity," *Current Opinion in Clinical Nutrition and Metabolic Care*, vol. 13, no. 1, pp. 87–92, 2010.

[84] M. A. Noaishi, M. M. Afify, and A. A. Abd Allah, "Study the inhalation exposure effect of pesticides mixture in the white rat," *Nature & Science*, vol. 11, no. 7, pp. 45–54, 2013.

[85] H. Falcão and A. M. Japiassú, "Albumin in critically ill patients: controversies and recommendations," *Revista Brasileira de Terapia Intensiva*, vol. 23, no. 1, pp. 87–95, 2011.

[86] E. Cataudella, G. Malaguarnera, C. Gagliano et al., "Pesticides exposure and the management of acute hepatic injury," *Acta Medica Mediterranea*, vol. 28, no. 3, pp. 245–252, 2012.

[87] J.-M. Collombet, "Nerve agent intoxication: recent neuropathophysiological findings and subsequent impact on medical management prospects," *Toxicology and Applied Pharmacology*, vol. 255, no. 3, pp. 229–241, 2011.

[88] A. Osman, S. A. Mastan, S. Rabia Banu, and P. Indira, "Sublethal effect of cypermethrin on acetylcholinesterase (AChE) activity and acetylcholine (Ach) content in selected tissues of Channa striatus (Bloch.)," *Journal of Toxicology and Environmental Health Sciences*, vol. 7, no. 4, pp. 31–37, 2015.

[89] M. Pohanka, "Inhibitors of acetylcholinesterase and butyrylcholinesterase meet immunity," *International Journal of Molecular Sciences*, vol. 15, no. 6, pp. 9809–9825, 2014.

[90] M. E. A. Elhalwagy, N. S. Darwish, D. A. Shokry et al., "Garlic and α lipoic supplementation enhance the immune system of albino rats and alleviate implications of pesticides mixtures," *International Journal of Clinical and Experimental Medicine*, vol. 8, no. 5, pp. 7689–7700, 2015.

[91] J. L. Franco, T. Posser, J. J. Mattos et al., "Zinc reverses malathion-induced impairment in antioxidant defenses," *Toxicology Letters*, vol. 187, no. 3, pp. 137–143, 2009.

[92] F. S. Larsen, J. Gottstein, and A. T. Blei, "Cerebral hyperemia and nitric oxide synthase in rats with ammonia-induced brain edema," *Journal of Hepatology*, vol. 34, no. 4, pp. 548–554, 2001.

[93] T. R. Scott, V. T. Kronsten, R. D. Hughes, and D. L. Shawcross, "Pathophysiology of cerebral oedema in acute liver failure," *World Journal of Gastroenterology*, vol. 19, no. 48, pp. 9240–9255, 2013.

[94] R. Penchalamma and D. P. Jacob, "Dimethoate on protein metabolic profiles in rat kidney," *Weekly Science Research Journal*, vol. 2, no. 11, pp. 2321–7871, 2014.

[95] C. R. Bosoi, X. Yang, J. Huynh et al., "Systemic oxidative stress is implicated in the pathogenesis of brain edema in rats with chronic liver failure," *Free Radical Biology and Medicine*, vol. 52, no. 7, pp. 1228–1235, 2012.

[96] A. Lemberg and M. A. Fernandez, "Hepatic encephalopathy, ammonia, glutamate, glutamine and oxidative stress," *Annals of Hepatology*, vol. 8, no. 2, pp. 95–102, 2009.

[97] J. S. Bajaj, "The role of microbiota in hepatic encephalopathy," *Gut Microbes*, vol. 5, no. 3, pp. 397–403, 2014.

[98] T. Rahman, I. Hosen, M. M. T. Islam, and H. U. Shekhar, "Oxidative stress and human health," *Advances in Bioscience and Biotechnology*, vol. 3, no. 7, pp. 997–1019, 2012.

[99] Z. Badade, S. Rastogi, and S. Singh, "Antioxidant status and oxidative stress in organophosphate pesticide poisoning," *Journal of Dental and Medical Sciences*, vol. 7, no. 6, pp. 20–24, 2013.

[100] A. E.-A. A. Diab, E.-S. A. A. El-Aziz, A. A. Hendawy, M. H. Zahra, and R. Z. Hamza, "Antioxidant role of both propolis and ginseng against neurotoxicity of chlorpyrifos and profenofos

in male rats," *Life Science Journal-Acta Zhengzhou University Overseas*, vol. 9, pp. 987–1008, 2012.

[101] M. M. Ahmed and N. I. Zaki, "Assessment the ameliorative effect of pomegranate and rutin on chlorpyrifos-ethyl-induced oxidative stress in rats," *Nature and Science*, vol. 7, no. 10, pp. 49–61, 2009.

[102] A. M. Al-Othman, K. S. Al-Numair, G. E. El-Desoky et al., "Protection of α-tocopherol and selenium against acute effects of malathion on liver and kidney of rats," *African Journal of Pharmacy and Pharmacology*, vol. 5, no. 10, pp. 1263–1271, 2011.

[103] M. E. A. Elhalwagy and N. I. Zaki, "Comparative study on pesticide mixture of organophosphorus and pyrethroid in commercial formulation," *Environmental Toxicology and Pharmacology*, vol. 28, no. 2, pp. 219–224, 2009.

[104] T. M. Heikal, M. El-Sherbiny, S. A. Hassan, A. Arafa, and H. Z. Ghanem, "Antioxidant effect of selenium on hepatotoxicity induced by chlorpyrifos in male rats," *International Journal of Pharmacy and Pharmaceutical Sciences*, vol. 4, no. 4, pp. 603–609, 2012.

[105] D. L. Baconi, M. Bârcă, G. Manda, A.-M. Ciobanu, and C. Bălălău, "Investigation of the toxicity of some organophosphorus pesticides in a repeated dose study in rats," *Romanian Journal of Morphology and Embryology*, vol. 54, no. 2, pp. 349–356, 2013.

[106] A. Newairy and H. Abdou, "Effect of propolis consumption on hepatotoxity and brain damage in male rats exposed to chlorpyrifos," *African Journal of Biotechnology*, vol. 12, no. 33, pp. 5232–5243, 2013.

[107] O. Owoeye, F. V. Edem, B. S. Akinyoola, S. Rahaman, E. E. Akang, and G. O. Arinola, "Histological changes in liver and lungs of rats exposed to dichlorvos before and after vitamin supplementation," *European Journal of Anatomy*, vol. 16, no. 3, pp. 190–198, 2012.

14

Estimation of the Mechanism of Adrenal Action of Endocrine-Disrupting Compounds Using a Computational Model of Adrenal Steroidogenesis in NCI-H295R Cells

Ryuta Saito,[1,2,3] Natsuko Terasaki,[4] Makoto Yamazaki,[3] Naoya Masutomi,[4] Naohisa Tsutsui,[4] and Masahiro Okamoto[1]

[1]Graduate School of Bioresource and Bioenvironmental Sciences, Kyushu University, Higashi-ku, Fukuoka 812-8582, Japan
[2]Biology Research Laboratories, Mitsubishi Tanabe Pharma Corporation, Toda-shi, Saitama 335-8505, Japan
[3]DMPK Research Laboratories, Mitsubishi Tanabe Pharma Corporation, Toda-shi, Saitama 335-8505, Japan
[4]Safety Research Laboratories, Mitsubishi Tanabe Pharma Corporation, Kisarazu-shi, Chiba 292-0818, Japan

Correspondence should be addressed to Ryuta Saito; saitou.ryuuta@mc.mt-pharma.co.jp

Academic Editor: Steven J. Bursian

Adrenal toxicity is one of the major concerns in drug development. To quantitatively understand the effect of endocrine-active compounds on adrenal steroidogenesis and to assess the human adrenal toxicity of novel pharmaceutical drugs, we developed a mathematical model of steroidogenesis in human adrenocortical carcinoma NCI-H295R cells. The model includes cellular proliferation, intracellular cholesterol translocation, diffusional transport of steroids, and metabolic pathways of adrenal steroidogenesis, which serially involve steroidogenic proteins and enzymes such as StAR, CYP11A1, CYP17A1, HSD3B2, CYP21A2, CYP11B1, CYP11B2, HSD17B3, and CYP19A1. It was reconstructed in an experimental dynamics of cholesterol and 14 steroids from an *in vitro* steroidogenesis assay using NCI-H295R cells. Results of dynamic sensitivity analysis suggested that HSD3B2 plays the most important role in the metabolic balance of adrenal steroidogenesis. Based on differential metabolic profiling of 12 steroid hormones and 11 adrenal toxic compounds, we could estimate which steroidogenic enzymes were affected in this mathematical model. In terms of adrenal steroidogenic inhibitors, the predicted action sites were approximately matched to reported target enzymes. Thus, our computer-aided system based on systems biological approach may be useful to understand the mechanism of action of endocrine-active compounds and to assess the human adrenal toxicity of novel pharmaceutical drugs.

1. Introduction

Because steroid hormones play an important role in a wide range of physiological processes, the potential to disturb endocrine effects is a major concern in the development of novel pharmaceutical drugs such as etomidate and aminoglutethimide [1]. The adrenal gland is the most common target for toxicity in the endocrine system *in vivo*, because steroid hormones are primarily synthesized through enzymatic reactions in the adrenal cortex [2–5]. Indeed, in these studies based on chemically induced endocrine lesions observed *in vivo*, the most frequent site of reported effects was the adrenal gland. Therefore, the prediction of human adrenal toxicity based on the mechanism of on- or off-target actions in the early stages of drug development is important.

The NCI-H295R human adrenocortical carcinoma cell line has been used to elucidate mechanisms of adrenal steroidogenic disrupting compounds [1, 6]. The H295R cell line was established by Gazder and his collaborators in 1990 [7], which expresses all key steroidogenic enzymes and steroidogenesis-related proteins [7–9]. H295R cells have the physiological characteristics of zonally undifferentiated human fetal adrenal cells and the ability to produce steroid hormones found in the adult adrenal cortex [1, 7, 9]. *In vitro* bioassays using the H295R human cell line have been able to evaluate the effects of chemicals on steroid hormone production [10–15], steroidogenic enzyme activities [11, 16, 17], and the expression of steroidogenic genes [11, 18]. In transcriptome studies, the mechanisms of action of many steroidogenic disrupting compounds have been qualitatively assessed in terms of adrenal toxicity. However, gene expression does not always reflect the production of steroid hormones [19]. Furthermore, measuring a few specific steroid hormones may not be a useful approach to study the mechanisms of steroidogenic disrupting effects in complex pathways such as adrenal steroidogenesis. To systematically understand how exogenous compounds affect adrenal steroidogenesis, simultaneous determination of all detectable steroid hormones and integrative analysis of these complex data would be important. As an exploratory approach to analyze complex data, ToxClust developed by Zhang and colleagues in 2009 is able to visualize concentration-dependent response relationships in the characteristics of chemically induced toxicological effects [20]. However, this exploratory approach is unable to provide a quantitative understanding of the mechanism of action of adrenal toxicants or reveal systematic information about the effect of each enzymatic reaction, interactions, and feedback in the adrenal steroidogenesis pathway.

Systems biology based on computational models of biological processes and the comprehensive measurement of biological molecules is the most powerful approach to quantitatively understand the influence of each factor in complex biological pathways. In recent studies by our collaborators, a computational model of adrenal steroidogenesis has been developed in NCI-H295R cells, including the steroidogenic disrupting effects of metyrapone to inhibit enzymatic reactions of CYP11B1 [21, 22]. The model reproduces the dynamics of adrenal steroidogenesis in NCI-H295R cells and the influence of metyrapone. A current computational model of adrenal steroidogenesis was incorporated with a reaction of oxysterol synthesis as a bypass to consume cellular cholesterol [22]. In addition, all reactions in this model are described by a kinetic equation of the first-order reaction [22]. It is difficult to quantitatively evaluate the influence of each protein in the complicated system of adrenal steroidogenesis using the reported models, because it is simple and any biochemical and cellular biological information is not sufficient. For example, to clearly understand the cause of the change from the differentially dynamic patterns of steroid hormones, it is necessary to consider the substrate inhibition of steroidogenic enzyme because most of steroidogenic enzymes recognize multiple steroids as the enzymatic substrate. However, the substrate inhibition of steroidogenic enzyme cannot be described by the mathematical model based on kinetic equations of first-order reaction that does not consider Michaelis constant K_m expressing the affinity of the substrate. To quantitatively estimate the mechanism of steroidogenic disrupting compounds from comprehensive experimental data of adrenal steroidogenesis in NCI-H295R cells, the reported model should be improved according to the following two points. First, the kinetic equation of enzymatic reactions should be exchanged from the first-order equation to a steady-state kinetic equation based on the mechanism of

the enzymatic reaction. Because a mathematical model organized by first-order equations operates in a simple structure-dependent manner, it does not show complex behavior based on molecular interactions, feedback, or regulation. Second, intracellular localization processes of cholesterol should be incorporated as a considerable mechanism. Because intracellular cholesterol molecules are stored as cholesterol esters or widely distributed as membrane components, only a few cholesterol molecules localized on the mitochondrial inner membrane are available for the adrenal steroidogenesis pathway [23, 24]. Moreover, cholesterol-trafficking processes from the outer to inner mitochondrial membranes, which are regulated by steroidogenic acute regulatory (StAR) protein, are one of the rate-limiting steps in adrenal steroidogenesis [24]. By overcoming these limitations in the reported steroidogenesis model, systems analysis of adrenal steroidogenesis in H295R cells may be able to quantitatively estimate the mechanism of action of steroidogenic disrupting compounds.

In the present study, to quantitatively estimate the toxicological mechanism of endocrine-active compounds in adrenal steroidogenesis and to predict human adrenal toxicity of novel pharmaceutical drugs in the drug discovery phase, we developed a novel computational model of steroidogenesis in NCI-H295R cells. It includes cholesterol transport into intracellular regions from the extracellular space, the cholesterol translocation system in intracellular regions, including oxysterol synthesis, the metabolic pathway of adrenal steroidogenesis, and transport of steroid hormones. Global sensitivity analysis of this adrenal steroidogenesis model is able to evaluate the influence of each steroidogenic enzyme and related protein for each steroid hormone observed in an *in vitro* steroidogenesis assay of NCI-H295R cells. Furthermore, the mechanisms of action of steroidogenesis disrupting compounds for steroidogenic enzymes can be estimated by the optimization method to solve the reverse problem from the concentration changes of 12 steroid hormones measured by liquid chromatography/mass spectrometry in the steroidogenesis assay of NCI-H295R cells *in vitro*. Using this developed model of adrenal steroidogenesis and the analytical approach, the *in vitro* steroidogenesis assay of NCI-H295R cells can assess the human adrenal toxicity of a novel pharmaceutical drug based on quantitative understanding of its toxicological mechanism in adrenal steroidogenesis.

2. Materials and Methods

2.1. The Experimental Part

2.1.1. Cell Culture. NCI-H295R human adrenocortical carcinoma cells were purchased from the American Type Culture Collection (Cat# CRL-2128, Manassas, VA) and cultured at 37°C in a humidified atmosphere with 5% CO_2. The cells were maintained in a 1:1 mixture of Dulbecco's modified Eagle's medium (DMEM, GIBCO, Life Technologies, Carlsbad, CA) and F-12 medium (MP Biomedicals Inc., Irvine, CA) supplemented with 15 mM HEPES (Dojindo Laboratories, Kumamoto, Japan), 0.00625 mg/mL insulin (Sigma-Aldrich, Inc., St. Louis, MO), 0.00625 mg/mL transferrin

(Sigma-Aldrich Inc., St. Louis, MO), 30 nM sodium selenite (Wako Pure Chemical Industries Ltd., Osaka, Japan), 1.25 mg/mL bovine serum albumin (BSA, Sigma-Aldrich Inc., St. Louis, MO), 0.00535 mg/mL linoleic acid (Sigma-Aldrich Inc., St. Louis, MO), 2.5% Nu Serum (Becton, Dickinson and Company, Franklin Lakes, NJ), 100 U/mL penicillin (Meiji Seika Pharma, Tokyo, Japan), and 100 mg/L streptomycin (Meiji Seika Pharma, Tokyo, Japan).

2.1.2. Adrenal Steroidogenesis in Human Adrenal Corticocarcinoma NCI-H295R Cells. NCI-H295R cells were stimulated with adrenocorticotrophic hormone (ACTH), forskolin, and angiotensin II to initiate steroidogenesis. Changes in steroid concentrations over time were measured after stimulation in both cells and culture medium to construct a simulation model.

The cells were seeded at 6×10^5 cells/well in 6-well plates. After 3 days of culture, the culture medium was changed to stimulation medium consisting of DMEM/F-12 (1 : 1) medium supplemented with 0.00625 mg/mL insulin, 0.00625 mg/mL transferrin, 30 nM sodium selenite, 1.25 mg/mL BSA, 0.00535 mg/mL linoleic acid, 10% fetal bovine serum (GIBCO, Life Technologies, Carlsbad, CA), 100 U/mL penicillin, 100 mg/L streptomycin, 50 nM ACTH (Sigma-Aldrich Inc., St. Louis, MO), 20 μM forskolin (Sigma-Aldrich Inc., St. Louis, MO), and 100 nM angiotensin II (Calbiochem, Merck Millipore, Darmstadt, Germany). Culture media and cells were collected at 0, 8, 24, 48, and 72 h after stimulation. The cells were collected in 100 μL distilled water and sonicated to produce a cell lysate. The cultures were conducted in four wells/time point ($N = 4$).

The concentrations of 12 steroids, pregnenolone (PREG), 17α-hydroxypregnenolone (HPREG), dehydroepiandrosterone (DHEA), progesterone (PROG), 17α-hydroxyprogesterone (HPROG), androstenedione (DIONE), testosterone (TESTO), 11-deoxycorticosterone (DCORTICO), 11-deoxycortisol (DCORT), corticosterone (CORTICO), cortisol (CORT), and aldosterone (ALDO), in the medium and cell lysate were measured by LC/MS. Concentrations of estrone (E1) and 17β-estradiol (E2) were measured by enzyme-linked immunosorbent assays (Wako Pure Chemical Industries Ltd., Osaka, Japan). In addition, the concentration of cholesterol was measured using a commercial kit (Wako Pure Chemical Industries Ltd., Osaka, Japan) based on the cholesterol oxidase method.

2.1.3. Liquid Chromatography. A LC-VP series (Shimadzu, Kyoto, Japan) consisting of an SIL-HTc autosampler, LC-10ADvp Pump, CTO-10ACvp column oven, and DGU-14AM degasser was used to set the reverse-phase liquid chromatographic conditions. The column was a Cadenza CD-C18 column (100 × 2 mm i.d., 3 μm, Imtakt Corp., Kyoto, Japan) used at 45°C. The mobile phase included water/acetonitrile/formic acid 95/5/0.05 (v/v/v, Solvent A) and water/acetonitrile/formic acid 35/65/0.05 (v/v/v, Solvent B). The gradient elution programs were 0% B (0-1 min with an isocratic gradient), 0–40% B (1-2 min with a linear gradient), 40% B (2–7 min with an isocratic gradient), 40–100% B (7–12 min with a linear gradient), 100% B (12–14 min with

an isocratic gradient), 100–0% B (14-15 min with a linear gradient), and 0% B (15-16 min with an isocratic gradient) at a flow rate of 0.3 mL/min. The autosampler tray was cooled to 45°C and the injection volume was 5 μL. HPLC grade acetonitrile and formic acid were purchased from WAKO.

2.1.4. Mass Spectrometry. A triple quadrupole mass spectrometer API4000 (Applied Biosystems/MDS Sciex, Concord, Canada) coupled with an electrospray ionization source was operated in the positive ion mode. The optimized ion source conditions were as follows: collision gas, 6 psi; curtain gas, 40 psi; ion source gas 1, 50 psi; ion source gas 2, 80 psi; ion source voltage, 5500 V; ion source temperature, 600°C. Nitrogen was used as the collision gas in the multiple reaction monitoring (MRM) mode. The conditions of declustering potential, collision energy, and collision cell exit potential were optimized by every steroid. The transitions in MRM were as follows: PREG m/z 317 → 299, HPREG m/z 315 → 297, DHEA m/z 289 → 271, PROG m/z 315 → 109, HPROG m/z 331 → 109, DIONE m/z 287 → 97, DCORT m/z 331 → 123, DCORTICO m/z 347 → 161, CORTICO m/z 347 → 100, CORT m/z 363 → 309, ALDO m/z 361 → 343, and TESTO m/z 289 → 109. Mass spectroscopic data were acquired and quantified using the Analyst 1.4.2 software package (Applied Biosystems/MDS Sciex, Concord, Canada).

2.1.5. Estimation of the Cell Volume. Cell volume was estimated from the number of cells in the well and the average diameter of the cells. Cells were detached from the well using 0.025% trypsin (MP Biomedicals, Inc., Irvine, CA) in a 0.02% EDTA solution (Dojindo Laboratories, Kumamoto, Japan) at the start of preculture, start of stimulation, and at 24, 48, and 72 h after stimulation. The numbers and diameters of the cells were measured by a cell counter Vi-cell XR 2.01 (Beckman Coulter, Krefeld, Germany) after trypan blue staining. Parameters of the cell volume and number of cells were estimated to fit experimental time-course data using exponential curves.

2.1.6. Test Compounds in Validation Study. NCI-H295R cells were exposed to seven well-characterized inhibitors of steroidogenesis, and then the concentrations of the steroids in the culture medium were measured to estimate the enzyme inhibition to evaluate the performance of the simulation model. The adrenal steroidogenic inhibitors included aminoglutethimide (AGT, Bachem AG, Bubendorf, Switzerland), o,p′-DDD (DDD, Sigma-Aldrich Inc., St. Louis, MO), spironolactone (SP, Sigma-Aldrich Inc., St. Louis, MO), metyrapone (MP, Sigma-Aldrich Inc., St. Louis, MO), ketoconazole (KC, Wako Pure Chemical Industries, Ltd., Osaka, Japan), miconazole (MC, Wako Pure Chemical Industries, Ltd., Osaka, Japan), and daidzein (DZ, Sigma-Aldrich Inc., St. Louis, MO). The cells were also exposed to four adrenal toxicants whose adrenal toxicity is not mediated through steroidogenesis inhibition. The toxicants were acrylonitrile (AN, Wako Pure Chemical Industries, Ltd., Osaka, Japan), salinomycin (SM, Sigma-Aldrich, Inc., St. Louis, MO), thioguanine (TG, Tokyo Chemical Industry Co., Ltd., Tokyo, Japan), and fumaronitrile (FN, Wako Pure Chemical

Industries, Ltd., Osaka, Japan). All chemicals were dissolved in DMSO (Wako Pure Chemical Industries, Ltd., Osaka, Japan) and added to the culture medium at 1 : 1000 dilutions.

2.1.7. Validation Study Using Adrenal Toxicants. NCI-H295R cells were cultured for 3 days in 6-well plates and then stimulated with the above-mentioned compounds. Upon the start of stimulation, various concentrations of test chemicals were added to the cultures. After a further 3 days of culture with the chemicals, the concentrations of 12 steroids (PREG, HPREG, DHEA, PROG, HPROG, DIONE, DCORTICO, DCORT, CORTICO, CORT, ALDO, and TESTO) in the culture medium were measured by LC/MS/MS. The test concentrations of the chemicals were determined by dose-finding cytotoxicity assays. The cytotoxicity assay was conducted in 96-well plates using ATP content in cells as an endpoint (CellTiter-Glo™ Luminescent Cell Viability Assay, Promega). Concentrations that caused more than 20% cytotoxicity were not used in the steroidogenesis assay. The test concentrations of adrenal steroidogenesis inhibitors and other compounds are shown in Table 1.

2.1.8. Statistical Analysis. Comparisons were performed by the two-sample Welch's *t*-test with Bonferroni multiple testing correction for each steroid hormone species. Statistically significant steroid hormones were considered at adjusted *p* values of less than 0.01. Differential metabolic steroid profiles were classified by hierarchical cluster analysis. Pairwise distances between all compounds and all steroids were calculated by standardized Euclidean metric. This distance matrix was analyzed with Ward's method for hierarchical clustering. Statistical analysis was performed using MATLAB software (MathWorks, Inc., Natick, MA).

2.2. The Computational Part

2.2.1. Mathematical Modeling of Adrenal Steroidogenesis in NCI-H295R Cells. Steroid hormones secreted from human adrenal corticocarcinoma NCI-H295R cells are synthesized from cholesterol through the C_{21}-steroid hormone biosynthesis pathway. A mathematical model of adrenal steroidogenesis in NCI-H295R cells was constructed with cholesterol transport and the intracellular localization pathway, the oxysterol synthesis pathway as a bypass of steroidogenesis, the C_{21}-steroid hormone biosynthesis pathway as the main steroidogenesis pathway, passive transport of steroid hormones, and cell proliferation (Figure 1). In this model, two compartments, the intracellular space and culture medium, were incorporated as the available region. Equations and parameters of the cell proliferation and diffusional transport of steroid hormones have been proposed by previous studies [21, 22]. Cholesterol transport and the intracellular localization pathway including the oxysterol bypass were integrated using a part of the ACTH-stimulated cortisol secretion model described by Dempsher and colleagues [47]. The C_{21}-steroid hormone biosynthesis pathway includes 14 steroid hormones, PREG, HPREG, DHEA, PROG, HPROG, DIONE, TESTO, DCORTICO, DCORT, CORTICO, CORT, ALDO, E1, and E2, and 17 enzymatic reactions catalyzed by

nine steroidogenic enzymes, cholesterol side chain cleavage enzyme (CYP11A1), 17α-hydroxylase (CYP17H), $C_{17,20}$-lyase (CYP17L), 3β-hydroxysteroid dehydrogenase (HSD3B2), 21-hydroxylase (CYP21A2), 11β-hydroxylase (CYP11B1), 18-hydroxylase (CYP11B2), 17β-hydroxysteroid dehydrogenase (HSD17B3), and aromatase (CYP19A1). In this mathematical model of adrenal steroidogenesis in NCI-H295R cells, the flux velocities of molecular transportation and enzymatic reaction rates of steroidogenic enzymes were defined based on the first-order reaction and rapid-equilibrium enzyme kinetics, respectively. All equations in the mathematical model of adrenal steroidogenesis of NCI-H295R cells were described in a supplementary document (see Supplementary Material available online at http://dx.doi.org/10.1155/2016/4041827). The rate constants and the maximum activities were estimated by fitting to experimental time-course data of the concentrations of cholesterol and all steroids. Initial values of cholesterol and the 14 steroid concentrations were used in each experimentally measured value, and every steroid concentration was assumed to rapidly reach the equilibrium state between the culture medium and intracellular space. All fixed values of static parameters and initial values of variable parameters in this model were described in Tables S1 and S2 in a supplementary document, respectively.

2.2.2. Modeling and Simulation Environment. This computational model of adrenal steroidogenesis in NCI-H295R cells was developed on the *simBio* platform which is a general environment of biological dynamic simulation and computational model development [48]. ODEs were solved by the fourth-order Runge-Kutta method with a variable time step. The time step (*dt*) was adjusted to refer to the maximum absolute value of flux velocities or enzymatic reaction rates at each time point, and the range of the time step was from 1×10^{-5} to 10^{-2}. To confirm whether the range of the time step was suitable, the numerical error ratio was calculated by certain fixed time steps in the range of the time step, which was under 1×10^{-8} in every time step. The duration time of computational simulation of adrenal steroidogenesis in NCI-H295R cells was set at 72 h.

2.2.3. Parameter Optimization. To reconstruct experimental time-course patterns of the concentrations of cholesterol and the 14 steroids in the culture medium and intracellular space, we optimized every rate constant and maximum velocity of the steroidogenic enzymes. This parameter optimization problem was solved by the Levenberg-Marquardt method which is one of the nonlinear least squares methods [49–51]. The objective function of optimization was used as the following normalized least squares distance (NLSD):

$$\text{NLSD} = \sum_h \sum_i \sum_j \frac{\left(X_{h,i,j}^{\text{exp}} - X_{h,i,j}^{\text{sim}}\right)^2}{X_{h,i}^{\text{max}2}}, \tag{1}$$

where *h* is the compartment (culture medium or intracellular space), *i* is the molecular species (cholesterol and the 14 steroids), *j* is the time point (0, 8, 24, 48, and 72 h), $X_{h,i,j}^{\text{exp}}$ is the experimentally measured concentration of molecule

TABLE 1: Adrenal toxicities and actions of tested compounds.

Test chemical	Test concentrations (μM)	Pathological features of adrenal toxicity	Reported enzyme inhibitions	References
Acrylonitrile (AN)	0.1, 1, 10, and 100	Hemorrhagic adrenal necrosis	Not reported	[25]
Salinomycin (SM)	0.00001, 0.01, 0.1, 1, and 10	Damage to adrenal medullae	Not reported	[26]
Thioguanine (TG)	0.01, 1, 10, and 100	Hemorrhagic adrenal necrosis	Not reported	[25]
Fumaronitrile (FN)	0.1, 1, 10, and 100	Hemorrhagic adrenal necrosis	Not reported	[25]
Aminoglutethimide (AGT)	0.1, 1, 10, and 100	Hypertrophy, vascular degeneration	CYP11A1, CYP21A2, CYP11B1, and CYP11B2	[6, 27–30]
o,p'-DDD (DDD)	0.1, 1, 10, 25, and 100	Atrophy	CYP11A1, HSD3B2, CYP21A2, CYP11B1, and CYP11B2	[29, 31, 32]
Spironolactone (SP)	1, 10, 50, and 100	Hypertrophy	CYP17H, CYP17L, CYP11B1, and CYP11B2	[6, 33–35]
Metyrapone (MP)	0.1, 1, 10, and 100	Hypertrophy, vascular degeneration	CYP11A1, CYP11B1, and CYP11B2	[6, 29, 36–39]
Ketoconazole (KC)	0.1, 1, 10, and 100	Hypertrophy	CYP11A1, CYP17H, CYP17L, HSD3B2, CYP21A2, and CYP11B1	[6, 29, 40–43]
Miconazole (MC)	0.1, 1, 10, 25, 50, and 100	Hypertrophy	CYP11A1, CYP17H, CYP17L, CYP21A2, and CYP11B1	[41, 44, 45]
Daidzein (DZ)	0.1, 1, 10, and 100	Unknown	HSD3B2 and CYP21A2	[46]

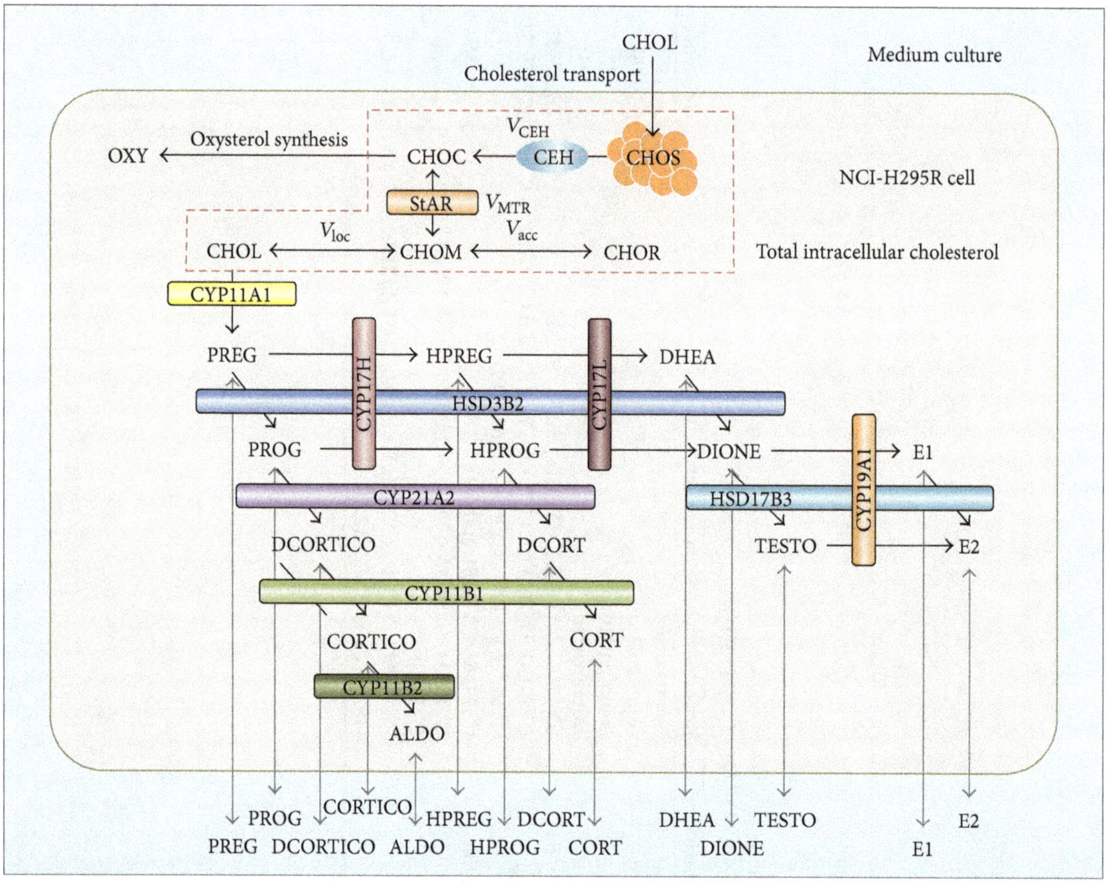

FIGURE 1: Schematic diagram of the mathematical model of adrenal steroidogenesis in NCI-H295R cells. Overview of the mathematical model of adrenal steroidogenesis in NCI-H295R cells, including cholesterol transport and intracellular localization, oxysterol synthesis, the C_{21}-steroid hormone biosynthesis pathway, passive diffusional transport of steroid hormones, and cell proliferation. CHOL: total cholesterol in medium culture, CHOS: stored cholesterol esters in the endoplasmic reticulum, CHOC: intracellular free cholesterol, CHOM: mitochondrial free cholesterol, CHON: mitochondrial free cholesterol close to CYP11A1 enzymes, CHOR: mitochondrial free cholesterol remote from CYP11A1 enzymes, PREG: pregnenolone, HPREG: 17α-hydroxypregnenolone, DHEA: dehydroepiandrosterone, PROG: progesterone, HPROG: 17α-hydroxyprogesterone, DIONE: androstenedione, DCORTICO: 11-deoxycorticosterone, DCORT: 11-deoxycortisol, CORTICO: corticosterone, CORT: cortisol, ALDO: aldosterone, TESTO: testosterone, E1: estrone, E2: 17β-estradiol, OXY: oxysterol, CEH: cholesterol ester hydrolase, StAR: steroidogenic acute regulatory protein, CYP11A1: P450 side chain cleavage enzyme, CYP17H: 17α-hydroxylase of CYP17, CYP17L: C_{17-20} lyase of CYP17, HSD3B2: 3β-hydroxysteroid dehydrogenase, CYP21A2: 21-hydroxylase, CYP11B1: 11β-hydroxylase, CYP11B2: 18-hydroxylase, HSD17B3: 17β-hydroxysteroid dehydrogenase, and CYP19A1: aromatase.

i in compartment h at time point j, $X_{h,i,j}^{sim}$ is the simulated concentration of molecule i in compartment h at time point j, and $X_{h,i}^{max}$ is the maximum concentration of molecule i in compartment h over all time points. Data points under the lower quantitation limit were excluded from the evaluation by the objective function.

Effects of every static model parameter for parameter optimization were calculated from differences of fitting the objective function using sensitivity analysis.

2.2.4. Quantitative Estimation of the Mechanism of Action of Adrenal Toxicants. Metabolic steroid profiling and differential patterns of the adrenal steroid hormones by chemical perturbation were reconstructed to optimize the relative activities of the steroidogenic enzymes. The input data for the quantitative mechanistic analysis of adrenal toxic compounds was a fold change (ratio) of the measured 12

steroid concentrations induced by drug exposure for 72 h. The two-step optimization method of the real-coded genetic algorithm (RCGA) was adopted as a global optimization method in the quantitative mechanistic analysis of adrenal toxic compounds. The operations of the crossover and generation alteration model in RCGA were used for the real-coded ensemble crossover (REX) and just generation gap (JGG) [52–55]. As the initial parameters of RCGA, maximum generation, population size, selection size of parent individuals, population size of child individuals, and termination criteria were 1000, 100, 6, 25, and under 0.1 of NLSD, respectively. The search space for the relative activities of the steroidogenic enzymes was from 1/100 to 100. To evaluate the fitness of each individual, the sum of squared residuals for fold changes of measured 12 steroid concentrations was used as the objective function. Nonlinear least squares optimization by the Levenberg-Marquardt method was used as a local search [49–51]. As the estimated mechanisms of actions of the adrenal toxic compounds, the relative activities of eight steroidogenic enzymes (CYP11A1, CYP17H, CYP17L, HSD3B2, CYP21A2, CYP11B1, CYP11B2, and HSD17B3) were optimized by the above-mentioned 2-step optimization method. Every optimization calculation was duplicated to check the numerical stability of the optimal parameters.

2.2.5. Global Dynamic Sensitivity Analysis. The property of every kinetic parameter in this computational model of steroidogenesis in NCI-H295R cells was evaluated by dynamic sensitivity analysis. The sensitivity ($S_{x,y}$) of kinetic parameter x for variable parameter y was defined by the following equation:

$$S_{x,y(t)} = \frac{\Delta y_{(t)}/y_{(t)}}{\Delta x/x}, \qquad (2)$$

where variable parameter y was the concentration of a steroid hormone in the cytosolic space of NCI-H295R cells. The perturbation for kinetic parameters was +10% ($\Delta x/x = 0.1$).

3. Results

3.1. Experimental Data on Adrenal Steroidogenesis

3.1.1. Adrenal Steroidogenesis of NCI-H295R Cells and the Mass Balance. All steroid hormones in the culture medium were significantly increased after 72 h of stimulation with 50 nM ACTH, 20 μM forskolin, and 100 nM angiotensin II (Figure 2(a)). Mass balances in steroidogenesis of NCI-H295R cells under nontreatment and control (stimulated) conditions are shown in Figures 2(b) and 2(c), respectively. Under stimulation, the dynamics of net mass in these experiments were unchanged, and accumulated cholesterol was converted to adrenal steroids.

3.1.2. Cytotoxicity of Adrenal Toxicants. Viabilities of cells treated with each compound were expressed as a relative value to the ATP level of the control. Effects of AN, SM TG, FN, AGT, DDD, SP, MP, KC, MC, and DZ on cell viability were determined to be valid under 80% of the relative ATP level at 7 days after treatment. AN, SM, TG, and FN showed cytotoxicity at over 100, 1, 10, and 10 μM, respectively. AGT, MP, and DZ did not affect cell viability at up to 100 μM. DDD, SP, KC, and MC induced less than 80% of cell viability at over 100, 50, 100, and 25 μM, respectively.

3.1.3. Differentially Steroid Profiling of Adrenal Toxicants. After NCI-H295R cells were exposed to each test compound during three days, the concentrations of 12 steroid hormones in the culture medium were simultaneously measured by LC/MS/MS. All effects of the compounds on adrenal steroidogenesis were evaluated at the concentration without any overt cytotoxicity. The differential metabolic steroid profiles of 11 adrenal toxic compounds were classified and visualized by using hierarchical clustering analysis (Figure 3).

Four adrenal toxicants without steroidogenic inhibition, AN, SM, TG, and FN, did not change the medium concentrations of all steroid hormones by more than 2-fold. Above-mentioned 4 compounds at every condition and 7 adrenal steroidogenic inhibitors at the low exposure concentration were gathered into a big cluster as nonchange group. The 7 steroidogenic inhibitors at the maximum exposure concentration showed the characteristic steroid profiles each, but 100 μM DZ and 10 μM SP were classified as a cluster. AGT drastically decreased the medium concentrations of PREG, HPREG, DHEA, PROG, DCORTICO, CORTICO, and ALDO at 100 μM. DDD dose-dependently decreased the medium concentrations of PROG, DCORTICO, CORTICO, CORT, and ALDO at >10 μM and decreased PREG, HPREG, DHEA, PROG, HPROG, DIONE, and DCORT at the maximum exposure concentration of 25 μM. SP increased PREG, HPREG, and DHEA and decreased PROG, DIONE, DCORTICO, DCORT, CORTICO, ALDO, and TESTO at 10 μM. MP dose-dependently decreased CORTICO, CORT, and ALDO and decreased DHEA, HPROG, DIONE, and TESTO at the maximum exposure concentration of 100 μM. KC drastically decreased the medium concentrations of PREG, HPREG, DHEA, HPROG, DIONE, DCORTICO, DCORT, CORTICO, CORTO, ALDO, and TESTO at 10 μM. MC increased the medium concentrations of PROG and decreased DIONE, DCORT, CORT, and TESTO at 10 μM. DZ increased PREG, HPREG, and DHEA and decreased DIONE, DCORTICO, DCORT, CORTICO, CORT, ALDO, and TESTO at 100 μM.

3.2. The Mathematical Modeling

3.2.1. Optimization of the Mathematical Model of Adrenal Steroidogenesis in NCI-H295R Cells. The mathematical model of adrenal steroidogenesis in NCI-H295R cells was optimized for several kinetic parameters of cholesterol transport, intracellular localization, the oxysterol pathway, and maximum velocity of steroidogenic enzymes to fit the experimental time-course data. All optimized kinetic parameters are shown in Table S1 in a supplementary document. The optimized mathematical model was reconstructed with the experimental dynamic patterns of cholesterol and the 14 steroid hormones in the intracellular space and culture medium. The fitness was 0.621761 of NLSD values as the fitting objective function. The simulation results and experimental data are shown in Figure 4.

Optimized kinetic parameters were calculated sensitivities for the NLSD value as the fitting score and are shown in Table S1 in a supplementary document. The highly sensitive parameters for fitting the NLSD score were the extracted nine kinetic parameters, $k_{\text{Cholesterol Transport}}$, k_f^{acc}, k_f^{loc}, k_b^{loc}, $V_{\text{max}}^{\text{CYP11A1}}$, K_m^{CYP11A1}, $V_{\text{maxA}}^{\text{CYP17H}}$, $V_{\text{maxA}}^{\text{HSD3B2}}$, and $V_{\text{maxA}}^{\text{CYP21A2}}$, which had higher than 3.0 fitting sensitivity.

3.3. The Validation Using the Adrenal Toxicants

3.3.1. Mechanistic Analysis of Adrenal Toxicants. Effects of adrenal toxic compounds on steroidogenic enzymes were quantitatively predicted from the change in the ratio of the measured medium concentrations of the 12 steroid

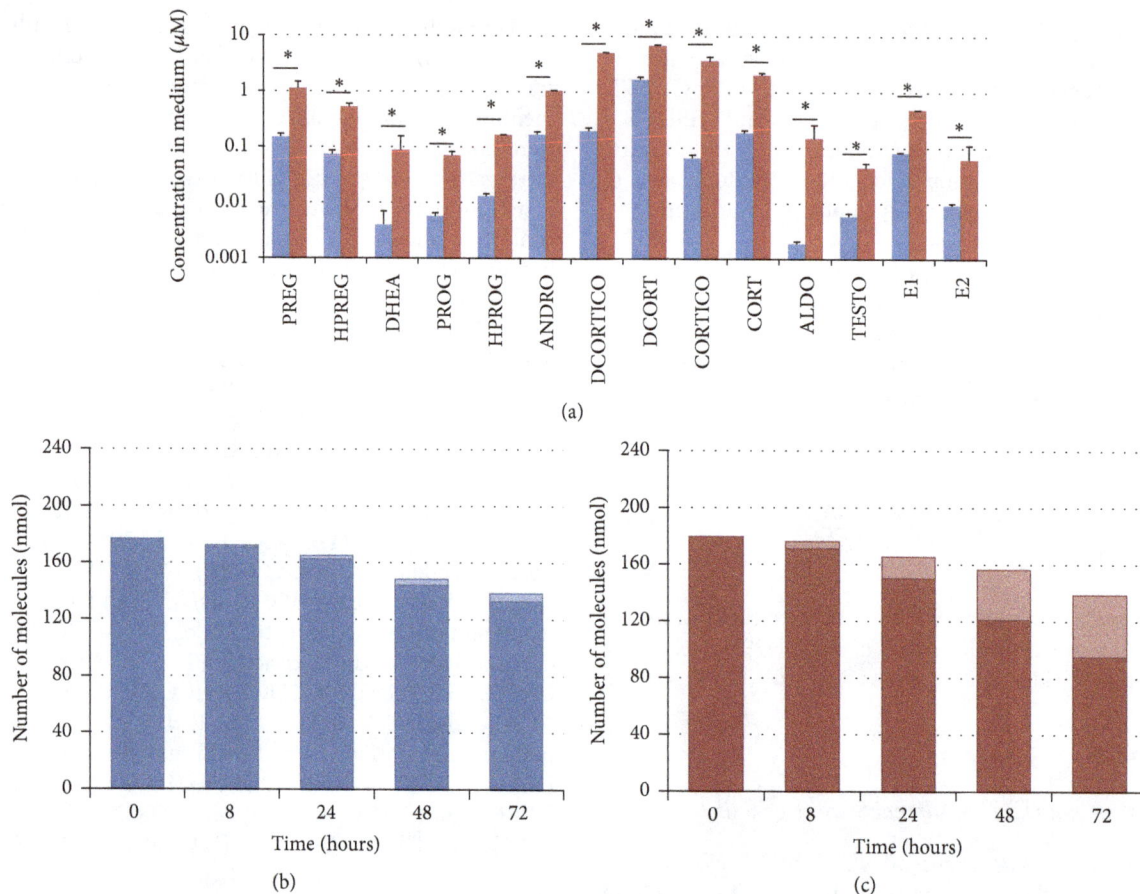

FIGURE 2: Experimental data of metabolic profiling of adrenal steroid hormones and the mass balance. Concentrations of steroid hormones secreted from NCI-H295R cells in the culture medium at 72 h after stimulation were compared with the untreated condition and the stimulated condition by 50 nM ACTH, 20 μM forskolin, and 100 nM angiotensin II (a). Net molecular amounts including cholesterol and steroid hormones in the culture medium and intracellular space are plotted at five time points (0, 8, 24, 48, and 72 h after stimulation) under the untreated condition (b) and the stimulated condition (c). In the bar graphs, dark and light bars indicate the amount of cholesterol and adrenal steroids, respectively. All data are shown as the mean $\pm$ SD (N = 4). $^*p$ values corrected by the familywise error rate <0.01. PREG: pregnenolone, HPREG: 17α-hydroxypregnenolone, DHEA: dehydroepiandrosterone, PROG: progesterone, HPROG: 17α-hydroxyprogesterone, DIONE: androstenedione, DCORTICO: 11-deoxycorticosterone, DCORT: 11-deoxycortisol, CORTICO: corticosterone, CORT: cortisol, ALDO: aldosterone, and TESTO: testosterone.

hormones at 72 h after drug exposure using the mathematical model of adrenal steroidogenesis in NCI-H295R cells. The reproducibility of the estimated results was confirmed by performing the test twice. The estimated effects of 11 adrenal toxic compounds on eight steroidogenic enzymes are shown in Figure 5. The adrenal toxic compounds without steroidogenic inhibition, such as vasculotoxic agents (AN, SM, TG, and FN), were not estimated for the target steroidogenic enzymes under noncytotoxic conditions. Every fitness values were under 0.05 of NLSD values used as the fitting objective function (Figures 5(a)–5(d)). Other steroidogenic inhibitors (AGT, DDD, SP, MP, KC, MC, and DZ) are described in detail below.

3.3.2. AGT. The mechanism of action of AGT in adrenal steroidogenesis was estimated by inhibition of CYP11A1, HSD3B2, CYP21A2, and CYP11B1 at 100 μM (estimated inhibitions were 77.0%, 78.0%, 81.1%, and 59.8%, resp.) (Figure 5(e)). AGT has been reported to inhibit CYP11A1,

CYP21A2, CYP11B1, and CYP11B2 [6, 27–30]. Our results were mostly consistent with the previous reports. In particular, CYP11A1 appeared to be inhibited strongly by AGT. In our study, HSD3B2 inhibition of AGT was shown by mechanistic analysis based on systems biology approaches as a novel mechanism of action of AGT. Inhibition of AGT by CYP11B2 was not estimated in our study. However, the concentration of ALDO in the culture medium decreased to 3.8% of the normal stimulated condition. Inhibition of AGT by CYP11B2 has been shown using sheep adrenal homogenates as well as a human adrenal homogenate from a patient with Cushing's syndrome [30]. The activity of 18-hydroxylase induced by CYP11B2 was determined as the conversion of corticosterone to 18-hydroxycorticosterone in the previous study. The cause of the discrepancy regarding the effect of AGT on CYP11B2 was suggested to be substrate inhibition, because the intracellular concentration of CORTICO was increased by over 10 times of that in the culture medium to reach 50 μM. Another possibility was poor quantitative

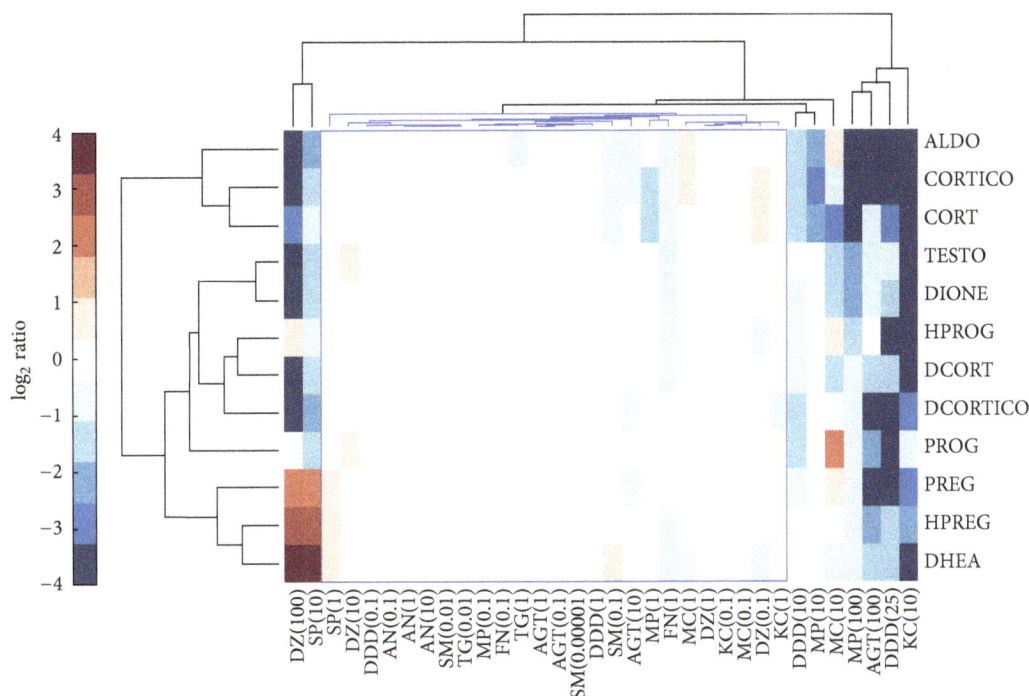

FIGURE 3: Hierarchical cluster analysis of differential metabolic profiles of 12 steroid hormones by exposure to adrenal toxicity compounds. Adrenal toxicants were classified by using the differential metabolic profiling of 12 steroid hormones. Concentrations of 12 adrenal steroids secreted from NCI-H295R cells were drastically changed by the exposure of adrenal steroidogenesis inhibitors. The 12 adrenal steroid hormones were quantitatively measured by LC-MS/MS simultaneously. Four adrenal vasculotoxic compounds: acrylonitrile: AN, fumaronitrile: FN, salinomycin: SM, and thioguanine: TG, were used as negative control compounds for adrenal steroidogenesis inhibitors. Seven adrenal steroidogenesis inhibitors: aminoglutethimide: AGT, o,p'-DDD: DDD, spironolactone: SP, metyrapone: MP, ketoconazole: KC, miconazole: MC, and daidzein: DZ, showed a characteristic steroid profile each and were classified as each independent singleton at the maximum exposure condition. Exposure concentrations of adrenal toxic compounds were described in brackets of the sample name and the units were prepared as μM. A blue cluster was classified as a group of nonchange samples including negative control compounds and low exposure conditions of adrenal steroidogenesis inhibitors. PREG: pregnenolone, HPREG: 17α-hydroxypregnenolone, DHEA: dehydroepiandrosterone, PROG: progesterone, HPROG: 17α-hydroxyprogesterone, DIONE: androstenedione, DCORTICO: 11-deoxycorticosterone, DCORT: 11-deoxycortisol, CORTICO: corticosterone, CORT: cortisol, ALDO: aldosterone, and TESTO: testosterone.

reliability of the experimental data, because the ALDO concentration was under the lower limit of quantification at 100 μM AGT. Hecker and colleagues reported that 3 μM AGT decreases PREG and PROG concentrations and increases the TESTO concentration [10]. However, AGT did not increase the TESTO concentration in our study. One possibility is that the concentration of TESTO was already enhanced by about 3.3-fold through stimulation with ACTH, forskolin, and angiotensin II.

3.3.3. DDD.

The mechanism of action of DDD in adrenal steroidogenesis was estimated by dose-dependent inhibition of CYP11A1, HSD3B2, CYP21A2, and CYP11B1 (estimated inhibitions at 25 μM were 87.0%, 86.9%, 76.9%, and 84.9%, resp.) (Figure 5(f)). DDD has been reported to inhibit CYP11A1, HSD3B2, CYP21A2, CYP11B1, and CYP11B2 [29, 31, 32]. Inhibition of DDD by CYP11B2 was not estimated in our study. However, the concentration of ALDO in the culture medium decreased to 3% of that in the normal stimulated condition. Inhibition of DDD by CYP11B2 has been shown using mitochondrial and microsomal fractions prepared by standard centrifugation procedures from a bovine adrenal

cortex homogenate [32]. The cause of the discrepancy regarding the inhibition of DDD by CYP11B2 could not be explained by same effect in the case of AGT.

3.3.4. SP.

The mechanism of action of SP in adrenal steroidogenesis was estimated by inhibition of HSD3B2, CYP21A2, and HSD17B3 (estimated inhibitions at 10 μM were 70.2%, 59.5%, and 59.3%, resp.) (Figure 5(g)). SP has been reported to inhibit CYP17H, CYP17L, CYP11B1, and CYP11B2 [6, 33–35]. The inhibitory effect of SP on the HSD3B2 enzyme was a novel mechanism of action. The main action of SP is as a mineralocorticoid receptor (MR) antagonist. SP has also been reported to exert some off-target effects by binding to androgen, glucocorticoid, and progesterone receptors [56–58]. SP has been shown to inhibit the production of ALDO and CORT from PREG induced by angiotensin II in H295R cells, but the specific MR antagonist eplerenone did not show the inhibitory effects [59]. Therefore, HSD3B2 inhibition by SP is not mediated via MR, and the action might be direct inhibition of HSD3B2 enzymes or a part of known off-target effects mediated through other nuclear hormone receptors. Regarding CYP17H and CYP17L, our results were consistent

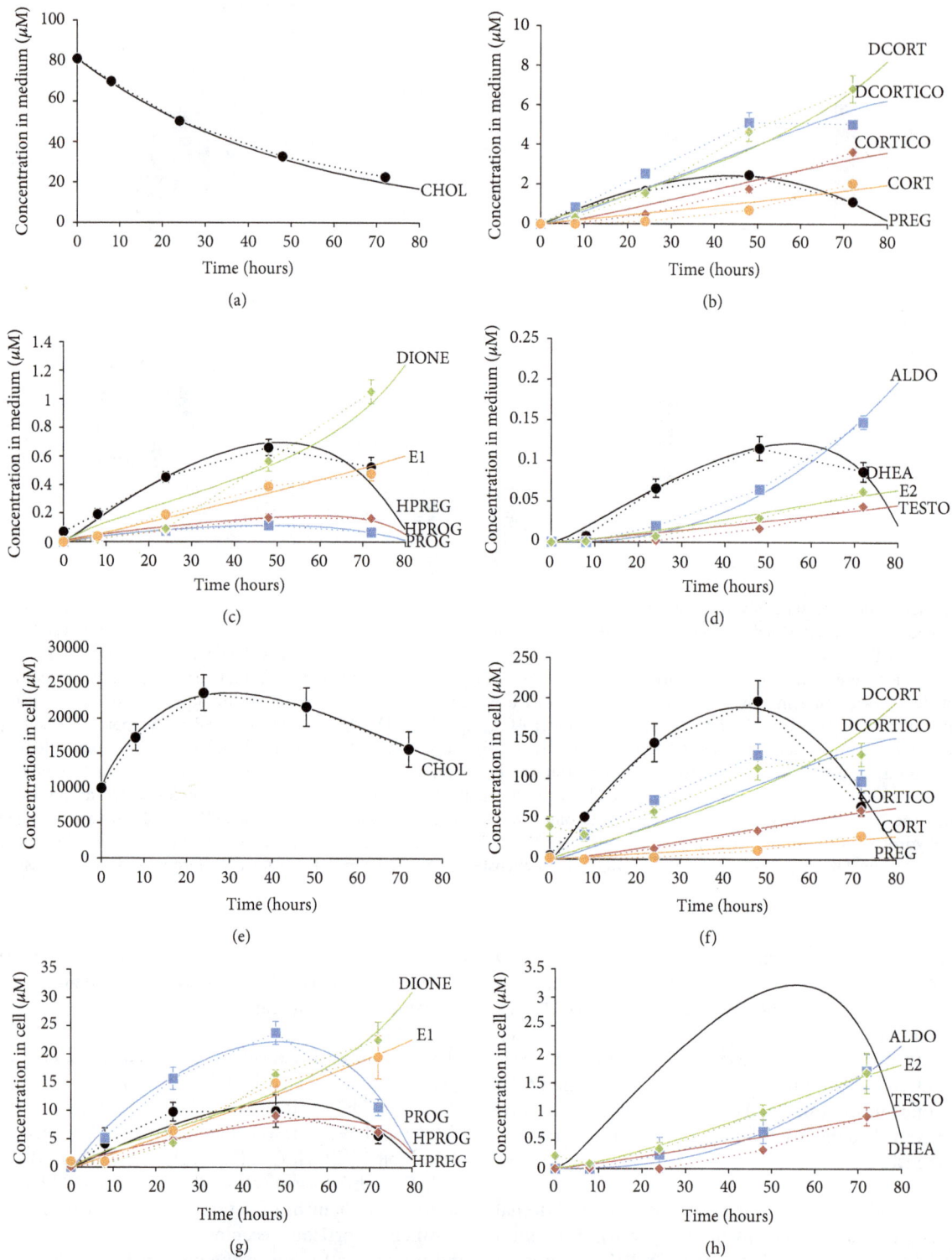

FIGURE 4: Comparison of time-course profiles of cholesterol and adrenal steroids produced by NCI-H295R cells between experimentally measured and simulated data. To intuitively confirm reconstruction of the measured experimental data in the developed simulation model of NCI-H295R cells, dynamics of cholesterol and adrenal steroids produced by NCI-H295R cells were plotted to overlay experimental data with the simulated results. Graphs show the dynamics of medium concentrations of cholesterol (a) and adrenal steroids ((b)–(d)) and intracellular concentrations of cholesterol (e) and adrenal steroids ((f)–(h)). Steroid hormones were categorized into three groups by concentration levels. Major steroids were PREG: pregnenolone, DCORTICO: 11-deoxycorticosterone, DCORT: 11-deoxycortisol, CORTICO: corticosterone, and CORT: cortisol ((b) and (f)). Moderate steroids were HPREG: 17α-hydroxypregnenolone, PROG: progesterone, HPROG: 17α-hydroxyprogesterone, DIONE: androstenedione, and E1: estrone ((c) and (g)). Minor steroids were DHEA: dehydroepiandrosterone, ALDO: aldosterone, TESTO: testosterone, and E2: 17β-estradiol ((d) and (h)). Experimental data are shown as symbols with dotted lines. All data represent the mean ± SD ($N = 4$). Simulation data are shown as solid lines.

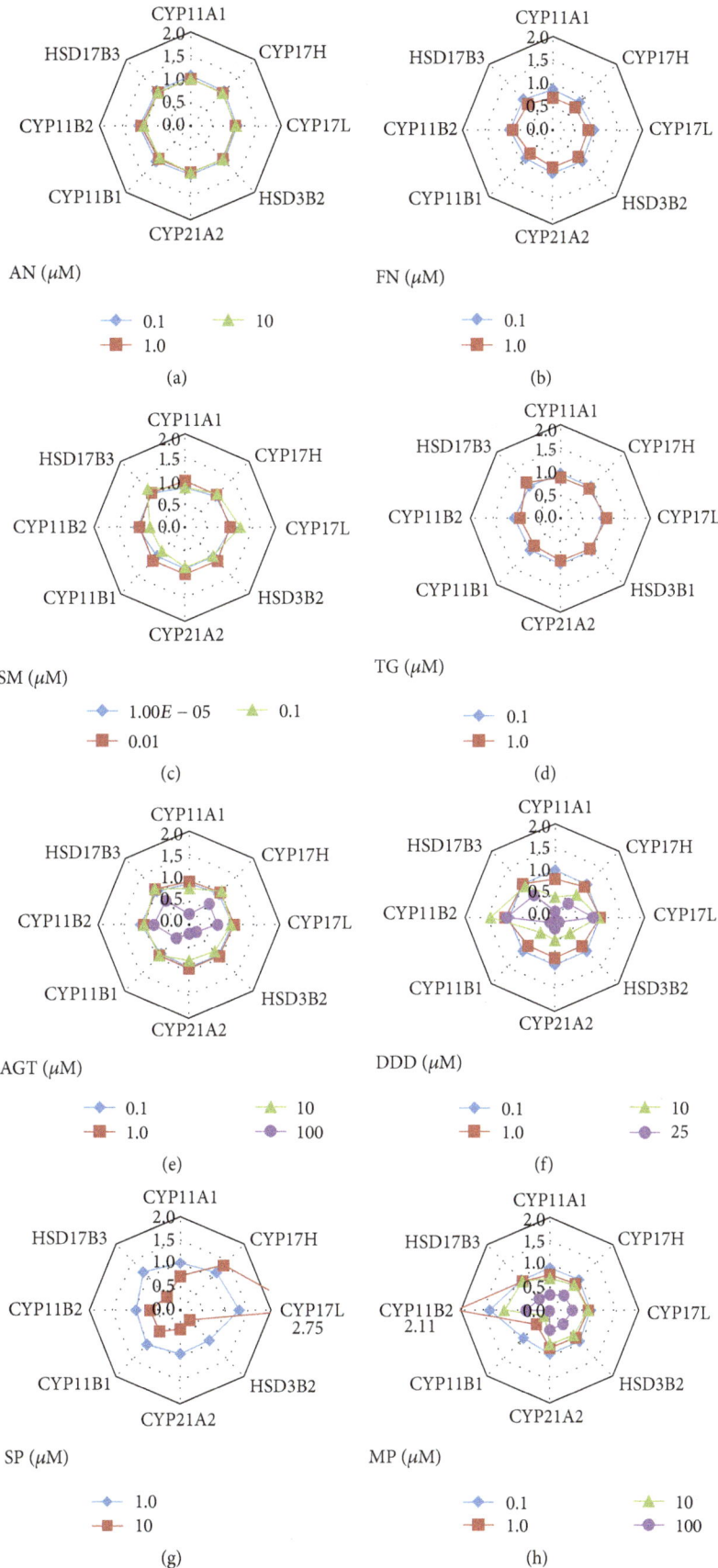

FIGURE 5: Continued.

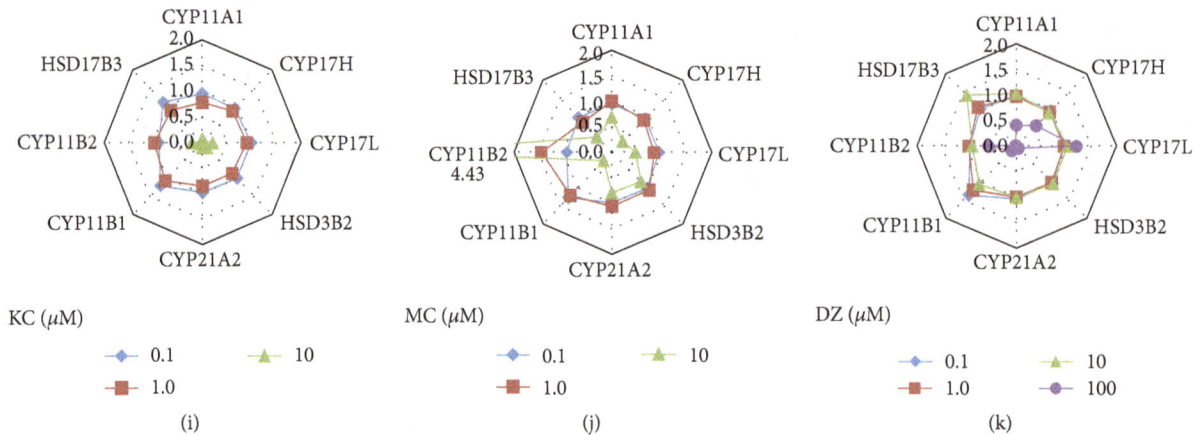

FIGURE 5: Estimated mechanism of action of adrenal toxicants by using the mathematical model of adrenal steroidogenesis in NCI-H295R cells. Mechanisms of action of adrenal toxicity compounds were quantitatively estimated from experimental results of differential steroid profiling using the mathematical model of adrenal steroidogenesis in NCI-H295R cells. The drug action was defined as a scaling factor of enzymatic activity in the simulation model. These scaling factors were optimized to fit experimental data by a hybrid optimization method of the RCGA and nonlinear least squares. Estimated drug actions by the exposure of vasculotoxic agents acrylonitrile: AN (a), fumaronitrile: FN (b), salinomycin: SM (c), and thioguanine: TG (d) and the steroidogenic inhibitors aminoglutethimide: AGT (e), o,p'-DDD: DDD (f), spironolactone: SP (g), metyrapone: MP (h), ketoconazole: KC (i), miconazole: MC (j), and daidzein: DZ (k) are shown as a spider radar chart. CYP11A1: P450 side chain cleavage enzyme, CYP17H: 17α-hydroxylase of CYP17, CYP17L: C_{17-20} lyase of CYP17, HSD3B2: 3β-hydroxysteroid dehydrogenase, CYP21A2: 21-hydroxylase, CYP11B1: 11β-hydroxylase, CYP11B2: 18-hydroxylase, and HSD17B3: 17β-hydroxysteroid dehydrogenase.

with previous reports [33, 34]. 7α-thiospironolactone, which is synthesized by deacetylation of SP, inhibits CYP17H and CYP17L [34]. The fact that there were no inhibitions of CYP17H or CYP17L in our study suggests that SP might not be deacetylated to 7α-thiospironolactone in NCI-H295R cells. Regarding CYP11B1 and CYP11B2, our results were unclear compared with a previous study. It has been shown that $30\,\mu$M SP inhibits CYP11B1 and CYP11B2 in human and bovine adrenal mitochondria [35]. The cause of CYP11B1 and CYP11B2 inhibition by SP could not be determined in our study, which might be due to the lower maximum exposure concentration of SP than that in the previous report. We could not examine SP concentrations over $10\,\mu$M because these concentrations were cytotoxic in NCI-H295R cells.

3.3.5. MP. The mechanism of action of MP in adrenal steroidogenesis was estimated by dose-dependent inhibition of CYP11B1 (estimated inhibitions at 1, 10, and $100\,\mu$M were 57.1%, 82.7%, and 98.2%, resp.) (Figure 5(h)). MP has been reported to inhibit CYP11B1 as its major effect and CYP11A1 and CYP11B2 as a weak effect [6, 29, 36–39]. The results were able to show that MP is a selective inhibitor of CYP11B1 in the previous report. However, the estimated effect of MP at a high concentration, $100\,\mu$M as the maximum exposure concentration, was unclear. According to the previous report, selectivity of MP for CYP11B1/CYP11B2 is about five times [39]. In addition, $20\,\mu$M MP has a slight inhibition effect on CYP11A1 in H295R cells [29].

3.3.6. KC. The mechanism of action of KC in adrenal steroidogenesis was estimated by inhibition of CYP11A1, CYP17H, CYP17L, HSD3B2, CYP21A2, CYP11B1, and

CYP11B2 (estimated inhibitions at $10\,\mu$M were 92.6%, 94.3%, 51.8%, 83.0%, 88.2%, 97.4%, and 79.8%, resp.) (Figure 5(i)). KC has been reported to inhibit CYP11A1, CYP17H, CYP17L, HSD3B2, CYP21A2, and CYP11B1 [6, 29, 40–43]. Our results were almost consistent with the previous reports. KC inhibits CYP11A1, CYP17H, CYP21A2, and CYP11B1 in NCI-H295R cells at $10\,\mu$M [29] and CYP17H, CYP17L, CYP21A2, and CYP11B1 in human adrenal mitochondria and Leydig cell microsomes at $2–5\,\mu$M [60, 61]. However, KC has shown only weak inhibition of HSD3B2 and HSD17B3 in Leydig cells at the millimolar level [60, 61]. Regarding CYP11B2 and HSD17B3, we considered that these estimated inhibitions of KC did have sufficient reliability in terms of quantitative prediction precision, because ALDO and TESTO concentrations were less than the lower limit of quantification at $10\,\mu$M KC.

3.3.7. MC. The mechanism of action of MC in adrenal steroidogenesis was estimated by inhibition of CYP17H, CYP17L, CYP11B1, and HSD17B3 (estimated inhibitions at $10\,\mu$M were 69.1%, 53.0%, 76.4%, and 57.1%, resp.) (Figure 5(j)). MC has been reported to inhibit not only CYP17H and CYP17L but also CYP11A1, CYP21A2, and CYP11B1 [41, 44, 45]. The results in the previous reports were able to estimate that MC is a CYP17 inhibitor. However, CYP11A1 inhibition by MC, probably instead of a reduction in StAR expression, was not clearly detected in our study using NCI-H295R cells, because there were no decreases in the concentrations of PREG and PROG in the culture medium. Indirect inhibition of CYP11A1 via the peripheral-type benzodiazepine receptor has been reported in mouse adrenocortical Y-1 cells treated with MC in the absence of stimuli by measuring PREG production [44]. On the other hand, reductions of StAR protein expression and/or transport activity without affecting total steroid synthesis or CYP11A1 and HSD3B2 enzyme expression or activities have been reported in $(BU)_2$cAMP-stimulated MA-10 Leydig tumor cells treated with MC by measuring PROG production [45]. Therefore, the effect of MC on the initial reaction in adrenal steroidogenesis from cholesterol should be different according to the cell type and stimulation condition. Inhibition of CYP21A2 and CYP11B1 by MC has been reported as decreases in the consumption of PROG and DCORTICO, respectively [41]. Inhibition of CYP11B1 was estimated by the action of MC in this study, but that of CYP21A2 was not detected. In the previous experimental report, inhibitory sites by MC might have been reflected by inhibition of CYP17H activity, because CYP21A2 activity was measured as a decrease in labeled PROG.

3.3.8. DZ.

The mechanism of action of DZ in adrenal steroidogenesis was estimated by inhibition of CYP11A1, HSD3B2, CYP21A2, CYP11B1, and HSD17B3 (estimated inhibitions at $100\,\mu M$ were 58.6%, 94.1%, 96.5%, 87.2%, and 98.1%, resp.) (Figure 5(k)). DZ has been reported to inhibit HSD3B2 and CYP21A2 [46]. The results of HSD3B2 and CYP21A2 were consistent with the previous report. However, inhibitions have not been reported for CYP11A1, CYP11B1, and HSD17B3. These estimated effects of DZ on CYP11B1 and HSD17B3 were unclear, because the concentrations of ALDO and TESTO were less than the lower limit of quantification at $100\,\mu M$. In addition, these enzymes act downstream of the strong action points of DZ, such as HSD3B2 and CYP21A2.

3.4. The Simulations and the Systematic Model Analysis

3.4.1. Dynamic Sensitivity Analysis of Adrenal Steroidogenesis.
To comprehensively understand the dynamics of adrenal steroidogenesis, dynamic sensitivities were calculated for steroid concentrations secreted by NCI-H295R cells using our constructed mathematical model of steroidogenesis. The results of dynamic sensitivity analysis at 72 h of duration and 6 h of interval time are presented as a heat-map in Figure 6.

The top 10 parameters of the total area under the curve of dynamic sensitivity for cholesterol and the 14 steroids in culture medium were V_{maxA}^{HSD3B2}, $V_{max}^{CYP11A1}$, $V_{maxA}^{CYP21A2}$, k_f^{loc}, k_b^{loc}, $K_m^{CYP11A1}$, V_{maxA}^{CYP17H}, $k_{Cholesterol\ Transport}$, k_f^{acc}, and $V_{maxB}^{CYP21A2}$ in order from the top. Cholesterol uptake ($k_{Cholesterol\ Transport}$), StAR protein ($k_f^{loc}$), and CYP11A1 ($V_{max}^{CYP11A1}$), which are determining factors of the capacity for steroidogenesis, promoted the production of mineralocorticoids (DCORTICO, CORTICO, and ALDO) and restrained the synthesis of glucocorticoids (DCORT and CORT) and sex steroids (DIONE, TESTO, and E1) because of the accumulation of intermediate molecules in steroidogenesis (PREG, HPREG, DHEA, PROG, and HPROG) only by self-activation. The dynamic patterns of the intermediate molecules in steroidogenesis were mainly dependent on the activity of CYP17H and HSD3B2 with PREG as the substrate of these enzymes, in which the dynamic sensitivities of V_{maxA}^{CYP17H} for HPREG, and HPROG and V_{maxA}^{HSD3B2} for PROG, HPROG, and DCORTICO

reversed the direction of sensitivity at 49–66 h after stimulation. The dynamic sensitivities of the maximum activities of HSD3B2 for PREG (V_{maxA}^{HSD3B2}) and CYP21A2 for PROG ($V_{maxA}^{CYP21A2}$) were related to all steroids at 72 h. Almost all model parameters had positive sensitivity for downstream steroids in the adrenal steroidogenic pathway and negative sensitivity for direct-binding steroids as substrates of the steroidogenic enzyme. The sensitivity of V_{max} in all steroidogenic enzymes was relatively higher than K_m for the same steroid substrate.

3.4.2. Simulation of the Metabolic Balance of Adrenal Steroidogenesis Pathway.
To clearly show the property of the metabolic shift between mineralocorticoid and glucocorticoid biosynthesis, we performed two-dimensional parameter scanning of the enzymatic activities of CYP17H and HSD3B2 (Figure 7). NCI-H295R cells lost the ability to produce all steroid hormones when enzymatic activities of CYP17H and HSD3B2 were changed by over 60% and 30%, respectively. Activation of CYP17H and/or HSD3B2 induced the metabolic shift that enhanced the glucocorticoid biosynthesis and deviated from the mineralocorticoid biosynthesis. On the other hand, inhibition of CYP17H and/or HSD3B2 induced the metabolic shift that enhanced the mineralocorticoid biosynthesis and deviated from the glucocorticoid biosynthesis. Moreover, the enzymatic activity of HSD3B2 regulated the metabolic balance of sex steroids and the precursors on adrenal steroidogenesis of NCI-H295R cells. E1, TESTO, and DIONE were produced by NCI-H295R cells when activating the enzymatic activity of HSD3B2. Conversely, E2 and DHEA were produced by NCI-H295R cells when suppressing the enzymatic activity of HSD3B2. The biosynthesis of downstream steroids in adrenal steroidogenesis pathway, such as mineralocorticoids and glucocorticoids, was almost completely terminated when the enzymatic activity of HSD3B2 was decreased by over 80%.

4. Discussion

4.1. Importance of 3β-HSD Activity in Adrenal Steroidogenesis.
Our systematic analysis using the mathematical model of adrenal steroidogenesis in NCI-H295R cells revealed that the enzymatic activity of 3β-HSD controls the dynamics of adrenal steroidogenesis. The activity of the StAR protein controls the net capacity of steroidogenesis in steroidogenic cells, which is the transport of cholesterol from the outer to inner mitochondrial membranes. Both the expression levels of StAR protein and mRNA are rapidly elevated in response to stimulation by tropic hormones such as ACTH [62, 63]. Another important factor in adrenal steroidogenesisis is the cholesterol side chain cleavage enzyme CYP11A1, the first rate-limiting and hormonally regulated step in the synthesis of all steroid hormones, which is conversion of cholesterol to pregnenolone in mitochondria [64]. According to our results of global sensitivity analysis (Supplementary Table 1 and Figure 6(d)), in addition to CYP11A1 and StAR proteins, 3β-HSD was one of the key regulators in adrenal steroidogenesis of NCI-H295R cells. And also, this result suggests that a significant regulatory mechanism in steroidogenesis

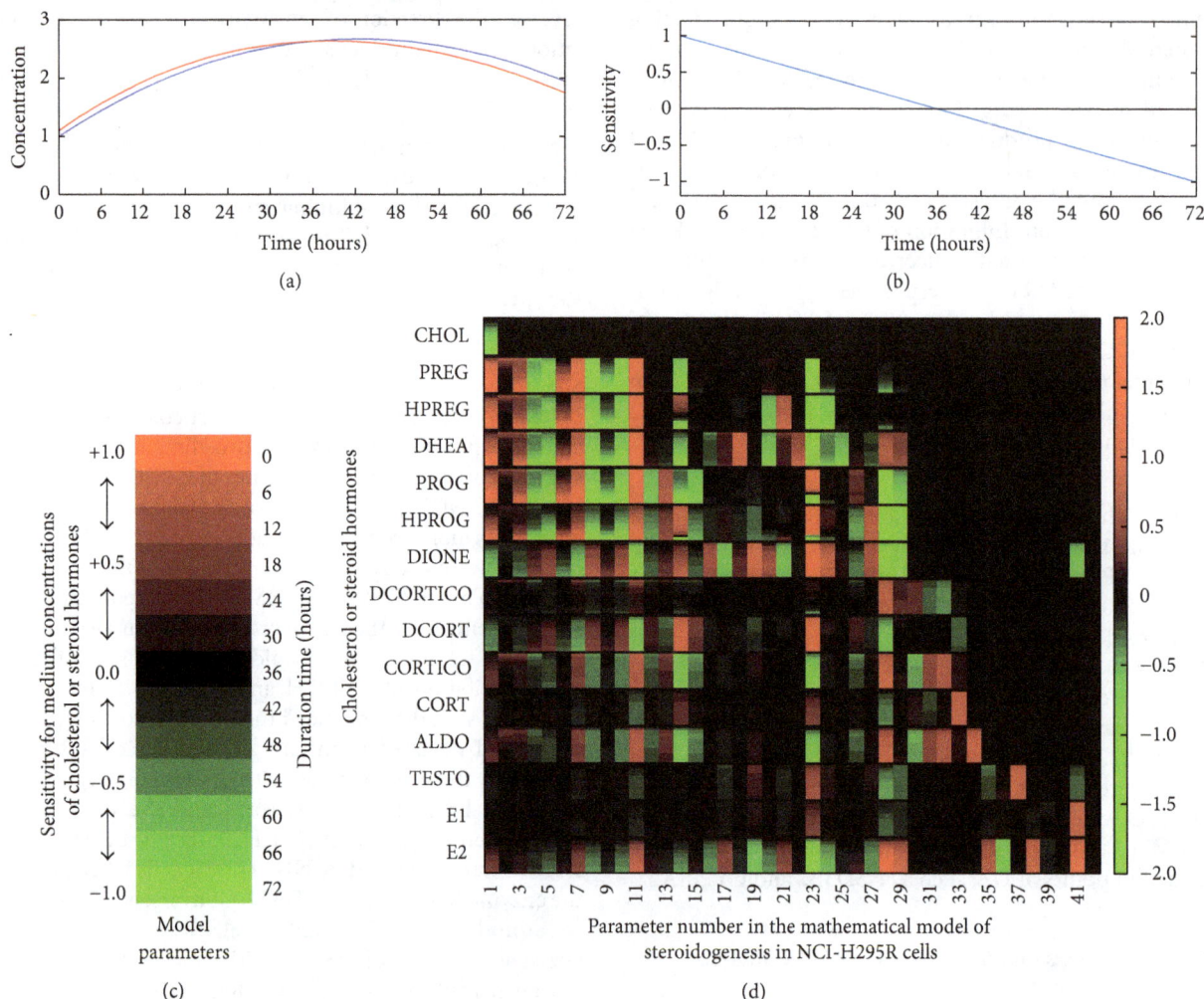

FIGURE 6: Heat-map of the global dynamic sensitivity analysis of adrenal steroid concentrations produced by NCI-H295R cells. The global dynamic sensitivity analysis is a powerful tool to comprehensively understand the dependencies of the model parameters in the mathematical model of the biological complex system. Dynamic sensitivities of model parameters in the mathematical model of adrenal steroidogenesis in NCI-H295R cells were calculated for all steroid concentrations in the culture medium every 6 h until 72 h after stimulation. To clarify the view of heat-map of global dynamic sensitivity analysis, imaginary data of the dynamics of steroid concentrations in the original model (blue line) and perturbed model for sensitivity analysis (red line) were prepared (a). Using this imaginary data, the calculated dynamic sensitivities (b) and the visualized dynamic sensitivity as one block of the heat-map (c) were shown, respectively. By the same method that explained using imaginary data, the large-scale data of the global dynamic sensitivity analysis on the mathematical model of adrenal steroidogenesis in NCI-H295R cells was comprehensively visualized as a big graph of heat-map (d). Parameter numbers in the horizontal axis are (1) $k^{\text{Choresterol Transport}}$, (2) k^{CEH}, (3) k_f^{MTR}, (4) k_b^{MTR}, (5) k_f^{acc}, (6) k_b^{acc}, (7) k_f^{loc}, (8) k_b^{loc}, (9) $k_{\text{Oxysterol Synthesis}}$, (10) K_m^{CYP11A1}, (11) $V_{\text{max}}^{\text{CYP11A1}}$, (12) K_{mA}^{CYP17H}, (13) K_{mB}^{CYP17H}, (14) $V_{\text{maxA}}^{\text{CYP17H}}$, (15) $V_{\text{maxB}}^{\text{CYP17H}}$, (16) $V_{\text{maxB}}^{\text{CYP17H}}$, (17) K_{mB}^{CYP17L}, (18) $V_{\text{maxB}}^{\text{CYP17L}}$, (19) $V_{\text{maxA}}^{\text{CYP17L}}$, (20) K_{mA}^{HSD3B2}, (21) K_{mB}^{HSD3B2}, (22) K_{mC}^{HSD3B2}, (23) $V_{\text{maxA}}^{\text{HSD3B2}}$, (24) $V_{\text{maxB}}^{\text{HSD3B2}}$, (25) $V_{\text{maxB}}^{\text{HSD3B2}}$, (26) K_{mA}^{CYP21A2}, (27) K_{mB}^{CYP21A2}, (28) $V_{\text{maxA}}^{\text{CYP21A2}}$, (29) $V_{\text{maxB}}^{\text{CYP21A2}}$, (30) K_{mA}^{CYP11B1}, (31) K_{mB}^{CYP11B1}, (32) $V_{\text{maxA}}^{\text{CYP11B1}}$, (33) $V_{\text{maxB}}^{\text{CYP11B1}}$, (34) k^{CYP11B2}, (35) K_{mA}^{HSD17B3}, (36) K_{mB}^{HSD17B3}, (37) $V_{\text{maxA}}^{\text{HSD17B3}}$, (38) $V_{\text{maxB}}^{\text{HSD17B3}}$, (39) K_{mA}^{CYP19A1}, (40) K_{mB}^{CYP19A1}, (41) $V_{\text{maxA}}^{\text{CYP19A1}}$, and (42) $V_{\text{maxB}}^{\text{CYP19A1}}$. PREG: pregnenolone, HPREG: 17α-hydroxypregnenolone, DHEA: dehydroepiandrosterone, PROG: progesterone, HPROG: 17α-hydroxyprogesterone, DIONE: androstenedione, DCORTICO: 11-deoxycorticosterone, DCORT: 11-deoxycortisol, CORTICO: corticosterone, CORT: cortisol, ALDO: aldosterone, and TESTO: testosterone.

pathway is very reasonable. StAR, CYP11A1, and 3β-HSD (isoforms 1 or 2 in humans) proteins generally respond to the same hormones that stimulate steroid production through common pathways such as cAMP signaling in adrenal glands and testes [65, 66]. Moreover, our data also support recent experimental evidence from clinical and *in vivo* studies, suggesting that the enzymatic activity of 3β-HSD plays

an important role in the regulation of mineralocorticoid synthesis in adrenal steroidogenesis and contributes to hypertension caused by abnormal overproduction of aldosterone [67–70]. Circadian clock-deficient Cry-null mice show salt-sensitive hypertension due to abnormally high synthesis of aldosterone, which is caused by constitutively high expression of HSD3B6 mRNA and protein in the adrenal cortex [67, 68].

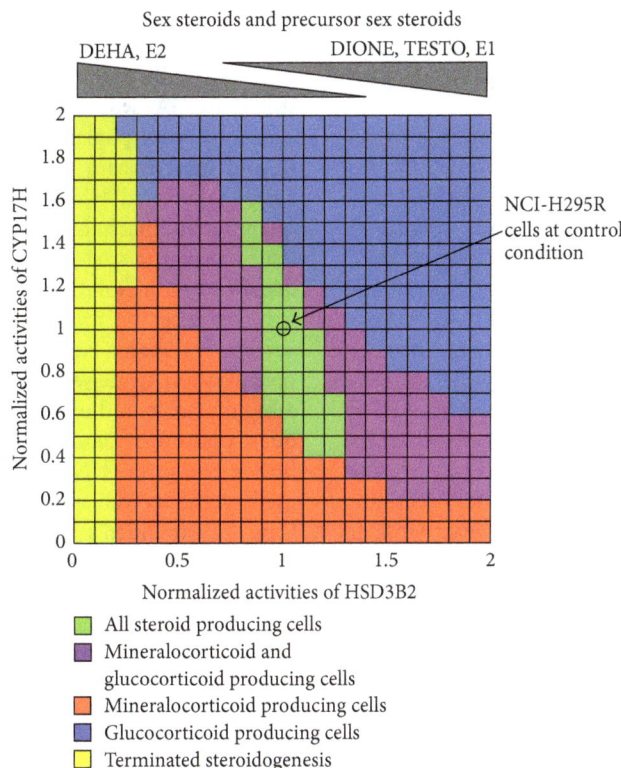

FIGURE 7: Metabolic categories of the steroidogenic cells determined by the balance of HSD3B2 and CYP17H activities. The two-dimensional parameter scanning analysis by the perturbation of two focused parameters clarifies the interaction and the relationship between the two parameters in the complex system. Functional cellular categories of steroidogenic cells were defined by the levels of mineralocorticoid (ALDO), glucocorticoids (DCORT and CORT), and androgens (DHEA and DIONE) at 72 h after stimulation. Enzymatic activities of HSD3B2 and CYP17 were normalized by standard values of the simulation model in NCI-H295R cells. Scanning ranges of HSD3B2 and CYP17 activities were 0–200%, each 10%. Green regions are all 14 steroids produced by NCI-H295R cells. Red, blue, and purple regions are mineralocorticoid producing cells, glucocorticoids-producing cells, and both corticoid-producing cells, respectively. Yellow regions are steroidogenesis of NCI-H295R cells terminated upstream of the adrenal steroidogenesis pathway.

Recent clinical observations have revealed predominant expression of HSD3B2 mRNA and protein in tumor cells of aldosterone-producing adenoma (APA), and HSD3B1 mRNA significantly correlated with CYP11B2 mRNA levels and plasma aldosterone concentrations in APA patients [69, 70]. However, the relationship is unclear and disputed in a small-scale clinical study indicating that genetic variation in HSD3B1 affects blood pressure and hypertension in APA patients [71]. The results of our simulation study suggest that 3β-HSD protein (human genes are HSD3B1 and HSD3B2) is one of the determination factors for the dynamic property of adrenal steroidogenesis. Our results support the clinical evidence of Doi and colleagues [69], and we believe that the HSD3B1 enzyme has a promising potential as novel drug target for endocrine hypertension.

4.2. Metabolic Shift of Adrenal Steroidogenesis and the Contributions of HSD3B2 and CYP17H. The metabolic properties of adrenal steroidogenesis in NCI-H295R cells were revealed by dynamic sensitivity analysis using the mathematical model (Figure 6). Mineralocorticoids, such as DCORTICO, CORTICO, and ALDO, and intermediate steroids upstream of

the adrenal steroidogenesis pathway, such as PREG, HPREG, DHEA, PROG, and HPROG, were accelerated by reactions of cholesterol import ($k_{\text{Cholesterol Transport}}$), StAR protein ($k_f^{\text{MTR}}$ and k_f^{loc}), and CYP11A1 ($V_{\text{max}}^{\text{CYP11A1}}$). On the other hand, glucocorticoids, such as DCORT and CORT, and sex hormones, such as DIONE, TESTO, and E1, were suppressed by these model parameters. Therefore, enhancement of the net adrenal steroidogenesis capacity, which supplies PREG precursor to the pathway, causes a production shift from glucocorticoids to mineralocorticoids by substrate inhibitions of CYP17H, HSD3B2, and CYP21A2 caused by accumulation of initial intermediate steroids such as PREG and PROG. Sensitivities of CYP17H ($V_{\text{maxA}}^{\text{CYP17H}}$) and HSD3B2 ($V_{\text{maxA}}^{\text{HSD3B2}}$) for the products were dynamically changed and these parameters determined the metabolic balance of downstream steroids in the adrenal steroidogenesis pathway. According to these results of dynamic sensitivity analysis of StAR, CYP11A1, CYP17H, and HSD3B2, we suggest that the enhancement of CYP17H and HSD3B2 activity during ACTH stimulation was important to shift the steroidogenic output away from ALDO biosynthesis towards CORT biosynthesis, as well as adrenal androgen production. This suggestion partially supports a comparative animal study in which molecular and cellular variations in CYP17H activity dramatically affect acute cortisol production, resulting in distinct physiological and behavioral responses [72].

Results of two-dimensional parameter scanning of the enzymatic activities of CYP17H and HSD3B2 quantitatively showed the detail of the metabolic relationship between mineralocorticoid and glucocorticoid biosynthesis (Figure 7). Particularly, the results showed that the balance of these enzymatic activities was very important for the typical function of NCI-H295R cells, namely, the ability to produce all steroid hormones. NCI-H295R cells lost this function when enzymatic activities of CYP17H and HSD3B2 were changed by over 60% and 30%, respectively. In addition, they became mineralocorticoid (ALDO) secreting cells when the enzymatic activity of CYP17H or HSD3B2 was inhibited by over 50% or glucocorticoid (DCORT and CORT) secreting cells when these enzymes were activated by over 50%. In particular, this analysis also showed that HSD3B2 was a key player in the adrenal steroidogenesis of NCI-H295R cells, because HSD3B2 inhibition by over 80% almost completely inhibited the biosynthesis of downstream steroids. The ratio of CYP17A1 to HSD3B2 mRNA expression levels has been related to several endocrine diseases with a low level in APAs [73] and high level in cortisol-producing adenomas [74]. Furthermore, the expression levels or enzymatic activities of CYP17A1 and HSD3B1 have been related to androgen production in polycystic ovary syndrome [75, 76]. These clinical studies support our simulation results indicating that the balance of enzymatic activity of CYP17H and HSD3B2 determines the shift in steroidogenic output to mineralocorticoids, glucocorticoids, or androgens.

4.3. Methodologies of Quantitative Mechanistic Analysis for Drug Discovery. According to our results obtained using the mathematical model of steroidogenesis in NCI-H295R cells, such as sensitivity analysis, comprehensive analysis based on systems biology is available to quantitatively estimate the mechanism of action of steroidogenic disrupting compounds from differential profiling of adrenal steroid hormones, because dynamic patterns of steroid hormones in adrenal steroidogenesis pathway are highly complex. Our proposed method of quantitative mechanistic analysis of steroidogenic inhibitors was able to predict known action sites in the adrenal steroidogenesis pathway at only one time point (72 h after drug exposure). Moreover, according to the results of sensitivity analysis (Figure 6), V_{max} of all steroidogenic enzymes was more sensitive than the K_m, because the intracellular concentrations of steroid hormones were almost maintained at sufficiently high levels compared with K_m values of steroidogenic enzymes. These results suggested that estimation of the mechanism of action of drugs is more effective and detectable when using the influences of V_{max} as the searching parameters such as our proposed method. Our data showed that the proposed method based on a systems biology model is a very powerful tool for exploratory screening of steroidogenic disrupting compounds.

RCGA as a solver of parameter estimation problems in systems biology has been applied to biological network identification of gene regulatory networks and metabolic pathways and optimization of biological processes using experimentally observed time-course data [77–82]. In this study, RCGA was useful to estimate the mechanism of action of novel pharmaceutical drug candidates for adrenal steroidogenesis as a new application of RCGA in systems biology. We had two issues when applying RCGA to the quantitative mechanistic analysis of drug actions. These issues were the vast calculation cost and multimodality of quasi-optimum solutions in solving the optimization problem, because the mathematical model in systems biology consists of many equations and parameters. A proposed optimization strategy using RCGA based on REX/JGG was a highly stable and efficient calculation method for a better quasi-optimum solution than the unimodal normal distribution crossover (UNDX)/minimum generation gap (MGG) method that is well applied in the engineering field. In addition, we expanded the RCGA optimization program based on REX/JGG to a hybrid method of GA and then applied a local search as recommended by Harada and Kobayashi [28, 83]. A final optimal solution was obtained with a good convergence property. Because these problems are general in systems biology studies, we suggest that the proposed hybrid method based on REX/JGG is a very useful tool for quantitative mechanistic analysis of novel pharmaceutical drugs, not limited to steroidogenic disrupting compounds.

5. Conclusions

The novel mathematical model of adrenal steroidogenesis was constructed in this study, including cholesterol transport and distribution, the C_{21}-steroid hormone pathway, steroid transport, and cell proliferation, which could reproduce adrenal steroidogenesis in NCI-H295R cells. According to the results of dynamic sensitivity analysis using the new model, HSD3B2 plays the most important role in the metabolic balance of adrenal steroidogenesis in NCI-H295R cells. Moreover, to quantitatively estimate mechanisms of action of adrenal toxic compounds, we analyzed differential metabolic profiles of 12 steroid hormones at 3 days after exposure to 11 adrenal toxic compounds, by using the new mathematical model and a hybrid optimization method of the RCGA and a local search (nonlinear least squares). We could estimate which steroidogenic enzymes were affected by these compounds using the hybrid optimization method. Vasculotoxic agents were estimated to have no effect according to the results obtained by our method. In terms of adrenal steroidogenic inhibitors, the predicted action sites were approximately matched to the target enzymes as reported in the literature. Thus, our computer-aided method based on a systems biology approach may be useful to analyze the mechanism of action of endocrine-disrupting compounds and to assess the human adrenal toxicity of novel pharmaceutical drugs based on steroid hormone profiling.

Conflict of Interests

The authors declare that there is no conflict of interests regarding the publication of this paper.

Authors' Contribution

Ryuta Saito, Natsuko Terasaki, and Naohisa Tsutsui designed the study. Naohisa Tsutsui and Naoya Masutomi supervised the experiments. Natsuko Terasaki performed all *in vitro* experiments and collected data. Makoto Yamazaki performed all measurements of steroids. Ryuta Saito conceived the *in silico* strategies, analyzed data, developed all programs and the mathematical model, and performed all simulation analyses with Masahiro Okamoto. Ryuta Saito, Natsuko Terasaki, Makoto Yamazaki, Naoya Masutomi, and Masahiro Okamoto wrote the paper.

Acknowledgments

The authors would like to thank Dr. Michael S. Breen and Dr. Miyuki Breen for helpful discussions concerning previous mathematical models of adrenal steroidogenesis. This work was partially supported by the Grant-in-Aid for Scientific Research on Innovative Areas, "Synthetic Biology" (No. 23119001 (MO)) from Ministry of Education, Culture, Sports, Science and Technology in Japan.

References

[1] P. W. Harvey, D. J. Everett, and C. J. Springall, "Adrenal toxicology: a strategy for assessment of functional toxicity to the adrenal cortex and steroidogenesis," *Journal of Applied Toxicology*, vol. 27, no. 2, pp. 103–115, 2007.

[2] W. E. Ribelin, "The effects of drugs and chemicals upon the structure of the adrenal gland," *Fundamental and Applied Toxicology*, vol. 4, no. 1, pp. 105–119, 1984.

[3] H. D. Colby and P. A. Longhurst, "Toxicology of the adrenal gland," in *Endocrine Toxicology*, C. K. Atterwill and J. D. Flack, Eds., pp. 243–281, Cambridge University Press, Cambridge, UK, 1992.

[4] H. D. Colby, "In vitro assessment of adrenocortical toxicity," *Journal of Pharmacological and Toxicological Methods*, vol. 32, no. 1, pp. 1–6, 1994.

[5] T. J. Rosol, J. T. Yarrington, J. Latendresse, and C. C. Capen, "Adrenal gland: structure, function, and mechanisms of toxicity," *Toxicologic Pathology*, vol. 29, no. 1, pp. 41–48, 2001.

[6] P. W. Harvey and D. J. Everett, "The adrenal cortex and steroidogenesis as cellular and molecular targets for toxicity: critical omissions from regulatory endocrine disrupter screening strategies for human health?" *Journal of Applied Toxicology*, vol. 23, no. 2, pp. 81–87, 2003.

[7] A. F. Gazdar, H. K. Oie, C. H. Shackleton et al., "Establishment and characterization of a human adrenocortical carcinoma cell line that expresses multiple pathways of steroid biosynthesis," *Cancer Research*, vol. 50, no. 17, pp. 5488–5496, 1990.

[8] W. E. Rainey, I. M. Bird, C. Sawetawan et al., "Regulation of human adrenal carcinoma cell (NCI-H295) production of C19 steroids," *The Journal of Clinical Endocrinology & Metabolism*, vol. 77, no. 3, pp. 731–737, 1993.

[9] B. Staels, D. W. Hum, and W. L. Miller, "Regulation of steroidogenesis in NCI-H295 cells: a cellular model of the human fetal adrenal," *Molecular Endocrinology*, vol. 7, no. 3, pp. 423–433, 1993.

[10] M. Hecker, J. L. Newsted, M. B. Murphy et al., "Human adrenocarcinoma (H295R) cells for rapid in vitro determination of effects on steroidogenesis: hormone production," *Toxicology and Applied Pharmacology*, vol. 217, no. 1, pp. 114–124, 2006.

[11] A. Oskarsson, E. Ulleràs, K. E. Plant, J. P. Hinson, and P. S. Goldfarb, "Steroidogenic gene expression in H295R cells and the human adrenal gland: adrenotoxic effects of lindane in vitro," *Journal of Applied Toxicology*, vol. 26, no. 6, pp. 484–492, 2006.

[12] U. Müller-Vieira, M. Angotti, and R. W. Hartman, "The adrenocortical tumor cell line NCI-H295R as an in vitro screening system for the evaluation of CYP11B2 (aldosterone synthase) and CYP11B1 (steroid-11β-hydroxylase) inhibitors," *The Journal of Steroid Biochemistry and Molecular Biology*, vol. 96, no. 3-4, pp. 259–270, 2005.

[13] K. Imagawa, S. Okayama, M. Takaoka et al., "Inhibitory effect of efonidipine on aldosterone synthesis and secretion in human adrenocarcinoma (H295R) cells," *Journal of Cardiovascular Pharmacology*, vol. 47, no. 1, pp. 133–138, 2006.

[14] M. Voets, U. Müller-Vieira, S. Marchais-Oberwinkler, and R. W. Hartmann, "Synthesis of amidinohydrazones and evaluation of their inhibitory effect towards aldosterone synthase (CYP11B2) and the formation of selected steroids," *Archiv der Pharmazie*, vol. 337, no. 7, pp. 411–416, 2004.

[15] F. K. Nielsen, C. H. Hansen, J. A. Fey et al., "H295R cells as a model for steroidogenic disruption: a broader perspective using simultaneous chemical analysis of 7 key steroid hormones," *Toxicology in Vitro*, vol. 26, no. 2, pp. 343–350, 2012.

[16] S. Ohno, S. Shinoda, S. Toyoshima, H. Nakazawa, T. Makino, and S. Nakajin, "Effects of flavonoid phytochemicals on cortisol production and on activities of steroidogenic enzymes in human adrenocortical H295R cells," *Journal of Steroid Biochemistry and Molecular Biology*, vol. 80, no. 3, pp. 355–363, 2002.

[17] R. F. Cantón, J. T. Sanderson, S. Nijmeijer, Å. Bergman, R. J. Letcher, and M. van den Berg, "In vitro effects of brominated flame retardants and metabolites on CYP17 catalytic activity: a novel mechanism of action?" *Toxicology and Applied Pharmacology*, vol. 216, no. 2, pp. 274–281, 2006.

[18] K. Hilscherova, P. D. Jones, T. Gracia et al., "Assessment of the effects of chemicals on the expression of ten steroidogenic genes in the H295R cell line using real-time PCR," *Toxicological Sciences*, vol. 81, no. 1, pp. 78–89, 2004.

[19] T. Gracia, K. Hilscherova, P. D. Jones et al., "The H295R system for evaluation of endocrine-disrupting effects," *Ecotoxicology and Environmental Safety*, vol. 65, no. 3, pp. 293–305, 2006.

[20] X. Zhang, J. L. Newsted, M. Hecker, E. B. Higley, P. D. Jones, and J. P. Giesy, "Classification of chemicals based on concentration-dependent toxicological data using ToxClust," *Environmental Science and Technology*, vol. 43, no. 10, pp. 3926–3932, 2009.

[21] M. S. Breen, M. Breen, N. Terasaki, M. Yamazaki, and R. B. Conolly, "Computational model of steroidogenesis in human H295R cells to predict biochemical response to endocrine-active chemicals: model development for metyrapone," *Environmental Health Perspectives*, vol. 118, no. 2, pp. 265–272, 2010.

[22] M. Breen, M. S. Breen, N. Terasaki, M. Yamazaki, A. L. Lloyd, and R. B. Conolly, "Mechanistic computational model of steroidogenesis in H295R cells: role of oxysterols and cell proliferation to improve predictability of biochemical response to endocrine active chemical-metyrapone," *Toxicological Sciences*, vol. 123, no. 1, pp. 80–93, 2011.

[23] F. B. Kraemer, "Adrenal cholesterol utilization," *Molecular and Cellular Endocrinology*, vol. 265-266, pp. 42–45, 2007.

[24] W. L. Miller, "Steroidogenic acute regulatory protein (StAR), a novel mitochondrial cholesterol transporter," *Biochimica et*

Biophysica Acta (BBA)—Molecular and Cell Biology of Lipids, vol. 1771, no. 6, pp. 663–676, 2007.

[25] S. Szabo and I. T. Lippe, "Adrenal gland: chemically induced structural and functional changes in the cortex," *Toxicologic Pathology*, vol. 17, no. 2, pp. 317–329, 1989.

[26] C. Chen-Pan, I.-J. Pan, Y. Yamamoto, T. Sakogawa, J. Yamada, and Y. Hayashi, "Prompt recovery of damaged adrenal medullae induced by salinomycin," *Toxicologic Pathology*, vol. 27, no. 5, pp. 563–572, 1999.

[27] R. J. Santen and R. I. Misbin, "Aminoglutethimide: review of pharmacology and clinical use," *Pharmacotherapy*, vol. 1, no. 2, pp. 95–120, 1981.

[28] M. J. Carella, N. V. Dimitrov, V. V. Gossain, L. Srivastava, and D. R. Rovner, "Adrenal effects of low-dose aminoglutethimide when used alone in postmenopausal women with advanced breast cancer," *Metabolism*, vol. 43, no. 6, pp. 723–727, 1994.

[29] M. K. Johansson, J. T. Sanderson, and B.-O. Lund, "Effects of 3-MeSO2-DDE and some CYP inhibitors on glucocorticoid steroidogenesis in the H295R human adrenocortical carcinoma cell line," *Toxicology in Vitro*, vol. 16, no. 2, pp. 113–121, 2002.

[30] Y. Touitou, A. Bogdan, J. C. Legrand, and P. Desgrez, "Aminoglutethimide and glutethimide: effects on 18-hydroxycorticosterone biosynthesis by human and sheep adrenals in vitro," *Acta Endocrinologica*, vol. 80, no. 3, pp. 517–526, 1975.

[31] M. M. Hart and J. A. Straw, "Studies on the site of action of o,p'-DDD in the dog adrenal cortex. 1. Inhibition of ACTH-mediated pregnenolone synthesis," *Steroids*, vol. 17, no. 1–5, pp. 559–574, 1971.

[32] M. Ojima, M. Saitoh, N. Itoh, Y. Kusano, S. Fukuchi, and H. Naganuma, "The effects of o,p'-DDD on adrenal steroidogenesis and hepatic steroid metabolism," *Nippon Naibunpi Gakkai zasshi*, vol. 61, no. 3, pp. 168–178, 1985.

[33] L. F. Canosa and N. R. Ceballos, "Effects of different steroid-biosynthesis inhibitors on the testicular steroidogenesis of the toad Bufo arenarum," *Journal of Comparative Physiology B*, vol. 171, no. 6, pp. 519–526, 2001.

[34] D. C. Kossor, S. Kominami, S. Takemori, and H. D. Colby, "Role of the steroid 17 alpha-hydroxylase in spironolactone-mediated destruction of adrenal cytochrome P-450," *Molecular Pharmacology*, vol. 40, no. 2, pp. 321–325, 1991.

[35] S. C. Cheng, K. Suzuki, W. Sadee, and B. W. Harding, "Effects of spironolactone, canrenone and canrenoate K on cytochrome P450, and 11β and 18 hydroxylation in bovine and human adrenal cortical mitochondria," *Endocrinology*, vol. 99, no. 4, pp. 1097–1106, 1976.

[36] K. Yanagibashi, M. Haniu, J. E. Shively, W. H. Shen, and P. Hall, "The synthesis of aldosterone by the adrenal cortex. Two zones (fasciculata and glomerulosa) possess one enzyme for 11β-, 18-hydroxylation, and aldehyde synthesis," *The Journal of Biological Chemistry*, vol. 261, no. 8, pp. 3556–3562, 1986.

[37] K. Morishita, H. Okumura, N. Ito, and N. Takahashi, "Primary culture system of adrenocortical cells from dogs to evaluate direct effects of chemicals on steroidogenesis," *Toxicology*, vol. 165, no. 2-3, pp. 171–178, 2001.

[38] S. W. J. Lamberts, E. G. Bons, H. A. Bruining, and F. H. de Jong, "Differential effects of the imidazole derivatives etomidate, ketoconazole and miconazole and of metyrapone on the secretion of cortisol and its precursors by human adrenocortical cells," *Journal of Pharmacology and Experimental Therapeutics*, vol. 240, no. 1, pp. 259–264, 1987.

[39] L. Yin, S. Lucas, F. Maurer, U. Kazmaier, Q. Hu, and R. W. Hartmann, "Novel imidazol-1-ylmethyl substituted 1,2,5,6-tetrahydropyrrolo[3,2,1-*ij*]quinolin-4-ones as potent and selective CYP11B1 inhibitors for the treatment of Cushing's syndrome," *Journal of Medicinal Chemistry*, vol. 55, no. 14, pp. 6629–6633, 2012.

[40] M. DiMattina, N. Maronian, H. Ashby, D. L. Loriaux, and B. D. Albertson, "Ketoconazole inhibits multiple steroidogenic enzymes involved in androgen biosynthesis in the human ovary," *Fertility and Sterility*, vol. 49, no. 1, pp. 62–65, 1988.

[41] M. Ayub and M. J. Levell, "Inhibition of human adrenal steroidogenic enzymes in vitro by imidazole drugs including ketoconazole," *Journal of Steroid Biochemistry*, vol. 32, no. 4, pp. 515–524, 1989.

[42] D. Engelhardt, M. M. Weber, T. Miksch, F. Abedinpour, and C. Jaspers, "The influence of ketoconazole on human adrenal steroidogenesis: incubation studies with tissue slices," *Clinical Endocrinology*, vol. 35, no. 2, pp. 163–168, 1991.

[43] S. Bhasin, S. Sikka, T. Fielder et al., "Hormonal effects of ketoconazole in vivo in the male rat: mechanism of action," *Endocrinology*, vol. 118, no. 3, pp. 1229–1232, 1986.

[44] D. M. Zisterer and D. C. Williams, "Calmidazolium and other imidazole compounds affect steroidogenesis in Y1 cells: lack of involvement of the peripheral-type benzodiazepine receptor," *Journal of Steroid Biochemistry and Molecular Biology*, vol. 60, no. 3-4, pp. 189–195, 1997.

[45] L. P. Walsh, C. N. Kuratko, and D. M. Stocco, "Econazole and miconazole inhibit steroidogenesis and disrupt steroidogenic acute regulatory (StAR) protein expression post-transcriptionally," *Journal of Steroid Biochemistry and Molecular Biology*, vol. 75, no. 4-5, pp. 229–236, 2000.

[46] S. Ohno, S. Shinoda, S. Toyoshima, H. Nakazawa, T. Makino, and S. Nakajin, "Effects of flavonoid phytochemicals on cortisol production and on activities of steroidogenic enzymes in human adrenocortical H295R cells," *The Journal of Steroid Biochemistry and Molecular Biology*, vol. 80, no. 3, pp. 355–363, 2002.

[47] D. P. Dempsher, D. S. Gann, and R. D. Phair, "A mechanistic model of ACTH-stimulated cortisol secretion," *American Journal of Physiology*, vol. 246, no. 4, part 2, pp. R587–R596, 1984.

[48] N. Sarai, S. Matsuoka, and A. Noma, "simBio: a Java package for the development of detailed cell models," *Progress in Biophysics and Molecular Biology*, vol. 90, no. 1–3, pp. 360–377, 2006.

[49] K. Levenberg, "A method for the solution of certain non-linear problems in least squares," *Quarterly of Applied Mathematics*, vol. 2, pp. 164–168, 1944.

[50] D. W. Marquardt, "An algorithm for least-squares estimation of nonlinear parameters," *SIAM Journal on Applied Mathematics*, vol. 11, no. 2, pp. 431–441, 1963.

[51] P. E. Gill and W. Murray, "Algorithms for the solution of the nonlinear least-squares problem," *SIAM Journal on Numerical Analysis*, vol. 15, no. 5, pp. 977–992, 1978.

[52] Y. Akimoto, R. Hasada, J. Sakuma, I. Ono, and S. Kobayashi, "Generation alternation model for real-coded GA using multi-parent: proposal and evaluation of just generation gap (JGG)," in *Proceedings of the 19th SICE Symposium on Decentralized Autonomous Systems*, pp. 341–346, Tokyo, Japan, January 2007.

[53] Y. Akimoto, Y. Nagata, J. Sakuma, I. Ono, and S. Kobayashi, "Proposal and evaluation of adaptive real-coded crossover AREX," *Transactions of the Japanese Society for Artificial Intelligence*, vol. 24, no. 6, pp. 446–458, 2009.

[54] S. Kobayashi, "The frontiers of real-coded genetic algorithms," *Journal of Japanese Society for Artificial Intelligence*, vol. 24, no. 1, pp. 147–162, 2009.

[55] Y. Akimoto, Y. Nagata, J. Sakuma, I. Ono, and S. Kobayashi, "Analysis of the behavior of MGG and JGG as a selection model for real-coded genetic algorithms," *Transactions of the Japanese Society for Artificial Intelligence*, vol. 25, no. 2, pp. 281–289, 2010.

[56] A. Struthers, H. Krum, and G. H. Williams, "A comparison of the aldosterone-blocking agents eplerenone and spironolactone," *Clinical Cardiology*, vol. 31, no. 4, pp. 153–158, 2008.

[57] K. Yamasaki, M. Sawaki, S. Noda et al., "Comparison of the Hershberger assay and androgen receptor binding assay of twelve chemicals," *Toxicology*, vol. 195, no. 2-3, pp. 177–186, 2004.

[58] C. Eil and S. K. Edelson, "The use of human skin fibroblasts to obtain potency estimates of drug binding to androgen receptors," *The Journal of Clinical Endocrinology & Metabolism*, vol. 59, no. 1, pp. 51–55, 1984.

[59] P. Ye, T. Yamashita, D. M. Pollock, H. Sasano, and W. E. Rainey, "Contrasting effects of eplerenone and spironolactone on adrenal cell steroidogenesis," *Hormone and Metabolic Research*, vol. 41, no. 1, pp. 35–39, 2009.

[60] B. D. Albertson, K. L. Frederick, N. C. Maronian et al., "The effect of ketoconazole on steroidogenesis: I. Leydig cell enzyme activity in vitro," *Research Communications in Chemical Pathology and Pharmacology*, vol. 61, no. 1, pp. 17–26, 1988.

[61] B. D. Albertson, N. C. Maronian, K. L. Frederick et al., "The effect of ketoconazole on steroidogenesis. II. Adrenocortical enzyme activity in vitro," *Research Communications in Chemical Pathology and Pharmacology*, vol. 61, no. 1, pp. 27–34, 1988.

[62] D. M. Stocco and B. J. Clark, "Regulation of the acute production of steroids in steroidogenic cells," *Endocrine Reviews*, vol. 17, no. 3, pp. 221–244, 1996.

[63] L. K. Christenson and J. F. Strauss III, "Steroidogenic acute regulatory protein (StAR) and the intramitochondrial translocation of cholesterol," *Biochimica et Biophysica Acta (BBA)—Molecular and Cell Biology of Lipids*, vol. 1529, no. 1–3, pp. 175–187, 2000.

[64] E. R. Simpson, "Cholesterol side-chain cleavage, cytochrome P450, and the control of steroidogenesis," *Molecular and Cellular Endocrinology*, vol. 13, no. 3, pp. 213–227, 1979.

[65] H. A. LaVoie and S. R. King, "Transcriptional regulation of steroidogenic genes: STARD1, CYP11A1 and HSD3B," *Experimental Biology and Medicine*, vol. 234, no. 8, pp. 880–907, 2009.

[66] F. Raucci, A. D'Aniello, and M. M. Di Fiore, "Stimulation of androgen production by d-aspartate through the enhancement of StAR, P450scc and 3β-HSD mRNA levels in vivo rat testis and in culture of immature rat Leydig cells," *Steroids*, vol. 84, pp. 103–110, 2014.

[67] M. Doi, Y. Takahashi, R. Komatsu et al., "Salt-sensitive hypertension in circadian clock-deficient Cry-null mice involves dysregulated adrenal Hsd3b6," *Nature Medicine*, vol. 16, no. 1, pp. 67–74, 2010.

[68] H. Okamura, M. Doi, Y. Yamaguchi, and J.-M. Fustin, "Hypertension due to loss of clock: novel insight from the molecular analysis of Cry1/Cry2-deleted mice," *Current Hypertension Reports*, vol. 13, no. 2, pp. 103–108, 2011.

[69] M. Doi, F. Satoh, T. Maekawa et al., "Isoform-specific monoclonal antibodies against 3β-hydroxysteroid dehydrogenase/isomerase family provide markers for subclassification of human primary aldosteronism," *The Journal of Clinical Endocrinology & Metabolism*, vol. 99, no. 2, pp. E257–E262, 2014.

[70] S. Konosu-Fukaya, Y. Nakamura, F. Satoh et al., "3β-hydroxysteroid dehydrogenase isoforms in human aldosterone-producing adenoma," *Molecular and Cellular Endocrinology*, vol. 408, pp. 205–212, 2015.

[71] G. C. Verwoert, J. Hofland, N. Amin et al., "Expression and gene variation studies deny association of human *HSD3B1* gene with aldosterone production or blood pressure," *American Journal of Hypertension*, vol. 28, no. 1, pp. 113–120, 2015.

[72] D. Hough, K. Storbeck, S. W. P. Cloete, A. C. Swart, and P. Swart, "Relative contribution of P450c17 towards the acute cortisol response: lessons from sheep and goats," *Molecular and Cellular Endocrinology*, vol. 408, pp. 107–113, 2015.

[73] I. Sakuma, S. Suematsu, Y. Matsuzawa et al., "Characterization of steroidogenic enzyme expression in aldosterone-producing adenoma: a comparison with various human adrenal tumors," *Endocrine Journal*, vol. 60, no. 3, pp. 329–336, 2013.

[74] A. Tong, A. Jia, S. Yan, Y. Zhang, Y. Xie, and G. Liu, "Ectopic cortisol-producing adrenocortical adenoma in the renal hilum: histopathological features and steroidogenic enzyme profile," *International Journal of Clinical and Experimental Pathology*, vol. 7, no. 7, pp. 4415–4421, 2014.

[75] A. Hirsch, D. Hahn, P. Kempná et al., "Metformin inhibits human androgen production by regulating steroidogenic enzymes HSD3B2 and CYP17A1 and complex I activity of the respiratory chain," *Endocrinology*, vol. 153, no. 9, pp. 4354–4366, 2012.

[76] B. Xu, L. Gao, Y. Cui et al., "SET protein up-regulated testosterone production in the cultured preantral follicles," *Reproductive Biology and Endocrinology*, vol. 11, article 9, 2013.

[77] S. Kikuchi, D. Tominaga, M. Arita, M. Takahashi, and M. Tomita, "Dynamic modeling of genetic networks using genetic algorithm and S-system," *Bioinformatics*, vol. 19, no. 5, pp. 643–650, 2003.

[78] N. Shikata, Y. Maki, M. Nakatsui et al., "Determining important regulatory relations of amino acids from dynamic network analysis of plasma amino acids," *Amino Acids*, vol. 38, no. 1, pp. 179–187, 2010.

[79] M. Nakatsui, T. Ueda, Y. Maki, I. Ono, and M. Okamoto, "Method for inferring and extracting reliable genetic interactions from time-series profile of gene expression," *Mathematical Biosciences*, vol. 215, no. 1, pp. 105–114, 2008.

[80] A. Komori, Y. Maki, M. Nakatsui, I. Ono, and M. Okamoto, "Efficient numerical optimization algorithm based on new real-coded genetic algorithm, AREX + JGG, and application to the inverse problem in systems biology," *Applied Mathematics*, vol. 3, no. 10, pp. 1463–1470, 2012.

[81] J. A. Roubos, G. van Straten, and A. J. B. van Boxtel, "An evolutionary strategy for fed-batch bioreactor optimization; concepts and performance," *Journal of Biotechnology*, vol. 67, no. 2-3, pp. 173–187, 1999.

[82] D. Sarkar and J. M. Modak, "Genetic algorithms with filters for optimal control problems in fed-batch bioreactors," *Bioprocess and Biosystems Engineering*, vol. 26, no. 5, pp. 295–306, 2004.

[83] K. Harada, K. Ikeda, J. Sakuma, I. Ono, and S. Kobayashi, "Hybridization of genetic algorithm with local search in multiobjective function optimization: recommendation of GA then LS," *Transactions of the Japanese Society for Artificial Intelligence*, vol. 21, no. 6, pp. 482–492, 2006.

15

Role of Bioadsorbents in Reducing Toxic Metals

Blessy Baby Mathew,[1] **Monisha Jaishankar,**[1] **Vinai George Biju,**[2]
and Krishnamurthy Nideghatta Beeregowda[1]

[1]*Department of Biotechnology, Sapthagiri College of Engineering, 14/5 Chikkasandra, Hesarghatta Main Road,*
Bangalore, Karnataka 560057, India
[2]*CUFE, Christ University, Kanmanike, Kumbalgodu, Bangalore, Karnataka 560074, India*

Correspondence should be addressed to Blessy Baby Mathew; blessym21@gmail.com

Academic Editor: Orish Ebere Orisakwe

Industrialization and urbanization have led to the release of increasing amounts of heavy metals into the environment. Metal ion contamination of drinking water and waste water is a serious ongoing problem especially with high toxic metals such as lead and cadmium and less toxic metals such as copper and zinc. Several biological materials have attracted many researchers and scientists as they offer both cheap and effective removal of heavy metals from waste water. Therefore it is urgent to study and explore all possible sources of agrobased inexpensive adsorbents for their feasibility in the removal of heavy metals. The objective was to study inexpensive adsorbents like various agricultural wastes such as sugarcane bagasse, rice husk, oil palm shell, coconut shell, and coconut husk in eliminating heavy metals from waste water and their utilization possibilities based on our research and literature survey. It also shows the significance of developing and evaluating new potential biosorbents in the near future with higher adsorption capacity and greater reusable options.

1. Introduction

In the last century many products such as medicines, disinfectants, laundry detergents, paints, surfactants, pesticides, dyes, preservatives, personal care products, and food additives have been found to be threatening to human as well as the environment [1, 2]. Various industries like fuel production units, atomic energy stations, electroplating and fertilizer industry, leather and electrical appliance manufactory, and iron enterprises generate enormous wastes containing large amount of toxic heavy metals discarded into the environment resulting in ecological imbalance. The pollutants and decaying organic matter in waste water take up the dissolved oxygen and excessive nutrients like phosphorus and nitrogen cause eutrophication which promotes excessive plant growth and reduces available oxygen in the water body. Bacteria, viruses, and disease-causing pathogens also pollute beaches and contaminate shellfish populations, leading to restrictions on human recreation and drinking water consumption. Metabolism dependent and independent processes can also result in the accumulation of large amount of metals [3] and trigger the free radical response leading to oxidative stress [4].

1.1. Biosorption. The removal of metals or nonmetals and tiny particulates from a solution by means of any biological component is known as biosorption [5]. Cellular products and living and nonliving biomass can be used for effective adsorption [3], but their cost-effectiveness and reusability factor still remains under question. There are various physical, chemical, and biological methods to remove metal ions from aqueous solutions. Some of the conventional techniques like filtration, membrane technology, and ion exchange are very expensive and chemical precipitation and electrochemical treatment prove to be ineffective especially when the concentration of metal ion is 1–100 mg/L. It also results in large sludge production [6]. Many biological materials have high eradication rate in decreasing the concentration of heavy metals from ppm to ppb level [3]. Few types of biosorbents bind onto heavy metals with no specific priority, whereas others are specific for certain types of metals [7, 8].

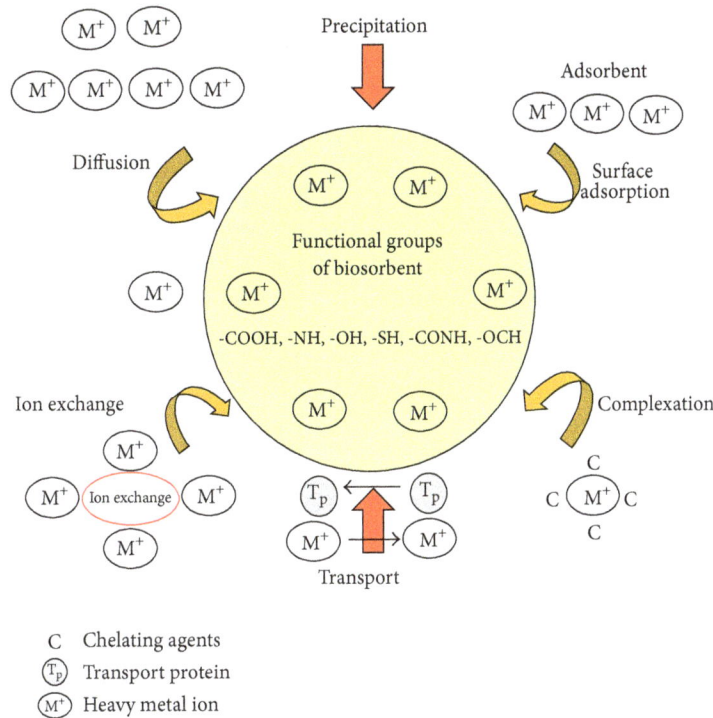

FIGURE 1: Biosorbent mechanisms.

This is one of the major reasons that research and studies on biosorption have become one of the most active work areas. In particular the low cost biosorbents obtained from agricultural and animal wastes are of major interest [9]. But the selection of biosorbent for a specific metal is a challenge and merely a hit and trial method, resulting from a series of experiments and in-depth research. We have attempted to carry out relevant researches on biosorption phenomena for the effective removal of metal ions using various agricultural wastes and to provide a summary of available information on a wide range of biosorbents through this paper as shown in Figure 1 [10].

1.2. Adsorption. A separation where in certain fluid elements are transferred to solid surface of the adsorbents is known as adsorption. Transfer of molecules from bulk solution to solid surface occurs based on concentration gradient. Here when a solid surface is exposed to a fluid phase, the molecules from the fluid phase accumulate or concentrate at the surface of a solid. All adsorption processes depend on mass transfer rates and solid-liquid equilibria [31]. The process is referred to as "desorption" if the mass transfer takes place in opposite direction. Highly porous materials are chosen as adsorbents, and adsorption occurs mostly on the pore walls or at particular sites within the particle. Difference in shape, molecular weight, or polarity makes the molecule stronger on the surface of other materials which makes separation easier. Solute diffusion rate in the capillary pores of adsorbent determines the overall adsorption rate. Rate of adsorption is equal to the square root of contact time with adsorbent.

1.2.1. Types of Adsorption Processes. Adsorption can be carried out as batch, semibatch, and continuous processes. When little quantities are to be treated, batch processes are generally carried out and the equilibrium distribution depends on the contact time in batch process [32]. Heavy metals in waste water include Cd, Cu, Zn, Cr, and Ni and most of the companies fail to solve the problems caused due to these discharge, as they lack proper technical knowledge and economic capabilities. The concentration of various heavy metals in waste water ranges from 10 ppm to 100 ppm [33]. Adsorbate and adsorbent experience certain attractive forces which bind them and these forces can be due to Van der Waals forces which are weak in nature or they may be due to chemical bonds which are strong in nature. On the basis of attraction and the strength of force prevailing between adsorbate and adsorbent, adsorption can be categorized into two.

(1) Physical Adsorption. Also known as physisorption, it occurs when the attractive forces present between adsorbate and adsorbent are weak like Van der Waals forces as in Figure 2. It has low enthalpy of adsorption (i.e., $\Delta H_{\text{adsorption}} =$ 20 to 40 KJ/mol) and occurs with development of multilayer of adsorbate on adsorbent. This phenomenon decreases with an increase in temperature and usually takes place at a lower temperature which is generally much below the boiling point of the adsorbate [34].

(2) Chemical Adsorption. Also known as chemisorption, it occurs when the attractive forces between the adsorbate and adsorbent are chemical forces of attraction or via chemical bond as in Figure 3. Here only a single layer formation of the

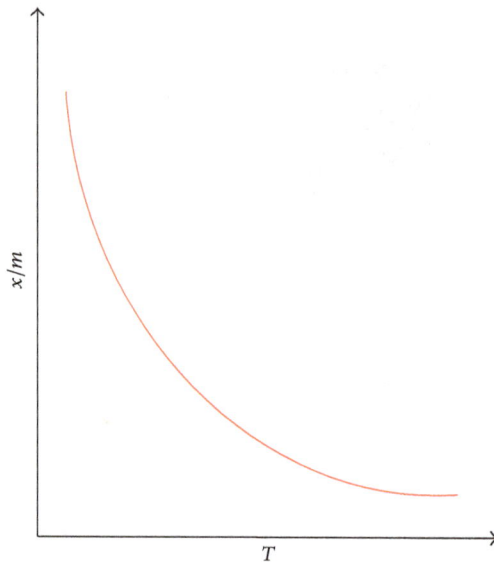

x = amount of absorbate
m = amount of absorbent

FIGURE 2: Physical adsorption versus temperature.

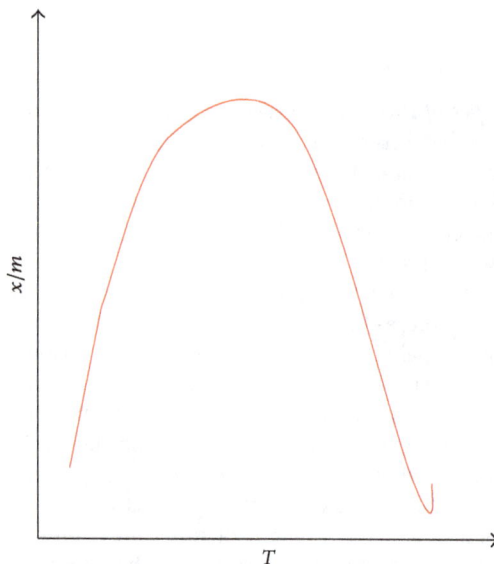

x = amount of absorbate
m = amount of absorbent

FIGURE 3: Chemical adsorption versus temperature.

adsorbate on adsorbent takes place and it has a high enthalpy of adsorption (i.e., $\Delta H_{adsorption}$ = 200 to 400 KJ/mol). This phenomenon first increases and then decreases with a rise in temperature [35].

1.3. Factors Affecting the Adsorption Process. Over the past 20 years there has been an exponential growth in the world's population. This has led to the environmental buildup of waste products, among which heavy metals are of major

concern. Heavy metals can be biodegradable which are being added to soil, water, and air in escalating amounts as well as nonbiodegradable. Some metals like zinc, magnesium, and copper are required for animal and plant life as micronutrients but the same would become more hazardous if they are taken up by plants or animals in large amounts [36]. The various factors on which the adsorption process depends are as follows.

1.3.1. Temperature. As the temperature increases, the adsorption capacity is found to decrease and vice versa. It is an exothermic process overall.

1.3.2. pH. As pH increases from 7.0 to 7.5, the retention capacity of the adsorbing surface increased significantly, whereas in lower pH the adsorption process was affected.

1.3.3. Pressure. With increase in pressure, adsorption increases up to a certain extent till saturation level is reached but after that no more adsorption takes place no matter how high the pressure is.

1.3.4. Adsorbent Activation. To provide higher number of vacant sites on surface of adsorbent, this can be done by breaking solid crystal in small pieces, heating charcoal at high temperature, breaking lump of solid into powder, or other methods suitable for particular adsorbent.

1.3.5. Surface Area of Adsorbent. As adsorption is a surface phenomenon it increases with increase in surface area. Thus for any big molecule with a higher surface area, the adsorption efficiency will increase. As we know, volume of an ideal gas at STP = 22.4 L = 22.4 dm^3 and the number of gaseous molecules present at STP = 6.023 $* 10^{23}$ molecules. Let us assume that Vmono is the adsorbed volume of gas at high pressure conditions so as to cover the surface with a uniform layer of gaseous molecules. Then assuming the total number of adsorbed gas molecules as N corresponding to volume V_{mono}, it can be given as

$$N = \left[\frac{V_{mono}}{22.4 \, dm^3 \, mol^{-1}} \right] \times 3.023 \times 10^{23} \, mol^{-1}. \quad (1)$$

1.4. Problems Associated with the Existing Technologies. The technologies which are being used at present for removal of metal ion from waste water are very expensive. They include ion exchange resin, solvent extraction, electrolytic and precipitation processes, electrodialysis, and membrane technology [37]. There are wide ranges of conventional technologies from granular activated carbon to reverse osmosis. These processes are, however, not economically feasible for small scale industries prevalent in developing economies due to large capital investment [38]. The most widely used method for removing heavy metals from waste water is by precipitation process but it results in the production of sludge containing high levels of heavy metals. Hence to purify the effluent prior to discharge there is a need for additional treatments like ion exchange, reverse osmosis, or adsorption process [39].

2. Technologies That Exist to Remove Metal Ions from Effluents

The removal of metal ions from effluents can be achieved by many methods. The technologies are divided into three types, namely, physical, chemical, and biological. The physical and chemical processes form the principal method of waste water treatment in industries. There were many merits and demerits caused due to high cost and disposal problems.

2.1. Physical Methods. Membrane filtration and adsorption are the physical methods. Membrane filtration processes include nanofiltration, reverse osmosis, and electrodialysis. Membrane fouling forms the major disadvantage of this membrane filtration. Since proper design of the adsorption process will create high quality treated effluents, adsorption process can be regarded as the best method for heavy metal removal from effluents.

2.2. Chemical Methods. To achieve the desired water quality in the most economical way, processes of different combinations were used. Electroflotation, electrokinetic coagulation, coagulation combined with flotation and filtration, conventional oxidation methods by oxidizing agents, irradiation, and electrochemical processes are the techniques which fall under chemical methods [40]. These chemical technologies are having many disposal problems and are very costly too. Even though these methods are efficient for removing the contaminants from waste water, they are commercially unattractive and very expensive. Some of the common problems are high electrical energy demand and consumption of chemical reagents.

2.3. Biological Methods. New separation methods are necessary to reduce heavy metal concentrations to environmentally tolerable levels at reasonable cost because most conventional methods are neither effective nor economical, especially when used for the reduction of heavy metal ions to low concentrations. This goal can be achieved through bioremoval [41–43]. The accumulation and concentration of heavy metals from aqueous solutions using biological materials is known as bioremoval [37] as shown in Figure 2 [44]. Many studies were done for the removal of heavy metals from solution by utilizing different agricultural products and byproducts. Several studies showed the efficacy of many organic waste components as sorbents for heavy metals [45–47]. If the adsorbent is inexpensive and does not require an additional pretreatment step before application, this process provides an outstanding alternative for treatment of contaminated water. But biological method is not favorable as it requires large area and has less design flexibility and lesser modes of operation and is constrained by sensitivity towards diurnal variation including certain chemical toxicity [48]. In contrast to other techniques adsorption has originated to be superior for water reuse in terms of primary cost, elasticity

and straightforwardness of design, ease of operation, and insensitivity to toxic pollutants and there is no production of dangerous materials [49]. Other than the above listed methods, the one method which is from the nature itself which would not just remove the metal ions but is also an example of effective usage of biowaste is bioadsorption, that is, the adsorption of any constituents, like metals, onto the surface of biological components. Selecting the most capable types of biomass from an enormously huge pool of readily accessible and cheap biomaterials was the first most important challenge for the biosorption field [50]. Full scale biosorption process requires the biological materials which have high metal binding capabilities and specific heavy metal selectivity. Biosorption mechanisms are understood to a limited extent. It may involve one process or a blend of processes like adsorption, electrostatic interaction, chelation, microprecipitation, and ion exchange [3, 51, 52]. These biomasses have been tested and reported to bind a variety of heavy metals to different extents. Microbial biosorption is another aspect under this which is carried out by different organisms like bacteria, fungus, and algae. Nearly 50 microbial strains of microorganisms, capable of degrading xenobiotics, have been isolated, such as *Pseudomonas, Mycobacterium, Alcaligenes,* and *Nocardia.* Microbial degradation of heavy metals assumes significance, since it provides an effective and economic means of disposing of toxic chemicals, particularly the environmental pollutants (Figure 4).

3. The Green Technology: Usage of Effective Bioadsorbents

3.1. Wheat Bran. Wheat bran acts as an efficient adsorbent for the heavy metal ions removal such as Pb(II), Cu(II), and Cd(II). Another study stated that significant adsorption in copper ions could be achieved by pretreatment with strong dehydrating agent like sulphuric acid (H_2SO_4) as the micropores and macropores conversion leads to increase in adsorption [53]. The maximum capacity achieved for 30 min was 51.5 mg/L (at pH 5) for Cu(II) ions. This method when used for lead ions showed maximum removal up to 82.8% at pH 6 after 2 h of equilibrium time [54] and for cadmium ions 101 mg/L at pH 5, efficient adsorption was seen at a contact time of 4 hrs. Langmuir, Freundlich, and Redlich-Peterson isotherm models were used to determine the adsorption capacity of wheat bran out of which Redlich-Peterson was found to be the best fitted model for adsorption.

3.2. Rice Husk. One of the agricultural wastes generated especially in rice producing countries, like Asia, is rice husk. Around 500 million metric tons of rice is produced around the world out of which rice husk constitutes 10 to 20%. Dry rice husk consists of 70 to 85% of organic matter, mainly sugars, lignin, cellulose, and so forth. It contains cellulose (32.24%), hemicelluloses (21.34%), lignin (21.44%), and mineral ash (15.05%) as well as high percentage of silica in its mineral ash, which is approximately 96.34% [55, 56]. Rice husk is chemically stable, has high mechanical strength, and is insoluble in water which makes it one of the best adsorbents

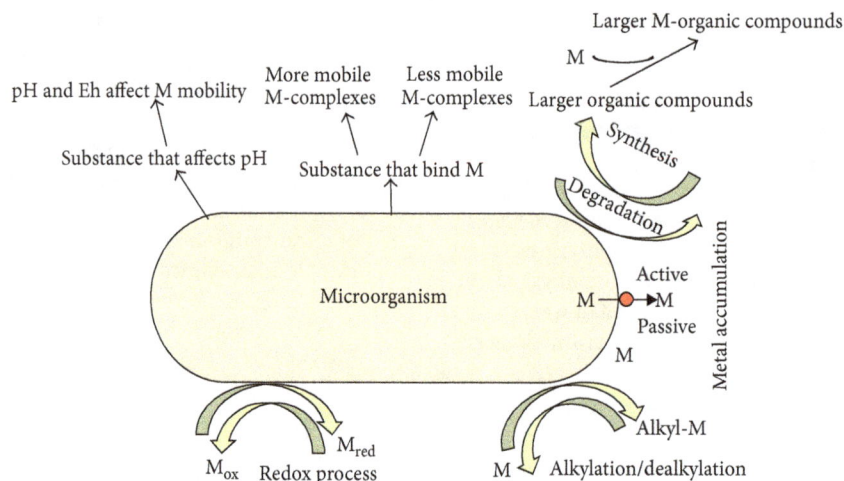

FIGURE 4: Metal accumulation process by microorganisms and its influence on metal mobility.

for heavy metal removal. The removal of heavy metals such as Cd, Pb, Zn, Cu, Co, Ni, and Au from rice husk was also studied [57]. Either modified or unmodified rice husk can be used for the treatment of heavy metals. Rice husk can be modified using hydrochloric acid or sodium carbonate [58] or by sodium hydroxide [59] or treated with epichlorohydrin [58]. Tartaric acid also can be used for modification [60, 61]. Pretreating rice husks helped in reducing cellulose crystallinity and rise in surface area or porosity and in removal of lignin and hemicelluloses by which adsorption capacity on heavy metals increased. Rice husk when treated with sodium carbonate and sodium carbonate or hydrochloric acid enhanced the cadmium adsorption capacity [58]. An adsorption site on the rice husk surface was protonated when it was treated with HCl and hence the heavy metals were left in the aqueous solution itself. The base soluble materials on rice husk were removed through NaOH treatment which also doubled the rate of cadmium adsorption (i.e., 7 mg/L) when compared to the rice husk adsorption of 4 mg/L. Some studies revealed that high reaction rate and improved cellulose hydrolysis can be achieved through pretreatment using dilute sulphuric acid [62]. Cellulose hydrolysis can be achieved through concentrated acids but they are corrosive and toxic, so they need to be recovered [63]. Another study showed the adsorption of copper and lead on rice husk modified using acids like citric acid, salicylic acid, tartaric acid, oxalic acid, mandelic acid, malic acid, and nitrilotriacetic acid [59]. Among these, rice husk heated with tartaric acid showed maximum adsorption. The effect of chelators on lead was also investigated which showed that when there was an increase in molar ratios of chelators like ethylenediaminetetraacetic acid and nitrilotriacetic acid there was a considerable raise in the adsorption of lead. Parameters like pH, initial concentration of adsorbent, particle size, and temperature affected the adsorption efficiency and it was found that modified rice husk had maximum capacity to adsorb copper and lead from aqueous solutions mainly when the pH was around 2-3 [60]. Rice husk treated with phosphate adsorbed maximum nickel and cadmium [64], whereas at a pH of 12, there was 90%

adsorption of chromium when rice husk carbon was used as adsorbent [65]. This was done by carbonizing rice husk with sulphuric acid and then activating it by CO_2 activation. 99% of hexavalent and 88% of total chromium were removed using this method. Rice husk showed 8.9 mg/g adsorption and commercial carbon showed 6.3 mg/g for chromium removal when column studies were done [66]. Another study using some of the dyes, Procion Red or Procion Yellow, showed that Procion Red dye treated rice husk removed 99.2% cadmium and 99.8% lead. Procion Yellow dye treated husk adsorbed 100% lead and 93.3% mercury. When waste water containing heavy metals was treated with rice husk it showed 79% chromium, 85% zinc, 80% copper, and 85% cadmium ions adsorption on the rice husk [67]. Another study with green algae as adsorbents resulted in 90% removal of heavy metals like Sr, Cd, Ni, Pb, Zn, Co, Cr, and As but could remove only 80% nickel [68]. Microporous and mesoporous activated carbon forms of rice husk were considered for the adsorption of chromium [69]. Rice husk was classified into two types and could be used as adsorbents on small waste water treatment plants and found adsorption about 100% for many heavy metals such as iron, manganese, zinc, copper, cadmium, and lead [70]. Raw rice husk was utilized for the removal of Cr(VI) and they concluded that an adsorbent dosage of 70 g/L for 2 hours at a pH 2 showed increase in the rate of adsorption and 66% of Cr(VI) was removed [71].

3.3. *Sugarcane Bagasse.* Sugar refining industry produces waste called bagasse pitch where the residual cane pulp is left over after sugar has been extracted. Cellulose, pentosan, and lignin are the components present in it [72]. The adsorption of cadmium and lead was studied on lignin obtained from sugarcane bagasse [73]. They found that ionic strength was inversely proportional to the adsorption capacity and reported that adsorption of lead followed Langmuir's model and temperature greater than 30°C worked best for cadmium removal. Lignin which was carboxymethylated had the ability to adsorb more amount of lead compared to cadmium. Temperature was found to be the most important as adsorption increased with increase in temperature. Single and multicomponent cadmium and zinc adsorption was done by using activated carbon prepared from bagasse [72], where a pH greater than 8 gave 100% adsorption of cadmium and zinc. 0.8 g/50 mL of adsorbent was necessary to remove 80%–100% of chromium at pH 1 but when they increased pH to 3, there was a decrease in adsorption efficacy by 15% [74]. According to another study the removal of hexavalent chromium from waste water using bagasse and coconut jute required low pH for maximum adsorption. Activated carbon obtained from jute had an adsorption efficiency of about 99.8% at pH 2. It was more stable at higher pH and hence it proved to be the most active adsorbent [75].

3.4. Fruit/Vegetable Waste.

The fruit/vegetable wastes like banana and orange peels were modified using acid and alkali solutions. The adsorption of $Cu2+$, $Zn2+$, $Co2+$, $Ni2+$, and $Pb2+$ onto the modified fruit/vegetable wastes was studied [76] Lead was adsorbed to the maximum and cobalt to the least. Banana showed an adsorption capacity of 7.97 ($Pb2+$), 6.88 ($Ni2+$), 5.80 ($Zn2+$), 4.75 ($Cu2+$), and 2.55 ($Co2+$) mg/L, when compared to orange peels which showed 7.75 ($Pb2+$), 6.01 ($Ni2+$), 5.25 ($Zn2+$), 3.65 ($Cu2+$), and 1.82 mg/L ($Co2+$). It was shown that adsorption capacity of acid treated peels was more efficient than alkali or water treated peels. NaOH and $Ca(OH)_2$ were used to regenerate the metal ions [77]. Saponified gels were prepared from orange peel constituents such as cellulose, hemicelluloses, pectin, limonene, and other lesser molecular weight compounds using $Ca(OH)_2$. Two different types of saponified gels were prepared using Ca^{+2} form and H^+ form and efficiency of both the saponified gels to remove heavy metals such as iron, lead, copper, zinc, cadmium, and manganese was analyzed. It was found that saponified gel prepared from Ca^{+2} can adsorb lead to the maximum compared to manganese and saponified gel prepared from H^+ can adsorb metals in the order of lead > iron > copper > zinc > manganese. Increase in pH increased the heavy metal adsorption. But in the case of Fe^{3+} it was not the same as it formed soluble complexes such as $Fe(OH)^+$, $Fe(OH)_2^+$, $Fe(OH)_2^{4+}$, and $Fe(OH)_4$ at pH 3. Significantly the study of both types of gels infers that they act as effective adsorbent in acidic solutions because of ion exchange mechanism. Acid treated fruit wastes such as cornelian cherry, apricot stone, and almond shell were able to adsorb maximum Cr(VI) at pH 1 [78]. They found out that the lower the concentration of metal ions, the higher the rate of adsorption. Their studies also concluded that cornelian cherry required an equilibrium time of 20 h when chromium concentration was 53 mg/L but when the concentration was increased to 203 mg/L the equilibrium time also rose to 70 h. $ZnCl_2$ treated olive stone showed maximum adsorption for cadmium and lead ions of about 85 mg/L [79], compared to untreated olive stone [80]. Citric acid treated orange peels showed maximum adsorption for cadmium. Cadmium adsorption increases due to the interaction between cellulose present in orange peels and citric acid as a result of the formation of ester linkage and introduction of carboxylic group [81]. Adsorption and recovery of cadmium from orange peels increase, when they are treated with acids of

high concentration [82]. Agricultural byproducts such as sugarcane, bagasse, peanut shells, macadamia, nut hulls, rice hulls, cottonseed hulls, corn cob, soybean hulls, almond shells, almond hulls, pecan shells, English walnut shells, and black walnut shells were also treated with citric acids to increase adsorption of copper [83]. All these byproducts were treated with NaOH and then with citric acid to increase adsorption of heavy metals. Among all the byproducts, citric acid treated soya bean hulls showed maximum adsorption for copper whereas English walnut shells and black walnut shells showed least adsorption as they are high density materials and lignin present in them blocks the reactive sites to citric acid resulting in minimum adsorption of copper. Another study reported that citric acid treated peanut shells showed maximum adsorption for metal ions such as copper, cadmium, nickel, zinc, and lead when compared to unmodified peanut shells. Peanut shells were treated with NaOH first and then with citric acid to obtain more active binding sites for metal adsorption. NaOH removes tannins and deesterifies which increases its capacity to adsorb metal ions. Vegetable wastes such as carrot residues were treated with HCl to eliminate the tannins, resins, reducing sugars, and colored materials which in turn increase its capacity to remove metal ions such as chromium, copper, and zinc [84]. Kinetic study revealed that 70% of metal ions were adsorbed within 10 min and maximum adsorption of chromium (45.09 mg/L), copper (32.74 mg/L), and zinc (29.61 mg/L) was seen at higher pH values of 4 for chromium and 5 for both zinc and copper ions.

3.5. Soya Bean Hulls, Cottonseed Hulls, Rice Bran, and Straw.

Soya beans were modified using citric acid and its adsorption efficiency for heavy metals. Copper ions were considered as typical metal ion for studying the adsorption of soybean hulls. 0.1 N NaOH was used to extract the hulls, and then it was modified at 120°C for 90 minutes using citric acid whose concentration ranged from 0.1 M to 1.2 M. Unmodified hulls showed an adsorption capacity of 0.39 m moles/g whereas citric acid modified hulls had an adsorption capacity of 0.68 to 2.44 m moles/g. Soya bean hulls when treated with NaOH and modified with 0.6 M citric acid could remove about 1.7 m moles of copper ions [85]. Reaction with citric acid showed an increase in carboxyl group on the hulls which in turn resulted in an increased uptake of copper ions. On the basis of dry weight, soya bean consisted of 109, 10.0, 36.4, 49.1, 676, 137, and <10 (mg/g) of protein, lipid ash, lignin, cellulose, hemicelluloses, and silica, respectively. Langmuir model was used to determine the adsorption efficiency. Soya bean and cottonseed hulls had higher adsorption efficacy when treated with NaOH and HCl when compared to water washed hulls [86]. When cotton seeds and soya bean hulls were heat treated they showed lower adsorption properties than water washed hulls. When the hulls were reprocessed after one adsorption/desorption cycle there was a decrease in adsorption capacity and so hulls were regarded as single use adsorbents.

3.6. Corncobs.

Corncobs were initially activated by high temperature carbonization but a certain study revealed that corncobs can also be activated by chemical methods using acids for copper adsorption [87]. Corncobs were treated with acids containing functional groups such as -OH, -COOH, and -COO at 150°C which reduced the pH from 5.2 to 2.7 and a maximum adsorption of copper (31.45 mg g/L) at a pH value of 4.5 was seen. The copper adsorption by corncobs decreased to 53%, 27%, and 19% in presence of interfering ions like Pb(II), Ca(II), and Zn(II), respectively. Hydrogen peroxide can be used to regenerate those acid treated corncobs and almost 90% of copper can be recovered. Corncob oxidation using nitric and citric acids showed significant areas for adsorption [88].

3.7. Tree Barks. Hydrochloric acid treated barks mainly sal (*Shorea robusta*), mango (*Mangifera indica*), and jackfruit (*Artocarpus integrifolia*) were used in removal of copper from aqueous solutions. Untreated barks had lesser capacity to chelate when compared to modified barks. The advantage of pretreating the barks was the overcome of those organic compounds which gave color to metal ion containing solution. Sal bark, mango, and jackfruit showed an adsorption capacity of 51.4 mg g/L, 42.6 mg g/L, and 17.4 mg g/L, respectively, for copper ions. Successful recovery of adsorbent can be obtained using HCl in higher concentration [89].

3.8. Neem Bark. It was found that *Azadirachta indica* bark (neem bark) has maximum adsorption capacity towards iron metal ions. The bark has different functional groups at the surface of adsorption site which makes it an efficient adsorbent for iron. Maximum adsorption was seen within 30 minutes of contact time and later the reaction slowed down as it approached to steady state. When neem and babool tree barks were kept in solution containing many metal ions, 80–90% of chromium, cadmium, and manganese were adsorbed within a contact period of 10 minutes at pH 2 [90]. The eucalyptus bark removed 99% of chromium(VI) and neem bark removed zinc metal ion within an equilibrium adsorption time of 35 minutes [91]. Due to less number of active adsorbent sites, the adsorption decreases as the contact time attains steady state and hence the removal of metal ions using neem bark acts as a low cost method for the treatment of toxic water containing iron metal ion [92].

3.9. Almond Shells. The ability of activated carbon prepared from almond shell to eradicate iron present in the synthetic solution proved that the ability of activated carbon to remove iron was very high. In this study the contact time was kept around 20 minutes and it was observed that there was an increase in iron uptake. Later when the contact time was increased above 20 minutes, there was no change in the percentage uptake of iron. Thus results indicated that 20 minutes was the optimum adsorption time for iron uptake. pH also showed its effect on iron adsorption. Adsorption of iron present in synthetic water onto almond shells increased as the pH increased from 1 to 9. But iron removal was found to be highest at a pH value of 5 for almond shells [93].

3.10. Peanut Shell. Peanut shell biomasses were used for the study of biosorption of chromium ions and copper ions from aqueous solutions. Biosorption was studied as a function of temperature, pH, and initial concentration of the biomass. Metals were studied separately for optimum sorption conditions. Different kinetic models were used to study the experimental data. These studies revealed that affinity of peanut shell towards Cu(II) and Cr(III) ions was very high. The adsorption capacity of copper and chromium was found to be 25.39 mg and 27.86 mg per gram of peanut shell biomass, respectively. These results proved that peanut shell can be used as an efficient low cost bioadsorbent for removing heavy metals in waste water. The effects of pH and cadmium concentration on adsorption were also analyzed. Results of batch experiments showed an adsorptive capacity of 87.72 mg/g for peanut shells. To study the adsorption equilibrium of peanut shells Langmuir isotherm model and Freundlich isotherm model were used [94].

3.11. Green Coconut Shell. Coconut shell is a byproduct which is composed of 35–45% and 23–43% of lignin and cellulose, respectively [95]. It acts as a strong potential adsorbent for metal ion adsorption and also cellulose contains carboxylic and phenolic acids which are polar functional groups which help in metal binding [96, 97]. At lower to higher range of metal concentrations (20–1000 mg/L), coconut shell has a capacity to adsorb cadmium ions. The study was concluded for the best adsorption of cadmium metal ion at a pH value of 7. The adsorption data for cadmium ion obtained was studied using isotherm models such as Freundlich and Langmuir adsorption models at 27°C.

3.12. Tamarind Pod Shells. Tamarind pod shells can be economically recycled for the treatment of water containing chromium metal ions. The shells were washed with distilled water in order to remove the dirt and other coloring substances by boiling the pod shells at 105°C. The rate of adsorption for different concentrations of Cr(VI) metal ions was done by varying the factors like agitation time, adsorbent dosage, and pH. The adsorption data was well fitted into Langmuir and Freundlich isotherm models. There was maximum adsorption of chromium onto the tamarind shells at pH 2 whereas the rate of adsorption decreased as the pH value increased. Equilibrium time for adsorption was considered using different concentrations of chromium metal ion solution and the time attained was about 60 minutes. Desorption of metal ion from shells was studied using acid and alkali solutions. Binding of metal ion to shells must be possibly by chemisorptions or ion exchange which was inferred during the desorption studies of metal ion [98].

3.13. Egg Shells. Egg shells act as a good adsorbent for the removal of toxic heavy metals. The waste egg shells were calcinated in the pretreatment process for effective adsorption of heavy metals. These calcined egg shells were used in the removal of heavy metals from waste water. There was 100% adsorption of cadmium and 99% adsorption of chromium for a contact time of about 10 minutes. Even natural egg shell can be used as adsorbent but it is more efficient for the removal of lead compared to cadmium and chromium. There was less adsorption of cadmium and chromium even when the contact time was increased to 60 min as the rate of reaction was slow for natural egg shell. Cadmium and chromium showed a rapid adsorption rate, when the pH was raised from 6.55 to 12.0 within the contact time of 20 s. Calcined egg shell can be used to treat heavy metals found in the electroplating waste water [99].

3.14. Silverleaf Nightshade. Silverleaf nightshade *(Solanum elaeagnifolium)* was used as a biosorbent by base modification using NaOH for the removal of metal ions such as lead, copper, nickel, cadmium, zinc, and chromium by means of batch experiments studies. The adsorption capability of silverleaf nightshade for lead, copper, nickel, cadmium, zinc, and chromium(III) was determined by considering the parameters such as pH, equilibrium time, and metal binding capacity. At pH 5 within a time period of 10 to 15 minutes and at pH 2 there was optimal adsorption of chromium(VI). When *Solanum elaeagnifolium* was base treated the concentrations of metal ions adsorbed were 20.6 mg/g, 13.1 mg/g, 6.5 mg/g, 18.9 mg/g, 7.0 mg/g, 208 mg/g, and 2.2 mg/g of lead(II), copper(II), nickel(II), cadmium(II), zinc(II), chromium(III), and chromium(VI), respectively. Metal ion recovery from the bioadsorbent was done by using hydrochloric acid. This indicates that silverleaf nightshade can be used in treating the waste water containing toxic metal ions and it is cost-effective when compared to other methods implied previously [100].

3.15. Banana Peel. Fruit wastes like banana peel were used as bioadsorbent. It was best suited for copper removal from waste water. The banana peels were cut, washed, dried, and then grounded into powder for using it as a bioadsorbent. Some of the parameters like particle size, pH, temperature, and agitation speed, and contact time were studied to check the efficiency of copper adsorption onto banana peel. A pH of 6 was found to be optimum for the removal of copper ions. The adsorption capacity was found to be 27.78 mg/g. Studies also showed that one gram of banana peel can remove 7.97 mg of lead ions at a pH of 5.5 [101].

3.16. Leca. Leca or light expanded clay aggregate was used to remove heavy metals. Lead and cadmium adsorption capability of light expanded clay aggregate at different pH, contact time, and adsorbent concentration was studied. The effluents from paint industry are rich in lead and cadmium so those effluents were considered to perform batch studies. The adsorption was analyzed by varying the amount of leca in the range of 1, 2, 3, 4, 5, 6, 7, 8, 9, and 10 g/L. The amount of lead adsorption was found to be 93.75% on 10 g/L of leca at a pH of 7 and that for cadmium at the same conditions was 89.7%. The experimental data agreed well with Freundlich adsorption isotherm and the appropriate contact time was 1 to 2 hours. Thus leca can be used as a low cost adsorbent for treatment of heavy metals especially lead and cadmium from industrial waste water [102].

3.17. Papaya Seeds. The current methods of removing heavy metals are very costly so there is need for low cost adsorbent for the removal of metals like copper ions present in the aqueous solutions. The effect of pH, mixing rate, contact time, and adsorbate concentration was analyzed using batch studies to examine the rate of adsorption of copper ions on papaya seeds. The adsorption kinetic data were estimated by second-order and pseudo-first-order kinetics and the data fitted Langmuir and Freundlich isotherms very well. The maximum rate of adsorption of copper was seen when the pH was maintained at 6 and solution stirred at 350 rpm. 212 mg/g was the adsorption capacity of the papaya seeds. Chemisorptions process was denoted as the rate limiting step in the process of adsorption and it was found out by using the pseudo-second-order kinetic model as the data correlated well with this model. Finally these studies proved that papaya seed can be used as an effective adsorbent for the removal of heavy metals such as copper ions, from waste water [103].

3.18. Black Tea Waste. Studies showed that black tea waste can be used to remove heavy metals like zinc, cadmium, and cobalt from waste water. When the contact time was 180 minutes all the three metals were adsorbed. The adsorption capacity of heavy metals on tea waste mainly depends on the pH. An optimum pH of 6 is chosen for maximum adsorption of cobalt, cadmium, and zinc. Around 13.77 mg/g of Cd, 15.39 mg/g of Co, and 12.24 mg/g of Zn were adsorbed when only half gram of black tea waste was used. Experimental data fits well with the Freundlich and Langmuir isotherms. Hence tea waste can be used as one of the best and efficient adsorbents for waste water treatment [104].

3.19. Coffee Residues. The spent coffee grounds produced by instant coffee industry as a waste can be economically reused for the adsorption of toxic metal ions like copper, zinc, cadmium, and lead. The study was conducted with the aid of batch adsorption method in order to study the effect of parameters such as pH, metal ion concentration, adsorbent concentration, and temperature on metal adsorption. The best suited isotherm model was Langmuir adsorption isotherm in which the data was well fitted. Adsorption of metal ions to coffee residues was disturbed by flocculation at the adsorption site due to high density. So the formation of solid flocculent was treated by dispersant which showed increase in the maximum adsorption of metal ions. Using dilute acid solution the adsorption property was well maintained from the loss of change in the sites in column adsorption studies. It was reported that coffee grounds could remove the metal ions at the level of μgL^{-1}. Using potentiometric titration the acid base chemistry and stoichiometry of H^+ ion were studied for tea leaves and coffee grounds. Hence the study concluded that tea and coffee residues can be used to remove trace metal ions from water [105]. Table 1 shows the specific metal adsorption capacity of various agricultural wastes where several authors evaluated the adsorption efficiency for various heavy metals by using different isotherm models which shows the interaction pattern between the adsorbate and adsorbent. An increase in temperature led to a decrease in the amount of metal adsorbed, regardless of the residue employed for adsorption process. The activation procedure was the same for many adsorbents but the coir fibers showed higher adsorption capacity (263 mg/g), followed by

TABLE 1: Comparison of adsorption capacity of various agricultural wastes.

Agricultural waste	Metal	Adsorption capacity (mg/g)	Reference
Wheat bran	Pb	69–87	[11]
Rice bran	Cu	27.81	[12]
Black gram husk	Pb, Cd, Zn, Cu, Ni	19.56–49.97	[13]
Dal husk	Cr(VI), Fe(III)	96.05, 66.63	[14]
Coffee waste	Pb	63	[15]
Exhausted coffee	Cr(VI)	1.42	[16]
Coffee husk	Cu	7.5	[17]
Tea residue	Cu/Pb	48–65	[18]
Almond shell	Pb	8.08, 28.18	[19]
Nut shell	Cr(VI)	1.47	[16]
Walnut shell	Cr(VI)	1.33	[16]
Chestnut shell	Cu	12.56	[20]
Peanut shell	Cu	21.25	[21]
Peanut hull	Cu/Pb	0.18, 0.21	[22]
Mango peel	Cu	46.09	[23]
Grape bagasse	Pb	0.428	[24]
Barley straw	Cu/Pb	4.64, 23.2	[19]
Saw dust	Cr(VI)	10.01, 16.05	[25, 26]
Coir fibers	Pb	263	[27]
Pumpkin waste	Cr(VI), Pb	68	[28]
Sugar beet pulp	Cu	31.4	[29]
Pea waste	Cr(VI)	21.2	[30]

dal husk (96.05 mg/g), wheat bran (69 mg/g), pumpkin waste (68 mg/g), and coffee waste (63 mg/g). The least adsorption was shown by peanut hull (0.18–0.21 mg/g), grape bagasse (0.428 mg/g), walnut shell (1.33 mg/g), nut shell (1.47 mg/g), and exhausted coffee (1.42 mg/g). The surface area of any adsorbent is the deciding factor for its efficiency; that is, the higher the surface area, the higher the adsorption.

3.20. Sawdust. Studies were carried out on adsorption of chromium from the electroplating waste water [48]. Phosphate treated saw dust showed an increased adsorption of chromium when compared to the unmodified one. Ajmal et al., 1996, also reported that the adsorption of chromium depends on pH. A pH value of 2 and less than that was shown to be optimum for maximum removal of chromium from aqueous solution. Synthetic waste water and electroplating waste water containing about 50 mg/L of chromium were used in column process as well as in batch studies and these adsorbents showed 100% adsorption of chromium. 0.01 M NaOH was used to recover chromium ions. Activated carbon prepared from coconut tree saw dust was used to study the removal of chromium from aqueous solution through batch experiments [106]. Initial Cr(VI) concentration, carbon concentration, agitation time, and pH were the factors considered to study the adsorption process and the data was modeled using Langmuir and Freundlich adsorption isotherms. At an initial pH of 3.0 the adsorption capacity of the adsorbents with a particle size 125–250 μm was found to be 3.46 mg/g using Langmuir isotherm. Acidic pH was optimum for maximum heavy metal removal [107].

Low cost adsorbents such as those discussed above are strongly recommended in industries for waste water treatment applications due to their local obtainability, technical viability, and engineering applicability. But before fermentation, acid-hydrolyzation of the agricultural wastes is done by breaking down the cellulose and lignin to produce bioethanol using microbes. If acid-hydrolysis is not done, it can result in lower yield. Other methods by which the biowastes could be treated are vacuum distillation, hydrotreatment, solvent extraction, thin film evaporation, and so forth. The contaminants can also be removed by using the right combination of heat and pressure at ambient conditions. In composting, enormous amount of readily organic matter which can be easily degraded is added to a contaminant that is further tailed by an aerobic incubation at a temperature ranging from 20 to 60°C. This becomes slightly labour intensive as the carbon and nitrogen ratios need to be adjusted frequently. This helps in converting the waste organic matter of used leaves, shells, husks, and peels to useful soil modifications by employing aerobic and anaerobic microbes which promotes the growth of certain bacteria, fungi, and actinomycetes. Land farming is another alternative method where the contaminated agricultural wastes or soil can be spread on fields to plow and fertilize the agricultural land which can be later redeveloped cost-effectively by planting heavy metal tolerant weeds and by using certain phytochelators. Heavy metals can also be precipitated as sulfates, carbonates, or hydroxide sulfides from the waste soil and water. Bioventing on the other hand promotes *in situ* biodegradation of biodegradable pollutants. This can also help in cleaning up of aquifers that are contaminated by solvents such as trichloroethylene which can be degraded only by cometabolic processes using enzymes. But some approaches can be costly which can be managed well by development of protein hydrolysates and by using activated carbon along with the agricultural wastes. The latest development in the green technology is biosorption of heavy metals by nonliving biomass of aquatic plant species such as *Hydrilla verticillata, Salvinia herzogii, Potamogeton lucens, Eichhornia crassipes, Ceratophyllum demersum*, and *Ludwigia stolonifera*. Another method employs microbes from the same site of pollution to accumulate heavy metals. These metals act as feed which is taken up for the microbial growth, metabolism, and living. The microbes release these heavy metals after a long time, but in a very lower concentration when compared to what they had initially absorbed. This process is known as bioaccumulation. The absorption of the toxic substances such as a metal is at a rate faster than that at which the substance is lost by catabolism and excretion. Other biological treatments using mixed microbial cultures and white rot fungi for decolorization of dyes are also common [108–111].

4. Conclusion

The existing technologies for waste water treatment have major problems such as costs involved in the construction of waste water treatment plants which are high; that is, they are uneconomical, consume lot of space, are commercially unattractive, and have disposal problems. Reports suggest that there is a bulk production of chemicals from various waste water treatment plants and requirement for a high electrical energy input. Handling of the dry sludge also becomes difficult and as well nature capacity to treat water remains unutilized. So there was a need for some alternative method which can overcome all these problems and treat the waste water in an appropriate way. Thus making use of bioadsorbents is an effective method to adsorb toxic heavy metals from effluents not polluting the ground water and at the same time utilizing the discarded open waste in the environment for a useful purpose of waste water treatment. This method not only requires minimal energy input, less labour, and low investment, but also proves to be cost-effective, but additional information about the pore size distribution of adsorbent, molecular size of metal ions, functional groups present on surface of adsorbent, initial pH, temperature, particle size of adsorbent, and so forth are critical details which influence the efficiency of adsorption processes. Several waste reduction programs should be held to reuse and recycle the wastes with an aim of zero waste production.

Disclosure

The manuscript has been prepared by the consent of coauthors.

Competing Interests

The authors would like to declare that there is no conflict of interests for publication of this article.

Acknowledgments

The authors are grateful to the Department of Biotechnology, Sapthagiri College of Engineering, Bangalore, for providing all lab facilities.

References

[1] K. Kümmerer, "The presence of pharmaceuticals in the environment due to human use—present knowledge and future challenges," *Journal of Environmental Management*, vol. 90, no. 8, pp. 2354–2366, 2009.

[2] M. Jaishankar, T. Tseten, N. Anbalagan, B. B. Mathew, and K. N. Beeregowda, "Toxicity, mechanism and health effects of some heavy metals," *Interdisciplinary Toxicology*, vol. 7, no. 2, pp. 60–72, 2014.

[3] J. Wang and C. Chen, "Biosorption of heavy metals by *Saccharomyces cerevisiae*: a review," *Biotechnology Advances*, vol. 24, no. 5, pp. 427–451, 2006.

[4] B. B. Mathew, A. Tiwari, and S. K. Jatawa, "Free radicals and antioxidants: a review," *Journal of Pharmacy Research*, vol. 4, no. 12, 2011.

[5] G. M. Gadd, "Interactions of fungi with toxic metals," *New Phytologist*, vol. 124, no. 1, pp. 25–60, 1993.

[6] B. Volesky, "Detoxification of metal-bearing effluents: biosorption for the next century," *Hydrometallurgy*, vol. 59, no. 2-3, pp. 203–216, 2001.

[7] B. Volesky and Z. R. Holan, "Biosorption of heavy metals," *Biotechnology Progress*, vol. 11, no. 3, pp. 235–250, 1995.

[8] M. Jaishankar, B. B. Mathew, M. S. Shah, T. P. Krishnamurthy, and S. K. R. Gowda, "Biosorption of few heavy metal ions using agricultural wastes," *Journal of Environment Pollution and Human Health*, vol. 2, no. 1, pp. 1–6, 2014.

[9] S. E. Bailey, T. J. Olin, R. M. Bricka, and D. D. Adrian, "A review of potentially low-cost sorbents for heavy metals," *Water Research*, vol. 33, no. 11, pp. 2469–2479, 1999.

[10] N. Gaur, G. Flora, M. Yadav, and A. Tiwari, "A review with recent advancements on bioremediation-based abolition of heavy metals," *Environmental Science: Processes & Impacts*, vol. 16, no. 2, pp. 180–193, 2014.

[11] Y. Bulut and Z. Baysal, "Removal of Pb(II) from wastewater using wheat bran," *Journal of Environmental Management*, vol. 78, no. 2, pp. 107–113, 2006.

[12] X. S. Wang and J. P. Chen, "Biosorption of Congo red from aqueous solution using wheat bran and rice bran: batch studies," *Separation Science and Technology*, vol. 44, no. 6, pp. 1452–1466, 2009.

[13] A. Saeed, M. Iqbal, and M. W. Akhtar, "Application of biowaste materials for the sorption of heavy metals in contaminated aqueous medium," *Pakistan Journal of Scientific and Industrial Research*, vol. 45, no. 3, pp. 206–211, 2002.

[14] V. R. Parate and M. I. Talib, "Study of metal adsorbent prepared from tur dal (Cajanuscajan) husk: a value addition to agrowaste , iosr journal of environmental science," *IOSR Journal of Environmental Science, Toxicology and Food Technology*, vol. 8, no. 9, pp. 43–54, 2014.

[15] F. Boudrahem, F. Aissani-Benissad, and H. Aït-Amar, "Batch sorption dynamics and equilibrium for the removal of lead ions from aqueous phase using activated carbon developed from coffee residue activated with zinc chloride," *Journal of Environmental Management*, vol. 90, no. 10, pp. 3031–3039, 2009.

[16] Y. Orhan and H. Büyükgüngör, "The removal of heavy metals by using agricultural wastes," *Water Science & Technology*, vol. 28, no. 2, pp. 247–255, 1993.

[17] W. E. Oliveira, A. S. Franca, L. S. Oliveira, and S. D. Rocha, "Untreated coffee husks as biosorbents for the removal of heavy metals from aqueous solutions," *Journal of Hazardous Materials*, vol. 152, no. 3, pp. 1073–1081, 2008.

[18] B. M. W. P. K. Amarasinghe and R. A. Williams, "Tea waste as a low cost adsorbent for the removal of Cu and Pb from wastewater," *Chemical Engineering Journal*, vol. 132, no. 1-3, pp. 299–309, 2007.

[19] E. Pehlivan, T. Altun, S. Cetin, and M. I. Bhanger, "Lead sorption by waste biomass of hazelnut and almond shell," *Journal of Hazardous Materials*, vol. 167, no. 1-3, pp. 1203–1208, 2009.

[20] Z.-Y. Yao, J.-H. Qi, and L.-H. Wang, "Equilibrium, kinetic and thermodynamic studies on the biosorption of Cu(II) onto chestnut shell," *Journal of Hazardous Materials*, vol. 174, no. 1-3, pp. 137–143, 2010.

[21] C.-S. Zhu, L.-P. Wang, and W.-B. Chen, "Removal of Cu(II) from aqueous solution by agricultural by-product: peanut hull," *Journal of Hazardous Materials*, vol. 168, no. 2-3, pp. 739–746, 2009.

[22] F. D. Oliveira, A. C. Soares, O. M. Freitas, and S. A. Figueiredo, "Copper, nickel and zinc removal by peanut hulls: Batch and column studies in mono, tri-component systems and with real effluent," *Global Nest Journal*, vol. 12, no. 2, pp. 206–214, 2010.

[23] M. Iqbal, A. Saeed, and I. Kalim, "Characterization of adsorptive capacity and investigation of mechanism of Cu2+, Ni2+ and Zn2+ adsorption on mango peel waste from constituted metal solution and genuine electroplating effluent," *Separation Science and Technology*, vol. 44, no. 15, pp. 3770–3791, 2009.

[24] N. V. Farinella, G. D. Matos, and M. A. Z. Arruda, "Grape bagasse as a potential biosorbent of metals in effluent treatments," *Bioresource Technology*, vol. 98, no. 10, pp. 1940–1946, 2007.

[25] P. S. Bryant, J. N. Petersen, J. M. Lee, and T. M. Brouns, "Sorption of heavy metals by untreated red fir sawdust," *Applied Biochemistry and Biotechnology*, vol. 34-35, no. 1, pp. 777–788, 1992.

[26] V. P. Dikshit, "Removal of chromium (VI) by adsorption using sawdust," *National Academy Science Letters-India*, vol. 12, no. 12, pp. 419–421, 1989.

[27] K. Kadirvelu and C. Namasivayam, "Agricultural by-product as metal adsorbent: sorption of lead(II) from aqueous solution onto coirpith carbon," *Environmental Technology*, vol. 21, no. 10, pp. 1091–1097, 2000.

[28] A. I. Okoye, P. M. Ejikeme, and O. D. Onukwuli, "Lead removal from wastewater using fluted pumpkin seed shell activated carbon: adsorption modeling and kinetics," *International Journal of Environmental Science & Technology*, vol. 7, no. 4, pp. 793–800, 2010.

[29] Z. Aksu and İ. A. İşoğlu, "Removal of copper(II) ions from aqueous solution by biosorption onto agricultural waste sugar beet pulp," *Process Biochemistry*, vol. 40, no. 9, pp. 3031–3044, 2005.

[30] J. Anwar, U. Shafique, Waheed-uz-Zaman et al., "Removal of chromium from water using pea waste—a green approach," *Green Chemistry Letters and Reviews*, vol. 3, no. 3, pp. 239–243, 2010.

[31] B.-C. Pan, H. Qiu, L. V. Lu, Q.-J. Zhang, Q.-X. Zhang, and W.-M. Zhang, "Critical review in adsorption kinetic models," *Journal of Zhejiang University Science A*, vol. 10, pp. 716–724, 2009.

[32] A. Mishra and B. D. Tripathi, "Utilization of fly ash in adsorption of heavy metals from wastewater," *Toxicological and Environmental Chemistry*, vol. 90, no. 6, pp. 1091–1097, 2008.

[33] M. F. De Boodt, "Application of the sorption theory to eliminate heavy metals from waste waters and contamined soils. In interaction at the soil colloid- soil solutions interface," in *Interactions at the Soil Colloid—Soil Solution Interface*, G. H. Bolt, M. F. De Boodt, M. H. B. Hayes, and M. B. McBride, Eds., vol. 190 of *NATO ASI Series E: Applied Sciences*, pp. 293–320, Springer, Berlin, Germany, 1991.

[34] J. P. Fraissard, *Physical Adsorption: Experiment, Theory, and Applications*, vol. 491, Springer Science & Business Media, Berlin, Germany, 1997.

[35] B. M. W. Trapnell and D. O. Hayward, *Chemisorption*, Butterworths, Oxford, UK, 1964.

[36] C. Appel and L. Ma, "Heavy metals in the environment concentration, pH and surface charge effects on Cd and Pb sorption in three tropical soils," *Journal of Environmental Quality*, vol. 21, pp. 581–589, 2002.

[37] J. Van Staden and W. A. Stirk, "Removal of heavy metals from solution using dried brown seaweed material," *Botanica Marina*, vol. 43, no. 5, pp. 467–473, 2000.

[38] M. Horsfall and A. I. Spiff, "Studies on the Effect of pH on the Sorption of Pb^{2+} and Cd^{2+} ions from aqueous Solutions by *Caladium bicolor* (Wild cocoyam) Biomass," *Electronic Journal of Biotechnology*, vol. 7, no. 3, pp. 313–323, 2004.

[39] M. Ulmanu, E. Marañón, Y. Fernández, L. Castrillón, I. Anger, and D. Dumitriu, "Removal of copper and cadmium ions from diluted aqueous solutions by low cost and waste material adsorbents," *Water, Air, and Soil Pollution*, vol. 142, no. 1–4, pp. 357–373, 2003.

[40] G. Prasad, K. K. Pandey, and V. N. Singh, "Mixed adsorbents for Cu(II) removal from aqueous solutions," *Environmental Technology Letters*, vol. 7, no. 1-12, pp. 547–554, 1986.

[41] L. Addour, D. Belhocine, N. Boudries, Y. Comeau, A. Pauss, and N. Mameri, "Zinc uptake by *Streptomyces rimosus* biomass using a packed-bed column," *Journal of Chemical Technology and Biotechnology*, vol. 74, no. 11, pp. 1089–1095, 1999.

[42] S. Al-Asheh and Z. Duvnjak, "Sorption of heavy metals by canola meal," *Water, Air, and Soil Pollution*, vol. 114, no. 3-4, pp. 251–276, 1999.

[43] S. Klimmek, H.-J. Stan, A. Wilke, G. Bunke, and R. Buchholz, "Comparative analysis of the biosorption of cadmium, lead, nickel, and zinc by algae," *Environmental Science & Technology*, vol. 35, no. 21, pp. 4283–4288, 2001.

[44] M. Ledin and K. Pedersen, "The environmental impact of mine wastes—roles of microorganisms and their significance in treatment of mine wastes," *Earth-Science Reviews*, vol. 41, no. 1, pp. 67–108, 1996.

[45] R. W. Henderson, D. S. Andrews, G. R. Lightsey, and N. A. Poonawala, "Reduction of mercury, copper, nickel, cadmium, and zinc levels in solution by competitive adsorption onto peanut hulls, and raw and aged bark," *Bulletin of Environmental Contamination and Toxicology*, vol. 17, no. 3, pp. 355–359, 1977.

[46] M. Friedman and A. C. Waiss Jr., "Mercury uptake by selected agricultural products and by-products," *Environmental Science and Technology*, vol. 6, no. 5, pp. 457–458, 1972.

[47] J. M. Randall, V. Garrett, R. L. Bermann, and A. C. Waiss Jr., "Use of bark to remove heavy metal ions from waste solutions," *Forest Products Journal*, vol. 24, no. 9, pp. 80–84, 1974.

[48] M. Ajmal, R. A. K. Rao, and R. Ahmad, "Adsorption studies of heavy metals on tectona grandis: removal and recovery of Zn (II) from electroplating wastes," *Journal of Dispersion Science and Technology*, vol. 32, no. 6, pp. 851–856, 2011.

[49] G. McKay, M. S. Otterburn, and A. G. Sweeney, "Kinetics of colour removal from effluent using activated carbon," *Journal of the Society of Dyers and Colourists*, vol. 96, no. 11, pp. 576–579, 1980.

[50] D. Kratochvil and B. Volesky, "Advances in the biosorption of heavy metals," *Trends in Biotechnology*, vol. 16, no. 7, pp. 291–300, 1998.

[51] F. Veglio' and F. Beolchini, "Removal of metals by biosorption: a review," *Hydrometallurgy*, vol. 44, no. 3, pp. 301–316, 1997.

[52] K. Vijayaraghavan and Y.-S. Yun, "Bacterial biosorbents and biosorption," *Biotechnology Advances*, vol. 26, no. 3, pp. 266–291, 2008.

[53] A. Özer, D. Özer, and A. Özer, "The adsorption of copper(II) ions on to dehydrated wheat bran (DWB): determination of the equilibrium and thermodynamic parameters," *Process Biochemistry*, vol. 39, no. 12, pp. 2183–2191, 2004.

[54] A. Özer and H. B. Pirinçci, "The adsorption of Cd(II) ions on sulphuric acid-treated wheat bran," *Journal of Hazardous Materials*, vol. 137, no. 2, pp. 849–855, 2006.

[55] I. A. Rahman, J. Ismail, and H. Osman, "Effect of nitric acid digestion on organic materials and silica in rice husk," *Journal of Materials Chemistry*, vol. 7, no. 8, pp. 1505–1509, 1997.

[56] I. A. Rahman and J. Ismail, "Preparation and characterization of a spherical gel from a low-cost material," *Journal of Materials Chemistry*, vol. 3, no. 9, pp. 931–934, 1993.

[57] T. G. Chuah, A. Jumasiah, I. Azni, S. Katayon, and S. Y. T. Choong, "Rice husk as a potentially low-cost biosorbent for heavy metal and dye removal: an overview," *Desalination*, vol. 175, no. 3, pp. 305–316, 2005.

[58] U. Kumar and M. Bandyopadhyay, "Sorption of cadmium from aqueous solution using pretreated rice husk," *Bioresource Technology*, vol. 97, no. 1, pp. 104–109, 2006.

[59] Y. Gou, S. Yang, W. Fu et al., "Adsorption of malachite green on micro- and mesoporous rice husk-based active carbon," *Dyes and Pigments*, vol. 56, no. 3, pp. 219–229, 2003.

[60] K. K. Wong, C. K. Lee, K. S. Low, and M. J. Haron, "Removal of Cu and Pb by tartaric acid modified rice husk from aqueous solutions," *Chemosphere*, vol. 50, no. 1, pp. 23–28, 2003.

[61] K. K. Wong, C. K. Lee, K. S. Low, and M. J. Haron, "Removal of Cu and Pb from electroplating wastewater using tartaric acid modified rice husk," *Process Biochemistry*, vol. 39, no. 4, pp. 437–445, 2003.

[62] A. Esteghlalian, A. G. Hashimoto, J. J. Fenske, and M. H. Penner, "Modeling and optimization of the dilute-sulfuric-acid pretreatment of corn stover, poplar and switchgrass," *Bioresource Technology*, vol. 59, no. 2-3, pp. 129–136, 1997.

[63] M. von Sivers and G. Zacchi, "A techno-economical comparison of three processes for the production of ethanol from pine," *Bioresource Technology*, vol. 51, no. 1, pp. 43–52, 1995.

[64] M. Ajmal, R. A. K. Rao, S. Anwar, J. Ahmad, and R. Ahmad, "Adsorption studies on rice husk: removal and recovery of Cd(II) from wastewater," *Bioresource Technology*, vol. 86, no. 2, pp. 147–149, 2003.

[65] N. Balasubramanian, T. V. Ramakrishna, and K. Srinivasan, "Studies on chromium removal by rice husk carbon," *Indian Journal of Environmental Health*, vol. 30, no. 4, pp. 376–387, 1988.

[66] R. Suemitsu, R. Uenishi, I. Akashi, and M. Nakano, "The use of dyestuff-treated rice hulls for removal of heavy metals from waste water," *Journal of Applied Polymer Science*, vol. 31, no. 1, pp. 75–83, 1986.

[67] E. Munaf and R. Zein, "The use of rice husk for removal of toxic metals from waste water," *Environmental Technology*, vol. 18, no. 3, pp. 359–362, 1997.

[68] D. Roy, P. N. Greenlaw, and B. S. Shane, "Adsorption of heavy metals by green algae and ground rice hulls," *Journal of Environmental Science And Health—Part A: Environmental Science And Engineering And Toxicology*, vol. 28, no. 1, pp. 37–50, 1993.

[69] Y. Guo, J. Qi, S. Yang, K. Yu, Z. Wang, and H. Xu, "Adsorption of Cr(VI) on micro- and mesoporous rice husk-based active carbon," *Materials Chemistry and Physics*, vol. 78, no. 1, pp. 132–137, 2003.

[70] A. A. M. Daifullah, B. S. Girgis, and H. M. H. Gad, "Utilization of agro-residues (rice husk) in small waste water treatment plans," *Materials Letters*, vol. 57, no. 11, pp. 1723–1731, 2003.

[71] S. Ibrahim, N. A. Khan, and P. Subramaniam, "Rice husk as an adsorbent for heavy metal," in *Proceedings of the International Conference on Water and Wastewater (Asia Water)*, Kuala Lumpur, Malaysia, 2004.

[72] D. Mohan and K. P. Singh, "Single- and multi-component adsorption of cadmium and zinc using activated carbon derived from bagasse—an agricultural waste," *Water Research*, vol. 36, no. 9, pp. 2304–2318, 2002.

[73] W. S. Peternele, A. A. Winkler-Hechenleitner, and E. A. G. Pineda, "Adsorption of Cd(II) and Pb(II) onto functionalized formic lignin from sugar cane bagasse," *Bioresource Technology*, vol. 68, no. 1, pp. 95–100, 1999.

[74] I. Ali, M. Asim, and T. A. Khan, "Low cost adsorbents for the removal of organic pollutants from wastewater," *Journal of Environmental Management*, vol. 113, pp. 170–183, 2012.

[75] V. K. Aggarwal, S. Chand, and P. Kumar, "Removal of Hexavalent Chromium from the Wastewater by Adsorption," *Indian Journal of Environmental Health*, vol. 36, no. 3, pp. 151–158, 1994.

[76] G. Annadurai, R. S. Juang, and D. J. Lee, "Adsorption of heavy metals from water using banana and orange peels," *Water Science and Technology*, vol. 47, no. 1, pp. 185–190, 2003.

[77] R. P. Dhakal, K. N. Ghimire, and K. Inoue, "Adsorptive separation of heavy metals from an aquatic environment using orange waste," *Hydrometallurgy*, vol. 79, no. 3-4, pp. 182–190, 2005.

[78] E. Demirbas, M. Kobya, E. Senturk, and T. Ozkan, "Adsorption kinetics for the removal of chromium (VI) from aqueous solutions on the activated carbons prepared from agricultural wastes," *Water SA*, vol. 30, no. 4, pp. 533–539, 2004.

[79] M.-R. Huang, Q.-Y. Peng, and X.-G. Li, "Rapid and effective adsorption of lead ions on fine poly(phenylenediamine) microparticles," *Chemistry—A European Journal*, vol. 12, no. 16, pp. 4341–4350, 2006.

[80] I. Kula, M. Uğurlu, H. Karaoğlu, and A. Çelik, "Adsorption of Cd(II) ions from aqueous solutions using activated carbon prepared from olive stone by $ZnCl_2$ activation," *Bioresource Technology*, vol. 99, no. 3, pp. 492–501, 2008.

[81] W. E. Marshall, L. H. Wartelle, D. E. Boler, M. M. Johns, and C. A. Toles, "Enhanced metal adsorption by soybean hulls modified with citric acid," *Bioresource Technology*, vol. 69, no. 3, pp. 263–268, 1999.

[82] A. B. Pérez-Marín, V. M. Zapata, J. F. Ortuño, M. Aguilar, J. Sáez, and M. Lloréns, "Removal of cadmium from aqueous solutions

by adsorption onto orange waste," *Journal of Hazardous Materials*, vol. 139, no. 1, pp. 122–131, 2007.

[83] L. H. Wartelle and W. E. Marshall, "Citric acid modified agricultural by-products as copper ion adsorbents," *Advances in Environmental Research*, vol. 4, no. 1, pp. 1–7, 2000.

[84] B. Nasernejad, T. E. Zadeh, B. B. Pour, M. E. Bygi, and A. Zamani, "Camparison for biosorption modeling of heavy metals (Cr (III), Cu (II), Zn (II)) adsorption from wastewater by carrot residues," *Process Biochemistry*, vol. 40, no. 3-4, pp. 1319–1322, 2005.

[85] W. E. Marshall, L. H. Wartelle, D. E. Boler, M. M. Johns, and C. A. Toles, "Enhanced metal adsorption by soybean hulls modified with citric acid," *Bioresource Technology*, vol. 69, no. 3, pp. 263–268, 1999.

[86] W. E. Marshall and M. M. Johns, "Agricultural by-products as metal adsorbents: sorption properties and resistance to mechanical abrasion," *Journal of Chemical Technology and Biotechnology*, vol. 66, no. 2, pp. 192–198, 1996.

[87] M. Nasiruddin Khan and M. Farooq Wahab, "Characterization of chemically modified corncobs and its application in the removal of metal ions from aqueous solution," *Journal of Hazardous Materials*, vol. 141, no. 1, pp. 237–244, 2007.

[88] R. Leyva-Ramos, L. A. Bernal-Jacome, and I. Acosta-Rodriguez, "Adsorption of cadmium(II) from aqueous solution on natural and oxidized corncob," *Separation and Purification Technology*, vol. 45, no. 1, pp. 41–49, 2005.

[89] B. R. Reddy, N. Mirghaffari, and I. Gaballah, "Removal and recycling of copper from aqueous solutions using treated Indian barks," *Resources, Conservation and Recycling*, vol. 21, no. 4, pp. 227–245, 1997.

[90] V. P. Kudesia, *Water Pollution*, Pragati Prakashan Meerut, Meerut, India, 1980.

[91] V. Sarin and K. K. Pant, "Removal of chromium from industrial waste by using eucalyptus bark," *Bioresource Technology*, vol. 97, no. 1, pp. 15–20, 2006.

[92] N. Kannan and T. Veemaraj, "Kinetics of adsorption for the removal of zinc (II) ions from aqueous solution using indigenously prepared jack fruit seed and commercial activated carbons," *Indian Journal of Environmental Protection*, vol. 30, no. 5, pp. 366–373, 2010.

[93] G. Anusha, "Removal of iron from waste water using bael fruit," *International Proceedings of Chemical, Biological & Environmental Engineering*, vol. 6, pp. 258–260, 2011.

[94] A. Witek-Krowiak, R. G. Szafran, and S. Modelski, "Biosorption of heavy metals from aqueous solutions onto peanut shell as a low-cost biosorbent," *Desalination*, vol. 265, no. 1-3, pp. 126–134, 2011.

[95] O. A. Carrijo, R. S. Liz, and N. Makishima, "Fiber of green coconut shell as agricultural substratum," *Brazilian Horticulture*, vol. 20, pp. 533–535, 2002.

[96] J. T. Matheickal, Q. Yu, and G. M. Woodburn, "Biosorption of cadmium(II) from aqueous solutions by pre-treated biomass of marine alga *DurvillAea potatorum*," *Water Research*, vol. 33, no. 2, pp. 335–342, 1999.

[97] G. H. Pino, L. M. Souza De Mesquita, M. L. Torem, and G. A. S. Pinto, "Biosorption of cadmium by green coconut shell powder," *Minerals Engineering*, vol. 19, no. 5, pp. 380–387, 2006.

[98] N. Ahalya, R. D. Kanamadi, and T. V. Ramachandra, "Biosorption of Chromium (VI) by Tamarindus indica pod shells," *Journal of Environmental Science Research International*, vol. 1, pp. 77–81, 2008.

[99] H. J. Park, S. W. Jeong, J. K. Yang, B. G. Kim, and S. M. Lee, "Removal of heavy metals using waste eggshell," *Journal of Environmental Sciences*, vol. 19, no. 12, pp. 1436–1441, 2007.

[100] T. H. Baig, A. E. Garcia, K. J. Tiemann, and Gardea-Torresdey, "Adsorption of heavy metal ions by the biomass of Solanum Elaeagnifolium (silverleaf night shade)," in *Proceedings of the Conference on Hazardous Waste Research*, pp. 131–142, 1999.

[101] G. Annadurai, H. S. Juang, and D. J. Lee, "Adsorption of heavy metal from water using banana and orange peels," *Water Science and Technology*, vol. 47, pp. 185–190, 2002.

[102] M. Malakootian, J. Nouri, and H. Hossaini, "Removal of heavy metals from paint industry's wastewater using Leca as an available adsorbent," *International Journal of Environmental Science and Technology*, vol. 6, no. 2, pp. 183–190, 2009.

[103] Z. A. Zakaria, E. E. Abdul Hisam, M. S. Rofiee et al., "*In vivo* antiulcer activity of the aqueous extract of *Bauhinia purpurea* leaf," *Journal of Ethnopharmacology*, vol. 137, no. 2, pp. 1047–1054, 2011.

[104] R. R. Mohammed, "Removal of Heavy Metals from Waste Water Using Black Teawaste," *Arabian Journal for Science and Engineering*, vol. 37, no. 6, pp. 1505–1520, 2012.

[105] H. D. Utomo, *The adsorption of heavy metals by waste tea and coffee residues [Ph.D. thesis]*, University of Otago, 2007.

[106] K. Selvi, S. Pattabhi, and K. Kadirvelu, "Removal of Cr(VI) from aqueous solution by adsorption onto activated carbon," *Bioresource Technology*, vol. 80, no. 1, pp. 87–89, 2001.

[107] W. Alan, *Hazardous Elements in Soil*, Cambridge University Press, Cambridge, UK, 1994.

[108] L. Crawford Ronald and L. Crawford Don, *Bioremediation: Principles and Applications*, 2005.

[109] K. M. S. Surchi, "Agricultural wastes as low cost adsorbents for Pb removal: kinetics, equilibrium and thermodynamics," *International Journal of Chemistry*, vol. 3, no. 3, article 103, 2011.

[110] B. Dhir and R. Kumar, "Adsorption of heavy metals by salvinia biomass and agricultural residues," *International Journal of Environmental Research*, vol. 4, no. 3, pp. 427–432, 2010.

[111] K. A. Adegoke and O. S. Bello, "Dye sequestration using agricultural wastes as adsorbents," *Water Resources and Industry*, vol. 12, pp. 8–24, 2015.

16

The Effect of Parathion on Red Blood Cell Acetylcholinesterase in the Wistar Rat

Naofumi Bunya,[1] Keigo Sawamoto,[1] Hanif Benoit,[2] and Steven B. Bird[2]

[1]*Sapporo Medical University, Sapporo 060-8556, Japan*
[2]*Department of Emergency Medicine, University of Massachusetts Medical School, Worcester, MA 01655, USA*

Correspondence should be addressed to Steven B. Bird; steven.bird@umassmemorial.org

Academic Editor: Orish Ebere Orisakwe

Organophosphorus (OP) pesticide poisoning is a significant problem worldwide. Research into new antidotes for these acetylcholinesterase inhibitors, and even optimal doses for current therapies, is hindered by a lack of standardized animal models. In this study, we sought to characterize the effects of the OP pesticide parathion on acetylcholinesterase in a Wistar rat model that included comprehensive medical care. *Methods.* Male Wistar rats were intubated and mechanically ventilated and then poisoned with between 20 mg/kg and 60 mg/kg of intravenous parathion. Upon developing signs of poisoning, the rats were treated with standard critical care, including atropine, pralidoxime chloride, and midazolam, for up to 48 hours. Acetylcholinesterase activity was determined serially for up to 8 days after poisoning. *Results.* At all doses of parathion, maximal depression of acetylcholinesterase occurred at 3 hours after poisoning. Acetylcholinesterase recovered to nearly 50% of baseline activity by day 4 in the 20 mg/kg cohort and by day 5 in the 40 and 60 mg/kg cohorts. At day 8, most rats' acetylcholinesterase had recovered to roughly 70% of baseline. These data should be useful in developing rodent models of acute OP pesticide poisoning.

1. Introduction

Organophosphorus (OPs) pesticides were developed in the 1930s. By the year 2000, approximately 1 billion pounds of pesticides was used annually in the United States, with worldwide use estimated to by more than 5.5 billion pounds [1]. OP pesticides irreversibly bind to and inhibit acetylcholinesterase (AChE). AChE is an enzyme that catalyzes the breakdown of acetylcholine (Ach) to choline and acetic acid. During neurotransmission, ACh is released from the presynaptic neuron into the synaptic cleft and binds to ACh receptors on the postsynaptic membrane, thereby propagating the signal from the nerve. AChE (which is located at the neuromuscular junction, central and peripheral nervous tissues, and red blood cells) terminates the nerve signal transmission by hydrolyzing ACh [2]. Therefore, AChE inhibition by OP pesticides leads to a widely dispersed accumulation of ACh. This increase in ACh manifests acutely as the cholinergic syndrome: bradycardia; central respiratory failure; and bronchorrhea and bronchospasm [3–5]. To examine the time course of AChE after OP poisoning, we needed to overcome this acute cholinergic syndrome. For this reason, the rats needed to be supported with a mechanical ventilator and comprehensive medical therapy.

In part because the OP pesticides are used to such a large degree in developing countries, there is significant mortality due to OP pesticide poisoning. The World Health Organization has estimated that more than 3 million people suffer from pesticide poisoning each year, with a case fatality rate of up to 10% [6]. These numbers do not take into account estimates that self-poisoning with pesticides accounts for more than 250,000 deaths per year worldwide, accounting for about one-third of the world's suicides [7]. Aside from acute mortality, it is now known that significant morbidity such as muscle weakness and neurocognitive dysfunction occurs after OP pesticide poisoning [8–10].

Part of the difficulty in studying both the acute and chronic effects of OP pesticides is the lack of animal models of OP poisoning and infrequent reporting of AChE activity and variable dosing and formulation of various pesticides [11, 12]. The aim of this investigation was to determine the effect of AChE of various doses of the highly toxic OP pesticide parathion, in order to determine the LD50 of parathion in a validated OP pesticide poisoning rodent model utilizing comprehensive intensive care therapy.

2. Material and Methods

Male Wistar rats weighing 200–350 gm (Charles River Laboratories, Wilmington, MA) were housed in pairs, maintained on 12 : 12 light : dark cycle, and provided food and water *ad libitum*. Parathion-ethyl (Sigma-Aldrich, St. Louis, MO) was administered at three different doses: 20 mg/kg, 40 mg/kg, and 60 mg/kg. The scientific literature is not consistent when determining the LD50 of toxic OPs in animal models. For instance, various strains of rodents have been used; the OP pesticide has been administered by various routes; and most importantly, comprehensive medical therapy (including mechanical ventilation) has rarely been utilized. It is worth noting that the LD50 for parathion has been reported to be as low as 2 mg/kg in the rat [13, 14].

Rats were briefly anesthetized for 1-2 minutes with isoflurane. Once anesthetized, endotracheal intubation was performed using a 14- or 16-gauge Teflon catheter. An internal jugular catheter of PE-50 tubing was placed and tunneled subcutaneously to between the scapulae. A 24-gauge catheter was also placed in a tail vein. General anesthesia was maintained with 2–4% isoflurane and oxygenation saturation, heart rate, noninvasive blood pressure, and temperature (with feedback to a heating pad) were monitored. Mechanical ventilation was performed using various rodent ventilators (Harvard Apparatus, Braintree, MA) with intermittent capnography. Once ventilation was stabilized, parathion was administered via the jugular vein catheter at a dose of 20 mg/kg (20 rats), 40 mg/kg (35 rats), or 60 mg/kg (37 rats).

When bradycardia developed (defined as a decrease in heart rate of 50% from baseline) atropine was given as a bolus dose of either 0.1 or 0.6 mg/kg followed by a continuous infusion of either 40 or 250 mcg/kg/h via the jugular vein. In order to mimic a human poisoning scenario, where comprehensive medical therapy is used, 0.125 mg/kg of midazolam (Patterson Veterinary Supply, Devens, MA) was given subcutaneously and every 4 hours. Pralidoxime chloride (2-PAM, Sigma-Aldrich, St. Louis, MO) was administered at a dose of either 15 mg/kg or 90 mg/kg every 6 hours via tail vein. The higher doses of atropine and pralidoxime were based upon recent guidance from the NIH to use species-specific modifications of human medication doses [15]. The pralidoxime dosing interval was chosen based upon typical dosing regimens used in the United States. Because pralidoxime is standard therapy in the United States, the Institutional Animal Care and Use Committee of the University of Massachusetts Medical School only approved this study with the utilization of pralidoxime. Maintenance intravenous fluid of normal saline (1.5 mL/kg/h continuously) via tail vein route was given and the body temperature of 37-38 degrees Celsius was maintained throughout.

Twenty-four hours after poisoning the ventilator was stopped and the rats were extubated. In order to counteract the continued cholinergic signs atropine was infused continuously via the tunneled jugular catheter for another

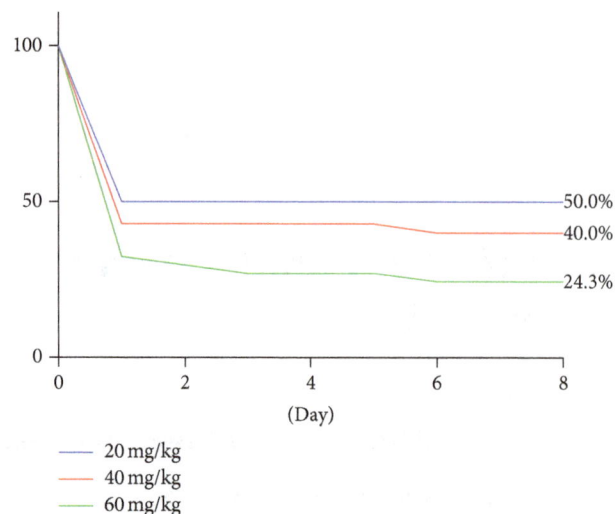

FIGURE 1: Kaplan-Meier survival curves for various doses of intravenous parathion.

24–48 hours in an infusion chamber (Instech, Plymouth Meeting, PA). At day 3 or 4 after poisoning (dependent upon a rat's condition), the animal was moved to normal housing container. Not all rats survived the poisoning model, but survivors were euthanized at day 8 after poisoning.

Animal ChE Test System Model 610 (EQM Research, Cincinnati, OH) was used to measure AChE from blood expressed from the tail vein. The Animal ChE Test System is a validated desktop AChE measurement system that allows AChE determination from just 10 μL of blood. The AChE reagent is >95% specific due to the addition of a specific inhibitor of plasma butyrylcholinesterase (PChE), As1397 (10-(a-diethylaminopropionyl)-phenothiazine). In order to minimize any interactions between parathion, pralidoxime, and AChE, all blood samples were analyzed immediately upon obtaining the blood.

All statistical analyses were performed with GraphPad Prism software version 4 (GraphPad Software, San Diego, CA).

3. Results

Of the 20 rats given 20 mg/kg parathion, 10 survived to day 8. At 40 mg/kg, 14 rats out of 35 survived, and at 60 mg/kg parathion 9 rats out of 37 survived. Figure 1 is a Kaplan-Meier survival curve after poisoning with various doses of parathion.

Of the rats that did not survive parathion doses from 20 to 60 mg/kg, nearly all (93%) were dead within 24 hours of poisoning or proximate to the time of extubation (within 1 to 2 hours). One rat was dead at day 6 in the 40 mg/kg parathion group. Two rats were dead at day 3 and one rat was dead at day 6 in the 60 mg/kg parathion group. Because nonsurviving rats typically died within 24 hours of poisoning, no further AChE data could be obtained. However, AChE activity was neither lower nor more rapidly inhibited in the nonsurvivors. Furthermore, these animals generally looked very weak but

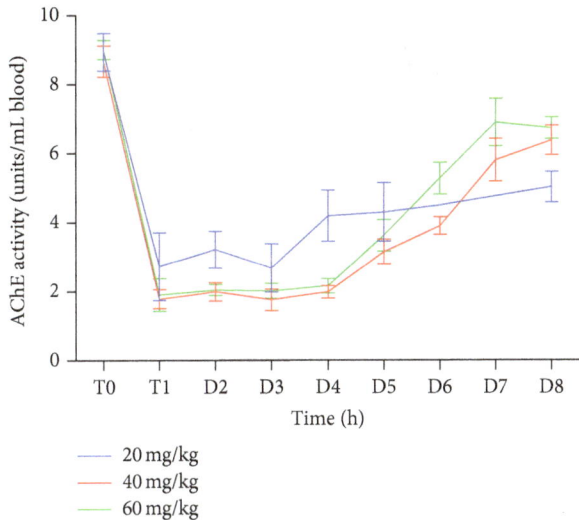

FIGURE 2: AChE activity after poisoning with various doses of IV parathion.

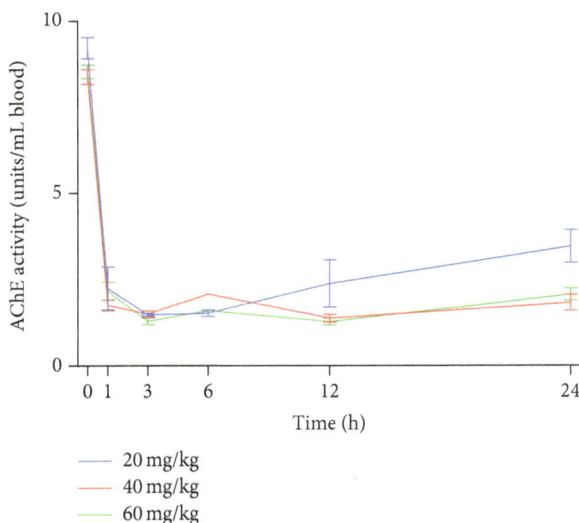

FIGURE 3: AChE activity over the first 24 hours after poisoning with various doses of IV parathion.

did not appear to have more cholinergic signs than surviving rats.

AChE activity over a period of 8 days after poisoning for all parathion doses in surviving rats is shown in Figure 2. AChE recovered to nearly 50% of baseline activity by day 4 in the 20 mg/kg cohort and by day 5 in the 40 and 60 mg/kg cohorts. At day 8, most rats' AChE recovered to roughly 70% of baseline.

Figure 3 shows AChE activity over the first 24 hours after parathion poisoning in all rats and for parathion doses from 20 mg/kg to 60 mg/kg. All rats were grouped together regardless of the pralidoxime dose received (either 15 or 90 mg/kg), as there was no statistically significant difference observed in AChE activity based upon dose of pralidoxime (data not shown).

For all doses studied, AChE decreases to the lowest point at 3 hours after parathion poisoning. Rats in the 20 mg/kg parathion group began to recover AChE at 12 hours, whereas rats in the 40 and 60 mg/kg groups recovered AChE to a statistically significant degree at 24 hours after poisoning. However, the area under the curve (AUC) of AChE activity over 24 hours was not statistically different among the 20, 40, or 60 mg/kg parathion cohorts.

4. Discussion

Data from these studies demonstrate that in this rat model AChE activity is inhibited very quickly and in a dose dependent manner, with a nadir of AChE occurring at approximately 3 hours after poisoning regardless of the dose of parathion administered. In animals that were alive 8 days after poisoning, AChE had only returned to approximately 70% of the baseline activity, regardless of the parathion dose used. Furthermore, there was no difference observed in AChE activity in animals that received either 15 mg/kg or 90 mg/kg 2-PAM.

This seeming indifference to the dose of 2-PAM is not unexpected. The true value of 2-PAM in the treatment of acute OP poisoning is the subject of significant debate. Mechanistically, pralidoxime dose reactivates OP-inhibited AChE and improves neuromuscular transmission in *ex vivo* models [16, 17]. However, while pralidoxime has for years been considered standard therapy for acute OP poisoning and has been shown to be beneficial in some animal models [18] and human studies of OP poisoning [19], these results are not universal. For instance, several clinical trials of pralidoxime have failed to show benefit (or trended towards harm) in patients acutely poisoned with OP pesticides [20–23]. While the possible reasons for why pralidoxime may or may not be beneficial in humans poisoned by OP pesticides are beyond the scope of this paper, there are certainly many factors simultaneously at play, including the time from poisoning to treatment; the type of OP pesticide (e.g., dimethyl versus diethyl OP); the lipophilicity of the OP pesticide; and the dose of pralidoxime. Furthermore, there may be a threshold dose and effect for pralidoxime, and using doses above this threshold does not improve AChE reactivation.

Few animal models of acute OP pesticide poisoning exist. This has been particularly true with rodents, and no previous studies have looked at comprehensive medical therapy to include mechanical ventilation. This study is important as it allows us to obtain biochemical and survival data in rodents treated identically to poisoned humans. Developing these important animal models has been hindered by the variability of the models and the lack of studying or reporting meaningful data in these models. For example, depending on the age, gender, and rodent species used, the oral LD50 of parathion has been reported to be between 2 mg/kg and 30 mg/kg [14]. Such extreme variability makes it virtually impossible to draw any meaningful conclusions or to develop a realistic animal model. We chose our doses of parathion to span these reported LD50s. Furthermore, LD50s have been reported in animals exposed to parathion without any medical therapy. But in order to test new therapies, it is important to know what the LD50 is in animals given comprehensive medical therapy. Lastly, nearly all animal studies of OP pesticide poisoning fail to report AChE activity. Thus, until now the true LD50 of parathion *during medical treatment* has been unknown.

However, rodent and other models serve a critically important purpose with acetylcholinesterase inhibitor research. The US Food and Drug Administration employs what has been termed the "animal rule" in order to approve therapies aimed at reducing or preventing serious or life-threatening conditions caused by exposure to a "permanently disabling toxic agent," such as OP pesticides, in which human efficacy trials are not possible or ethical [12]. Based on this animal rule, the FDA may rely exclusively on animal efficacy studies to provide evidence of therapeutic [24]. While the animal rule is relatively new and underutilized for drug deployment, it was invoked by the FDA in 2003 for the approval of pyridostigmine bromide as a pretreatment for nerve agent exposure in military personnel [25].

As expected with any toxin, there was a dose dependent decrease in survival in this model, even with critical care support. At a parathion dose of 20 mg/kg, exactly one-half of animals survived to 24 hours and to 8 days after poisoning. At a dose of 60 mg/kg parathion 24.3% of animals survived: thus the LD75 for IV parathion is approximately 60 mg/kg. This is important, as is toxicology survival research in animal models: a toxin dose of greater than a single LD50 is needed in order to detect clinically and statistically meaningful results with a minimal number of animals. It appears that 3x LD50 of parathion (i.e., 60 mg/kg intravenously) may be a reasonable dose for further survival studies.

5. Conclusion

In the Wistar rat, parathion inhibits AChE in a dose dependent manner, with the AChE nadir occurring at approximately 3 hours after IV parathion administration regardless of the parathion dose used. Using comprehensive critical care therapy, including mechanical ventilation, atropine, pralidoxime, and midazolam, the IV LD50 for parathion is approximately 20 mg/kg. These data will be useful for investigators developing models of acute OP poisoning and studying treatment algorithms for acute poisoning.

Competing Interests

The authors declare that there are no competing interests regarding the publication of this paper.

References

[1] M. C. R. Alavanja, "Introduction: pesticides use and exposure extensive worldwide," *Reviews on Environmental Health*, vol. 24, no. 4, pp. 303–309, 2009.

[2] P. Taylor and Z. Radic, "The cholinesterases: from genes to proteins," *Annual Review of Pharmacology and Toxicology*, vol. 34, pp. 281–320, 1994.

[3] M. Eddleston and D. N. Bateman, "Pesticides," *Medicine*, vol. 40, no. 3, pp. 147–150, 2012.

[4] S. B. Bird, R. J. Gaspari, and E. W. Dickson, "Early death due to severe organophosphate poisoning is a centrally mediated process," *Academic Emergency Medicine*, vol. 10, no. 4, pp. 295–298, 2003.

[5] E. W. Dickson, S. B. Bird, R. J. Gaspari, E. W. Boyer, and C. F. Ferris, "Diazepam inhibits organophosphate-induced central respiratory depression," *Academic Emergency Medicine*, vol. 10, no. 12, pp. 1303–1306, 2003.

[6] J. Jeyarathnam, "Acute pesticide poisoning: a major global health problem," *World Health Statistics Quarterly*, vol. 43, no. 3, pp. 139–144, 1990.

[7] D. Gunnell, M. Eddleston, M. R. Phillips, and F. Konradsen, "The global distribution of fatal pesticide self-poisoning: systematic review," *BMC Public Health*, vol. 7, article 357, 2007.

[8] C. Rosenbaum and S. B. Bird, "Non-muscarinic therapeutic targets for acute organophosphorus poisoning," *Journal of Medical Toxicology*, vol. 6, no. 4, pp. 408–412, 2010.

[9] S. M. Ross, I. C. McManus, V. Harrison, and O. Mason, "Neurobehavioral problems following low-level exposure to organophosphate pesticides: a systematic and meta-analytic review," *Critical Reviews in Toxicology*, vol. 43, no. 1, pp. 21–44, 2013.

[10] M. F. Bouchard, J. Chevrier, K. G. Harley et al., "Prenatal exposure to organophosphate pesticides and IQ in 7-year-old children," *Environmental Health Perspectives*, vol. 119, no. 8, pp. 1189–1195, 2011.

[11] M. Eddleston, J. M. Street, I. Self et al., "A role for solvents in the toxicity of agricultural organophosphorus pesticides," *Toxicology*, vol. 294, no. 2-3, pp. 94–103, 2012.

[12] E. F. R. Pereira, Y. Aracava, L. J. DeTolla Jr. et al., "Animal models that best reproduce the clinical manifestations of human intoxication with organophosphorus compounds," *Journal of Pharmacology and Experimental Therapeutics*, vol. 350, no. 2, pp. 313–321, 2014.

[13] H. W. Chambers, E. Meek, and J. E. Chambers, "Chemistry of organophosphorus insecticides," in *Haye's Handbook of Pesticide Toxicology*, R. Krieger, Ed., Academic Press, Cambridge, Mass, USA, 3rd edition, 2010.

[14] Pesticide Information Profiles-Parathion, 2016, http://extoxnet.orst.edu/pips/parathio.htm.

[15] S. Reagan-Shaw, M. Nihal, and N. Ahmad, "Dose translation from animal to human studies revisited," *The FASEB Journal*, vol. 22, no. 3, pp. 659–661, 2008.

[16] H. Thiermann, P. Eyer, F. Worek, and L. Szinicz, "Effects of oximes on muscle force and acetylcholinesterase activity in isolated mouse hemidiaphragms exposed to paraoxon," *Toxicology*, vol. 214, no. 3, pp. 190–197, 2005.

[17] H. Thiermann, L. Szinicz, P. Eyer, T. Zilker, and F. Worek, "Correlation between red blood cell acetylcholinesterase activity and neuromuscular transmission in organophosphate poisoning," *Chemico-Biological Interactions*, vol. 157-158, pp. 345–347, 2005.

[18] S. B. Bird, T. D. Sutherland, C. Gresham, J. Oakeshott, C. Scott, and M. Eddleston, "OpdA, a bacterial organophosphorus hydrolase, prevents lethality in rats after poisoning with highly toxic organophosphorus pesticides," *Toxicology*, vol. 247, no. 2-3, pp. 88–92, 2008.

[19] K. S. Pawar, R. R. Bhoite, C. P. Pillay, S. C. Chavan, D. S. Malshikare, and S. G. Garad, "Continuous pralidoxime infusion versus repeated bolus injection to treat organophosphorus pesticide poisoning: a randomised controlled trial," *The Lancet*, vol. 368, no. 9553, pp. 2136–2141, 2006.

[20] S. Syed, S. A. Gurcoo, A. Farooqui, W. Nisa, K. Sofi, and T. M. Wani, "Is the World Health Organization-recommended dose of pralidoxime effective in the treatment of organophosphorus poisoning? A randomized, double-blinded and placebo-controlled trial," *Saudi Journal of Anaesthesia*, vol. 9, no. 1, pp. 49–54, 2015.

[21] N. A. Buckley, M. Eddleston, Y. Li, M. Bevan, and J. Robertson, "Oximes for acute organophosphate pesticide poisoning," *The Cochrane Database of Systematic Reviews*, no. 2, Article ID CD005085, 2011.

[22] R. Rahimi, S. Nikfar, and M. Abdollahi, "Increased morbidity and mortality in acute human organophosphate-poisoned patients treated by oximes: a meta-analysis of clinical trials," *Human & Experimental Toxicology*, vol. 25, no. 3, pp. 157–162, 2006.

[23] M. Eddleston, P. Eyer, F. Worek et al., "Pralidoxime in acute organophosphorus insecticide poisoning—a randomised controlled trial," *PLoS Medicine*, vol. 6, no. 6, Article ID e1000104, 2009.

[24] K. L. Bergman, "The animal rule: the role of clinical pharmacology in determining an effective dose in humans," *Clinical Pharmacology & Therapeutics*, vol. 98, no. 4, pp. 365–368, 2015.

[25] P. Aebersold, "FDA experience with medical countermeasures under the animal rule," *Advances in Preventive Medicine*, vol. 2012, Article ID 507571, 11 pages, 2012.

17

Pattern and Epidemiology of Poisoning in the East African Region

Dexter Tagwireyi,[1] Patience Chingombe,[1] Star Khoza,[2] and Mandy Maredza[3]

[1]Drug and Toxicology Information Service (DaTIS), School of Pharmacy, College of Health Sciences, University of Zimbabwe, P.O. Box A178, Avondale, Harare, Zimbabwe
[2]Department of Clinical Pharmacology, College of Health Sciences, University of Zimbabwe, P.O. Box A178, Avondale, Harare, Zimbabwe
[3]School of Public Health, Faculty of Health Sciences, University of Witwatersrand, Johannesburg, South Africa

Correspondence should be addressed to Dexter Tagwireyi; dextagwireyi@gmail.com

Academic Editor: Steven J. Bursian

The establishment and strengthening of poisons centres was identified as a regional priority at the first African regional meeting on the Strategic Approach to International Chemicals Management (SAICM) in June 2006. At this meeting, the possibility of a subregional poisons centre, that is, a centre in one country serving multiple countries, was suggested. The WHO Headquarters following consultation with counterparts at the WHO Regional Office for Africa (AFRO) and the SAICM Africa Regional Focal Point successfully submitted a proposal to the SAICM Quick Start Programme (QSP) Trust Fund Committee for a feasibility study into a subregional poisons centre in the Eastern Africa subregion. However, before such a study could be conducted it was deemed necessary to carry out a literature review on the patterns and epidemiology of poisoning in this region so as to inform the feasibility study. The current paper presents the results of this literature review. The literature search was done in the months of June and July 2012 by two independent reviewers with no language or publication date restrictions using defined search terms on PUBMED. After screening, the eventual selection of articles for review and inclusion in this study was done by a third reviewer.

1. Background

The establishment and strengthening of poisons centres was identified as a regional priority at the first African regional meeting on the Strategic Approach to International Chemicals Management (SAICM) in June 2006. At this meeting, the possibility of a subregional poisons centre, that is, a centre in one country serving multiple countries, was suggested. However, at its fifth meeting in January 2010, the SAICM Africa Core Group, which comprises representatives from all subregions, noted a continuing lack of progress on this issue and requested that proposals be developed to address this. The World Health Organization (WHO) has had a long-standing programme of work directed at assisting countries to establish and strengthen poisons centres. As such, WHO Headquarters following consultation with counterparts at the WHO Regional Office for Africa (AFRO) and the SAICM

Africa Regional Focal Point successfully submitted a proposal to the SAICM Quick Start Programme (QSP) Trust Fund Committee for a feasibility study into a subregional poisons centre in the Eastern Africa subregion. The results of this feasibility study have since been published elsewhere [1]. In addition, a summary of the project has also been recently published [2]. However, before the feasibility study could be done and in order to get a better understanding of the problem of poisoning in this region, a systematic literature review on the patterns and epidemiology of poisoning in the Eastern African subregion (as defined by UNOSTAT) was carried out. This paper presents the results of this work. A recent impact review of the SAICM QSP programme mentioned the literature review on poisoning in Africa as one of the useful outputs of the QSP projects; however it was also stated in that same review that although a lot of useful information was gathered by the projects, this information is not readily available through the SAICM Secretariat. As a result of the above and the perceived usefulness of the data gathered during this review, it was decided to publish this work in an open access journal. It is hoped that this literature review will provide a valuable source for clinicians, toxicologists, and researchers alike who may wish to acquire a quick overview of issues relating to poisoning in the East African region. In addition, this paper is aimed at making literature on poisoning in Africa more readily accessible to the scientific and health communities, especially given the fact that toxicovigilance systems in Africa are still nascent [3] and thus such systematic data is hardly available.

The countries covered in the review were Burundi, Comoros, Djibouti, Eritrea, Ethiopia, Kenya, Madagascar, Malawi, Mauritius, Mozambique, Rwanda, Seychelles, Tanzania, Uganda, Zambia, and Zimbabwe.

2. Methods

In order to describe the patterns and epidemiology of poisoning in the subregion, a literature search was conducted. The literature search was done in the months of June and July 2012 by two independent reviewers with no language or publication date restrictions. For the literature search, MEDLINE (via PubMed) was searched using the following search strategy: (epidemiology OR incidence OR prevalence OR patterns) AND (poisoning OR snakebite OR scorpion sting OR pesticide OR organophosphate poisoning OR envenomation OR toxicity OR intoxication) AND africa OR (burundi OR comoros OR djibouti OR eritrea OR ethiopia OR kenya OR madagascar OR malawi OR mauritius OR mozambique OR rwanda OR seychelles OR tanzania OR uganda OR zambia OR zimbabwe). The same search strategy was used on Google Scholar. Where no scholarly articles were identified for a country, a further literature search using "poisoning" and the name of the country was done on https://www.google.co.zw/.

Potential articles for inclusion were identified after screening titles and abstracts. The final articles were included in the review after reading the full articles. Relevant references from these articles that were not identified via the bibliographic searches were sought for and the articles analysed. From the identified articles, epidemiological parameters such as case fatality rates, mortality rates, prevalence, and incidence were identified and reported. In addition, National Health Profiles from the study countries were evaluated to identify statistics on poisoning incidences or related parameters. Members of a project Steering Group largely composed of poisons centre specialists from Ghana, South Africa, Kenya, and Zimbabwe, as well as the UK and the World Health Organization, were also requested to suggest any grey literature that they may be aware of and the investigators also provided a list of literature that they were aware of. Case reports were also included in the review. The eventual selection of articles for review and inclusion was done by a third reviewer.

3. Results

Table 1 shows the characteristics of the studies included in this review. Although the main aim of the study was to describe epidemiological parameters, poisoning case reports are mentioned for the different countries. The results are presented according to countries.

3.1. Burundi. WHO has estimated that there were 7.8 deaths per 100,000 persons due to unintentional poisoning in 2004 [4]. No published studies of the epidemiology of poisoning in Burundi were found.

3.2. Comoros. WHO has estimated that there were 1.7 deaths per 100,000 persons due to unintentional poisoning in 2004 [4]. No published studies of the epidemiology of poisoning in Comoros were found.

3.3. Djibouti. WHO has estimated that there were 3.9 deaths per 100,000 people due to unintentional poisoning in 2004 [4]. Literature on the patterns and epidemiology of poisoning in Djibouti were scanty. There was a prospective descriptive study of childhood acute accidental poisoning with kerosene in Djibouti done by Benois and colleagues [5]. Of the 17 cases involved, 35% were asymptomatic and were discharged with 41% developing pneumonia. Seignot and others [6] also reported on a fatal envenomation in a 44-year-old male who was bitten by an African viper (*Echis carinatus*) in Djibouti. Larréché et al. [7] conducted a retrospective study of snakebite victims for the period from October 1994 to May 2006. In this study, the authors compared the normalisation of the haemostasis disorders with early administration of antivenin versus delayed administration. Aigle and colleagues [8] also described a prospective study of stingray stings between July 2008 and July 2009. A total of twelve stings were treated during the study period. There were however no specific studies describing the epidemiology of poisoning in general in the country.

3.4. Eritrea. WHO has estimated that there were 3.7 deaths per 100,000 persons due to unintentional poisoning in 2004 [4]. No published studies of the epidemiology of poisoning in Eritrea were found.

3.5. Ethiopia. WHO has estimated that there were 3.5 deaths per 100,000 persons due to unintentional poisoning in 2004 [4]. A number of papers have been published concerning poisoning in Ethiopia. Aseffa and colleagues [10] reported on an outbreak of food poisoning resulting from *Salmonella Newport*. This occurred between December 31, 1991, and January 4, 1992, and involved students at a Medical College in the country. Out of 344 students, 79 (23%) had clinical symptoms of food poisoning from the bacteria. The main symptoms of the food poisoning episode were malaise, diarrhoea, and abdominal cramps. There were no fatalities in this outbreak. Aga and Geyid [18] also reported on an outbreak of food poisoning resulting from eating food contaminated with *Datura stramonium* during the period of July and August 1984. In their paper, the authors reported on 688 cases seen at

TABLE 1: Literature review of poisoning in the Eastern Africa subregion.

Country	Authors (year)	Study setting	Study period	Type of study	Outcome of interest	Number of cases reviewed	Main results
Burundi	WHO (2009) [4]	National statistics	2004	Burden of disease estimation	Mortality from unintentional poisoning	—	7.8 deaths per 100,000 persons
Comoros	WHO (2009) [4]	National statistics	2004	Burden of disease estimation	Mortality from unintentional poisoning		1.7 deaths per 100,000 persons
Djibouti	WHO (2009) [4]	National statistics	2004	Burden of disease estimation	Mortality from unintentional poisoning		3.9 deaths per 100,000 persons
Djibouti	Benois et al. (2009) [5]	French Military Hospital, Djibouti	18 mths, 2006-7	Prospective descriptive study	Childhood kerosene poisoning	17	11 (64.7%) with pulmonary signs, 7 (41%) with pneumonia, and 6 (35%) asymptomatic
Djibouti	Seignot et al. (1992) [6]	Hopital d'Instruction des Armees		Case report	Snakebite (*Echis carinatus*)	1	Fatal outcome
Djibouti	Larréché et al. (2011) [7]	Intensive care unit of French Military Hospital, in Djibouti	Oct 1994–May 2006	Retrospective case review	Effectiveness of delayed antivenom administration in Snakebite with African viperidae	73	64 (76%) given antivenom; 68 (93%) had coagulopathy; administration of antivenom effective in correcting coagulopathy even if given >24 hours after bite
Djibouti	Aigle et al. (2010) [8]		July 2008–July 2009	Prospective case series	Stingray stings		12 stings treated during study period
Eritrea	WHO (2009) [4]	National statistics	2004	Burden of disease estimation	Mortality from unintentional poisoning		3.7 deaths per 100,000 persons
Ethiopia	WHO (2009) [4]	National statistics	2004	Burden of disease estimation	Mortality from unintentional poisoning		3.5 deaths per 100,000 persons
Ethiopia	Abebe (1991) [9]	Gondar College of Medical Sciences Students Clinic		Retrospective case review	Organophosphate poisoning	50	Case fatality rate was 20% 94% of cases were attempted suicide
Ethiopia	Aseffa et al. (1994) [10]		31 Dec–4 Jan 1992	Prospective case series	Food poisoning (*Salmonella Newport*)	344	79 (23%) of students had clinical symptoms of food poisoning
Ethiopia	Alem et al. (1999) [11]	Butajira rural district	Nov 1994–Jan 1995	Community based cross-sectional survey	Suicide attempts among adults	332	Poisoning (42.4%) was second most common method of attempting suicide; strong detergents and rodenticides most commonly used by women

TABLE 1: Continued.

Country	Authors (year)	Study setting	Study period	Type of study	Outcome of interest	Number of cases reviewed	Main results
Ethiopia	Abula and Wondmikun (2006) [12]	Gondar University Teaching Hospital	Jul 2001–Jun 2004	Retrospective case review	Acute poisoning	102	Poisoning accounted for 0.45% of emergency room admissions; organophosphates accounted for 41.5% of poisoning cases; case fatality rate 2.4%
Ethiopia	Melaku et al. (2006) [13]	Tikur Anbessa Specialised Teaching Hospital	1985–2000	Retrospective review of admissions to ICU	Acute poisoning	3548	168 (4.7%) admissions and 44 (3.9%) deaths due to organophosphate poisoning
Ethiopia	Desalew et al. (2011) [14]	Tikur Anbessa Specialised Teaching Hospital	Jan 2007–Dec 2008	Retrospective study	Acute adult poisoning	116	Most (96.5%) of the cases were intentional self-harm cases with household cleaning agents being the leading toxicants used (43.1%) followed by organophosphates (21.6%); the case fatality rate from this study was reported to be 8.6%
Ethiopia	Azazh (2011) [15]	Tikur Anbessa Specialised Teaching Hospital	Jan 2007	Case report	Organophosphate poisoning	1	N/A
Ethiopia	Selassie (1998) [16]	Jimma Hospital	Jan 1996–Jan 1997	Prospective study of admissions	Organophosphate poisoning	23	Male : female ratio was 1 : 2.83; most common clinical findings were vomiting and abdominal pain; no deaths; average time to reach hospital was 18 hours
Ethiopia	Makita et al. (2012) [17]	Debre Zeyit, Ethiopia	N/A	Mathematical modelling	Staphylococcal poisoning	N/A	Authors estimated that the annual incidence rate of staphylococcal poisoning in the area was 20 per 1000 people (90% CI: 13.9–26.9)
Ethiopia	Aga and Geyid (1992) [18]	Clinics	July–August 1984	Burden of disease estimation	Datura stramonium	688	Case fatality rate was 1.31%
Kenya	WHO (2009) [4]	National statistics	2004	Burden of disease estimation	Mortality from unintentional poisoning		3.4 deaths per 100,000 persons
Kenya	Charters (1957) [19]	Hospital	1949–52	Case reports	Mushroom poisoning	3	Clinical signs and symptoms described
Kenya	Davidson (1970) [20]	Hospital		Case report	Snakebite (Naja mossambica pallid)	1	Patient survived
Kenya	Mwangemi (1976) [21]	Wajir District Hospital	Dec 1973–Dec 1975	Retrospective case review	Snakebite	38	Case fatality rate was 2.6%
Kenya	Greenham (1978) [22]	Garissa Provincial Hospital	Nov 1976	Case report	Snakebite	1	Clinical picture of snakebite resulting from the spitting cobra (Naja mossambica pallida) in a 5-year-old child

TABLE 1: Continued.

Country	Authors (year)	Study setting	Study period	Type of study	Outcome of interest	Number of cases reviewed	Main results
Kenya	Smith et al. (1979) [23]	Gabra nomads	?	Case series	Botulism	300	Attack rate for the entire community of 300 was 3% and 62% for the funeral attenders
Kenya	Kahuho (1980) [24]	Intensive care unit in Kenyatta National Hospital	Aug 1972–Apr 1978	Retrospective case review	Drug and other chemicals poisoning	72	Case fatality rate among nomads was 50% Incidence of 33.7 cases per 1000 admissions Case fatality rate was 36.1% (52% for children under 5 years)
Kenya	Ngindu et al. (1982) [25]	Three hospitals in Machakos district	?	Case series	Aflatoxicosis	20	60% case fatality rate
Kenya	Snow et al. (1994) [26]	Kilifi District, Mombasa	1994	Community based retrospective survey	Snakebite	4712 households	Annual rate of snakebite estimated to be 150 per 100,000 people; only 19% of the victims were bitten by potentially venomous snakes; no deaths
Kenya	Coombs et al. (1997) [27]	(i) Kakamega and western Kenya, (ii) Lake Baringo and Laikipia, (iii) Kilifi and Malindi, and (iv) northern Kenya		Community based cross-sectional survey	Snakebite		The overall average frequency of snakebite was 13.8 per 100,000 people per year and the minimum rate of snakebite mortality was 0.45/100,000/year
Kenya	CDC (2004) [28]	Eastern and central provinces	Apr 2004–Jul 2004	Case series	Aflatoxicosis	317	39.4% case fatality rate
Kenya	Guantai et al. (1993) [29]	19 Kenyan District and provincial hospitals and Kenyatta National Hospital	3 years	Retrospective case review of paediatric poisonings	Poisoning	1904 in total, of which 40% were children <15 years	In the under five years group paraffin, drugs, and organophosphates accounted for 41.09, 23.81, and 15.17% of poisoning cases, respectively
Kenya	Lang et al. (2008) [30]	Kilifi District Hospital	Jan 2005–Dec 2006	Retrospective case review of paediatric poisonings	Accidental paraffin poisoning	48	Incidence of children hospitalised with paraffin poisoning was 17 in 100,000 Case fatality rate was 2%
Kenya	Musumba et al. (2004) [31]	Hospital		Case report	Salicylate poisoning	3	
Kenya	Mbakaya et al. (1994) [32]	Hospital	1998/1990	Retrospective case review	Pesticide poisoning	455	455 cases of organochlorine poisoning
Kenya	BBC news 20 Nov (2000) [33]	Media report	2000		Methanol poisoning	>640 cases	512 poisonings, plus 130 deaths from drinking chang'aa; it is also noted that more than 80 people died in 1998
Kenya	Ministry Environment (2011) [34]	National chemicals profile	2005		Methanol poisoning		50 deaths

Table 1: Continued.

Country	Authors (year)	Study setting	Study period	Type of study	Outcome of interest	Number of cases reviewed	Main results
Kenya	Nyamu et al. (2012) [35]	Kenyatta National Hospital	Jan 2002 to June 2003	Study of admissions	Poisoning	458 cases	Most common poisoning was due to pesticides, accounting for 43% of admissions, followed by household products at 24%
Madagascar	WHO (2009) [4]	National statistics	2004	Burden of disease estimation	Mortality from unintentional poisoning		2.9 deaths per 100,000 people
Madagascar	Vicens et al. (1986) [36]	Various hospitals	1982	Laboratory investigation of cases of botulism and analysis of suspected food	Food-induced botulism	20	Botulinum toxin Type E identified on bioassay
Madagascar	Domergue (1989) [37]	Hospital		Case reports	Snakebite (Colubrida opisthoglypha)	2	
Madagascar	Habermehl et al. (1994) [38]			Outbreak report	Severe ciguatera/ciguatera-like poisoning	>500	Case fatality rate was 20%
Madagascar	Ramialiharisoa et al. (1994) [39]	Hospital	Mar 1991–Jul 1992	Observational	Spider bite (latrodectism)	10	Case fatality rate was 10%
Madagascar	Ramialiharisoa et al. (1996) [40]; Ramialiharisoa et al. (1997) [41]	Vohipeno		Outbreak report	Ciguatera/ciguatera-like poisoning	600	310 patients admitted, 4 deaths
Madagascar	Ranaivoson et al. (1994) [42]		Dec 1994	Outbreak report	Seafood (sea turtle) poisoning	60	The poisoning attack rate was 48% The case fatality rate was 7.7%
Madagascar	Boisier et al. (1994) [43]	Hospital		Prospective observational	Seafood (Carcharhinus leucas) poisoning	200	The poisoning attack rate was 100% The case fatality rate was 30%
Madagascar	Champetier De Ribes et al. (1998) [44]	National surveillance	Jan 1993–Jan 1998	Prospective epidemiological study	Seafood poisoning	19 episodes	1789 people poisoned; 70% of episodes were due to consumption of sea turtle or shark; there were 102 deaths (case fatality rate of 6%)
Madagascar	Ribes et al. (1999) [45]	560 villages with 585,000 people along the Madagascar coast	1996-1997	Community based knowledge, attitude, and practice (KAP) survey	Seafood poisoning	380 cases of poisoning recalled over 1930–1996	Sharks were responsible for most serious poisoning (48%), in addition to other fishes (37%) and marine turtles (11%); neurological and gastrointestinal features predominated in shark poisonings

TABLE 1: Continued.

Country	Authors (year)	Study setting	Study period	Type of study	Outcome of interest	Number of cases reviewed	Main results
Madagascar	Robinson et al. (1999) [46]	Tulear Province with 41 villages spread along 300 km of coast with about 34,000 inhabitants	Jun–July 1996	Community based KAP survey	Seafood poisoning	84	Cases reported over period 1931–1995, involving fish, sharks, and turtles; case fatality rate of 16.7%
Madagascar	Ravaonindrina et al. (2001) [47]		July 1998	Case series	Puffer fish poisoning	4	One death; tetrodotoxin identified.
Malawi	WHO (2009) [4]	National statistics	2004	Burden of disease estimation	Mortality from unintentional poisoning		0.9 deaths per 100,000 persons
Malawi	O'Reilly and Heikens (2011) [48]	Hospital		Case report	Organophosphate poisoning	1	Survived
Malawi	Chibwana et al. (2001) [49]	Queen Elizabeth Central Hospital	1 year	Prospective observational	Childhood poisoning	144	Most (82%) of admissions were due to accidental poisoning Case fatality rate was 7.6%
Malawi	Dzamalala et al. (2006) [50]	Queen Elizabeth Central Hospital and University of Malawi College of Medicine Mortuaries	Jan 2000–Dec 2003	Retrospective audit of suicides autopsied	Deliberate self-harm leading to death (suicides)	84	Pesticide poisoning accounted for 66 cases (79%) of suicide
Malawi	Yu et al. (2009) [51]	Central referral hospital	?	Retrospective case review	Childhood injury		Poisoning accounted for 15.1% of child injuries in the study
Mauritius	WHO (2009) [4]	National statistics	2004	Burden of disease estimation	Mortality from unintentional poisoning		0.1 deaths per 100,000 persons
Mauritius	Glaizal et al. (2011) [52]	?	March 2010	Case reports	Ciguatera/ciguatera-like poisoning	4	Clinical poisoning, with recurrence 1 year later
Mozambique	WHO (2009) [4]	National statistics	2004	Burden of disease estimation	Mortality from unintentional poisoning		3.4 deaths per 100,000 persons
Mozambique	Ministry of Health (1984) [53]	Nampula province	Aug–Oct	Community based cross-sectional survey	Spastic paraparesis (mantakassa/konzo) caused by cassava consumption	1102	Highest incidence rate was 34 per 1000 inhabitants in one village
Mozambique	Cliff et al. (1986) [54]	Acordos de Lusaka village, Memba District	1981	?	Konzo caused by cassava consumption	?	Incidence rate was 34 cases per 1000 people

TABLE 1: Continued.

Country	Authors (year)	Study setting	Study period	Type of study	Outcome of interest	Number of cases reviewed	Main results
Mozambique	Casadei et al. (1990) [55]	Acordos de Lusaka village, Memba District	1982	?	Spastic paraparesis caused by cassava consumption	?	Incidence rate was 4 cases per 1000 persons
Mozambique	Cliff and Coutinho (1995) [56]	Provincial Hospital in Chimoio	Jun–Aug 1992	Case series	Acute cassava intoxication	70	0.14% case fatality rate 74% children under 15 years; 17% women and 9% men
Mozambique	Cliff et al. (1997) [57]	In Mujocjo, Nacacana, Moconi, and Terreni A Chieftaincies in Mogincual district, Mozambique	July 1993	Community based cross-sectional survey	Spastic paraparesis caused by cassava consumption	72	The highest prevalence rate was 30/1000 in Mujocojo Chieftaincy
Mozambique	Cliff et al. (1999) [58]	Mogincual district	July 1993		Ankle clonus, thiocyanate, linamarin and sulphate excretion	397	Proportion of children with clonus ranged from 4% to 22%; geometric mean thiocyanate, linamarin, and inorganic sulphate concentrations were 163 and 60 μmol/L and 4.4 mmol/L, respectively Proportion of schoolchildren with ankle clonus was 8% to 17%; 27 new cases of konzo were found; cassava flour samples were found to contain 26 to 186 ppm of cyanogen.
Mozambique	Ernesto et al. (2002) [59]	Memba and Mogincual districts: 3 communities	Oct 1999	Community based survey	Konzo and cyanogen in flour	27	
Rwanda	WHO (2009) [4]	National statistics	2004	Burden of disease estimation	Mortality from unintentional poisoning		1.3 deaths per 100,000 persons
Seychelles	WHO (2009) [4]	National statistics	2004	Burden of disease estimation	Mortality from unintentional poisoning		0 deaths per 100,000 persons
Seychelles	Lagraulet (1975) [60]			Case report	Poisoning with fish toxin		
Seychelles	Myers et al. (2009) [61]	Seychelles Child Development Study		Prospective longitudinal study	Effects of methyl mercury exposure	779	Recent postnatal exposure at 107 months of age was adversely associated with four endpoints, but no consistent pattern
Uganda	WHO (2009) [4]	National statistics	2004	Burden of disease estimation	Mortality from unintentional poisoning		11.4 deaths per 100,000 persons
Uganda	Bwibo (1969) [62]	New Mulago Hospital	Jan 1963–Dec 1968	Retrospective case review	Accidental poisoning in children	130	Admission rate for accidental poisoning in children was 0.65% Case fatality rate was 5.4%; household chemicals accounted for largest number of poisonings

TABLE 1: Continued.

Country	Authors (year)	Study setting	Study period	Type of study	Outcome of interest	Number of cases reviewed	Main results
Uganda	Cardozo and Mugerwa (1972) [63]	Mulago Hospital, Kampala	Jan–Dec 1970	Retrospective hospital based case review	Acute poisoning	70	48 cases were children, accounting for 0.75% of total paediatric admissions for the period; most admissions were for kerosene ingestion 22 cases were adults, accounting for 0.35% of the total admissions; pesticide poisoning was the most common cause
Uganda	Kinyanda et al. (2004) [64]	Kampala	Nov 2001–Oct 2002	Case-control study	Deliberate self-harm (DSH)	100 cases of DSH; 300 controls	Poisoning was the most important method used in DSH (65%). Organophosphates accounted for the highest proportion (45%) with medications accounting for (35%)
Uganda	Malangu (2008) [65]	Two Hospitals in Kampala	Jan–June 2005	Retrospective hospital based case review	Acute poisoning	276	Agrochemicals (42.4%) were responsible for most of the admitted cases that presented for treatment, followed by household chemicals (22.1%), carbon monoxide (20%), snakebites (14.1%), and food poisoning (1.4%) The overall case fatality rate was 1.4%, due to alcohol, carbon monoxide, and organophosphates
Uganda	Office of the President (2009) [66]	Nationwide	2009	Press release	Methanol poisoning	27	19 deaths
Uganda	Digital Journal (2010) [67]	Southwest Uganda	2010	Media report	Methanol poisoning	189	89 deaths
United Republic of Tanzania	WHO (2009) [4]	National statistics	2004	Burden of disease estimation	Mortality from unintentional poisoning		6.6 deaths per 100,000 persons
United Republic of Tanzania	Rwiza (1991) [68]	Usangi Government Hospital	Jun 1981	Hospital based case series	*Datura stramonium* food contamination	10	No fatalities recorded
United Republic of Tanzania	Yates et al. (2010) [69]	Snake Park Clinic, Meserani	Apr 2007–Dec 2009	Clinic based prospective case series	Management of snakebites	85	42 cases received antivenom; the case fatality rate was 1% (1 death in a 12-year-old), while 7% had a skin graft or amputation of a limb or digit
United Republic of Tanzania	Mbakaya et al. 1994 [32]	Hospitals	1989/1990	Retrospective case review	Pesticide poisoning	736	736 cases of organochlorine poisoning during study period
United Republic of Tanzania	Howlett et al. (1990, 1992) [70, 71]	Tarime District	1985	Case review	Konzo associated with cassava consumption		118 cases including 2 verified deaths

TABLE 1: Continued.

Country	Authors (year)	Study setting	Study period	Type of study	Outcome of interest	Number of cases reviewed	Main results
United Republic of Tanzania	Mlingi et al. (1991) [72]	Msasi District	1988	Case review	Konzo associated with cassava consumption	3	
United Republic of Tanzania	Mlingi et al. (2011) [73]	Mbinga District Mtwara Region	2001/2002 & 2002/2003		Konzo associated with cassava consumption	24 cases (Mbinga) 214 cases (Mtwara)	69% used poisoning, predominantly using antimalarials and pesticides
United Republic of Tanzania	Ndosi et al. (2004) [74]	Muhimbili Hospital, Dar Es Salaam		Prospective study of suicides	Poisoning	100 suicides	
Zambia	WHO (2009) [4]	National statistics	2004	Burden of disease estimation	Mortality from unintentional poisoning		4.8 deaths per 100,000 persons
Zambia	Gill (1979) [75]	Hospitals in Chingola and Chililabombwe	Dec 1975–Jan 1978	Case series	Mushroom poisoning	14	The case fatality rate 14%
Zambia	Bhushan et al. (1979) [76]	University Teaching Hospital, Lusaka	1978	Retrospective hospital based case review	Accidental poisoning	378	Case fatality rate of 0.5% with paraffin poisoning accounting for the largest proportion of admissions (57.1%), food poisoning (18.3%), household poisons (11%), and medicines (10.8%)
Zambia	Gernaat et al. (1998) [77]	St. Paul's Hospital, Nchelenge	4 years	Combined retrospective and prospective study of admissions	Poisoning	6412	Main prevalence of snakebite was in ages of 4–14 yrs
Zambia	Sinclair et al. (1989) [78]	Hospital	16 months	Case series of nontraumatic coma	Poisoning	170	Organophosphate poisoning, a significant cause
Zimbabwe	WHO (2009) [4]	National statistics	2004	Burden of disease estimation	Mortality from unintentional poisoning		8 deaths per 100,000 people
Zimbabwe	Nhachi and Kasilo (1992) [79]	Six referral hospitals in Zimbabwe	1980–1989	Retrospective hospital case review	Admitted cases of poisoning	6018	Case fatality rate was 15%
Zimbabwe	Tagwireyi et al. (2002) [80]	Eight referral hospitals in Zimbabwe	Jan 1998–Dec 1999	Retrospective hospital case review	Admitted cases of poisoning	2764	Case fatality rate was 4.4% for all cases
Zimbabwe	Tagwireyi et al. (2006) [81]	Six district hospitals and one provincial hospital	Jan 1998–Dec 1999	Retrospective hospital case review	Admitted cases of poisoning	711 district hospital cases and 341 provincial cases	Case fatality rate was 4.8% (district hospitals) and 4.7% (provincial hospital)
Zimbabwe	Dong and Simon (2001) [82]	Parirenyatwa hospital	Jan 1995–Nov 2000	Retrospective hospital case review	Organophosphate poisoning	599	Most cases were due to deliberate self-poisoning (74%) The case fatality rate was 8.3% Admissions increased by 320% over the 6 years

TABLE 1: Continued.

Country	Authors (year)	Study setting	Study period	Type of study	Outcome of interest	Number of cases reviewed	Main results
Zimbabwe	Kasilo et al. (1991) [83]	Six referral hospitals	1980–1989	Retrospective hospital case review	Organophosphate poisoning	606	Most cases were due to deliberate self-poisoning (75%) The case fatality rate in the series was 8%
Zimbabwe	Nhachi (1988) [84]	One referral hospital and one district hospital	Jan 1981–Dec 1986	Retrospective hospital case review	Organophosphate poisoning	161 (urban); 11 (rural)	Most cases (83%) were intentional poisoning from urban and for rural centre most (70%) were accidental Case fatality rate 14% (urban)
Zimbabwe	Nyazema (1984) [85]	Two central hospitals and Government Analyst Laboratory	1971–1982	Retrospective case review	Number of cases of traditional medicine poisoning	?	297 cases admitted to Harare hospital for the period from 1971 to 1982
Zimbabwe	Kasilo and Nhachi (1992) [86, 87]	Six referral hospitals	1980–1989	Retrospective hospital case review	Traditional medicines poisoning	1456	Case fatality rate was 6%
Zimbabwe	Tagwireyi and Ball (2002) [88]	Parirenyatwa Central Hospital	Jan 1995–Dec 1999	Retrospective hospital case review	Traditional medicines poisoning in adults	16	No deaths reported
Zimbabwe	Tagwireyi et al. (2002) [89]	Eight referral hospitals in Zimbabwe	Jan 1998–Dec 1999	Retrospective hospital case review	Traditional medicines poisoning in adults	63	Case fatality rate was 9.5%
Zimbabwe	Tagwireyi and Ball (2002) [88]	Parirenyatwa Central Hospital	Jan 1995–Dec 1999	Retrospective hospital case review	Elephant's Ear poisoning	15	Clinical presentation and management of Elephant's Ear poisoning was described No deaths were reported
Zimbabwe	Flegg (1981) [90]		Mar 1980–Mar 1981	Retrospective hospital case review	Mushroom poisoning	50	Case fatality rate was 12% 97.5% admissions due to accidental poisoning
Zimbabwe	Tagwireyi et al. (2002) [91]	Eight referral hospitals in Zimbabwe	Jan 1998–Dec 1999	Retrospective hospital case review	Acute poisoning in children (0–12 yrs)	761	Household chemicals especially paraffin responsible for largest proportion of admissions (43.2%) Case fatality rate was 3.1%
Zimbabwe	Chitsike (1994) [92]	Intensive care unit, Parirenyatwa Hospital	1990–1991	Retrospective hospital case review	Severe acute poisoning in children	42	Household chemicals especially paraffin responsible for largest proportion of admissions (26.2%) Case fatality rate of 21%
Zimbabwe	Kasilo and Nhachi (1992) [86, 87]	Six referral hospitals	1980–1989	Retrospective hospital case review	Acute poisoning in children (0–15 yrs)	2873	Most cases accidental (93.4%) Household chemicals especially paraffin responsible for largest proportion of admissions (27.2%) The case fatality rate of 4.9%
Zimbabwe	Blaylock (1982) [93]	Triangle District Hospital	Jan 1975–Jun 1981	Retrospective hospital case review	Snakebite	250	Case fatality rate of 0.4%
Zimbabwe	Geddes and Thomas (1985) [94]		?	Case report	Snakebite	1	Patient survived

TABLE 1: Continued.

Country	Authors (year)	Study setting	Study period	Type of study	Outcome of interest	Number of cases reviewed	Main results
Zimbabwe	Kasilo and Nhachi (1993) [95, 96]	Six referral hospitals	1980–1989	Retrospective hospital case review	Snakebite	995	Case fatality rate was 1.8%
Zimbabwe	Muguti et al. (1994) [97]	Mpilo Central Hospital	Jan 1990–Jun 1992	Retrospective hospital case review	Snakebite	83	Case fatality rate was 5%
Zimbabwe	Nhachi and Kasilo (1994) [98, 99]	Six referral hospitals	Jan 1991–Dec 1992	Prospective	Snakebite poisoning	274	Case fatality rate was 1.8%
Zimbabwe	Muguti and Dube (1998) [100]	Mpilo Central Hospital	?	Case report	Snakebite from the vine snake (*Thelotornis capensis oatessi*)	1	Patient survived
Zimbabwe	Tagwireyi et al. (2004, 2011) [101, 102]	Eight referral hospitals	Jan 1998–Dec 1999	Retrospective hospital case review	Snakebite	273	Case fatality rate was 2.9%
Zimbabwe	Nhachi and Kasilo (1994) [98, 99]	Six referral hospitals	1980–1989	Retrospective hospital case review	Household chemical poisoning	1192	Majority of the cases (61.3%) occurred in the 0–5 years age group Case fatality rate of 13%
Zimbabwe	Tagwireyi et al. (2006) [103]	Eight referral hospitals	Jan 1998–Dec 1999	Retrospective hospital case review	Paraffin (Kerosene) poisoning	327	Most exposure instances (91.7%) occurred accidentally, with only 6.7% resulting from deliberate ingestion of the chemical The case fatality rate was 0.3%
Zimbabwe	Bergman (1997) [104, 105]	Rural clinics in Gwanda South District	Sep 1991–Sep 1993	Prospective hospital and clinic based survey	*Parabuthus transvaalicus* scorpionism		Case fatality rate was 0.3%; the mortality rate in the district was 2.8 per 100 000 per year
Zimbabwe	Saunders and Morar (1990) [106]			Case report	Scorpion sting	1	Patient survived without any specific scorpion antivenin administration
Zimbabwe	Nhachi and Kasilo (1993) [107]	Six referral hospitals	1980–1989	Retrospective hospital case review	Scorpion and insects poisoning	92	In scorpion sting/bite admissions, bees (44.6%), wasps (8.7%), and spiders (8.7%) accounted for most of the exposure instances No fatalities were recorded
Zimbabwe	Tagwireyi and Ball (2011) [108]	Eight referral hospitals	1998–1999	Retrospective hospital case review	Scorpion envenomation	29	No fatalities
Zimbabwe	Kasilo and Nhachi (1994) [109]	Six referral hospitals	1980–1989	Retrospective hospital case review	Food poisoning	487	Case fatality rate was 2.5%
Zimbabwe	Tagwireyi et al. (2000) [110]	A provincial hospital	1999	Case report	Cantharidin poisoning due to blister beetle ingestion	1	Patient survived
Zimbabwe	Nhachi et al. (1992) [111]	Six referral hospitals	1980–1989	Retrospective hospital case review	Therapeutic drugs poisoning	1061	Pharmaceutical poisoning admissions resulted from mainly accidental exposure (63.5%) The case fatality rate was 3.9%

TABLE 1: Continued.

Country	Authors (year)	Study setting	Study period	Type of study	Outcome of interest	Number of cases reviewed	Main results
Zimbabwe	Queen et al. (1999) [112]		May 1987–April 1995	Retrospective hospital case review	Chloroquine overdose	?	Preponderance of females taking chloroquine in overdose, compared to other overdoses and toxic exposure, was reported (OR 1.99; 95% CI 1.31–3.04; $p < 0.001$) Case fatality rate of 40%
Zimbabwe	McKenzie (1996) [113]		Nov 1990–Oct 1994	Retrospective hospital case review	Chloroquine overdose	29	Case fatality rate of 20.7%
Zimbabwe	Ball et al. (2002) [114]	Eight referral hospitals	Jan 1998–Dec 1999	Retrospective hospital case review	Chloroquine poisoning	544 (chloroquine 279)	Case fatality rate due to chloroquine poisoning significantly higher than that of poisoning due to other drugs (5.7% versus 0.7%; $p < 0.0001$)
Zimbabwe	Tagwireyi et al. (2006) [81]	Six referral hospitals and one provincial hospital	Jan 1998–Dec 1999	Retrospective hospital case review	Differences and similarities in poisoning admissions in urban and rural health centres	711 (district hospital); 341 (provincial hospital)	Case fatality rate for district hospitals was 4.8% Case fatality rate for provincial hospital was 4.7%
Zimbabwe	Tagwireyi et al. (2006) [115]	Eight referral hospitals	Jan 1998–Dec 1999	Retrospective hospital case review	Pesticide poisoning	914	Almost half (49.1%) resulted from oral exposure to rodenticides, 42.2% from anticholinesterase-type pesticides (AChTP) The case fatality rate was 6.8%
Zimbabwe	Kasilo and Nhachi (1993) [96]	Six referral hospitals	1980–1989	Retrospective hospital case review	Metal poisoning	40	Copper accounted for the largest proportion (27.5%)

the study clinics exhibiting unusual signs and symptoms, with 33 requiring hospitalisation for intensive medical care. Nine deaths were reported (case fatality rate of 1.31%). Poisoning was identified as the second most common method of attempted suicide in a district of Ethiopia, accounting for 42.4% of the 332 lifetime suicide attempt respondents [11] from a community based survey which covered a total of 5259 houses with 12 531 residents above 15 years of age. Poisoning was second only to hanging which was reported in 48% of the suicide attempts. The authors reported that poisoning was used more commonly by women than by men with strong detergents and rodenticides being the most frequently used poisons.

Poisoning from organophosphates was also identified as an important cause of poisoning from studies in Ethiopia. Abebe [9] reported a high case fatality rate of 20% resulting from organophosphate poisoning in 50 Ethiopian patients. In a prospective study reported by Selassie [16], a total of 23 cases of organophosphate poisoning were admitted during the period from January 1996 to January 1997. The male to female ratio was reported as 1 : 2.83 with the most common clinical findings being vomiting and abdominal pains. There were no deaths reported in this study. A study by Melaku and colleagues [13] reported that organophosphate poisoning accounted for 4.7% (168/3548) of medical intensive care unit (MICU) admissions over a 15-year period (1985 to 2000) at Tikur Anbessa Specialised Teaching Hospital in Ethiopia [13]. Based on results of a retrospective study of acute poisoning admissions to Gondar University Teaching Hospital, Abula and Wondmikun [12] reported that organophosphate poisoning comprised 41.5% of all acutely poisoned patients with a case fatality rate of 2.4%. Desalew and colleagues [14] also identified organophosphates as an important cause of poisoning in adults in their study where they reviewed medical case files of 116 acutely poisoned adult patients (greater than 13 years) presenting to Tikur Anbessa Specialised University Hospital for the period from January 2007 to December 2008. From the results of their study, most (96.5%) of the cases were intentional self-harm cases with household cleaning agents being the leading toxicants used (43.1%) followed by organophosphates (21.6%) and phenobarbitone (10.3%). The case fatality rate from this study was reported to be 8.6% with most deaths occurring from organophosphate (5) and phenobarbitone (3) ingestion. Most patients stayed only one day in hospital (76%). The only study that reported on incidence of poisoning in Ethiopia was a risk assessment of staphylococcal poisoning due to consumption of informally marketed milk and home-made yoghurt in Debre Zeyit, Ethiopia [17]. Based on a mathematical model, the authors estimated that the annual incidence rate of staphylococcal poisoning in the area was 20 (90% CI: 13.9–26.9) per 1000 people.

3.6. Kenya. WHO has estimated that there were 3.4 deaths per 100,000 people due to unintentional poisoning in 2004 [4]. Literature from Kenya shows the existence of case reports on a wide range of poisonings including mushroom poisoning [19], snakebite from spitting cobra [20, 22], and salicylate poisoning [31]. Moreover, there are a couple of papers that have given epidemiological data on poisoning

outbreaks in the country. Smith and colleagues [23] reported on an outbreak of botulism in Kenyan nomads. The authors reported that 300 Gabra were involved in the outbreak. The outbreak is said to have begun with a young adult female who prepared some sour milk traditionally in a gourd using camel milk. Sixteen people attended her funeral. Of these ten (10) fell sick in four days following the funeral and five of them died. Of the six who did not fall sick, three had taken tea with fresh camel's milk and the remaining three took nothing. Investigations including laboratory analyses showed that the sour milk had been contaminated with *Clostridium botulinum* Type A. Thus the attack rate for the entire community of 300 was 3%, and 62% for the funeral attenders. Ngindu et al. [25] also reported on an outbreak of aflatoxicosis where 20 patients with hepatitis were admitted to three hospitals in Machakos district of Kenya with a very high case fatality rate of 60%. From this report, there was laboratory evidence of aflatoxicosis with maize contaminated with levels as high as 12,000 parts per billion and liver tissue necropsy giving levels of up to 89 parts per billion. More recently, an outbreak of acute hepatotoxicity was identified among people living in Kenya's eastern and central provinces in April 2004. In this particular outbreak, by July 20, 2004, the case fatality rate among the 317 cases was 39.4% (125 deaths had occurred). This was defined as one of the largest and most severe outbreaks of aflatoxicosis documented worldwide [28].

Apart from epidemiological data from outbreaks, a number of hospital based toxicoepidemiological studies have also been reported in the literature for Kenya. Mwangemi [21] reviewed the case notes of snakebite victims admitted to the Wajir District Hospital in Northeastern Province of Kenya for the period of 1974 to 1975. They identified a total of 38 patients. The case fatality rate was 2.6%, an adult male had his leg amputated, and 2 children required massive blood transfusions. The remaining 34 patients made good clinical recovery and were allowed to go home after 1-2 weeks [21].

Kahuho [24] also did a retrospective study of patients admitted with drug and other chemical poisonings in the intensive care unit of Kenyatta National Hospital between August 1972 and April 1978. During this period, there were a total of 72 poisoned patients out of 2135 admissions. Of these 28 (case fatality rate of 36.1%) died. Organophosphates accounted for the highest number of deaths, followed by unknown chemicals. There were 25 (34.7%) children aged below 5 years of whom 13 died. Most of the admissions were as a result of exposure to organophosphates (33.3%) of whom 45.9% died. Another retrospective review in the same hospital, this time looking at hospital admissions during 2002-2003, identified 463 cases of which 458 had complete case notes [35]. The largest age category was young adults (21–30 years), accounting for 38% of cases, with children under five years accounting for 23.4% of cases. Pesticide poisoning was the cause of 43% of poisoning admissions, with a predominance of organophosphates and rodenticides. In children under five, poisoning with household products accounted for 66.4% of cases, and almost all of these were due to paraffin ingestion.

A three-year retrospective review of admissions to 19 hospitals identified 1904 cases of poisonings [29]. The study focused on children, who accounted for 40%. In the under-five-year age group, paraffin, drugs, and organophosphates accounted for 41.09, 23.81, and 15.17% of poisoning cases, respectively.

A hospital based case review by Mbakaya et al. [32] identified 455 cases of poisoning due to organochlorines. This was despite the discontinued use of this pesticide in the countries where it was imported from. The authors attributed the continual use of the pesticide in Kenya to weak regulatory structures that enabled the importation and usage of pesticides no longer in use in the countries of origin.

From another hospital based retrospective case review, Lang and colleagues [30] reported a case fatality rate of 2% and an incidence of 17 per 100,000 for paraffin poisoning in children aged 0 to 13 years.

Snow et al., 1994 [26], undertook a community based retrospective survey of 4712 households on snakebite. The questionnaire was designed to cover circumstances of the bite, morbidity, sequelae, treatment, and perceptions. The data collected were for bites that had occurred in 1993. There were a total of 121 bites reported by the field staff. Of these 21 were in nonresidents of the study area and a further 22 were excluded from the analyses since further investigations revealed that they had been bitten prior to 1993. The annual rate of snakebite among the population was estimated to be 150/100,000 persons per annum. Of the 66 victims with whom in-depth interviews were done, most were male (57%) and most bites occurred in the night (55%). In addition, most of the bites (73%) were to the feet. Only 26 (39%) of the interviewees could reliably describe the snake that bit them. Only 19% of the victims were bitten by potentially venomous snakes with the puff adder being the most commonly identified venomous species. There were no deaths reported from this study for 1993.

Coombs and colleagues [27] collected primary data on the incidence and severity of and species responsible for snakebites in 4 areas of Kenya: (i) Kakamega and western Kenya, (ii) Lake Baringo and Laikipia, (iii) Kilifi and Malindi, and (iv) northern Kenya. The overall average frequency of snakebite was 13.8 per 100,000 persons per year (range 1.9–67.9). The minimum rate of snakebite mortality was 0.45/100,000/year. Thirty-four of the 50 units visited reported no knowledge of death from snakebite in the last 5 years. Possible reasons for the low estimates are discussed. Traditional treatments were common, especially the use of herbal remedies and incisions at the wound site.

Cases of methanol poisoning have become quite rampant in Kenya due to illicit alcohol production. Media reports indicate that, between 1998 and 2005, more than 250 people died due to methanol poisoning in the country. In 1998 more than 80 people died in Nairobi after drinking chang'aa (traditional brew). Similarly, hospital admissions at Kenyatta National Hospital indicate that, in 2000, 512 people were admitted for chang'aa intoxication. Of these, 137 died (case fatality rate of 27%) and 20 became blind with others becoming visually impaired and physically disabled [33]. Fifty more deaths due to methanol poisoning were reported in Machakos in 2005 [34]. In response to this emergency, local

brews were legalized through the Alcoholic Drinks Control Act 2010 to ensure quality control [116].

3.7. Madagascar. WHO has estimated that there were 2.9 deaths per 100,000 people due to unintentional poisoning in 2004 [4]. From published literature, the pattern of poisoning in Madagascar appears to be skewed toward poisoning from natural toxins with case reports of poisoning by puffer fish [47], snakebite by *Madagascarophis (Colubrida opisthoglypha)* [37], and food-induced botulism [36]. Moreover, outbreaks after ingestion of sea food have been reported and do provide some good epidemiological data. Habermehl and others [38] reported on a single outbreak of severe ciguatera/ciguatera-like poisoning in Madagascar after ingestion of shark meat. In this outbreak, more than 500 people were poisoned of whom 98 died with a case fatality rate of 20%. Boisier and colleagues also reported on another mass poisoning after ingestion of a shark *(Carcharhinus leucas)* [43]. In this episode, a case fatality rate of 30% was reported among the 200 poisoned inhabitants of Manakara, a medium-sized town on the southeast coast of Madagascar. Similarly, Ramialiharisoa and others [40, 41] reported on a single outbreak of shark poisoning which occurred in Vohipeno, east coastal region of Madagascar, where 600 people were affected. In this outbreak, four deaths occurred and clinical symptoms of 310 cases admitted in the hospital suggested a ciguatera/ciguatera-like poisoning. The sea turtle has also resulted in mass food poisoning in the Antalaha district of Madagascar [42]. This poisoning episode which affected about 60 people had an attack rate of 48% and a case fatality rate of 7.7%. In total, between January 1993 and January 1998, 19 outbreaks of food poisonings occurred as a result of sea food consumption [44]. These outbreaks affected 1789 people of whom 102 died (case fatality rate of 6%). Consumption of shark and turtle meat accounted for 70% of cases. Ribes and coworkers [45] conducted a knowledge, attitude, and practice (KAP) survey concerning seafood poisoning. This was carried out in 560 villages with 585,000 people along the Madagascar coast. From the survey, there were 175 serious and 205 mild seafood poisonings after consumption of fish, shark, and turtle meals during the period of 1930 to 1996. Sharks were responsible for the most serious poisonings (48%), in addition to other fishes (37%) and marine turtles (11%). Neurological and gastrointestinal features predominated in shark poisonings. Robinson et al. [46] reported on a KAP survey concerning seafood poisonings conducted in Tulear Province with 41 villages spread along 300 km of coast with some 34,000 inhabitants.

Apart from the case reports and outbreaks highlighted above, Ramialiharisoa and colleagues [39] reported on a case series of 10 cases of envenomation by two spiders of the *Latrodectus* genus treated in the Intensive Care Unit of Antananarivo Hospital. In this study which spanned from March 1991 to July 1992, the case fatality rate was 10%.

It is worth noting that there was no literature found on other causes of poisoning apart from those of natural origin.

3.8. Malawi. WHO has estimated that there were 0.9 deaths per 100,000 persons due to unintentional poisoning in 2004

[4]. Epidemiological and other data concerning poisoning in Malawi is very limited. Apart from a case report of 12-day-old baby who survived an episode of organophosphate poisoning [48], we managed to identify only three other studies. The first was by Chibwana and colleagues [49] who conducted a one-year prospective study looking at children admitted with poisoning to Queen Elizabeth Central Hospital. They reported a total of 144 admissions of which 118 (82%) were accidental. The case fatality rate in the study was 7.6% with six of the 11 deaths resulting from traditional medicine intoxication. Yu and colleagues [51] reported that poisoning accounted for 15.1% of child injury using medical records at a central referral hospital in Malawi. Dzamalala and colleagues [50] did a retrospective audit of suicides autopsied at Queen Elizabeth Central Hospital and University of Malawi College of Medicine mortuaries between January 2000 and December 2003. Of the 84 suicide cases, the major mode of suicide was chemical poisoning using an agricultural pesticide ($n = 66$; 79%).

3.9. Mauritius. WHO has estimated that there were 0.1 deaths per 100,000 persons due to unintentional poisoning in 2004 [4]. Glaizal and colleagues [52] reported on 4 cases of French tourists who suffered ciguatera or ciguatera-like poisoning after visiting Mauritius. Apart from this case report, there was no other data in the medical literature of poisoning in the country.

3.10. Mozambique. WHO has estimated that there were 3.4 deaths per 100,000 people due to unintentional poisoning in 2004 [4]. In Mozambique all published literature available to us on poisoning was related to cyanide poisoning resulting from ingestion of cassava, a condition also known as Konzo. Cliff et al. [54] reported an incidence of 34 cases of this poisoning per 1000 in Acordos de Lusaka village, Memba District, in 1981. Casadei et al. [55] reported an incidence of 4 cases per 1000 in Acordos de Lusaka village, Memba District, in 1982. The Mozambique Ministry of Health [53] reported on what was perhaps the first recorded epidemic of Konzo in Mozambique. This work was done in the Nampula province of the country. Briefly, after reports of an epidemic of spastic paraparesis, the Ministry sent out mobile brigades of paramedical workers to search actively for these cases in the province. The brigade members were mostly sanitary agents or nurses and travelled by motorcycle or on foot. They began active detection in August until end of October by which time the epidemic was over and there were few new cases. Active case detection was based on close collaboration with community leaders who were asked to identify patients with difficulty in walking since the last rainy season. The main findings in the study were that there were 1102 patients identified, with the highest incidence rate being 34 per 1000 inhabitants in one village. From the results, 65% of the notified cases were children under 15 years, with males predominating. At over 15 years, females predominated with most cases aged between 20 and 40 years. Although most of the women were lactating, there were no cases of the disease among their babies.

Cliff and Coutinho [56] reported on an epidemic of acute intoxication resulting from ingestion of a newly introduced

cassava during drought in Mozambique. This study was done at a Provincial Hospital in Chimoio during the period June 1992–August 1992. The authors reported on a total of 70 cases, of whom 74% were children under 15 years; 17% were women and 9% men. There was one death in a 3-year-old thought to be due to aspiration pneumonia during coma.

Cliff et al. [57] reported on an epidemic of symmetric paraparesis associated with cassava consumption and cyanide exposure (Konzo). This study was conducted in Mujocjo, Nacacana, Moconi, and Terreni A Chieftaincies in Mogincual district, Mozambique. In carrying out the study, community leaders were requested to call patients for examination in all sites except Moconi. Patients were interviewed and given a basic neurological examination. Konzo was diagnosed when patients had a symmetrical spastic abnormality of gait without signs of spinal disease. A priest was also asked to include the Christian community. Urine samples were also collected for thiocyanate, linamarin, and inorganic sulphate measurements from the first 30 children who appeared in each site. The study was conducted in July 1993. The main finding was that 72 patients were diagnosed with konzo. The highest prevalence rate was 30/1000 in Mujocojo Chieftaincy. Of the 72 patients, all had eaten bitter cassava; 89% were between 5 and 44 years. Males predominated in children under 15 years (60%) and women in adults (59%). There were no cases in children below 4 years.

Cliff and colleagues [58] also reported on a project where they examined 397 children for ankle clonus in three districts previously affected by konzo. The study found that the proportion of children with clonus ranged from 4% to 22%. Geometric mean thiocyanate, linamarin, and inorganic sulphate concentrations were 163 and 60 μmol/L and 4.4 mmol/L, respectively.

The last study that was identified in the literature was that of Ernesto and colleagues [59] who examined all schoolchildren in three communities in Memba and Mogincual Districts for ankle clonus. The proportion of schoolchildren with ankle clonus varied from 8 to 17% and 27 new cases of konzo were found. Of these, 17 were children, eight were women, and the remaining two were men. Cassava flour samples were found to contain 26 to 186 ppm of cyanogen. Mean concentrations of urinary thiocyanate in schoolchildren ranged from 225 to 384 μmol/L.

3.11. Rwanda. WHO has estimated that there were 1.3 deaths per 100,000 persons due to unintentional poisoning in 2004 [4]. Save for a newspaper article reporting on an outbreak of food poisoning after a Seventh Day Adventist church gathering, there is no literature on the epidemiology of poisoning in Rwanda. In the above case one news agency reported that at least 205 members of the Seventh Day Adventist Church in Gasaka Sector, Nyamagabe District, were receiving treatment at various health centres in Kigeme after consuming contaminated food [117]. Another news agency reporting on the same episode reported 50 admissions [118].

3.12. Seychelles. There is no WHO estimate for deaths due to unintentional poisoning [4]. There was only one study for Seychelles by Lagraulet [60] who reported on ichthyotoxism (poisoning by a fish toxin) in the Seychelles Islands. Apart from the aforementioned, the only other publications found in the literature related to pre- and postnatal exposure to methylmercury and the Seychelles Child Development Study, for example, Myers et al., 2009 [61].

3.13. Uganda. WHO has estimated that there were 11.4 deaths per 100,000 people due to unintentional poisoning in 2004 [4]. In 1969, Bwibo [62] described cases of accidental poisoning in children based on data from a children's ward of New Mulago Hospital for the period of January 1963 to December 1968, inclusive. From the study, a total of 130 children were admitted with accidental poisoning of which seven died (case fatality rate: 5.4%). The admission rate for the study period was 0.65%. Household chemicals which included kerosene, pesticides, and other poisons used in homes and gardens accounted for the largest proportion of admitted cases (43.1%). For the household chemicals, kerosene was the leading cause of accidental poisoning. With respect to patient demographics, almost all the cases occurred in children under 5 years old (93.1%), with more males (58%) than females. Of the seven deaths, 5 occurred in boys. All the deaths but one were as a result of medicaments.

Cardozo and Mugerwa [63] described the pattern of acute poisoning among Ugandans based on figures obtained from admissions of these cases to Mulago Hospital in Kampala, Uganda. This was a retrospective survey of all cases of acute poisoning admitted during a one-year period, January to December, 1970. The authors looked at all cases admitted to the general wards, but excluded all cases of alcohol poisoning in adults, as well as snakebite and bee stings. There were a total of 70 cases admitted during the study period of which 48 were in children aged 10 years and below. Of these children all the cases were as a result of accidental poisoning with most of the admissions resulting from kerosene ingestion (35.4%) and pesticides accounting for 18.8% of the cases and medicaments only 3 cases. The children represented 0.75% of total paediatric admissions for the period. In adults, almost half of all the cases resulted from pesticide exposure (10 cases). For the adult cases, there was no difference in gender distribution overall. This was 0.35% of the total admissions in adults.

Lubwama [119] reported on five cases of human salmonella food poisoning in Uganda.

Malangu [65] did a retrospective study of acute poisoning cases admitted to two hospitals in Kampala, Uganda, for the period of January 2005 to June 2005. From this study, the author found a total of 276 patients who were admitted to the hospitals. From the cases seen, the mean age was 26.6 years with 71% being males. From the work, agrochemicals (42.4%) were responsible for most of the admitted cases that presented for treatment, followed by household chemicals (22.1%), carbon monoxide (20.0%), snakebites (14.1%), and food poisoning (1.4%). The overall case fatality rate was 1.4% with 75% of those who died being of the male gender. Alcohol accounted for half of all the deaths with carbon monoxide and organophosphate pesticides accounting for 25% each.

Kinyanda and colleagues [64] conducted a case-control study in which 100 cases of deliberate self-harm (DSH) and 300 controls matched on age and sex were recruited from three general hospitals in Kampala. In order to obtain their data, they utilised a structured interview using a modified version of the European Parasuicide Study Interview Schedule 1. From their study they found that poisoning was the most important method used in DSH (65%). Of this category, organophosphate pesticides accounted for the highest proportion (45%) with medications accounting for (35%)—especially diazepam and chloroquine. From their work, they found that pesticides were the preferred method of DSH among males, while medications and other poisons were the preferred methods among females.

Several media reports indicate a high prevalence of methanol poisoning in Uganda. In 2009, the Minister of Health issued a press release on methanol poisoning within the country following a series of deaths that were due to unknown causes in different parts of the country. Following investigations which included interviews with relatives of the deceased and analysis of blood samples of survivors, it was found that a total of 27 people were affected throughout the country and each had ingested alcohol packed in sachets. Nineteen of these individuals died and blood levels of the survivors showed high levels of methanol [66]. Several other deaths have been reported through the media, with 89 people from Kabale and Kamwenge districts in southwest Uganda confirmed dead allegedly due to methanol poisoning in 2010. A further 100 people were hospitalised, including a two-year-old child [67].

3.14. United Republic of Tanzania. WHO has estimated that there were 6.6 deaths per 100,000 people due to unintentional poisoning in 2004 [4]. Data relating to poisoning in the published literature is also limited for Tanzania. A study by Rwiza [68] reported on a case series of ten agitated and psychotic patients with other classical signs of atropine poisoning who were admitted to Usangi hospital, Tanzania, after ingesting stiff-porridge made from millet which had been contaminated with seeds of *Datura stramonium* (Jimson weed). All the patients were treated and survived the episode. In this particular series, 7 of the patients were from the same family while the other three lived in separate homes. In the paper, the author alludes to the fact that records of the Chief Government Chemist reported that a similar type of food poisoning had occurred in at least eight other regions over the preceding seven years. The clinical presentation and management of poisoning from *Datura stramonium* are discussed in this paper.

In another study, Yates and colleagues [69] prospectively reviewed patients who, between April 2007 and the end of 2009, received treatment for snakebite envenomation at the Snake Park clinic in Meserani, Tanzania. The authors reported on 85 cases. The mean age was 23 years with a male to female ratio of 1.4. Most of the bites (77%) occurred after dark and during the rainy season (88%). In 32 of the cases, identification of the culprit snake responsible for the bite was not possible. Forty-two cases received antivenom. The case fatality rate was 1% (1 death in a 12-year-old). The authors also reported that 7% of the cases needed a skin graft or amputation of a limb or digit. In cases where the culprit snake was identified, the puff adder was identified in most of the cases.

A hospital based case review by Mbakaya et al. [32] indicated that poisoning due to organochlorine use accounted for 736 cases of poisoning in Tanzania between 1988 and 1990.

A few studies have been published on poisoning related to ingestion of cassava in Tanzania. In the first outbreak, Howlett and colleagues [70, 71] reported 39 cases of Konzo out of the 50 people clinically examined. Thirty of these were male and nine were female aged between 4 and 46 years. Nineteen of the cases were from six families with another 5 cases all from one family. Further investigation of this outbreak revealed 116 cases and 2 deaths due to Konzo. Mlingi and colleagues [72] report on 3 cases of Konzo that occurred in 1988 in Mtanda village, south of Tanzania. Mlingi and colleagues [73] further report on outbreaks of Konzo that occurred in Tanzania in 2001–2003. During this period, twenty-four cases of Konzo occurred in Mbinga District, Ruvuma region (2001-2002), while 214 konzo cases occurred in Mtwara Region in 2002-2003.

A prospective hospital based study of suicides in Dar Es Salaam, Tanzania, indicates that poisoning is a common method of committing suicide with 69% of subjects employing this method [74]. In this study, 28% of subjects used antimalarials (mostly chloroquine) to poison themselves, while 12% of subjects poisoned themselves with pesticides (chlorfenvinphos and diazinon). In the latter, chemicals were identified in 8 out of the 12 cases. The source of poisoning in this study could not be identified for 29 of the subjects.

3.15. Zambia.
WHO has estimated that there were 4.8 deaths per 100,000 persons due to unintentional poisoning in 2004 [4]. Bhushan and coworkers [76] reported on a retrospective analysis of 378 cases of accidental poisoning by ingestion or inhalation in children admitted to the University Teaching Hospital, Lusaka, Zambia, in 1978. The authors reported a case fatality rate of 0.5%. Paraffin poisoning accounted for the largest proportion of admissions (57.1%), followed by food poisoning (18.3%), household poisons (11%), and medicines (10.8%). Sinclair and colleagues [78] also highlight organophosphorus poisoning as one of the key causes of nontraumatic coma in Zambia.

Gill [75] presented a case series of fourteen cases of mushroom poisoning which presented to the hospitals of Chingola and Chililabombwe on the Zambian copper belt during the period from December 1975 to January 1978. In this case series, 2 patients died, making the case fatality rate 14%. In a combined retrospective and prospective 4-year study of 6412 children consecutively admitted to St. Paul's Hospital, Nchelenge, northeast Zambia, Gernaat and colleagues [77] found that snakebite was a significant cause of injury in 4–14-year-olds.

3.16. Zimbabwe.
WHO has estimated that there were 8 deaths per 100,000 people due to unintentional poisoning in 2004 [4]. For Zimbabwe a number of papers have been published in the area of poisoning. In order to make for easy reading, the literature concerning poisoning in Zimbabwe is separated into various sections related to the type of group covered by the study under separate headings.

3.16.1. Published Work on Epidemiology of Poisoning in General. By the time of the review, three studies had been conducted in an attempt to describe the overall patterns of poisoning in Zimbabwe regardless of the toxic substances involved and most of what is known today concerning poisoning in Zimbabwe emanates from these two studies. The first was done by Nhachi and Kasilo [79] and this was a retrospective study that looked at all poisoning admissions to six major referral hospitals in the country over a ten-year period (January 1980–December 1989) [79]. The hospitals that were involved included Parirenyatwa, Harare Central, United Bulawayo, Mpilo, Mutare, and Gweru hospitals. Of a total of 6018 cases of poisoning evaluated, the main agents associated with acute poisoning admissions to the hospitals were traditional medicines (22.9%), household chemicals (18.8%), snake and insect envenomation (17.1%), orthodox medicines (16.7%), and insecticides (14.8%). The overall case fatality rate in this study was reported to be 15% with the main agents associated with fatality being pesticides, traditional medicines, and orthodox medicines in descending order.

Tagwireyi and colleagues also did a retrospective case review and looked at all poisoning admissions to eight major referral hospitals in Zimbabwe over a two-year period covering the years 1998-1999 [80]. The study sample for this work included all the hospitals covered by Nhachi and Kasilo, but also added two other referral hospitals, that is, Bindura and Gwanda Hospitals. In this work, the authors reported a total of 2764 admissions resulting from toxic exposure to different toxins and toxicants. They reported a smaller proportion of poisoning cases resulting from accidental exposure (48.9%) than that reported by Nhachi and Kasilo (61.2%; [79]). In addition the spectrum of agents responsible for most admissions had changed with pesticides (32.8%) and pharmaceuticals (20.2%) accounting for most admissions. Household chemicals (15.7%), animal envenomation (11.8%), and natural toxins (6.8%) were also important causes of poisoning. In addition, the case fatality rate from this study which was 4.4 deaths per 100 admissions was much lower than that reported by Nhachi and Kasilo [79]. The work by Tagwireyi and colleagues [80, 89, 91] showed that the patterns of poisoning in Zimbabwe had changed over the last decade or so, with the authors attempting to explain some of these differences.

Tagwireyi and colleagues [81] also reported on the epidemiology of poisoning admissions to six district hospitals in one province of Zimbabwe. The authors compared the epidemiology at these health centres with that of the Provincial hospital serving the districts. They found that the patterns of poisoning were not the same in terms of toxic agents responsible for most cases of poisoning. The case fatality rates were however similar for the district hospitals and the provincial hospital at 4.8% and 4.7%, respectively.

3.16.2. Poisoning in Children. Concerning poisoning in children, Kasilo and Nhachi [86] presented and analysed a total of 2873 cases of children aged between 0 and 15 years. From this report, the authors found that the majority of the cases of childhood poisoning were accidental in nature (93.2%) with most cases occurring in the 0–5-year age group (75.4%). They also reported a case fatality rate of 4.9% with most of the deaths resulting from suicide among the 11–15-year age group and accidental poisonings among the 0–10 years old group. From their study, most of the poisoning patients were male (53.1%). The commonest toxic agents involved included household products (27.2%), traditional medicines (23%), venoms from snakebites and insect stings (16%), and therapeutic agents or pharmaceuticals (12.4%).

Chitsike [92] reported on a retrospective study of forty-two cases of acute poisoning admitted to a paediatric Intensive Care Unit at Parirenyatwa over a two-year period (1990-1991, inclusive). This study was different to that conducted by Kasilo and Nhachi in that it looked only at the severe cases of poisoning in children who required intensive care. However, as was the case with the former study, Chitsike also found that household products as exemplified by paraffin (26.2% of cases), traditional medicines (14.3%), and pharmaceuticals were the commonest causes of poisoning in children. As expected from the intensive care unit, the case fatality rate in the series by Chitsike was much higher than that reported by Kasilo and Nhachi [86], being 21%.

Tagwireyi and colleagues [91] reported on a total of 761 cases (aged 0–12 years) of childhood poisoning admitted to eight study hospitals of which 97.5% (742) were accidental with the majority of the cases (>80% of all childhood poisoning admissions) occurring before the age of 5 years. In addition, over 56.0% of the cases occurred in males. Cases of deliberate self-poisoning occurred in children aged 10 years and above, similar to the study by Kasilo and Nhachi [86]. The main agents responsible for poisoning admissions were household chemicals, especially paraffin (43.2%), pesticides (23.1), natural toxins which included traditional medicines (13.9%), and animal envenomation which included snakebite and scorpion sting (11.6%). The case fatality rate in this work was 3.1%.

3.16.3. Pesticide Poisoning.
Zimbabwe has a largely agrarian based economy and consequently depends heavily on the use of pesticides. However, despite the importance of pesticide poisoning in the country, there is sparse data relating to important epidemiological characteristics of pesticide poisoning with only a handful of studies having been published. The first report pertaining specifically to pesticide poisoning after independence in 1980 was done by Nhachi [84]. In this work, Nhachi compared a total of 161 cases of organophosphate poisoning cases admitted to Parirenyatwa hospital (for the period from January 1981 to June 1986) with 30 cases recorded at Shamva hospital (over 11 months). The study revealed that while the bulk of cases admitted to Parirenyatwa hospital were intentional poisonings (83% of cases), those admitted to the rural hospital were mainly accidental (70%). The author attributed this to "social factors" as exemplified by greater social pressures resulting from urbanisation. The case fatality rate for cases admitted to the urban hospital was 14% whereas the rural hospital did not record any fatalities during the 11-month study period.

Later, Kasilo and coworkers [83] published a subanalysis of a larger study on the pattern of poisoning in urban Zimbabwe [79]. This work described the pattern of organophosphate poisoning in Zimbabwe and found that these pesticides accounted for 10.1% (606 cases) of all the admissions to their study hospitals with most of these cases resulting from deliberate self-poisoning (75%), and 21% being accidental. The case fatality rate was 8%. The authors also reported that most admissions occurred in the 21–30-year age group (42% of all cases).

Dong and Simon [82] carried out a study to examine organophosphate poisoning in Zimbabwe by determining the trends of organophosphate admissions in an urban Zimbabwean hospital. Over a period of six years (1995 to 2000), they found 599 cases of organophosphate exposure, of which the male and female admission rates were similar (48% were male). The authors reported that suicide was the predominant cause of organophosphate poisoning accounting for 74% of the admissions. The case fatality rate in the series was reported as 8.3%. Dong and Simon [82] concluded that organophosphate poisoning is increasing rapidly with an increase in admissions of 320% over the six years of the study.

More recently, Tagwireyi and colleagues [115] arguing in the introduction to their paper that too much emphasis had been placed on individual pesticides, especially organophosphates in all past publications, reported on the epidemiology of pesticide poisoning in general, regardless of pesticide type. The authors found that of the 914 single pesticide exposure in their study, almost half (49.1%), resulted from oral exposure to rodenticides and 42.2% from anticholinesterase-type pesticides (AChTP), mostly organophosphates which were responsible for over 90% of admissions from AChTP. Accidental and deliberate self-poisoning (27.1% and 58.6%, resp.) accounted for most cases with only 8 homicides. The case fatality rate (CFR) in deaths/100 admissions was 6.8%. They revealed an important aspect pertaining to pesticide poisoning, which had not been highlighted before, that most of the cases of pesticide poisoning now resulted from exposure to the illegal rat poisons, popularly known as "mushonga yemakonzo," which were being sold in street corners in Zimbabwe. The authors from their results recommended that stricter control should be done of these substances.

3.16.4. Pharmaceutical Poisoning.
Concerning poisoning from orthodox medicines, Nhachi and colleagues [111] carried out a subanalysis of their data on the patterns of poisoning admissions to major referral hospitals in Zimbabwe. The authors reported that pharmaceutical poisoning admissions to the study hospitals resulted from mainly accidental exposure (63.5%). In addition, analgesics (22% of all pharmaceutical admissions), sedatives and hypnotics (13.2%), antipsychotics (11.6%), and antimalarials (9.3%) were the major groups of drugs implicated, with the case fatality rate in the study being 3.9 deaths per 100 admissions (3.9%).

Queen and colleagues [112] reported on an increasing incidence of poisoning admissions involving chloroquine, suggesting that the pattern reported by Nhachi and coworkers may have changed. The authors looked at the pattern of serious chloroquine overdose based on a retrospective examination of all toxicology cases recorded at the Parirenyatwa Hospital Casualty Department resuscitation room for the period from May 1, 1987, to April 30, 1995. They found a statistically significant rise in the number of chloroquine overdose cases presenting to the resuscitation room during the study period from nil cases in 1987/1988 to 33 in 1994/1995 ($p = 0.001$), with a case fatality rate of 40%. In addition, a preponderance of females taking chloroquine in overdose, compared to other overdoses and toxic exposure, was reported (OR 1.99; 95% CI 1.31–3.04; $p < 0.001$). Queen and colleagues [112] postulated that this gender distribution could have been related to the use of high doses of chloroquine to induce abortion and recommended further investigation into this issue.

Another study looking specifically at aspects of poisoning from pharmaceuticals was done by McKenzie [113]. The author described the features of chloroquine poisoning by carrying out a retrospective review of all cases of confirmed acute chloroquine poisoning admitted to intensive care units at Harare and Parirenyatwa central hospitals for the period from November 1990 to October 1994. Of the 29 cases identified, 69% (20) were female and 31% (9) were male with a case fatality rate of 20.7%. The common clinical features in the patients were similar to those documented in the literature and included respiratory failure, depressed level of consciousness, hypothermia, hypotension, cardiac arrest, and hypokalaemia.

Ball and colleagues [114] reported on a retrospective hospital record review to describe the epidemiology of chloroquine poisoning compared with that of other medicines. They selected all records of admissions to the eight referral hospitals due to poisoning with single pharmaceutical agents and separated these into those involving either chloroquine or other medicines. Case characteristics were compared and a retrospective cohort study was performed to investigate the association of pregnancy with chloroquine overdose. From their analysis, of 544 cases, antimalarials accounted for the largest proportion of admissions (53.1%), with chloroquine accounting for 96.2% (279 cases) of these. The cases of chloroquine poisoning were then compared with the remaining 265 cases. The authors found that a greater proportion of patients took chloroquine deliberately (80.3% versus 68.7%; $p < 0.05$) and that case fatality rate due to chloroquine poisoning was significantly higher than that of poisoning due to other drugs (5.7% versus 0.7%; $p < 0.0001$). They also found that patients admitted with chloroquine poisoning (188 cases) were twice as likely to be found pregnant (relative risk = 2.3, 95% CI = 1.2–4.5) than similar women admitted due to other medicines (157 cases). The authors concluded that chloroquine is the most common cause of pharmaceutical poisoning admission at referral hospitals in Zimbabwe.

3.16.5. *Household Chemical Poisoning.* Concerning household chemical poisoning, Nhachi and Kasilo [98] carried out a retrospective analysis to evaluate the epidemiology of poisoning by household chemicals based on their data on admissions at Zimbabwe's six main urban hospitals over a 10-year period (1980–1989). They reported that a total of 1192 household chemicals poisoning cases were recorded, and this constituted a fifth of all poisoning cases recorded during the study period. In line with international literature on the subject, the researchers found that the majority of the cases (61.3%) occurred in the 0–5-year age group, with the 16–25- and 26–30-year age groups accounting for 11% and 5.2%,

respectively. The authors also reported as expected that the bulk of the cases (66.8%) resulted from accidental exposure to the chemicals. They reported a case fatality rate resulting from household chemical exposure of 13% with most of the deaths being suicides. Paraffin (kerosene) was the most common poisoning agent accounting for 68% of the cases. This was followed by rat poisons (5.8%), bleaches (5.1%), and caustic soda (3.3%). The authors concluded that incidence of poisoning with household chemicals could be reduced by health education directed to parents emphasising the importance of safe storage of paraffin and other household chemicals and by legislation to stop retailers from selling paraffin for domestic use in second-hand containers.

More recently, Tagwireyi and coworkers [103] reported on a total of 327 admissions due to oral exposure to paraffin which represented 11.8% of all the poisoning admissions to the eight study hospitals. In accordance to literature from other countries, most exposure instances (91.7%) occurred accidentally, with only 6.7% resulting from deliberate ingestion of the chemical. Over 85% of cases were in the 0–5-year age range and less than 10% were above the age of 12 years. The median age on admission was found to be much higher for deliberate self-poisoning (23 yrs; IQR 19–26 yrs) compared to that for accidental poisoning (1.5 yrs; IQR 1-2 yrs). The authors also examined the drug management of paraffin poisoning and found that over three-quarters of patients received an antibiotic either alone or in combination with another antibiotic or drug. Paracetamol (24.3%) was the next most commonly encountered treatment. The case fatality rate was 0.3 deaths per 100 admissions (95% Confidence Interval 0.0–1.7).

3.16.6. *Animal Envenomation—Snakebite.* Concerning snakebite, there have only been a handful of studies on the epidemiology and other related factors of snakebite, most of which have been based on data from single hospitals or case reports. Blaylock [93] described various clinicoepidemiological aspects of this type of envenomation based on clinical observations from retrospective data of 250 snakebite cases admitted to a hospital in the south-eastern lowveld of Zimbabwe (Triangle hospital) over six and a half years (January 1975 to June 1981). He presented data on the clinical presentations, types of snakes, and treatment given to snakebitten patients attending the hospital with a case fatality rate of 0.4%.

Geddes and Thomas [94] reported on a case report of a boomslang bite in a 30-year-old snake-handler who was bitten around the shoulder blade area. This patient was successfully treated with the South African Institute of Medical Research (SAIMR) monovalent boomslang antivenin.

Kasilo and Nhachi [95] reported on the pattern of snakebite in Zimbabwe from 995 cases of snakebite. The authors noted a mortality rate of 1.8% in the series as well as the fact that antibiotics were the most commonly used treatment for snakebite and were often used irrationally. In addition, they reported that most snakebites occurred in patients aged between 16 and 20 years. The authors reported that the few records of the types of snakes associated with envenomation were, in order of frequency, cobra, adders (puff and night), mamba, and boomslang. They concluded from their results that prevention and prompt treatment of snake envenomation were a priority for the reduction of incidence of poisoning.

As no studies had been done in the past reporting on snakebite admissions to rural/district hospitals where one would expect it to be rife, Nhachi and Kasilo [99] reported a series of 274 cases of snakebite admitted to hospitals in the eight provinces of Zimbabwe. This was and is the only prospective study on snakebite conducted in Zimbabwe in the area of clinical toxicology. This study was done over a period of 2 years (January 1991 to December 1992). From this work, only five deaths (1.8% of the total cases) were reported. The majority of snakebites (63%) occurred at night (between 6.30 p.m. and midnight) and over 74% took place during the hot rainy season. Of the snakes identified in the bites, the cobra was identified in 37% of cases, the puff adder in 20% of cases, and the black and green mamba in 18% of the cases. In line with their earlier study, Nhachi and Kasilo noted that treatment of snake envenomation consisted mainly of the administration of antibiotics (151 cases). Analgesics (144 cases), antivenom tropical snake polyvalent (ATT) (89 cases), antitoxoid tetanus (TT) (61 cases), antihistamines (47 cases), and traditional medicines (43 cases) were also used.

Muguti and colleagues [97] reported a retrospective analysis of 83 consecutive patients treated for snakebite at one of the central hospitals in Zimbabwe (Mpilo) for the period from January 1990 to June 1992. In this study, the authors also reported that antibiotics were the most commonly used medication for snakebite, in addition to presenting data on the most frequently bitten areas and clinical features. The mortality rate was 5%, which was attributed to the lack of antivenom at the hospital during the study period [97]. Muguti and Dube [100] published what is perhaps the only published clinical case report of a bite from the vine snake (*Thelotornis capensis oatessi*) in Zimbabwe for which antivenom was not available [100]. In this case report, the patient survived the bite after vigorous supportive therapy.

Tagwireyi and colleagues also recently reported on the patterns and epidemiology of snakebite admissions to the eight major referral hospitals included in their main study [101]. In their work, these researchers reported on a total of 273 snakebite admissions. Of these the type of snake involved in the bites was recorded in 14.6% of the cases with 62.5% involving puff adders and 22.9% involving cobras and mambas. As with all other studies on snakebite in Zimbabwe, the gender distribution was similar. Again, in line with reports from other studies in Zimbabwe, most of the bites (>80%) occurred during the summer months of November to April. The case fatality rate from snakebite was also comparable to earlier studies being 2.9%. These results were recently later published in a full paper by the same authors [102].

3.16.7. Animal Envenomation—Scorpion Sting. Saunders and Morar [106] reported on a case of scorpion envenomation, thought to have resulted from a scorpion of the genus *Parabuthus* judging from the clinical picture of the patient. In their case report the patient survived without any specific scorpion antivenin administration. In a ten-year retrospective study of all cases of poisoning to six major referral

hospitals in Zimbabwe, Nhachi and Kasilo [107] reported that only five cases of scorpion sting were admitted to the study hospitals, with no further details on the cases. They also reported that, of the 92 cases of insect and scorpion sting/bite admissions, bees (44.6%), wasps (8.7%), and spiders (8.7%) accounted for most of the exposure instances. No fatalities were recorded in this series indicating that scorpion sting and insect bites were rarely fatal in Zimbabwe.

Bergman [104] described the epidemiological and clinical features of scorpion stings in Gwanda South District. He collected a case series of consecutive scorpion sting victims presenting to Manama Hospital and all seven rural health centres in Gwanda South District, Zimbabwe, between September 1991 and September 1993. Bergman reported 244 cases, of which 184 were *Parabuthus transvaalicus*, Purcell, 1899. From this work, the author identified seventeen patients with severe *P. transvaalicus* scorpionism and published a case series of these patients and their clinical picture [105]. From this study, Bergman described the clinical features of *P. transvaalicus* scorpionism for the first time. He noted that they resembled those of *P. granulatus* scorpionism which, however, has significant sympathetic nervous system stimulation, the distinguishing features being visual disturbances, anxiety, restlessness, and raised blood pressure. The case fatality rate was 0.3% in the study by Bergman and mortality rate in the district was 2.8 per 100,000 per year. Tagwireyi and Ball [108] also reported on a case series of scorpion sting admissions to major referral hospitals in Zimbabwe. In this paper, there were no fatalities reported.

3.16.8. Traditional Medicine Poisoning. Nyazema [85] carried out a study to determine the number of cases of poisoning due to traditional medicines as recorded at Parirenyatwa, Harare Central hospitals, and the Government Analyst Laboratory. The author reported a total of 297 cases admitted to Harare hospital for the period from 1971 to 1982. Specific numbers were not given in the text for the number of cases recorded at the other two institutions. Moreover, although the author stated in his paper that the mortality at Harare hospital increased twofold, no specific figures were given. Nyazema [120] also reported on results of a study of the records of four hospitals from 1971 to 1982, carried out to see how many people had been poisoned with herbal remedies. As one of the main findings, the author noted that the number had increased since 1971. In addition, the author interviewed a total of 50 traditional healers concerning record-keeping and knowledge of toxicity. Kasilo and Nhachi [87] then reported on a subanalysis of a total of 1456 cases of traditional medicine poisoning from their 10-year retrospective study of all poisonings. They reported that poisoning from traditional medicines represented 23% (the biggest single group) of all poisoning cases. Almost two-thirds (67%) of the patients were male and most of the admitted patients were under 5 years of age (53%). Of the traditional medicine poisoning cases, 61% of poisonings were associated with treatment of an ailment and 8% were accidental poisonings, while 2.2% resulted from deliberate self-poisoning. The authors reported a case fatality rate of 6% from their study. They found that the main reasons for seeking treatment with traditional medicines were for depressed fontanelle and fever in children and diarrhoea and abdominal pain in adults. Treatment in all poisoned patients consisted mainly of supportive therapy and included the induction of vomiting with ipecacuanha in children.

Tagwireyi and Ball [88] after noting a paucity of information regarding the clinical presentation of poisoning associated with use of traditional medicines ("muti") in Zimbabwe, conducted a small case series describing the common adverse effects of poisoning and relating these with the reasons for taking the traditional medicines. They looked at all records of admissions for traditional medicine poisoning to Parirenyatwa hospital over the period 1995 to 1999, inclusive. From a total of 16 cases, Tagwireyi and Ball reported that the main reason for taking traditional medicines was to treat abdominal pain (five cases). They also found that, of these five cases, most suffered from toxic effects related to the genitourinary system, mainly dysuria (4 of 5 cases) and haematuria (5 of 5 cases). Due to the small numbers in their series, the researchers suggested that further studies were needed to ascertain if "muti" taken for abdominal pains contains a nephrotoxic agent.

Tagwireyi and colleagues [89] then followed up on their earlier study by carrying out a retrospective review of all cases of poisoning with traditional medicines at eight main referral hospitals in Zimbabwe (January 1998–December 1999, inclusive) to describe the most common signs and symptoms, reasons for taking the medicine, and management of poisoning in adults. From a series of 63 cases, they found that in line with their earlier work, where the reasons for taking the traditional medicine were known, most cases had taken it for either abdominal pains or aphrodisiac purposes. Nonspecific adverse effects including vomiting, abdominal pains, and diarrhoea were the most commonly encountered. Again in line with their earlier work, Tagwireyi et al. showed that a large proportion of patients with traditional medicine poisoning also suffered from genitourinary tract adverse outcomes especially haematuria and dysuria. In their work the authors speculated that the nephrotoxic effects seen could be due to a number of things including heavy metal contamination of traditional medicines, cantharides, and inherent nephrotoxic effects of the phytomedicines themselves. The authors suggested that further research was required to elucidate the toxic components responsible for the observed ill effects and whether these effects are due to the medicines themselves or to coexisting illnesses. The case fatality rate in this series was 9.5%. The exact culprit agents associated with deaths were not identified.

3.16.9. Plant and Mushroom Poisoning. In view of "a large proportion" of calls to the national Drug and Toxicology Information Service as well as a lack of published data on the toxicoepidemiology and management of Elephant's Ear plant (which is in the Araceae family of plants), Tagwireyi and Ball [121] did a small retrospective series of all cases of Elephant's Ear ingestion. Their study looked at hospital medical records from Parirenyatwa hospital for the period of January 1995–December 1999, inclusive. In their work, the authors reviewed 15 cases of Elephant's Ear plant ingestion and described the

clinical signs and symptoms associated with the exposure. In line with international literature, they also noted that almost all cases occurred in children aged 4 years and below (only one case was in an adult aged 17 years). There were no fatalities in this study.

Mushroom poisoning occurs mainly during the rainy season when these fungi grow. There are a large number of fungi in the world but perhaps the most toxic of these belong to the *Amanita* family of fungi. Flegg [90] reported on 50 cases of mushroom poisoning admissions to Harare hospital for the period from March 1980 to March 1981. As expected, the author found that the bulk of the admissions occurred during the rainy season with 80% of the cases occurring between December 1980 and January 1981. In the paper, the author described the clinical course of all the cases noting that most (80%) of the cases presented with either gastrointestinal symptoms, neurologic symptoms, or both. The case fatality rate in this study was 12% with six deaths. Of these, the postmortem results were available in four and showed evidence of haemorrhage in many organs including the lungs, pericardium, gastrointestinal tract, and urinary tract. In two cases, centrilobular liver necrosis and acute tubular necrosis of the kidneys were present. The author accounted that *Amanita phalloides* had been responsible for all the deaths. The author then went on to describe the identification, toxic chemistry, pharmacokinetics, clinical features, diagnosis, and treatment of poisoning from *Amanita phalloides* mushrooms.

3.16.10. Food Poisoning. Concerning food poisoning, Kasilo and Nhachi [109] reported on 487 cases of food poisoning. In their study, the authors identified mushroom (47%), food-borne, and other related toxins (37%) as the major cases of food poisoning. The case fatality rate in this study was reported as 2.5%. Tagwireyi and colleagues [110] reported a unique case of food poisoning after the ingestion of a poisonous insect *(Mylabris dicincta)*, commonly referred to as the "blister beetle." They gave a detailed case report of this toxic ingestion in a four-year-old girl whom the authors speculated could have mistaken the beetles for the edible *Eulopidae mashona*. The patient presented with classical signs and symptoms of cantharidin poisoning with blistering in the mouth, hypersalivation, haematuria, and abdominal pains. The authors described the management administered to this patient with the consultation of the national poisons information centre. The patient survived the episode and was discharged after nine days of admission. In their paper, the authors presented an overview of the clinical effects of cantharidin toxicity as well as its treatment.

3.16.11. Poisoning from Metals. Kasilo and Nhachi [96] reported on 40 cases of heavy metal poisoning from their retrospective study of six referral hospitals in Zimbabwe (although it is interesting to note that 5 of these were cases of cyanide poisoning). The authors identified eight different metals as culprit agents in the poisoning cases of which copper accounted for the largest proportion (27.5%). The majority of the cases (70%) were in the 18–60-year age range. From the study it is not clear what the case fatality rate was although the authors stated that 5 cases (12.5%) were suicides (they did not stipulate whether these were attempted/failed suicides or completed/successful suicides).

4. Conclusions

The present paper sought to highlight important aspects of the patterns and epidemiology of poisoning in the Eastern African region. From the results presented above, it is evident that pesticides are an important cause of poisoning in the region. In addition, snakebite is also a cause for concern. Also of note was the fact that island countries had patterns of poisoning very different to landlocked countries.

Competing Interests

The authors declare that there are no competing interests regarding the publication of this paper.

Acknowledgments

The authors would like to acknowledge the SAICM steering committee which was overseeing this QSP project and was responsible for reviewing every aspect of the literature review.

References

[1] C. Marks, N. van Hoving, N. Edwards et al., "A promising poison information centre model for Africa," *The African Journal of Emergency Medicine*, vol. 6, no. 2, pp. 64–69, 2016.

[2] WHO, *Improving the Availability of Poison Centre Services in Africa*, World Health Organisation, Geneva, Switzerland, 2015, http://www.who.int/ipcs/poisons/centre/WEB_WHO_PHE_PoisonCentre.pdf.

[3] P. G. Bertrand, H. A. M. Ahmed, R. Ngwafor, and C. Frazzoli, "Toxicovigilance systems and practices in Africa," *Toxics*, vol. 4, no. 3, article 13, 2016.

[4] WHO, *Death and DALY Estimates for 2004 by Cause for Countries: Persons, All Ages by Country*, 2009, http://apps.who.int/gho/data/node.main.1009?lang=en.

[5] A. Benois, F. Petitjeans, L. Raynaud, E. Dardare, and H. Sergent, "Clinical and therapeutic aspects of childhood kerosene poisoning in Djibouti," *Tropical Doctor*, vol. 39, no. 4, pp. 236–238, 2009.

[6] P. Seignot, J. P. Ducourau, P. Ducrot, G. Angel, L. Roussel, and M. Aubert, "Fatal poisoning by an African viper's bite (*Echis carinatus*)," *Annales Françaises d'Anesthésie et de Réanimation*, vol. 11, no. 1, pp. 105–110, 1992.

[7] S. Larréché, G. Mion, A. Mayet et al., "Antivenin remains effective against African Viperidae bites despite a delayed treatment," *The American Journal of Emergency Medicine*, vol. 29, no. 2, pp. 155–161, 2011.

[8] L. Aigle, C. Lions, and F. Mottier, "Management of bluespotted stingray injuries in Djibouti from July 2008 to July 2009," *Médecine Tropicale*, vol. 70, no. 3, pp. 259–263, 2010.

[9] M. Abebe, "Organophosphate pesticide poisoning in 50 Ethiopian patients," *Ethiopian Medical Journal*, vol. 29, no. 3, pp. 109–118, 1991.

[10] A. Aseffa, G. Mengistu, and M. Tiruneh, "Salmonella newport: outbreak of food poisoning among college students due to

[11] A. Alem, D. Kebede, L. Jacobsson, and G. Kullgren, "Suicide attempts among adults in Butajira, Ethiopia," *Acta Psychiatrica Scandinavica*, vol. 100, no. S397, pp. 70–76, 1999.

[12] T. Abula and Y. Wondmikun, "The pattern of acute poisoning in a teaching hospital, north-west Ethiopia," *Ethiopian Medical Journal*, vol. 44, no. 2, pp. 183–189, 2006.

[13] Z. Melaku, M. Alemayehu, K. Oli, and G. Tizazu, "Pattern of admissions to the medical intensive care unit of Addis Ababa University Teaching Hospital," *Ethiopian Medical Journal*, vol. 44, no. 1, pp. 33–42, 2006.

[14] M. Desalew, A. Aklilu, A. Amanuel, M. Addisu, and T. Ethiopia, "Pattern of acute adult poisoning at Tikur Anbessa specialized teaching hospital, a retrospective study, Ethiopia," *Human & Experimental Toxicology*, vol. 30, no. 7, pp. 523–527, 2011.

[15] A. Azahz, "Severe organophosphate poisoning with delayed cholinergic crisis, intermediate syndrome and organophosphate induced delayed polyneuropathy on succession," *Ethiopian Journal of Health Science*, vol. 21, no. 3, pp. 203–208, 2011.

[16] P. Selassie, "Organophosphate poisoning in Jimma," *Ethiopian Journal of Health Sciences*, vol. 8, no. 1, pp. 47–52, 1998.

[17] K. Makita, F. Desissa, A. Teklu, G. Zewde, and D. Grace, "Risk assessment of staphylococcal poisoning due to consumption of informally-marketed milk and home-made yoghurt in Debre Zeit, Ethiopia," *International Journal of Food Microbiology*, vol. 153, no. 1-2, pp. 135–141, 2012.

[18] A. Aga and A. Geyid, "An outbreak of acute toxicity caused by eating food contaminated with Datura stramonium," *Ethiopian Journal of Health Development*, vol. 6, pp. 25–31, 1992.

[19] A. D. Charters, "Mushroom poisoning in Kenya," *Transactions of the Royal Society of Tropical Medicine and Hygiene*, vol. 51, no. 3, pp. 265–270, 1957.

[20] R. A. Davidson, "Case of African cobra bite," *The British Medical Journal*, vol. 4, no. 736, p. 660, 1970.

[21] P. M. Mwangemi, "Poisonous snake bite—a reappraisal," *East African Medical Journal*, vol. 53, no. 11, pp. 657–659, 1976.

[22] R. Greenham, "Spitting Cobra (*Naja mossambica pallida*) bite in a Kenyan child," *Transactions of the Royal Society of Tropical Medicine and Hygiene*, vol. 72, no. 6, pp. 674–675, 1978.

[23] D. H. Smith, G. L. Timms, and M. Refai, "Outbreak of botulism in Kenyan nomads," *Annals of Tropical Medicine and Parasitology*, vol. 73, no. 2, pp. 145–148, 1979.

[24] S. K. Kahuho, "Occasional report: drug poisoning in the intensive Intensive Care Unit, Kenyatta National Hospital," *East African Medical Journal*, vol. 57, no. 7, pp. 490–494, 1980.

[25] A. Ngindu, P. R. Kenya, D. M. Ocheng et al., "Outbreak of acute hepatitis caused by aflatoxin poisoning in Kenya," *The Lancet*, vol. 319, no. 8285, pp. 1346–1348, 1982.

[26] R. W. Snow, R. Bronzan, T. Roques, C. Nyamawi, S. Murphy, and K. Marsh, "The prevalence and morbidity of snake bite and treatment-seeking behaviour among a rural Kenyan population," *Annals of Tropical Medicine and Parasitology*, vol. 88, no. 6, pp. 665–671, 1994.

[27] M. D. Coombs, S. J. Dunachie, S. Brooker, J. Haynes, J. Church, and D. A. Warrell, "Snake bites in Kenya: a preliminary survey of four areas," *Transactions of the Royal Society of Tropical Medicine and Hygiene*, vol. 91, no. 3, pp. 319–321, 1997.

[28] Centers for Disease Control and Prevention (CDC), "Outbreak of aflatoxin poisoning—eastern and central provinces, Kenya,

contaminated undercooked eggs," *Ethiopian Medical Journal*, vol. 32, no. 1, pp. 1–6, 1994.

January–July 2004," *Morbidity and Mortality Weekly Report*, vol. 53, no. 34, pp. 790–793, 2004.

[29] C. K. Maitai, I. O. Kibwage, A. N. Guantai, J. N. Ombega, and F. A. Ndemo, "A retrospective study of childhood poisoning in Kenya in 1991– 93," *East and Central African Journal of Pharmaceutical Sciences*, vol. 1, no. 1, pp. 7–10, 1998.

[30] T. Lang, N. Thuo, and S. Akech, "Accidental paraffin poisoning in Kenyan children," *Tropical Medicine & International Health*, vol. 13, no. 6, pp. 845–847, 2008.

[31] C. O. Musumba, A. O. Pamba, P. A. Sasi, M. English, and K. Maitland, "Salicylate poisoning in children: report of three cases," *East African Medical Journal*, vol. 81, no. 3, pp. 159–163, 2004.

[32] C. Mbakaya, G. Ohayo-Mitoko, V. Ngowi et al., "The status of pesticide usage in East Africa," *African Journal of Health Sciences*, vol. 1, article 37, 1994.

[33] BBC News, 2000, http://news.bbc.co.uk/2/hi/africa/1032331.stm.

[34] Ministry of Environment and Mineral Resources Kenya, *Kenya National Profile to Assess the Chemicals Management*, 2011, http://cwm.unitar.org/national-profiles/publications/cw/np/np_pdf/Kenya_National_Profile_final.pdf.

[35] D. G. Nyamu, C. K. Maitai, L. W. Mecca, and E. M. Mwangangi, "Trends of acute poisoning cases occurring at the Kenyatta National Hospital, Nairobi, Kenya," *East and Central African Journal of Pharmaceutical Sciences*, vol. 15, no. 2, pp. 29–34, 2012.

[36] R. Vicens, N. Rasolofonirina, and P. Coulanges, "First human cases of food-induced botulism in Madagascar," *Archives de l'Institut Pasteur de Madagascar*, vol. 52, no. 1, pp. 11–21, 1986.

[37] C. A. Domergue, "A venomous snake of Madagascar. 2 case reports of bites by Madagascarophis (Colubrida opisthoglypha)," *Archives de l'Institut Pasteur de Madagascar*, vol. 56, no. 1, pp. 299–311, 1989.

[38] G. G. Habermehl, H. C. Krebs, P. Rasoanaivo, and A. Ramialiharisoa, "Severe ciguatera poisoning in Madagascar: a case report," *Toxicon*, vol. 32, no. 12, pp. 1539–1542, 1994.

[39] A. Ramialiharisoa, L. De Haro, J. Jouglard, and M. Goyffon, "Latrodectism in Madagascar," *Medecine Tropicale*, vol. 54, no. 2, pp. 127–130, 1994.

[40] A. Ramialiharisoa, R. Rafenoherimanana, L. de Haro, and J. Jouglard, "Collective poisoning of ciguateric type after ingestion of shark in Madagascar. Data collected by the Antananarivo medical team," *Presse Médicale*, vol. 25, no. 29, article 1350, 1996.

[41] A. Ramialiharisoa, L. Razafindraktoto, and P. Rasoanaivo, "Shark poisoning in Madagascar: a case report," *African Journal of Health Sciences*, vol. 4, no. 1, pp. 33–34, 1997.

[42] G. Ranaivoson, G. Champetier de Ribes, E. R. Mamy, G. Jeannerod, P. Razafinjato, and S. Chanteau, "Mass food poisoning after eating sea turtle in the Antalaha district," *Archives de l'Institut Pasteur de Madagascar*, vol. 61, no. 2, pp. 84–86, 1994.

[43] P. Boisier, G. Ranaivoson, N. Rasolofonirina et al., "Fatal ichthyosarcotoxism after eating shark meat. Implications of two new marine toxins," *Archives de l'Institut Pasteur de Madagascar*, vol. 61, no. 2, pp. 81–83, 1994.

[44] G. Champetier De Ribes, G. Ranaivoson, N. Ravaonindrina et al., "Un problème de santé réémergent à Madagascar: les intoxications collectives par consommation d'animaux marins. Aspects épidémiologiques, cliniques et toxicologiques des épisodes notifiés de janvier 1993 à janvier 1998," *Archives de l'Institut Pasteur de Madagascar*, vol. 64, pp. 71–76, 1998.

[45] G. C. Ribes, S. Ramarokoto, S. Rabearintsoa et al., "Seafood poisoning in Madagascar: current state of knowledge and results of a retrospective study of the inhabitants of coastal villages," *Sante*, vol. 9, no. 4, pp. 235–241, 1999.

[46] R. Robinson, R. G. Champetier, G. Ranaivoson, M. Rejely, and D. Rabeson, "KAP study (knowledge-attitude-practice) on seafood poisoning on the southwest coast of Madagascar," *Bulletin de la Société de Pathologie Exotique*, vol. 92, no. 1, pp. 46–50, 1999.

[47] N. Ravaonindrina, T. H. Andriamaso, and N. Rasolofonirina, "Puffer fish poisoning in Madagascar: four case reports," *Archives de l'Institut Pasteur de Madagascar*, vol. 67, no. 1-2, pp. 61–64, 2001.

[48] D. A. O'Reilly and G. T. Heikens, "Organophosphate poisoning in a 12-day-old infant: case report," *Annals of Tropical Paediatrics*, vol. 31, no. 3, pp. 263–267, 2011.

[49] C. Chibwana, T. Mhango, and E. M. Molyneux, "Childhood poisoning at the Queen Elizabeth Central Hospital, Blantyre, Malawi," *East African Medical Journal*, vol. 78, no. 6, pp. 292–295, 2001.

[50] C. P. Dzamalala, D. A. Milner, and N. G. Liomba, "Suicide in Blantyre, Malawi (2000–2003)," *Journal of Clinical Forensic Medicine*, vol. 13, no. 2, pp. 65–69, 2006.

[51] K. L. Yu, C. N. Bong, M. C. Huang et al., "The use of hospital medical records for child injury surveillance in northern Malawi," *Tropical Doctor*, vol. 39, no. 3, pp. 170–172, 2009.

[52] M. Glaizal, L. Tichadou, G. Drouet, M. Hayek-Lanthois, and L. De Haro, "Ciguatera contracted by French tourists in Mauritius recurs in Senegal," *Clinical Toxicology*, vol. 49, no. 8, p. 767, 2011.

[53] Ministry Of Health-Mozambique, "Mantakassa: an epidemic of spastic paraparesis associated with chronic cyanide intoxication in a cassava staple area of Mozambique. 1. Epidemiology and clinical and laboratory findings in patients. Ministry of Health, Mozambique," *Bulletin of the World Health Organization*, vol. 62, no. 3, pp. 477–484, 1984.

[54] J. Cliff, S. Essers, and H. Rosling, "Ankle clonus correlating with cyanide intake from cassava in rural children from Mozambique," *Journal of Tropical Pediatrics*, vol. 32, no. 4, pp. 186–189, 1986.

[55] E. Casadei, J. Cliff, and J. Neves, "Surveillance of urinary thiocyanate concentration after epidemic spastic paraparesis in Mozambique," *Journal of Tropical Medicine and Hygiene*, vol. 93, no. 4, pp. 257–261, 1990.

[56] J. Cliff and J. Coutinho, "Acute intoxication from newly-introduced cassava during drought in Mozambique," *Tropical doctor*, vol. 25, no. 4, p. 193, 1995.

[57] J. Cliff, D. Nicala, F. Saute et al., "Konzo associated with war in Mozambique," *Tropical Medicine & International Health*, vol. 2, no. 11, pp. 1068–1074, 1997.

[58] J. Cliff, D. Nicala, F. Saute et al., "Ankle clonus and thiocyanate, linamarin, and inorganic sulphate excretion in school children in communities with konzo, Mozambique," *Journal of Tropical Pediatrics*, vol. 45, no. 3, pp. 139–142, 1999.

[59] M. Ernesto, A. P. Cardoso, D. Nicala et al., "Persistent konzo and cyanogen toxicity from cassava in northern Mozambique," *Acta Tropica*, vol. 82, no. 3, pp. 357–362, 2002.

[60] J. Lagraulet, "Ichtyotoxism in the Seychelles Islands," *Bulletin de la Societé de Pathologie Exotique et de ses Filiales*, vol. 68, p. 115, 1975.

[61] G. J. Myers, S. W. Thurston, A. T. Pearson et al., "Postnatal exposure to methyl mercury from fish consumption: a review and new data from the Seychelles Child Development Study," *NeuroToxicology*, vol. 30, no. 3, pp. 338–349, 2009.

[62] N. O. Bwibo, "Accidental poisoning in children in Uganda," *British Medical Journal*, vol. 4, no. 683, pp. 601–602, 1969.

[63] L. J. Cardozo and R. D. Mugerwa, "The pattern of acute poisoning in Uganda," *East African Medical Journal*, vol. 49, no. 12, pp. 983–988, 1972.

[64] E. Kinyanda, H. Hjelmeland, and S. Musisi, "Deliberate self-harm as seen in Kampala, Uganda," *Social Psychiatry and Psychiatric Epidemiology*, vol. 39, no. 4, pp. 318–325, 2004.

[65] N. Malangu, "Acute poisoning at two hospitals in Kampala-Uganda," *Journal of Forensic and Legal Medicine*, vol. 15, no. 8, pp. 489–492, 2008.

[66] "Uganda Office of the President 2009 Press release on methanol poisoning," http://www.digitaljournal.com/article/291234#ixzz2Dbx447JW.

[67] DIGITAL JOURNAL, Home-made brew laced with methanol kills 89 in Uganda, April 2010, http://digitaljournal.com/article/291234#ixzz2Dbx447JW.

[68] H. T. Rwiza, "Jimson weed food poisoning. An epidemic at Usangi rural government hospital," *Tropical and Geographical Medicine*, vol. 43, no. 1-2, pp. 85–90, 1991.

[69] V. M. Yates, E. Lebas, R. Orpiay, and B. J. Bale, "Management of snakebites by the staff of a rural clinic: the impact of providing free antivenom in a nurse-led clinic in Meserani, Tanzania," *Annals of Tropical Medicine and Parasitology*, vol. 104, no. 5, pp. 439–448, 2010.

[70] W. P. Howlett, G. R. Brubaker, N. Mlingi, and H. Rosling, "Konzo, an epidemic upper motor neuron disease studied in Tanzania," *Brain*, vol. 113, no. 1, pp. 223–235, 1990.

[71] W. Howlett, G. Brubaker, N. Mlingi, and H. Rosling, "A geographical cluster of konzo in Tanzania," *Journal of Tropical and Geographical Neurology*, vol. 2, pp. 102–108, 1992.

[72] N. Mlingi, S. Kimatta, and H. Rosling, "Konzo, a paralytic disease observed in southern Tanzania," *Tropical Doctor*, vol. 21, no. 1, pp. 24–25, 1991.

[73] N. L. V. Mlingi, S. Nkya, S. R. Tatala, S. Rashid, and J. H. Bradbury, "Recurrence of konzo in southern Tanzania: rehabilitation and prevention using the wetting method," *Food and Chemical Toxicology*, vol. 49, no. 3, pp. 673–677, 2011.

[74] N. K. Ndosi, M. P. Mbonde, and E. Lyamuya, "Profile of suicide in Dar es Salaam," *East African Medical Journal*, vol. 81, no. 4, pp. 207–211, 2004.

[75] G. V. Gill, "Mushroom poisoning in Zambia," *East African Medical Journal*, vol. 56, no. 4, pp. 178–181, 1979.

[76] V. Bhushan, C. Chintu, and K. Gupta, "Accidental poisoning in children in Lusaka," *Medical Journal of Zambia*, vol. 13, no. 4, pp. 61–63, 1979.

[77] H. B. P. E. Gernaat, W. H. J. C. Dechering, and H. W. A. Voorhoeve, "Clinical epidemiology of paediatric disease at Nchelenge, north-east Zambia," *Annals of Tropical Paediatrics*, vol. 18, no. 2, pp. 129–138, 1998.

[78] J. R. Sinclair, D. A. K. Watters, and A. Baghsaw, "Non-traumatic coma in Zambia," *Tropical Doctor*, vol. 19, no. 1, pp. 6–10, 1989.

[79] C. F. B. Nhachi and O. M. J. Kasilo, "The pattern of poisoning in urban Zimbabwe," *Journal of Applied Toxicology*, vol. 12, no. 6, pp. 435–438, 1992.

[80] D. Tagwireyi, D. E. Ball, and C. F. B. Nhachi, "Poisoning in Zimbabwe: a survey of eight major referral hospitals," *Journal of Applied Toxicology*, vol. 22, no. 2, pp. 99–105, 2002.

[81] D. Tagwireyi, D. E. Ball, and C. F. B. Nhachi, "Differences and similarities in poisoning admissions between urban and rural health centers in Zimbabwe," *Clinical Toxicology*, vol. 44, no. 3, pp. 233–241, 2006.

[82] X. Dong and M. A. Simon, "The epidemiology of organophosphate poisoning in urban Zimbabwe from 1995 to 2000," *International Journal of Occupational and Environmental Health*, vol. 7, no. 4, pp. 333–338, 2001.

[83] O. J. Kasilo, T. Hobane, and C. F. B. Nhachi, "Organophosphate poisoning in urban Zimbabwe," *Journal of Applied Toxicology*, vol. 11, no. 4, pp. 269–272, 1991.

[84] C. F. B. Nhachi, "An evaluation of organophosphate poisoning cases in an urban setting in Zimbabwe," *East African Medical Journal*, vol. 65, no. 9, pp. 588–592, 1988.

[85] N. Z. Nyazema, "Poisoning due to traditional remedies," *Central African Journal of Medicine*, vol. 30, no. 5, pp. 80–83, 1984.

[86] O. M. J. Kasilo and C. F. B. Nhachi, "A pattern of acute poisoning in children in urban Zimbabwe: ten years experience," *Human & Experimental Toxicology*, vol. 11, no. 5, pp. 335–340, 1992.

[87] O. M. J. Kasilo and C. F. B. Nhachi, "The pattern of poisoning from traditional medicines in urban Zimbabwe," *South African Medical Journal*, vol. 82, no. 3, pp. 187–188, 1992.

[88] D. Tagwireyi and D. E. Ball, "'Muti' poisoning in Zimbabwe," *Tropical Doctor*, vol. 32, no. 1, pp. 41–42, 2002.

[89] D. Tagwireyi, D. E. Ball, and C. F. B. Nhachi, "Traditional medicine poisoning in Zimbabwe: clinical presentation and management in adults," *Human & Experimental Toxicology*, vol. 21, no. 11, pp. 579–586, 2002.

[90] P. J. Flegg, "Mushroom poisoning," *The Central African Journal of Medicine*, vol. 27, no. 7, pp. 125–129, 1981.

[91] D. Tagwireyi, D. Ball, and C. Nhachi, "Childhood poisoning in Zimbabwe," *Journal of Toxicology. Clinical Toxicology*, vol. 40, p. 336, 2002.

[92] I. Chitsike, "Acute poisoning in a paediatric intensive care unit in Harare," *The Central African Journal of Medicine*, vol. 40, no. 11, pp. 315–319, 1994.

[93] R. S. Blaylock, "Snake bites at Triangle Hospital January 1975 to June 1981," *Central African Journal of Medicine*, vol. 28, pp. 1–10, 1982.

[94] J. Geddes and J. E. P. Thomas, "Boomslang bite—a case report," *The Central African Journal of Medicine*, vol. 31, no. 6, pp. 109–112, 1985.

[95] O. M. J. Kasilo and C. F. B. Nhachi, "A retrospective study of poisoning due to snake venom in Zimbabwe," *Human & Experimental Toxicology*, vol. 12, no. 1, pp. 15–18, 1993.

[96] O. M. J. Kasilo and C. F. B. Nhachi, "Survey of chemical (mostly metals) poisoning cases as reflected in hospital admissions in urban Zimbabwe," *Bulletin of Environmental Contamination and Toxicology*, vol. 50, no. 2, pp. 260–265, 1993.

[97] G. I. Muguti, A. Maramba, and C. T. Washaya, "Snake bites in Zimbabwe: a clinical study with emphasis on the need for antivenom," *The Central African Journal of Medicine*, vol. 40, no. 4, pp. 83–88, 1994.

[98] C. F. B. Nhachi and O. M. J. Kasilo, "Household chemicals poisoning admissions in Zimbabwe's main urban centres," *Human & Experimental Toxicology*, vol. 13, no. 2, pp. 69–72, 1994.

[99] C. F. B. Nhachi and O. M. J. Kasilo, "Snake poisoning in rural Zimbabwe—a prospective study," *Journal of Applied Toxicology*, vol. 14, no. 3, pp. 191–193, 1994.

[100] G. I. Muguti and M. Dube, "Severe envenomation by a 'pet' vine snake," *The Central African Journal of Medicine*, vol. 44, no. 9, pp. 232–234, 1998.

[101] D. Tagwireyi, D. E. Ball, and C. F. B. Nhachi, "Snakebite admissions to major hospitals in zimbabwe," *Journal of Toxicology. Clinical Toxicology*, vol. 42, no. 5, p. 766, 2004.

[102] D. Tagwireyi, C. F. Nhachi, and D. E. Ball, "Snakebite admissions in Zimbabwe: pattern, clinical presentation and management," *The Central African Journal of Medicine*, vol. 57, no. 5–8, pp. 17–22, 2011.

[103] D. Tagwireyi, D. E. Ball, and C. F. B. Nhachi, "Toxicoepidemiology in Zimbabwe: admissions resulting from exposure to paraffin (Kerosene)," *Clinical Toxicology*, vol. 44, pp. 103–107, 2006.

[104] N. J. Bergman, "Scorpion sting in Zimbabwe," *South African Medical Journal*, vol. 87, no. 2, pp. 163–167, 1997.

[105] N. J. Bergman, "Clinical description of *Parabuthus transvaalicus* scorpionism in Zimbabwe," *Toxicon*, vol. 35, no. 5, pp. 759–771, 1997.

[106] C. R. Saunders and A. B. Morar, "Beware the scorpion *Parabuthus*," *The Central African Journal of Medicine*, vol. 36, no. 4, pp. 114–115, 1990.

[107] C. F. B. Nhachi and O. M. J. Kasilo, "Poisoning due to insect and scorpion stings/bites," *Human & Experimental Toxicology*, vol. 12, no. 2, pp. 123–125, 1993.

[108] D. Tagwireyi and D. E. Ball, "Hospital admissions due to scorpion sting in zimbabwe," *Journal of Applied Sciences in Southern Africa*, vol. 17, no. 2, pp. 1–9, 2011.

[109] O. M. J. Kasilo and C. F. B. Nhachi, "Food poisoning admissions in referral hospitals in Zimbabwe: a retrospective study," *Human & Experimental Toxicology*, vol. 13, no. 2, pp. 77–82, 1994.

[110] D. Tagwireyi, D. E. Ball, P. J. Loga, and S. Moyo, "Cantharidin poisoning due to 'Blister Beetle' ingestion," *Toxicon*, vol. 38, no. 12, pp. 1865–1869, 2000.

[111] C. F. B. Nhachi, T. Habane, P. Satumba, and O. M. J. Kasilo, "Aspects of orthodox medicines (therapeutic drugs) poisoning in urban Zimbabwe," *Human & Experimental Toxicology*, vol. 11, no. 5, pp. 329–333, 1992.

[112] H. F. Queen, C. Tapfumaneyi, and R. J. Lewis, "The rising incidence of serious chloroquine overdose in Harare, Zimbabwe: emergency department surveillance in the developing world," *Tropical Doctor*, vol. 29, no. 3, pp. 139–141, 1999.

[113] A. G. McKenzie, "Intensive therapy for chloroquine poisoning. A review of 29 cases," *South African Medical Journal*, vol. 86, no. 5, pp. 597–599, 1996.

[114] D. E. Ball, D. Tagwireyi, and C. F. B. Nhachi, "Chloroquine poisoning in Zimbabwe: a toxicoepidemiological study," *Journal of Applied Toxicology*, vol. 22, no. 5, pp. 311–315, 2002.

[115] D. Tagwireyi, D. E. Ball, and C. F. B. Nhachi, "Toxicoepidemiology in Zimbabwe: pesticide poisoning admissions to major hospitals," *Clinical Toxicology*, vol. 44, no. 1, pp. 59–66, 2006.

[116] A. Akida, M. Isinta, F. Ndiawo, D. Agedo, and J. Tsinanga, "(P2-54) legislation shaped by an emergency: methanol poisoning experience at Kenyatta National Hospital, Kenya," *Prehospital and Disaster Medicine*, vol. 26, pp. s161–s162, 2011.

[117] The New Times, "Over 200 hospitalised after food poisoning," 2012, http://www.newtimes.co.rw/news/index.php?i=15008&a=54217.

[118] The Rwanda Express, "50 Residents admitted over food poisoning," 2012, http://rwandaexpress.blogspot.com/2012/06/rwanda-50-residents-admitted-over-food.html.

[119] S. W. Lubwama, "Human *Salmonella serotypes* in Uganda, 1967–1982," *East African Medical Journal*, vol. 62, no. 4, pp. 260–265, 1985.

[120] N. Z. Nyazema, "Herbal toxicity in Zimbabwe," *Transactions of the Royal Society of Tropical Medicine and Hygiene*, vol. 80, no. 3, pp. 448–450, 1986.

[121] D. Tagwireyi and D. E. Ball, "The management of Elephant's Ear poisoning," *Human & Experimental Toxicology*, vol. 20, no. 4, pp. 189–192, 2001.

18

Possible Protective Effect of Diacerein on Doxorubicin-Induced Nephrotoxicity in Rats

Marwa M. M. Refaie,[1] Entesar F. Amin,[1] Nashwa F. El-Tahawy,[2] and Aly M. Abdelrahman[1]

[1]*Department of Pharmacology, Faculty of Medicine, El-Minia University, El-Minia 61111, Egypt*
[2]*Department of Histology, Faculty of Medicine, El-Minia University, El-Minia 61111, Egypt*

Correspondence should be addressed to Marwa M. M. Refaie; marwamonier@yahoo.com

Academic Editor: Maria Teresa Colomina

Nephrotoxicity is one of the limiting factors for using doxorubicin (DOX). Interleukin 1 has major role in DOX-induced nephrotoxicity, so we investigated the effect of interleukin 1 receptor antagonist diacerein (DIA) on DOX-induced nephrotoxicity. DIA (25 and 50 mg/kg/day) was administered orally to rats for 15 days, in the presence or absence of nephrotoxicity induced by a single intraperitoneal injection of DOX (15 mg/kg) at the 11th day. We measured levels of serum urea, creatinine, renal reduced glutathione (GSH), malondialdehyde (MDA), total nitrites (NO_x), catalase, and superoxide dismutase (SOD). In addition, caspase-3, tumor necrosis factor alpha (TNFα), nuclear factor kappa B (NFκB) expressions, and renal histopathology were assessed. Our results showed that DOX-induced nephrotoxicity was ameliorated or reduced by both doses of DIA, but diacerein high dose (DHD) showed more improvement than diacerein low dose (DLD). This protective effect was manifested by significant improvement in all measured parameters compared to DOX treated group by using DHD. DLD showed significant improvement of creatinine, MDA, NO_x, GSH, histopathology, and immunohistochemical parameters compared to DOX treated group.

1. Introduction

Drug-induced nephrotoxicity is a major cause of acute kidney injury [1]. DOX is one of the key chemotherapeutic drugs for cancer treatment, but its use is limited by chronic and acute toxic side effects [2]. DOX is an antibiotic anthracycline that was isolated from a pigment of *Streptomyces peucetius* in the early 1960s and it had been employed for more than 30 years in the battle against cancer, but it is now chemically synthesized [3]. The exact mechanism of DOX-induced nephrotoxicity is not yet completely understood. Renal DOX-induced toxicity may be part of a multiorgan damage mediated mainly through free radical formation eventually leading to membrane lipid peroxidation [4]. Induction of apoptosis and modulation of NO_x are mechanisms that are involved in toxic adverse effects associated with DOX therapy [5]. In addition, DOX has a direct renal damaging effect as it accumulates preferentially in the kidney. DOX has toxic effects on other organs such as heart and liver which may lead to modulation of blood supply to the kidney and alter xenobiotic detoxification processes, respectively,

thus indirectly contributing to DOX-induced nephropathy [6].

DIA is a new anti-inflammatory, analgesic, and antipyretic drug that was developed specially for the treatment of osteoarthritis [7]. It is highly effective in relieving the symptoms of osteoarthritis and may be able to modify the course of the disease [7]. DIA acts by inhibiting the production of interleukin 1 by human monocytes [8]. Interleukin 1 is a proinflammatory and proapoptotic agent that induces cytokine production by activating NFκB and mitogen activated protein kinase signaling [9]. A major cause of DOX-induced nephrotoxicity is the production of reactive oxygen species which induce cytokines, including interleukin 1 [6, 9, 10]. The aim of the present study was to study the effect of the interleukin 1 receptor antagonist diacerein (DIA) on DOX-induced nephropathy.

2. Materials and Methods

2.1. Chemicals. DIA powder was from Eva Pharma Company and it was dissolved in 1% carboxymethylcellulose. DOX hydrochloride 10 mg vial (Pharmacia Italia, SPA, Italy), polyclonal rabbit/antirat caspase-3, TNFα, and NFκB antibody (Lab Vision, USA), biotinylated goat anti-rabbit secondary antibody (Transduction Laboratories, USA), urea, GSH, SOD, and catalase kits (Biodiagnostic, Egypt), and creatinine (Humen, Germany) were purchased.

2.2. Animals. Adult male Wistar rats weighing about 250–350 g were obtained from the Animal Research Centre, Giza, Egypt. Animals were kept in standard housing conditions in cages and were left to acclimatize for one week. Rats were supplied with laboratory chow and tap water. This work was conducted in the Pharmacology Department, Faculty of Medicine, El-Minia University, Egypt, and the animal experimental protocol was approved by the faculty board.

2.3. Experimental Design. Rats were randomly assigned into 6 groups ($n = 6$ each) as follows.

> Group I received vehicle (1% carboxymethylcellulose) for 15 days and ip saline at day 11.
>
> Group II was treated with DLD (25 mg/kg/d orally) for 15 days and ip saline at day 11.
>
> Group III was treated with DHD (50 mg/kg/d orally) and ip saline at day 11.
>
> Group IV was treated with vehicle for 15 days and DOX (15 mg/kg) at day 11.
>
> Group V was treated with DLD (25 mg/kg/d orally) for 15 days + ip injection of DOX (15 mg/kg) at day 11.
>
> Group VI was treated with DHD (50 mg/kg/d orally) for 15 days + ip injection of DOX (15 mg/kg) at day 11. The doses of DOX and DIA were based on the previous studies [4, 11].

2.4. Evaluation of Renal Function. After 4 days of DOX injection, each rat was weighed then anesthetized with ip injection of urethane (25% in a dose of 1.6 gm/kg) and then sacrificed.

Venous blood samples were collected from the jugular vein.

Serum was collected for biochemical analysis of urea [12] and creatinine [13]. They were determined using colorimetric diagnostic kits according to the manufacturer's instructions.

After sacrifice, both kidneys were rapidly excised and weighed.

A longitudinal section of the left kidney and one half was fixed in 10% formalin then embedded in paraffin for histopathological and immunohistochemical examinations. The rest of the kidneys were snap frozen in liquid nitrogen and kept at −80°C.

2.5. Evaluation of GSH. GSH spectrophotometric kit was used. Briefly, the method is based on the fact that sulfhydryl group of GSH reacts with 5, 5′-dithiobis (2-nitrobenzoic acid) (Ellman's reagent) and produces a yellow colored 5-thio-2-nitrobenzoic acid which was measured colorimetrically

at 405 nm using Beckman DU-64 UV/VIS spectrophotometer, USA. Results were expressed as mmol/g tissue [14].

2.6. Evaluation of Renal Catalase Levels. Assessment of renal catalase antioxidant enzyme activity was determined from the rate of decomposition of H_2O_2 at 510 nm after the addition of tissue homogenate as described by colorimetric kit. The results were expressed as unit/g tissue [15].

2.7. Evaluation of SOD Levels. The assessments of SOD levels were based on the ability of the enzyme to inhibit the phenazine methosulfate-mediated reduction of nitroblue tetrazolium dye and the results were expressed as unit/g tissue [16].

2.8. Assessment of Renal Lipid Peroxides

2.8.1. Principle. The renal contents of lipid peroxides were assayed by a spectrophotometric method based on the reaction between MDA and thiobarbituric acid [17].

2.8.2. Procedure. The absorbance values of the samples and the blank were determined at 535 nm using a (Beckman DU-64 spectrophotometer, USA) and then blank absorbance value was subtracted from the sample absorbance value. From a standard curve, MDA concentration in the unknown sample was extrapolated from the corresponding absorbance using the regression line from the standard curve and expressed as nmol/gm tissue by multiplying in the tissue dilution factor.

2.9. Assessment of NO_x Levels

2.9.1. Principle. Nitric oxide (NO) in the form of nitrite was determined with spectrophotometric method using Griess reagent systems. The stable oxidation end products of NO, nitrite (NO_2^-), and nitrate (NO_3^-) were used as indicators of NO production. NO_x was measured after the reduction of nitrate to nitrite by copperized cadmium granules in glycine buffer at pH 9.7. Quantification of NO_2^- was based on the Griess reaction, in which a chromophore with a strong absorbance at 540 nm is formed by the reaction of nitrite with a mixture of N-naphthylene diamine and sulfanilamide [18]. The absorbance of the sample and the blank were measured at 545 nm using (Beckman DU-64 spectrophotometer, USA). The blank absorbance is then subtracted from the sample absorbance.

From a standard curve, NO_x content in the unknown sample was extrapolated from the corresponding absorbance using the regression line from the standard curve and expressed as nmol/g tissue.

2.10. Histological Examination. Renal tissue was fixed in 10% formalin, embedded in paraffin, sectioned by a microtome at 5 μm thickness and stained with hematoxylin and eosin for routine histopathological assessment.

TABLE 1: Effect of DLD (25 mg/kg/day) and DHD (50 mg/kg/day) on serum creatinine, serum urea, MDA, and NO_x levels in DOX -induced nephrotoxicity (15 mg/kg).

Group	Creatinine (mg/dL)	Urea (mg/dL)	MDA (nmol/g tissue)	NO_x (nmol/g tissue)
Control	0.8828 ± 0.07291	50.26 ± 4.450	42.27 ± 2.202	179.5 ± 11.98
DLD	0.7395 ± 0.06486	51.75 ± 1.721	44.77 ± 2.098	272.8 ± 22.35
DHD	0.9540 ± 0.08678	53.73 ± 2.989	52.02 ± 5.036	295.0 ± 20.25
DOX	1.475 ± 0.0522^a	251.8 ± 12.23^a	250.9 ± 16.37^a	1114 ± 64.29^a
DOX/DLD	1.211 ± 0.0660^{ab}	241.7 ± 13.17^a	51.86 ± 4.461^b	322.8 ± 11.33^{ab}
DOX/DHD	1.153 ± 0.0209^{ab}	69.74 ± 4.161^b	46.79 ± 1.39^b	228.5 ± 18.83^b

Values are representation of 4–6 observations as means ± SEM. Results are considered significantly different when $P < 0.05$. [a] Significant difference compared to control; [b] significant difference compared to DOX group.

TABLE 2: Effect of DLD (25 mg/kg/day) and DHD (50 mg/kg/day) on GSH, catalase, and SOD in DOX (15 mg/kg) induced nephrotoxicity.

Group	GSH (mmol/g tissue)	Catalase (unit/g tissue)	SOD (unit/g tissue)
Control	10.32 ± 0.2999	92.10 ± 2.835	829.7 ± 5.182
DLD	10.22 ± 0.5530	91.53 ± 1.860	832.0 ± 6.915
DHD	9.085 ± 0.3000	91.80 ± 2.127	826.6 ± 7.575
DOX	4.814 ± 0.1630^a	72.49 ± 3.662^a	657.6 ± 15.28^a
DOX/DLD	8.678 ± 0.1985^{ab}	80.48 ± 4.108	722.7 ± 41.13^a
DOX/DHD	9.215 ± 0.2814^b	8627 ± 4.496^b	807.3 ± 16.96^b

Values are representation of 4–6 observations as means ± SEM. Results are considered significantly different when $P < 0.05$. [a] Significant difference compared to control; [b] significant difference compared to DOX group.

2.10.1. Morphometric Study. The renal tissues were examined in random microscopic areas semiquantitatively under 40 high power fields and the number of changes was assessed by the counting of 3 nonoverlapped fields for the same slide of each animal. The frequency and the severity of lesions in the kidneys were assessed semiquantitatively as follows: Score −: assigned normal, Score +: in between normal and mild, Score ++ (mild level): less than 25% of the examined fields revealed histological alterations, Score +++ (moderate level): less than 50% of the examined fields revealed histological alterations, and Score ++++ (severe level): less than 75% of the total fields examined revealed histological alterations [19].

2.11. Immunohistochemical Examination. The caspase-3, TNFα, and NFκB immunolabeled cells were counted. In each animal, 3 sections were examined and the cells were counted in 3 adjacent nonoverlapping fields levels. Immunohistochemical staining was performed for caspase-3, TNFα, and NFκB using polyclonal rabbit/antirat antibody according to previously published protocol [20, 21], respectively.

2.12. Statistical Analysis. Data was analyzed by one way ANOVA followed by Dunnett multiple comparison test. The values are represented as means ± SEM. Statistical analysis was done using GraphPad Prism software (version 5). The differences were considered significant when the calculated P value is less than 0.05.

3. Results

3.1. Effect of DIA on Urea and Creatinine in DOX Treated Rats. Table 1 shows the results of the effect of DIA on serum creatinine and urea. Rats receiving a single dose of DOX (15 mg/kg, ip) showed a significant increase in serum creatinine and urea levels compared to control group. Both doses of DIA resulted in significant decrease in serum creatinine compared to DOX treated rats. DIA 50 mg/kg/day but not 25 mg/kg/day resulted in significant decrease in serum urea compared to DOX treated rats.

3.2. Effect of DIA on MDA and NO_x Levels in DOX-Induced Nephrotoxicity. Renal MDA was evaluated as an indicator of kidney lipid peroxidation and nitrites and nitrates as an indicator of renal NO_x levels (Table 1). DOX (15 mg/kg) significantly increased renal MDA and NO_x levels compared to control group. Administrating both doses of DIA to DOX treated rats significantly decreased MDA and NO_x compared to DOX treated group.

3.3. Effect of DIA on GSH, SOD, and Catalase Levels in DOX-Induced Nephrotoxicity. Treatment with DOX (15 mg/kg) caused significant decrease in renal GSH, SOD, and catalase levels compared with untreated control group (Table 2). Concomitant treatment of DOX with DIA significantly increased the levels of renal GSH, SOD, and catalase compared to DOX treated group.

3.4. Histological Results. The histological study of the rat renal cortical tissue of control group (Figure 1(a)), DLD (25 mg/kg/day) group (Figure 1(b)), and DHD (50 mg/kg/day) group (Figure 1(c)) showed normal architecture of renal glomeruli and tubules. DOX treated group (Figure 1(d)) showed marked enlargement of some vascular glomeruli which tightly fill the renal corpuscles. Most renal corpuscular and tubular

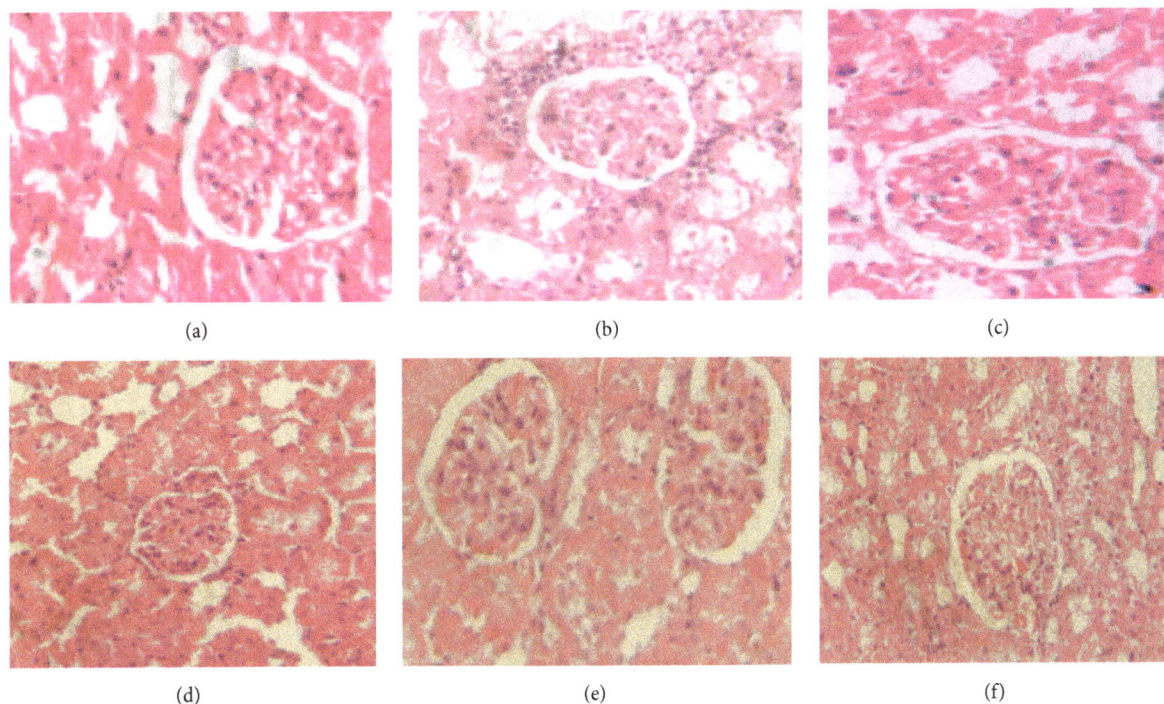

(a)

(b)

(c)

(d)

(e)

(f)

FIGURE 1: Photomicrographs of renal cortex of (a), (b), and (c), control, DLD, and DHD groups, respectively, showing normal lobular organization of the renal cortex; normal renal glomeruli and tubules. (d) DOX treated group showing markedly enlarged and congested vascular renal glomeruli and cytoplasmic vacuolations of corpuscular cells. Inflammatory cell infiltrations are observed. (e) DOX/DLD group showing less cytoplasmic vacuolations of the renal corpuscular cells and tubular cells. (f) DOX/DHD showing apparent normal renal cortex. H&E ×400. Bar = 20 μ.

TABLE 3: Scoring of morphological changes observed in control and experimental groups by light microscope ($n = 6$).

Findings	Control group	DLD group	DHD group	DOX treated group	DOX/DLD group	DOX/DHD group
(i) Glomerular vacuolations	−	−	−	++++	+	+
(ii) Enlarged renal corpuscles	−	−	−	++++	+	−
(iii) Tubular cells vacuolations	−	+	−	++++	+	+
(iv) Lumen widening	−	−	−	++++	+	−
(v) Distortion and Degeneration	−	−	−	++++	+	−
(vi) Casts	−	−	−	−	−	−

Animal groups tested are control untreated group, animals treated with diacerein (25 mg/kg/day, DLD) and diacerein (50 mg/kg/day, DHD), respectively, and animals treated with doxorubicin (DOX, 15 mg/kg), or with DOX together with low or high dose of diacerein (DOX/DLD or DOX/DHD), respectively. Normal (−), in-between normal and mild (+), mild (++), moderate (+++), and severe (++++) [9].

cells showed abundant cytoplasmic vacuolations and tubular distortion. Interstitial inflammatory cells infiltrations were observed. DOX + DLD group (Figure 1(e)) showed amelioration of the damaging effects of DOX. There were less tubular distortion, narrow Bowman's spaces, and fewer cytoplasmic vacuolations of renal corpuscle and tubular cells were also observed. DOX + DHD group (Figure 1(f)) had more obvious decrease in the morphological changes caused by DOX exposure.

3.5. Morphometric Results. The severity of the morphological changes was assessed semiquantitatively; DOX exposed group showed increase in the glomerular and tubular morphological changes at the light microscopic levels when compared with control group. These changes were suppressed by the administration of both doses of DIA, but the high dose showed marked improvement than the low dose (Table 3).

3.6. Immune-Histochemical Results. Administration of DOX caused significant increase in the immunoreactivity of caspase-3, NFκB, and TNFα (Figures 2, 3, and 4 and Table 4) respectively, which were highly expressed in both renal glomeruli and tubules cytoplasmically and in some nuclei. Administration of both doses of DIA concomitantly with DOX decreased the expression of them, compared to DOX group. Administration of both doses of DIA in vehicle treated rats alone and control groups showed no expression.

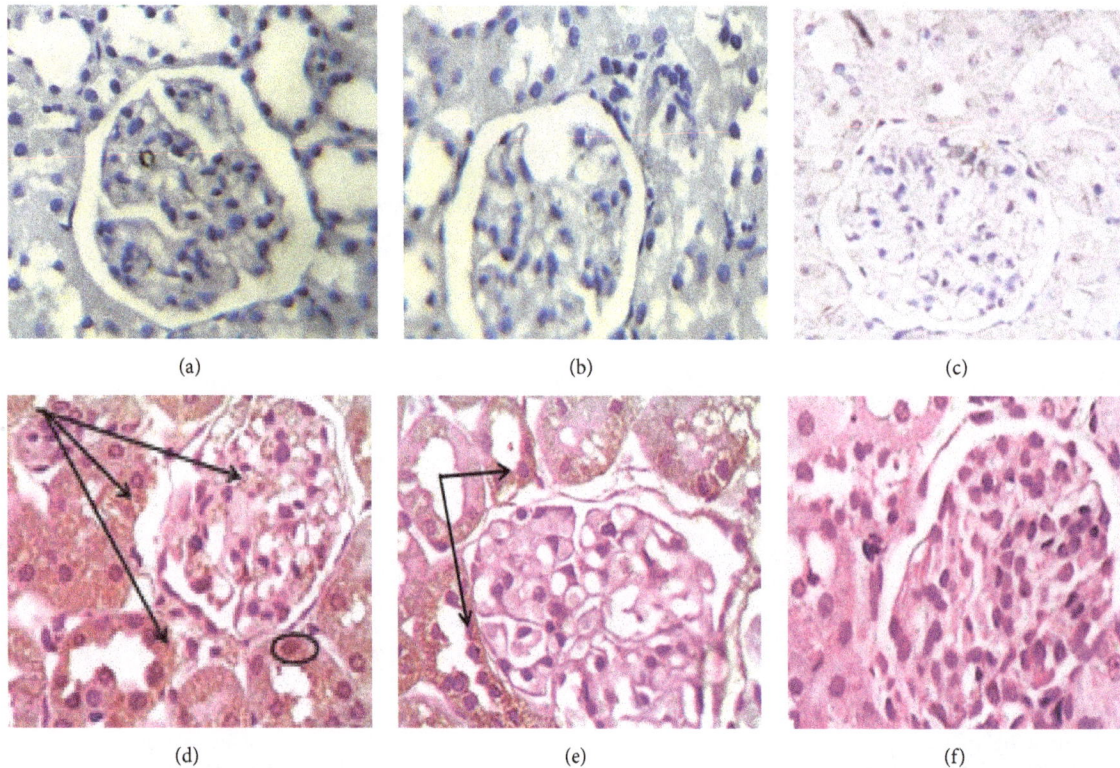

(a)   (b)   (c)

(d)   (e)   (f)

FIGURE 2: Photomicrographs of renal cortex immune stained for caspase-3 of (a), (b), and (c), control, DLD, and DHD groups, respectively, showing negative immunoreactivity. (d) DOX treated group showing extensive expression in the renal glomeruli and renal tubules. (e) DOX/DLD group showing moderate expression within the glomeruli and the renal tubules. (f) DOX/DHD group showed marked improvement with no expression in glomeruli and renal tubules. The expression is mainly cytoplasmic, but with some immunopositive nuclei. Immunohistochemistry counter stained with H&E ×400. Bar = 20 μ.

TABLE 4: The effect of DLD and DHD doses on caspase-3, TNFα, and NFκB immune expressions.

Group	Caspase-3	TNFα	NFκB
Control	0.42 ± 0.80	0.40 ± 0.78	0.40 ± 0.88
DLD	0.60 ± 0.88	0.60 ± 0.80	0.60 ± 0.80
DHD	0.40 ± 0.40	2.40 ± 0.40	0.40 ± 0.40
DOX	58.60 ± 8.90[a]	80.60 ± 8.90[a]	58.60 ± 8.90[a]
DOX/DLD	30.20 ± 7.90[a/b]	35.20 ± 7.90[a/b]	25.20 ± 7.90[a/b]
DOX/DHD	10.00 ± 6.90[b]	5.00 ± 4.90[b]	10.00 ± 6.90[b]

Animal groups tested are control untreated group, animals treated with low or high doses of DIA alone (DLD or DHD), respectively, and animals treated with DOX or with DOX together with low or high dose of DIA (DOX/DLD or DOX/DHD), respectively.
[a]Significant from control group; [b]significant from doxorubicin group.

4. Discussion

Anticancer therapy usually demolishes the physiological homoeostasis and affects multiple organs during treatment process. Effective anticancer therapy with anthracyclines as DOX is limited because of its toxicity to various organs including kidneys [6]. Nephrotoxic action of DOX is also considered to be via drug-induced free radical generation [22]. The formation of free radicals induces the production of proinflammatory cytokines as interleukin 1 initiating the biological effects associated with inflammation [23]. This directed our attention to investigate the role of DIA which is interleukin 1 receptor antagonist as a possible nephroprotective agent against DOX-induced renal damage.

Induction of DOX nephrotoxicity was detected in our study by significant elevation of serum urea and creatinine levels which were confirmed by toxic histopathological changes compared to control group. Urea and serum creatinine are the most sensitive markers of nephrotoxicity implicated in the diagnosis of renal injury [24, 25]. The nephrotoxic effect of DOX is characterized by decreasing glomerular filtration rate leading to a rise in serum urea and creatinine. Our results are in good agreement with the previous studies [22, 26].

Improvement of DOX-induced nephrotoxicity was previously tried by compounds that partially succeeded in preserving normal renal function and structure probably through their antioxidant and anti-inflammatory effects as caffeic acid phenethyl ester [27], *Zingiber officinale* Roscoe [28], and *Solanum torvum* [26] so that we investigated the role of another antioxidant and anti-inflammatory drug as DIA on DOX-induced nephrotoxicity.

DIA could significantly decrease serum urea and creatinine compared to DOX treated group. That is due to the anti-inflammatory and antioxidant effects of DIA which

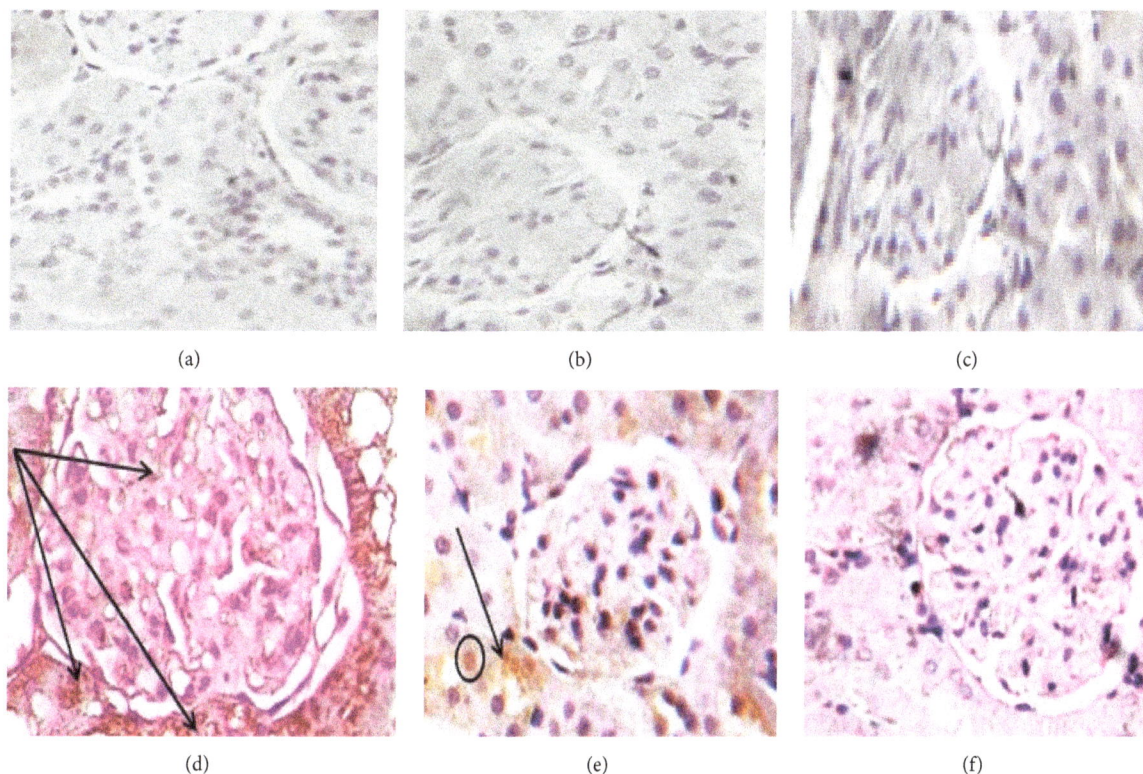

FIGURE 3: Photomicrographs of renal cortex immune stained for NFκB of (a), (b), and (c), control, DLD, and DHD groups, respectively, showing negative immunoreactivity. (d) DOX treated group showing extensive expression in the renal glomeruli and renal tubules. (e) DOX/DLD group showing moderate expression within the glomeruli and the renal tubules. (f) DOX/DHD group showed marked improvement with no expression in glomeruli and renal tubules. The expression is mainly cytoplasmic but with some immunopositive nuclei. Immunohistochemistry counter stained with H&E ×400. Bar = 20 μ.

suppress DOX mediated oxidative stress, inflammation, and tissue damage. Our histopathological changes showed that DOX treated group presented with marked damage of renal tubules. This is in agreement with Rashid et al. [22] and Al-Saedi et al. [29] who showed the same histopathological findings.

Coadministration of DIA significantly improved the histopathological changes compared to DOX treated group. These results are in agreement with Zhao et al. [30] who detected the protective effect of rhein (the active metabolite of DIA) on acetaminophen induced hepatotoxicity and nephrotoxicity in rats. They found that serum urea and creatinine significantly decreased in rhein and acetaminophen coadministration compared to acetaminophen group and normalization of toxic histopathological changes.

The elevated levels of GSH could effectively provide thiol group for the possible GSH mediated detoxification reactions of GPx (glutathione peroxidase) and GST (glutathione-s-transferase) which is involved in the scavenging of O_2^- generated from the DOX [31]. Our findings are consistent with the previous reports that showed that GSH concentration is significantly decreased upon DOX treatment compared to control group [4, 22].

SOD extensively distributes in all cells and has a significant shielding role against oxidative injury induced by reactive oxygen species [22].

In our study, the activities of SOD and catalase significantly decreased in DOX treated rats in kidney as compared to control rats. The accumulation of these highly reactive free radicals leads to the reduction of the activity of SOD and catalase which in turn results in damaging effects in the form of loss of cell membrane integrity and function. The decrease in the SOD and catalase activities related to the increase in the intracellular levels of H_2O_2. Catalase has been reported to be responsible for the detoxification of H_2O_2, which is an effective inhibitor of SOD. Other researchers reported the same results [32, 33].

Coadministration of DIA significantly improved SOD, GSH, and catalase levels compared to DOX treated group. These results may be due to antioxidant effect of DIA which was approved previously by Tamura et al. [34] who indicated the inhibitory effect of DIA on indomethacin-induced gastric ulceration which could be mediated by the suppression of reactive oxygen species production based on its inhibition of neutrophil activation and antioxidant activity. In addition, Hu et al. [35] investigated the protective effects of rhein lysinate (RHL), against kidney impairment in senescence-prone inbred strain 10 (SAMP10) mice. Treatment of SAMP10 mice with RHL significantly increased the SOD and GPx levels in the kidneys.

Oxidative stress may damage cellular structures via lipid peroxidation of cellular membranes. $O_2^{\bullet-}$ reacts with lipid to

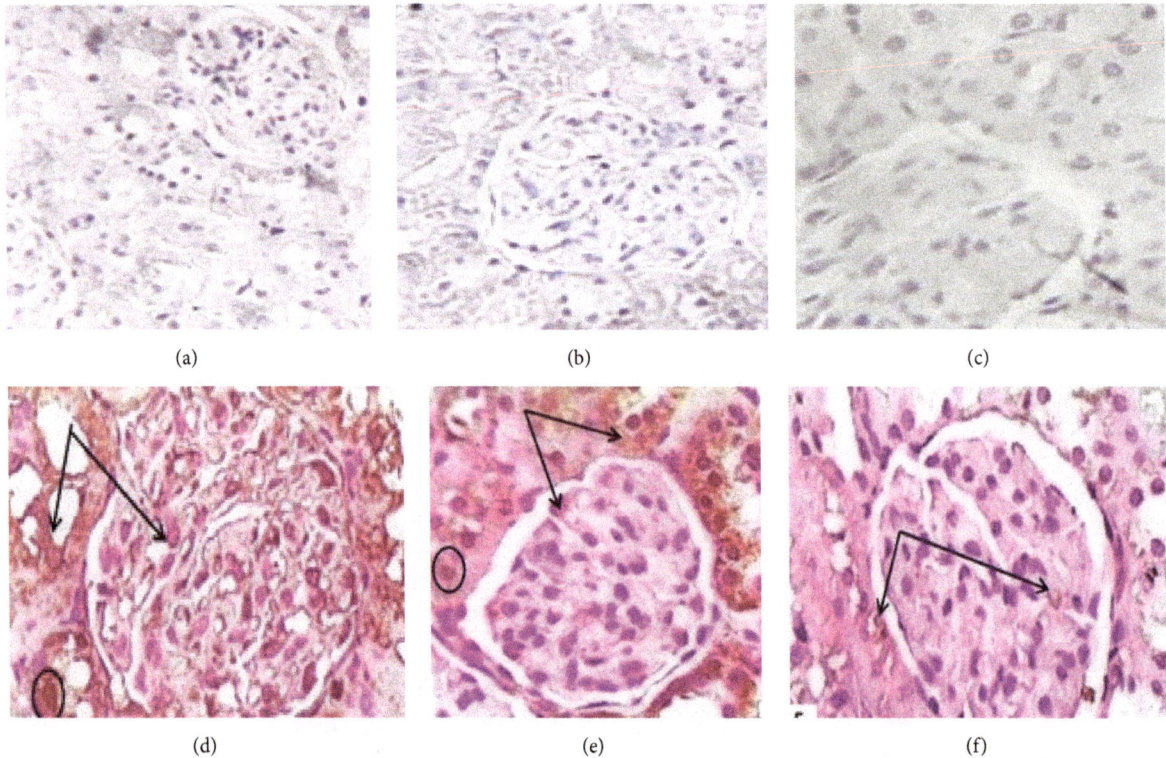

FIGURE 4: Photomicrographs of renal cortex immune stained for TNFα of: (a), (b), and (c), control, DLD, and DHD groups, respectively, showing negative immunoreactivity. (d) DOX treated group showing extensive expression in the renal glomeruli and renal tubules. (e) DOX/DLD group showing moderate expression within the glomeruli and the renal tubules. (f) DOX/DHD group showed marked improvement with no expression in glomeruli and renal tubules. The expression is mainly cytoplasmic, but with some immunopositive nuclei. Immunohistochemistry counter stained with H&E ×400. Bar = 20 μ.

form lipid peroxides followed by β-oxidation to form MDA [36]. That was detected in our study which showed significant increase of MDA level in DOX treated group compared to control group. These results are in agreement with El-Sheikh et al. [4] and Yagmurca et al. [27].

Another radical formatting mechanism in such an experimental protocol is NO_x producing system. The high production of NO_x results in peroxynitrite formation which is a potent and aggressive cellular oxidant and is involved in DOX toxicity [36]. The current findings showed that DOX administration significantly increased renal level of NO_x compared to control group and that is in agreement with other studies [26, 37].

Coadministration of DIA significantly decreased MDA and NO_x levels compared to DOX treated group. These results are in agreement with Zhao et al. [30] who detected the protective effect of rhein on acetaminophen induced nephrotoxicity in rats which was approved by significant decrease of MDA and NO_x on coadministration of rhein plus acetaminophen group compared to acetaminophen group. Our results are in agreement with Martel-Pelletier and Pelletier [38] who reported that NO is produced through the activity of inducible nitric oxide synthase and it is a major catabolic factor involved in the pathophysiology of OA. Interleukin 1β is a very potent stimulator of NO. Both DIA and rhein treatments markedly and significantly decreased

interleukin 1β-induced NO production. Our results are consistent with Hu et al. [35] who investigated the protective effects of rhein lysinate (RHL), against kidney impairment in senescence-prone inbred strain 10 (SAMP10) mice. Treatment of SAMP10 mice with RHL significantly decreased MDA levels in the kidneys.

DOX treatment induced p53 phosphorylation. Induction of p53 mediates cell apoptosis through activation of caspase-3 family of proteases and apoptotic cell death [39]. Our study is showing significant increase in caspase-3 expression in DOX treated group in comparison with control group.

Coadministration of DIA significantly decreased caspase-3 expression compared to DOX treated group. Our study is in consistence with Torina et al. [40] who showed that treatment with DIA once a day for 4 weeks after myocardial infarction improved ventricular remodeling by partial blockage of the proinflammatory cytokines which led to lower caspase-3 activity and NFκB p65 transcription B pathway.

DOX-induced superoxide anion production which was reported to be responsible for TNFα-induced nuclear factor (NF) activation that increases NF and TNFα over expression [41]. Our study showed significant increase in TNFα and NFκB expressions in DOX group compared to control group and the same results were found with Al-Saedi et al. [29].

Coadministration of DIA significantly decreased TNFα and NFκB expression compared to DOX treated group that is in agreement with Gadotti et al. [11] who showed that DIA inhibits neuropathic pain by decreasing proinflammatory cytokines as TNFα and NF$\kappa\beta$. Also, Hu et al. [42] hypothesized that the entity of diabetic nephropathy is inflammatory. The active metabolite of DIA is rhein which possesses anti-inflammatory activity and may be effective in suppressing the inflammatory cytokines contributing to the pathogenesis of diabetic nephropathy.

Moreover, Zhao et al. [30] demonstrated that rhein had protective effect in different models of nephropathy as IgA induced nephropathy, obstructive nephropathy, chronic allograft nephropathy, and high glucose and angiotensin II induced nephropathy. Oral administration of rhein (150 mg/kg/d) ameliorated renal lesions. Rhein was capable of protecting against renal injury by decreasing the activities of NFκB and caspase-3 in the early phase of glomerulosclerosis [43].

Our results are consistent with Meng et al. [44] who reported that rhein possesses various pharmacological activities, including anti-inflammatory, antioxidant, and antitumor. In their study, a model of hyperuricemia and nephropathy induced by adenine and ethambutol in mice was established. The results demonstrated that rhein significantly improved the symptoms of nephropathy through decreasing the production of proinflammatory cytokines, including interleukin 1β, prostaglandin E2, and TNFα. Yu et al. [45] aimed to explore the effect of rhein on sepsis-induced acute kidney injury by injecting lipopolysaccharide (LPS) and cecal ligation and puncture (CLP) in vivo and on LPS-induced HK-2 cells in vitro. Rhein effectively attenuated the severity of renal injury. Rhein could significantly decrease concentration of serum urea and creatinine and level of TNFα, NFκB, and IL-1β in two different mouse models of experimental sepsis.

5. Conclusion

In conclusion, DIA protected against DOX-induced nephrotoxicity in rats most probably due to its antioxidant and anti-inflammatory activities. However, DHD (50 mg/kg/day) showed more protective effect than DLD (25 mg/kg/day).

Conflict of Interests

The authors reported no conflict of interests regarding the publication of this paper.

References

[1] T. D. Dolin and J. Himmelfarb, "Drug-induced kidney disease," in *Pharmacotherapy: A Pathophysiologic Approach*, J. T. Dipiro, Ed., pp. 795–810, 7th edition, 2008.

[2] C. Carvalho, R. X. Santos, S. Cardoso et al., "Doxorubicin: the good, the bad and the ugly effect," *Current Medicinal Chemistry*, vol. 16, no. 25, pp. 3267–3285, 2009.

[3] J. L. Quiles, J. J. Ochoa, J. R. Huertas, M. Lopes Frias, and J. Mataix, "Olive oil and mitochondrial oxidative stress: studies on adriamycin toxicity, physical exercise and ageing," in *Olive Oil and Health*, J. L. Quiles, M. C. Ramirez-Tortosa, and P. Yaqoob, Eds., pp. 119–151, CABI Publishing, Oxford, UK, 2006.

[4] A. A. K. El-Sheikh, M. A. Morsy, M. M. Mahmoud, R. A. Rifaai, and A. M. Abdelrahman, "Effect of coenzyme-Q10 on doxorubicin-induced nephrotoxicity in rats," *Advances in Pharmacological Sciences*, vol. 2012, Article ID 981461, 8 pages, 2012.

[5] C. F. Thorn, C. Oshiro, S. Marshe et al., "Doxorubicin pathways: pharmacodynamics and adverse effects," *Pharmacogenetics and Genomics*, vol. 21, no. 7, pp. 440–446, 2011.

[6] R. Injac, M. Boskovic, M. Perse et al., "Acute doxorubicin nephrotoxicity in rats with malignant neoplasm can be successfully treated with fullerenol C60 (OH) 24 via suppression of oxidative stress," *Pharmacological Reports*, vol. 60, no. 5, pp. 742–749, 2008.

[7] M. Petrillo, F. Montrone, S. Adrizzone et al., "Endoscopic evaluation of diacetylrhein-induced gastric mucosal lesion," *Current Therapeutic Research*, vol. 49, pp. 10–15, 1991.

[8] J.-P. Pelletier, F. Mineau, J. C. Fernandes, N. Duval, and J. Martel-Pelletier, "Diacerhein and rhein reduce the interleukin 1β stimulated inducible nitric oxide synthesis level and activity while stimulating cyclooxygenase-2 synthesis in human osteoarthritic chondrocytes," *Journal of Rheumatology*, vol. 25, no. 12, pp. 2417–2424, 1998.

[9] B. Medhi, A. Prakash, P. K. Singh, R. Sen, and S. Wadhwa, "Diacerein: a new disease modulating agent in osteoarthritis," *Indian Journal of Physical Medicine and Rehabilitation*, vol. 18, no. 2, pp. 48–52, 2007.

[10] E. Ozbek, "Induction of oxidative stress in kidney," *International Journal of Nephrology*, vol. 2012, Article ID 465897, 9 pages, 2012.

[11] V. M. Gadotti, D. F. Martins, H. F. Pinto et al., "Diacerein decreases visceral pain through inhibition of glutamatergic neurotransmission and cytokine signaling in mice," *Pharmacology Biochemistry and Behavior*, vol. 102, no. 4, pp. 549–554, 2012.

[12] A. Vassault, D. Grafmeyer, J. de Graeve, R. Cohen, A. Beaudonnet, and J. Bienvenu, "Quality specifications and allowable standards for validation of methods used in clinical biochemistry," *Annales de Biologie Clinique*, vol. 57, no. 6, pp. 685–695, 1999.

[13] D. S. Young, L. C. Pestaner, and V. Gibberman, "Effects of drugs on clinical laboratory tests," *Clinical Chemistry*, vol. 21, no. 5, pp. 1D–432D, 1975.

[14] E. Beutler, O. Duron, and B. M. Kelly, "Improved method for the determination of blood glutathione," *The Journal of Laboratory and Clinical Medicine*, vol. 61, pp. 882–888, 1963.

[15] H. Aebi, "Catalase in vitro," *Methods in Enzymology*, vol. 105, pp. 121–126, 1984.

[16] M. Nishikimi, N. A. Rao, and K. Yagi, "The occurrence of superoxide anion in the reaction of reduced phenazine methosulfate and molecular oxygen," *Biochemical and Biophysical Research Communications*, vol. 46, no. 2, pp. 849–854, 1972.

[17] M. Mihara and M. Uchiyama, "Properties of thiobarbituric acid-reactive materials obtained from lipid peroxide and tissue homogenate," *Chemical and Pharmaceutical Bulletin*, vol. 31, no. 2, pp. 605–611, 1983.

[18] S. Söğüt, S. S. Zoroğlu, H. Özyurt et al., "Changes in nitric oxide levels and antioxidant enzyme activities may have a role in the pathophysiological mechanisms involved in autism," *Clinica Chimica Acta*, vol. 331, no. 1-2, pp. 111–117, 2003.

[19] D. Houghton, C. Plamp, J. Defehr, W. Bennett, G. Forter, and D. Gilbert, "Gentamicin and tobramycin nephrotoxicity," *The American Journal of Pathology*, vol. 98, no. 1, pp. 137–152, 1978.

[20] A. Côté, R. Silva, and A. C. Cuello, "Current protocols for light microscopy immunocytochemistry," in *Immunohistochemistry*

II, A. C. Cuello, Ed., pp. 147–168, John Wiley & Sons, Chichester, UK, 1993.

[21] T. Shirai, H. Yamaguchi, H. Ito, C. W. Todd, and R. B. Wallace, "Cloning and expression in *Escherichia coli* of the gene for human tumor necrosis factor," *Nature*, vol. 313, pp. 803–806, 1985.

[22] S. Rashid, N. Ali, S. Nafees et al., "Alleviation of doxorubicin-induced nephrotoxicity and hepatotoxicity by chrysin in Wistar rats," *Toxicology Mechanisms and Methods*, vol. 23, no. 5, pp. 337–345, 2013.

[23] C. A. Dinarello, "Interleukin 1 and interleukin 18 as mediators of inflammation and the aging process," *American Journal of Clinical Nutrition*, vol. 83, no. 2, pp. 447S–455S, 2006.

[24] R. Sallie, J. M. Tredger, and R. Williams, "Drugs and the liver," *Biopharmaceutics and Drug Disposition*, vol. 12, no. 4, pp. 251–259, 1991.

[25] N. Khan and S. Sultana, "Abrogation of potassium bromate-induced renal oxidative stress and subsequent cell proliferation response by soy isoflavones in Wistar rats," *Toxicology*, vol. 201, no. 1–3, pp. 173–184, 2004.

[26] M. Mohan, S. Kamble, P. Gadhi, and S. Kasture, "Protective effect of *Solanum torvum* on doxorubicin-induced nephrotoxicity in rats," *Food and Chemical Toxicology*, vol. 48, no. 1, pp. 436–440, 2010.

[27] M. Yagmurca, H. Erdogan, M. Iraz, A. Songur, M. Ucar, and E. Fadillioglu, "Caffeic acid phenethyl ester as a protective agent against doxorubicin nephrotoxicity in rats," *Clinica Chimica Acta*, vol. 348, no. 1-2, pp. 27–34, 2004.

[28] T. A. Ajith, M. S. Aswathy, and U. Hema, "Protective effect of *Zingiber officinale*roscoe against anticancer drug doxorubicin-induced acute nephrotoxicity," *Food and Chemical Toxicology*, vol. 46, no. 9, pp. 3178–3181, 2008.

[29] H. F. Al-Saedi, A. A. Al-Zubaidy, and Y. I. Khattab, "The possible effects of montelukast against doxorubicin-induced nephrotoxicity in rabbits," *International Journal of Advanced Research*, vol. 2, no. 11, pp. 723–729, 2014.

[30] J. J. Zhao, J. D. Rogers, S. D. Holland et al., "Pharmacokinetics and bioavailability of montelukast sodium (MK-0476) in healthy young and elderly volunteers," *Biopharmaceutics and Drug Disposition*, vol. 18, no. 9, pp. 769–777, 1997.

[31] N. Shinde, A. Jagtap, V. Undale, S. Kakade, S. Kotwal, and R. Patil, "Protective effect of Lepidium sativum against doxorubicin-induced nephrotoxicity in rats," *Research Journal of Pharmaceutical, Biological and Chemical Sciences*, vol. 1, no. 3, pp. 42–49, 2010.

[32] H.-K. Tu, K.-F. Pan, Y. Zhang et al., "Manganese superoxide dismutase polymorphism and risk of gastric lesions, and its effects on chemoprevention in a chinese population," *Cancer Epidemiology Biomarkers and Prevention*, vol. 19, no. 4, pp. 1089–1097, 2010.

[33] S. S. Al-Rejaie, "Effect of oleo-gum-resin on ethanol-induced hepatotoxicity in rats," *Journal of Medical Sciences*, vol. 12, no. 1, pp. 1–9, 2012.

[34] T. Tamura, T. Yokoyama, and K. Ohmori, "Effects of diacerein on indomethacin-induced gastric ulceration," *Pharmacology*, vol. 63, no. 4, pp. 228–233, 2001.

[35] G. Hu, J. Liu, Y.-Z. Zhen et al., "Rhein lysinate increases the median survival time of SAMP10 mice: protective role in the kidney," *Acta Pharmacologica Sinica*, vol. 34, no. 4, pp. 515–521, 2013.

[36] M. A. Morsy, S. A. Ibrahim, E. F. Amin, M. Y. Kamel, R. A. Rifaai, and M. K. Hassan, "Curcumin ameliorates methotrexate-induced nephrotoxicity in rats," *Advances in Pharmacological Sciences*, vol. 2013, Article ID 387071, 7 pages, 2013.

[37] H. M. Arafa, M. F. Abd-Ellah, and H. F. Hafez, "Abatement by naringenin of doxorubicin-induced cardiac toxicity in rats," *Journal of the Egyptian National Cancer Institute*, vol. 17, no. 4, pp. 291–300, 2005.

[38] J. Martel-Pelletier and J. Pelletier, "Effects of diacerein at the molecular level in the osteoarthritis disease process," *Therapeutic Advances in Musculoskeletal Disease*, vol. 2, no. 2, pp. 95–104, 2010.

[39] Y. M. Jang, S. Kendaiah, B. Drew et al., "Doxorubicin treatment in vivo activates caspase-12 mediated cardiac apoptosis in both male and female rats," *FEBS Letters*, vol. 577, no. 3, pp. 483–490, 2004.

[40] A. G. Torina, K. Reichert, F. Lima et al., "Diacerein improves left ventricular remodeling and cardiac function by reducing the inflammatory response after myocardial infarction," *PLOS ONE*, vol. 10, no. 3, Article ID e0121842, 2015.

[41] S. Chien, Y. Wu, Z. Chen, and W. Yang, "Naturally occurring anthraquinones: chemistry and therapeutic potential in autoimmune diabetes," *Evidence-Based Complementary and Alternative Medicine*, vol. 2015, Article ID 357357, 13 pages, 2015.

[42] C. Hu, X. D. Cong, D.-Z. Dai, Y. Zhang, G. L. Zhang, and Y. Dai, "Argirein alleviates diabetic nephropathy through attenuating NADPH oxidase, Cx43, and PERK in renal tissue," *Naunyn-Schmiedeberg's Archives of Pharmacology*, vol. 383, no. 3, pp. 309–319, 2011.

[43] Z.-Q. Ji, C.-W. Huang, C.-J. Liang, W.-W. Sun, B. Chen, and P.-R. Tang, "Effects of rhein on activity of caspase-3 in kidney and cell apoptosis on the progression of renal injury in glomerulosclerosis," *Zhonghua Yi Xue Za Zhi*, vol. 85, no. 26, pp. 1836–1841, 2005.

[44] Z. Meng, Y. Yan, Z. Tang et al., "Anti-hyperuricemic and nephroprotective effects of rhein in hyperuricemic mice," *Planta Medica*, vol. 81, no. 04, pp. 279–285, 2015.

[45] C. Yu, D. Qi, J. F. Sun, P. Li, and H. Y. Fan, "Rhein prevents endotoxin-induced acute kidney injury by inhibiting NF-κB activities," *Scientific Reports*, vol. 5, Article ID 11822, 2015.

19

Evaluation of "Dream Herb," *Calea zacatechichi*, for Nephrotoxicity Using Human Kidney Proximal Tubule Cells

Miriam E. Mossoba, Thomas J. Flynn, Sanah Vohra, Paddy Wiesenfeld, and Robert L. Sprando

Center for Food Safety and Applied Nutrition (CFSAN), Office of Applied Research and Safety Assessment (OARSA), Division of Toxicology (DOT), US Food and Drug Administration (US FDA), Neurotoxicology and In Vitro Toxicology Branch (NIVTB), 8301 Muirkirk Road, Laurel, MD 20708, USA

Correspondence should be addressed to Miriam E. Mossoba; miriam.mossoba@fda.hhs.gov

Academic Editor: Orish Ebere Orisakwe

A recent surge in the use of dietary supplements, including herbal remedies, necessitates investigations into their safety profiles. "Dream herb," *Calea zacatechichi*, has long been used in traditional folk medicine for a variety of purposes and is currently being marketed in the US for medicinal purposes, including diabetes treatment. Despite the inherent vulnerability of the renal system to xenobiotic toxicity, there is a lack of safety studies on the nephrotoxic potential of this herb. Additionally, the high frequency of diabetes-associated kidney disease makes safety screening of *C. zacatechichi* for safety especially important. We exposed human proximal tubule HK-2 cells to increasing doses of this herb alongside known toxicant and protectant control compounds to examine potential toxicity effects of *C. zacatechichi* relative to control compounds. We evaluated both cellular and mitochondrial functional changes related to toxicity of this dietary supplement and found that even at low doses evidence of cellular toxicity was significant. Moreover, these findings correlated with significantly elevated levels of nephrotoxicity biomarkers, lending further support for the need to further scrutinize the safety of this herbal dietary supplement.

1. Introduction

Calea zacatechichi (also called *Calea ternifolia* or "Dream Herb") is a flowering plant native to Central America and has a long tradition of use as a medicinal plant in indigenous cultures [1]. Exposure through inhalation (smoking) or ingestion (as tea) is primarily used to temporarily intensify lucid dreaming. It is also widely consumed to treat problems associated with the gastrointestinal and endocrine systems [2]. It has recently been marketed as a dietary supplement in the management of diabetes due to its ability to induce hypoglycemic effects [3–5] although its mechanism(s) of action remain unclear.

The oneirogenic and other biological effects of *C. zacatechichi* are attributed in part to their flavones and germacrolides components [6–10]. However, flavones represent a class of flavonoids that have been shown to carry cytotoxic effects in part through induction of cytochrome P450 enzyme expression [11–13]. In addition, germacrolides are part of the class of sesquiterpene lactones, which can also exhibit negative effects on both prokaryotic and mammalian cells [14]. The cytotoxicity of both flavonoids and sesquiterpene lactones has been exploited for use as therapy against cancer [15, 16].

Despite clear evidence that at least some of the biologically active components of *C. zacatechichi* have the potential to be cytotoxic, safety evaluations of whole forms of this herbal supplement are lacking, especially ones that focus on the kidney. The kidneys use a complex transport system to eliminate unwanted chemicals, regulate blood pressure and glucose levels, and maintain a balanced pH [17]. However, as the glomerular filtrate passes through the tubular system, the reabsorption of water and electrolytes by the proximal tubule cells can progressively concentrate chemicals in the lumen that do not get reabsorbed. Unfortunately, the proximal tubules can become exposed to toxic concentrations of such chemicals, even when blood concentrations are relatively lower, leaving the kidneys vulnerable to injury [17]. In the case of *C. zacatechichi*, it is unknown whether any of its components can be nephrotoxic, but given that it is marketed to diabetics, any preexisting diabetic nephropathy marked by glomerular or proximal tubule damage [18–20] could induce further kidney damage. Therefore, we focused our research on screening for the potential nephrotoxicity of *C. zacatechichi* using an *in vitro* model of human proximal tubule cells. We chose the HK-2 cell line as our human proximal tubule model for its robust performance in many *in vitro* toxicology studies [21–25]. We compared the effects of exposing HK-2 cells to *C. zacatechichi* and two control compounds, a known renal toxicant (cisplatin) and a known renal protectant (valproic acid), and evaluated their dose-dependent effects on cytotoxicity, mitochondrial injury, and four kidney-specific biomarkers of toxicity [26–28]: (1) Kidney Injury Molecule-1 (KIM-1), (2) Albumin, (3) Cystatin C, and (4) β2-microglobulin (B2M). KIM-1 is expressed in tubular epithelial cells in response to injury. Albumin, Cystatin C, and B2M are indicators of impaired reabsorption by the proximal tubules. In this study, we demonstrate that *C. zacatechichi* is capable of inducing both cellular and organellar toxicity in proximal tubule cells.

2. Materials and Methods

2.1. Characterization of Calea zacatechichi Extract. Voucher samples of *C. zacatechichi* deposited at the University of Mississippi, National Center for Natural Products Research (NCNPR) (NCNPR #2443), were authenticated using macroscopy and microscopy methods by an NCNPR botanist. A methanol-extract of *C. zacatechichi* was provided in lyophilized form by NCNPR and was stored in the dark at 4°C in a vacuum chamber. Dried extract of *C. zacatechichi* was analyzed by LC/QTof as described previously [29]. Compounds were putatively identified by matching exact mass of analytes with components of *C. zacatechichi* reported in the literature [8, 30–33].

2.2. Cell Culture and Treatments. HK-2 cells were grown, maintained, and treated in a manner similar to that described previously [29]. Stock treatment solutions of *C. zacatechichi*, nephrotoxicant (positive control) cis-diamineplatinum(II) dichloride (cisplatin) (Sigma-Aldrich, St. Louis, MO), and nephroprotectant (negative control) valproic acid (Sigma-Aldrich) were made by weighing out their powders, dissolving them in DMSO, and diluting this mixture with media for a final DMSO stock solution of 0.4% or less. Cells were incubated overnight and treated in triplicate for 24 hours at the dose range of 0–1000 μg/mL.

2.3. Cytotoxicity Assay. Treatment-related cytotoxicity was determined using the established CellTiter-Glo Cell Viability Assay (Promega, Madison, WI) following the manufacturer's recommendations. The premise of this luminescent assay is that ATP production is directly proportional to cell viability, as ATP is central to energy required for vital cellular

processes. Treated cells in black-wall, clear bottom 96-well plates were equilibrated to room temperature for 30 minutes, during which time water in the outer wells was replaced with approximately 100 uL of treatment or media only controls. Following that, an equal volume of CellTiter-Glo working solution was added to each well. Plates were placed on an orbital shaker for 2 minutes to induce cell lysis and then incubated for an additional 10 minutes before being read on an OMG Fluorostar plate reader (BMG LABTECH, Ortenberg, Germany) to measure the levels of luminescence emitted from each well.

2.4. Reactive Oxygen Species Assay. Quantification of reactive oxygen species (ROS) was determined using Promega's ROS-Glo H_2O_2 luminescence-based detection system and data were normalized to cell viability. Following 24 hrs of direct exposure to *C. zacatechichi*, cells were incubated with H_2O_2 substrate and detection reagent, as recommended in the manufacturer's instructions. Luminescence was read on an OMG Fluorostar plate reader.

2.5. Mitochondrial Membrane Potential Assay. Changes in mitochondrial membrane potential (MMP) were evaluated using the ratiometric dye JC-10 (Enzo, Farmingdale, NY). HK-2 cells that were directly exposed to *C. zacatechichi* were stained with 20 uM JC-10 (final concentration) for 2 hours, washed, and then read by plate reader (OMG Fluorostar). Excitation was set at 485 nm and emission at 520 and 590 nm was measured. We also verified that extract or media alone did not produce significant emission signals.

2.6. Nephrotoxicity Biomarker Assays. Culture supernatants from cells treated for 24 hours with *C. zacatechichi*, cisplatin, and valproic acid at doses of 333 and 111 μg/mL were evaluated for levels of biomarkers of kidney toxicity: Kidney Injury-1 (KIM-1), Albumin, Cystatin C, and beta-2-microglobulin (B2M) using the Human Kidney Toxicity kits (Bio-Rad, Hercules, CA). Following the manufacturer's protocol, plates were blocked, washed, and incubated with samples, standard solutions detection antibodies, before being given a final wash. Plates were read using a Luminex 200 instrument (Bio-Rad). Biomarker expression levels were normalized to cell viability.

2.7. Statistics. Microsoft Excel and Prism (GraphPad, San Diego, CA) were used for calculations and analyses of all data collected. Student's t-tests or 2-way ANOVAs were used to determine whether dose-matched treatment effects were statistically significant at P values less than 0.01 or 0.001 as indicated.

3. Results

3.1. Characterization of Calea zacatechichi Extract. LC-high resolution MS found 231 total molecular features in the *C. zacatechichi* extract. Of these, 24 features had exact mass consistent with that of reported components of *C. zacatechichi* (Figure 1). The major components based on peak volume,

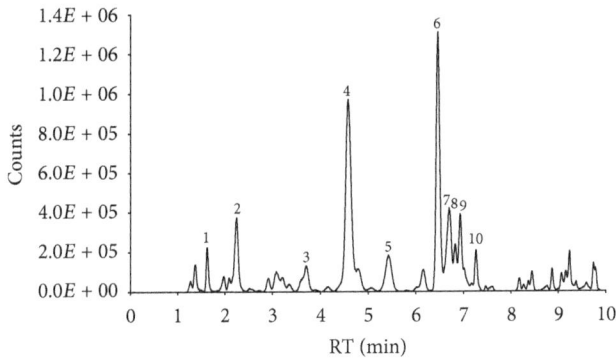

FIGURE 1: Extracted total compound chromatogram from chemical characterization of the *C. zacatechichi* extract by LC-high resolution mass spectroscopy. Putative compound identification was made by matching exact mass with that of known components of *C. zacatechichi* [8, 30–33]. (1) Ciliarin, (2) zexbrevin, (3) sesquiterpene lactone, (4) calein D, (5) 1-β-acetoxyzacatechinolide, (6) calein A, (7) 1-oxo-zacatechinolide, (8) calealactone E, (9) calealactone, and (10) acetoxycaleculatolide.

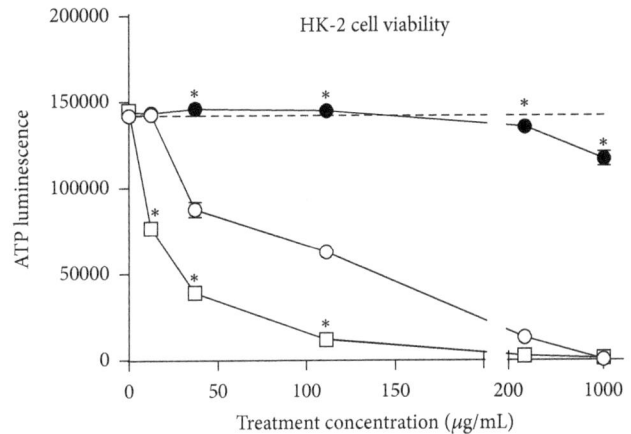

FIGURE 2: *C. zacatechichi* significantly decreases cell viability in a dose-dependent manner. HK-2 cells were treated with *C. zacatechichi* (open circles), cisplatin (open squares), or valproic acid (filled circles) at mean average concentrations (± SEM) ranging from 0 to 1000 μg/mL and cell viability was quantitatively assayed by ATP luminescence 24 hours after treatment. Dashed line indicates "no treatment" baseline ATP levels. ∗, cisplatin or valproic acid versus *C. zacatechichi*, $P < 0.001$.

calein A, ciliarin, acacetin, and calealactone C, accounted for about 50% of the known compounds and 8% of the total compounds [8, 30–33].

3.2. C. zacatechichi Strongly Inhibits HK-2 Cell Viability.

To investigate the nephrotoxicity of *C. zacatechichi*, we performed an ATP-based cell viability assay on HK-2 cells treated with a 6-dose concentration range from 0 to 1000 μg/mL for 24 hours. For comparison, we also treated cells for 24 hours with dose-matched concentrations of the known nephrotoxic compound, cisplatin, and the known nephroprotectant, valproic acid. We found that cisplatin induced a significant reduction in cell viability starting at the ~12 μg/mL dose tested ($P < 0.001$) and caused complete cell death at the maximum dose tested (Figure 2). Similarly, significant cytotoxicity of *C. zacatechichi* was detected starting at 37.0 μg/mL ($P < 0.001$) and still achieved complete cell death by 1000 μg/mL. For the range of doses tested, the cytotoxic effect of *C. zacatechichi* was directly proportional to the treatment dose and we calculated its lethal concentration 50 (LC_{50}) value to be 91.7 μg/mL, compared to 13.3 μg/mL for cisplatin. By contrast, valproic acid successfully maintained cell viability across the range of tested doses, except for the maximum dose of 1000 μg/mL, where cell viability dropped only slightly, as shown in Figure 2. As expected from a nephroprotectant, the calculated LC_{50} value of valproic acid is quite high at 3866 μg/mL, given the plateau shape of its cell viability curve.

3.3. Mitochondrial Toxicity Increases Proportionately with Higher Exposure to C. zacatechichi.

To begin studying early events of cellular toxicity, we evaluated how the mitochondria of HK-2 cells were affected by 24-hour treatments with *C. zacatechichi* relative to treatments with cisplatin or valproic acid. We first measured the levels of ROS produced in treated cells to indicate the levels of oxidative stress that was created in the intracellular environment of HK-2 cells. Using a luminescence assay of ROS detection, we found that *C. zacatechichi* treatment led to increasingly higher levels of ROS production in a manner that was directly proportional to the increasing treatment dose (Figure 3(a)). ROS production from cells treated with up to 333 μg/mL of *C. zacatechichi* was intermediary between those from the positive- and negative-control treated cells. At the 1000 μg/mL dose, however, *C. zacatechichi* induced ROS levels that surpassed those in cisplatin-treated cells ($P < 0.001$), as shown in Figure 3(a).

To gain a better understanding of (1) whether the elevated levels of ROS production actually correlated with mitochondrial injury and (2) to what extent injury took place, we performed a ratiometric assay using JC-10 dye to compare the relative levels of damaged and healthy mitochondria in treated HK-2 cells. Compared to the baseline ratio value of about 5, treatment with *C. zacatechichi* led to a uniquely sharp increase in the ratio of damaged to healthy mitochondria starting from the 12.3 μg/mL testing dose and achieved a maximum ratio value of about 50 when the treatment dose was increased to just 37.0 μg/mL (Figure 3(b)). This maximal relative level of mitochondrial damage was statistically significant ($P < 0.001$) and was well sustained for the remaining higher treatment doses of *C. zacatechichi*. By contrast, cisplatin induced mitochondrial damage at a much slower rate to achieve a ratio value of ~50 at 333 μg/mL. As expected, the mitochondrial injurious effects from valproic acid were minimal over the spectrum of treatment doses.

3.4. Proximal Tubule Cell Function Is Significantly Compromised by C. zacatechichi.

To address whether renal cell function would become compromised after treatment with *C. zacatechichi*, we evaluated cellular biomarkers that are strong indicators of nephrotoxicity [26–28]. We used a sensitive

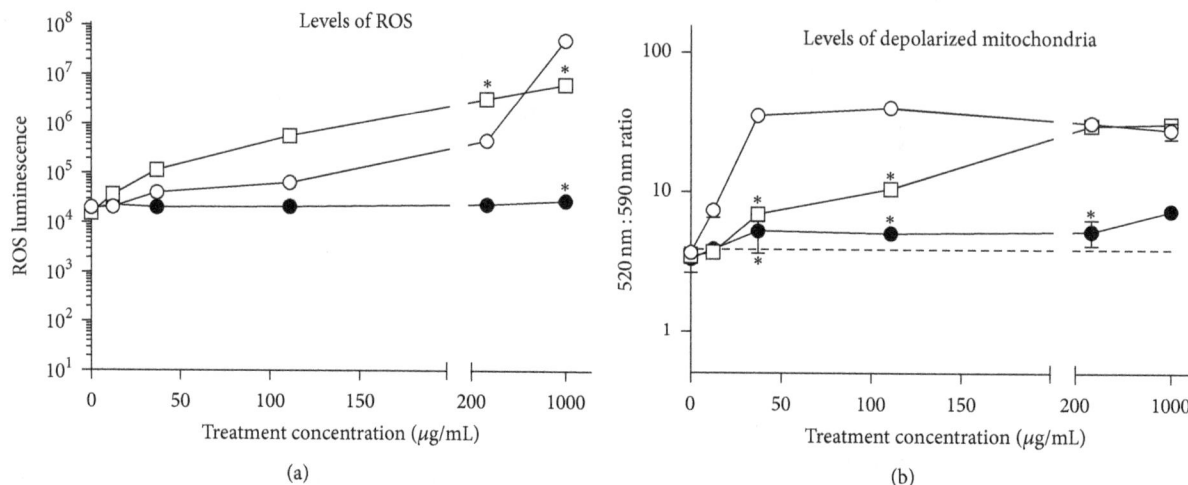

FIGURE 3: Cellular stress induced by *C. zacatechichi* is indicated by a surge in ROS and a rapid shift toward MMP loss. HK-2 cells treated for 24 hours with *C. zacatechichi* (open circles), cisplatin (open squares), or valproic acid (filled circles) were assayed for cellular levels of (a) normalized mean average ROS levels ($\pm$ SEM) as well as (b) changes in the relative amounts of mitochondria that undergo loss versus maintenance of membrane potential, calculated as a mean average ($\pm$ SEM) ratio of fluorescence emission at 520 versus 590 nm. *, cisplatin or valproic acid versus *C. zacatechichi*, $P < 0.001$.

multiplex approach to simultaneously detect differences in the levels of four FDA-qualified biomarkers: KIM-1, Albumin, Cystatin C, and B2M. We quantitated the concentrations of these analytes in the culture supernatants of HK-2 cells exposed to 111 or 333 μg/mL of *C. zacatechichi*, cisplatin, valproic acid, or untreated media for 24 hours (Figure 4). In agreement with our findings of cellular and mitochondrial toxicity, we found significantly elevated levels for nearly all of these markers ($P < 0.01$) in culture supernatants of HK-2 cells treated with *C. zacatechichi* compared to those treated with valproic acid or left untreated. The extent of biomarker elevation induced by *C. zacatechichi* never exceeded that of cisplatin. This trend was also observed at the lower treatment dose of 111 μg/mL, even though the actual concentrations of each biomarker were typically 10-fold less than in high-dose treatments, as shown in Figure 4.

4. Discussion

Although *C. zacatechichi* is not a controlled substance under United States federal law, it has been banned in the state of Louisiana as well as in Poland on the basis of its mind-altering effects [34, 35]. In our study, we used an *in vitro* human renal proximal tubule cell model to perform several assays that collectively evaluated the nephrotoxicity potential of *C. zacatechichi*. We used its alcohol extract to best model the tincture dietary supplements marketed in the United States. By comparing its toxicity profile to that of a highly toxic pure compound, cisplatin, and an innocuous pure compound, valproic acid, we established a stringent *in vitro* cell culture safety evaluation model system. Although we identified several of the chemical components of *C. zacatechichi*, we were focused on evaluating the toxicity of this herbal extract as a whole. *In vitro* testing not only provides a window into cell-specific effects [36] but also yields informative data

on the mechanism(s) of toxicity [37]. We chose to use the human renal proximal tubule epithelial cell line, HK-2, because the proximal tubule plays a critical role in controlling the clearance and reabsorption processes of xenobiotics and their metabolites [38, 39]. Proximal tubule epithelial cells encounter toxicants that are filtered and are an important component of overall nephrotoxicity that can lead to both acute and chronic kidney damage [40]. The HK-2 cell line is an appropriate choice for establishing a renal cell toxicology profile on *C. zacatechichi* for two main reasons. First, HK-2 cells are human derived and thus, data generated from this cell line are not confounded by differences between human and other species. Second, HK-2 cells closely recapitulate many aspects of the morphological and metabolic phenotype of proximal tubule cells *in vivo* [23, 41]. In our evaluation of cytotoxicity, we found striking similarities between our tested herbal extract and cisplatin at single dose treatment concentrations as low as approximately 37 μg/mL in the form of short-term exposure. Moreover, it appeared that the mechanism of action of *C. zacatechichi*'s active ingredients or renal-derived metabolites resembled those of the highly injurious cisplatin; elevated ROS levels and a severe loss of mitochondrial membrane potential were hallmarks of nephrotoxicity shared by these two substances. By contrast, valproic acid showed little or no toxicity potential until the highest dose of 1000 μg/mL was tested. The relatively high level of toxicity that was induced by *C. zacatechichi* within the 24 hours of direct exposure to HK-2 cells is of concern. However, since no data exist on the serum concentrations of *C. zacatechichi*'s active components, it is unclear how our chosen treatment doses compare to what kidney cells *in vivo* would be exposed to, especially postmetabolism by the gut and liver.

Although further studies would be needed to elucidate a more detailed mechanistic analysis of *C. zacatechichi*'s modes

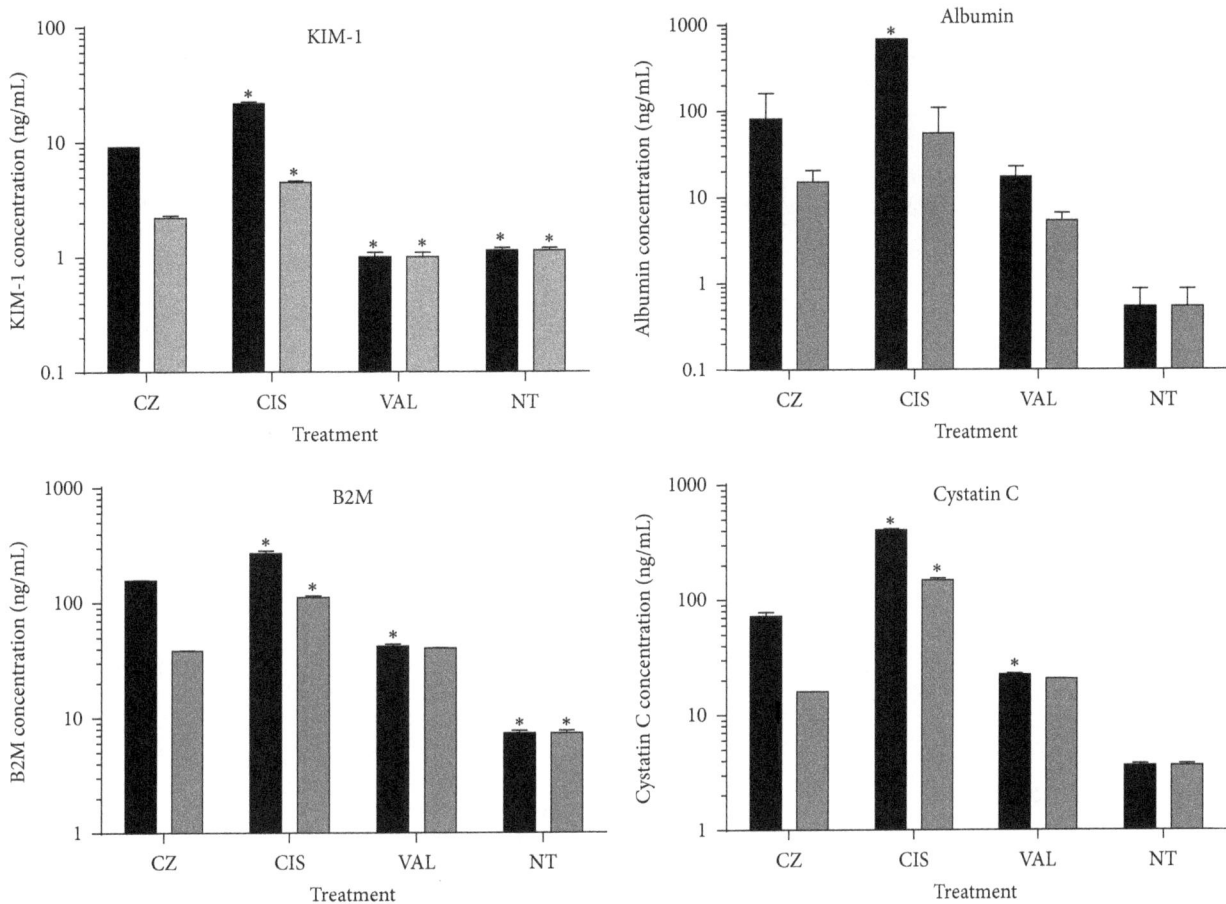

FIGURE 4: Biomarker signature of *C. zacatechichi*-associated nephrotoxicity. HK-2 cells were treated with *C. zacatechichi* (CZ), cisplatin (CIS), or valproic acid (VAL) or left untreated (NT). Treatment concentrations were either 333 μg/mL (black bars) or 111 μg/mL (gray bars). At 24 hours after treatment, HK-2 cell culture supernatants were harvested and assayed by Bio-Plex assay for average levels of KIM-1, Albumin, Cystatin C, and B2M (± SEM). Biomarker expression levels were normalized to cell viability. *, cisplatin or valproic acid versus *C. zacatechichi*, $P < 0.01$.

of action, we have found additional evidence of its potential to cause significant renal cell damage. Specifically, our panel of indicators of kidney injury showed that not only were these biomarkers elevated, but also the intensity of their elevation approached that measured in our assays following cisplatin treatment. The biomarkers we selected included those that have been qualified by the FDA to serve as official biomarkers of nephrotoxicity. They have gained attention recently as they have been shown to be solid correlates of *in vivo* nephrotoxicity [42]. Overall, our findings indicated that the cellular toxicity of *C. zacatechichi* was capable of producing elevations in all four biomarkers at the high treatment dose, but to a lesser extent than cisplatin.

Other toxicology studies on *C. zacatechichi* using *in vivo* model systems have not specifically evaluated nephrotoxicity endpoints but have still demonstrated its potential to have a range of side effects. In a rat model, for example, extracts of this herb were reported to inhibit edema and neutrophil migration [43]. In a feline model, it caused ataxia, vomiting, and unusual electroencephalogram (EEG) recordings [44]. In human volunteers, it resulted in significant increases in respiratory rates and decreases in reaction times [44].

In support of the idea that *C. zacatechichi* has the potential to cause cell injury, other groups have shown that extracts of this herb or its purified components can exert inhibitory effects on cells using *in vitro* model systems. For example, a recent toxicology study has shown that *C. zacatechichi* can inhibit the transcription factor NF-kappaB, which is critical to regulating cellular inflammation and other functions [45, 46]. A further understanding of *C. zacatechichi*'s mechanism(s) of action may be extrapolated from studies on other members of the *Calea* genus. For example, *C. platylepis*, *C. uniflora*, and *C. serrata* have been shown to possess potent antimicrobial, antifungal, and acaricidal activities, respectively [47–49]. In addition, *C. pinnatifida* was shown to have cytotoxic effects against a wide variety of human cell lines derived from a variety of organ systems, including kidney [50]. Moreover, studies on germacrolides, which are common components of most herbs in the *Calea* genus, including *C. zacatechichi*, have demonstrated the potential for antileishmania effects [8], inhibition of cellular differentiation [51], and cytotoxicity against human leukemia cells [52, 53].

Taken together, *C. zacatechichi* or its components may pose unwanted health effects, especially if long-term daily doses are taken to control hyperglycemia. Our *in vitro* HK-2 proximal tubule cell model depicted potentially nephrotoxic features of this herb at both the cellular and organellar levels. It would be pertinent to next perform an *in vivo* investigation of its systemic and organ-specific effects, including those on the other parts of the kidney.

Additional Points

Highlights. (i) *In vitro* exposure of human kidney cells to *Calea zacatechichi* is cytotoxic.

(ii) Mechanism of cytotoxicity may involve ROS production and mitochondrial injury.

(iii) Biomarkers of nephrotoxicity are elevated following *in vitro* exposure to *Calea zacatechichi*.

Abbreviations

ROS: Reactive oxygen species
MMP: Mitochondrial membrane potential
KIM-1: Kidney Injury Molecule-1
B2M: beta-2-microglobulin.

Competing Interests

The authors declare that they have no competing interests.

Acknowledgments

The authors are grateful to Dr. Ikhlas Khan and Dr. Vijayasankar Raman for generously providing *Calea zacatechichi* material. The authors sincerely thank Dr. Omari Bandele for initiating the HK-2 *in vitro* kidney model system at NIVTB. The authors also thank Dr. Yitong Liu and Ms. Shelia Pugh-Bishop for the helpful technical training in hepatotoxicology prior to the initiation of this study.

References

[1] J. L. Díaz, "Ethnopharmacology and taxonomy of Mexican psychodysleptic plants," *Journal of Psychedelic Drugs*, vol. 11, no. 1-2, pp. 71–101, 1979.

[2] S. O'Mahony Carey, "Psychoactive substances: a guide to ethnobotanical plants and herbs, synthetic chemicals, compounds and products," 2010.

[3] R. Román-Ramos, J. L. Flores-Sáenz, G. Partida-Hernandez, A. Lara-Lemus, and F. Alarcon-Aguilar, "Experimental study of the hypoglycemic effect of some antidiabetic plants," *Archivos de Investigacion Medica*, vol. 22, no. 1, pp. 87–93, 1991.

[4] F. J. Alarcon-Aguilara, R. Roman-Ramos, S. Perez-Gutierrez, A. Aguilar-Contreras, C. C. Contreras-Weber, and J. L. Flores-Saenz, "Study of the anti-hyperglycemic effect of plants used as antidiabetics," *Journal of Ethnopharmacology*, vol. 61, no. 2, pp. 101–110, 1998.

[5] A. Andrade-Cetto and M. Heinrich, "Mexican plants with hypoglycaemic effect used in the treatment of diabetes," *Journal of Ethnopharmacology*, vol. 99, no. 3, pp. 325–348, 2005.

[6] I.-Y. Lee, F. R. Fronczek, A. Malcolm, N. H. Fischer, and L. E. Urbatsch, "New germacranolides from Calea ternifolia and the molecular structure of 9α-hydroxy-11,13-dihydro-11α,13-epoxyatripliciolide-8β-o-[2- methylacrylate]," *Journal of Natural Products*, vol. 45, no. 3, pp. 311–316, 1982.

[7] N. H. Fischer, I.-Y. Lee, F. R. Fronczek, G. Chiari, and L. E. Urbatsch, "Three new furanone-type heliangolides from *Calea ternifolia* and the molecular structure of 8β-angeloyloxy-9α-hydroxycalyculatolide," *Journal of Natural Products*, vol. 47, no. 3, pp. 419–425, 1984.

[8] H. Wu, F. R. Fronczek, C. L. Burandt, and J. K. Zjawiony, "Antileishmanial germacranolides from *Calea zacatechichi*," *Planta Medica*, vol. 77, no. 7, pp. 749–753, 2011.

[9] M. V. Mariano, S. F. Antonio, and P. Joseph-Nathan, "Thymol derivatives from *Calea nelsonii*," *Phytochemistry*, vol. 26, no. 9, pp. 2577–2579, 1987.

[10] J. Cuatrecasas, "Prima flora colombiana: 3. Compositae—astereae," *Webbia*, vol. 24, no. 1, pp. 1–335, 1969.

[11] Y. J. Moon, X. Wang, and M. E. Morris, "Dietary flavonoids: effects on xenobiotic and carcinogen metabolism," *Toxicology in Vitro*, vol. 20, no. 2, pp. 187–210, 2006.

[12] W. Ren, Z. Qiao, H. Wang, L. Zhu, and L. Zhang, "Flavonoids: promising anticancer agents," *Medicinal Research Reviews*, vol. 23, no. 4, pp. 519–534, 2003.

[13] P. Hodek, P. Trefil, and M. Stiborová, "Flavonoids-potent and versatile biologically active compounds interacting with cytochromes P450," *Chemico-Biological Interactions*, vol. 139, no. 1, pp. 1–21, 2002.

[14] I. Merfort, "Perspectives on sesquiterpene lactones in inflammation and cancer," *Current Drug Targets*, vol. 12, no. 11, pp. 1560–1573, 2011.

[15] A. Ghantous, H. Gali-Muhtasib, H. Vuorela, N. A. Saliba, and N. Darwiche, "What made sesquiterpene lactones reach cancer clinical trials?" *Drug Discovery Today*, vol. 15, no. 15-16, pp. 668–678, 2010.

[16] M. K. Chahar, N. Sharma, M. P. Dobhal, and Y. C. Joshi, "Flavonoids: a versatile source of anticancer drugs," *Pharmacognosy Reviews*, vol. 5, no. 9, pp. 1–12, 2011.

[17] C. Klaassen, *Casarett & Doull's Toxicology: The Basic Science of Poisons*, McGraw-Hill Professional, 8th edition, 2013.

[18] Y. S. Kanwar, J. Wada, L. Sun et al., "Diabetic nephropathy: mechanisms of renal disease progression," *Experimental Biology and Medicine*, vol. 233, no. 1, pp. 4–11, 2008.

[19] S. P. Bagby, "Diabetic nephropathy and proximal tubule ROS: challenging our glomerulocentricity," *Kidney International*, vol. 71, no. 12, pp. 1199–1202, 2007.

[20] V. Vallon, "The proximal tubule in the pathophysiology of the diabetic kidney," *American Journal of Physiology—Regulatory Integrative and Comparative Physiology*, vol. 300, no. 5, pp. R1009–R1022, 2011.

[21] Y. Wu, D. Connors, L. Barber, S. Jayachandra, U. M. Hanumegowda, and S. P. Adams, "Multiplexed assay panel of cytotoxicity in HK-2 cells for detection of renal proximal tubule injury potential of compounds," *Toxicology in Vitro*, vol. 23, no. 6, pp. 1170–1178, 2009.

[22] S.-J. Sohn, S. Y. Kim, H. S. Kim et al., "In vitro evaluation of biomarkers for cisplatin-induced nephrotoxicity using HK-2 human kidney epithelial cells," *Toxicology Letters*, vol. 217, no. 3, pp. 235–242, 2013.

[23] P. Gunness, K. Aleksa, K. Kosuge, S. Ito, and G. Koren, "Comparison of the novel HK-2 human renal proximal tubular cell line with the standard LLC-PK1 cell line in studying drug-induced nephrotoxicity," *Canadian Journal of Physiology and Pharmacology*, vol. 88, no. 4, pp. 448–455, 2010.

[24] P. Jennings, S. Aydin, J. Bennett et al., "Inter-laboratory comparison of human renal proximal tubule (HK-2) transcriptome alterations due to Cyclosporine A exposure and medium exhaustion," *Toxicology in Vitro*, vol. 23, no. 3, pp. 486–499, 2009.

[25] N. D. Keirstead, M. P. Wagoner, P. Bentley et al., "Early prediction of polymyxin-induced nephrotoxicity with next-generation urinary kidney injury biomarkers," *Toxicological Sciences*, vol. 137, no. 2, Article ID kft247, pp. 278–291, 2014.

[26] F. Dieterle, F. Sistare, F. Goodsaid et al., "Renal biomarker qualification submission: a dialog between the FDA-EMEA and predictive safety testing consortium," *Nature Biotechnology*, vol. 28, no. 5, pp. 455–462, 2010.

[27] D. Eisinger, "Better tools for screening: early biomarkers of kidney toxicity," *Drug Discovery & Development*, vol. 16, no. 5, pp. 16–20, 2013.

[28] J. V. Bonventre, V. S. Vaidya, R. Schmouder, P. Feig, and F. Dieterle, "Next-generation biomarkers for detecting kidney toxicity," *Nature Biotechnology*, vol. 28, no. 5, pp. 436–440, 2010.

[29] M. E. Mossoba, T. J. Flynn, S. Vohra, P. L. Wiesenfeld, and R. L. Sprando, "Human kidney proximal tubule cells are vulnerable to the effects of *Rauwolfia serpentina*," *Cell Biology and Toxicology*, vol. 31, no. 6, pp. 285–293, 2015.

[30] F. Bohlmann and C. Zdero, "Neue germacrolide aus Calea zacatechichi," *Phytochemistry*, vol. 16, no. 7, pp. 1065–1068, 1977.

[31] P. K. Chowdhury, R. P. Sharma, G. Thyagarajan, W. Herz, and S. V. Govindan, "Stereochemisty of ciliarin, zexbrevin, and their relatives," *Journal of Organic Chemistry*, vol. 45, no. 24, pp. 4993–4997, 1980.

[32] W. Herz and N. Kumar, "Sesquiterpene lactones of *Calea zacatechichi* and *C. urticifolia*," *Phytochemistry*, vol. 19, no. 4, pp. 593–597, 1980.

[33] I. Köhler, K. Jenett-Siems, K. Siems et al., "In vitro antiplasmodial investigation of medicinal plants from El Salvador," *Zeitschrift für Naturforschung C*, vol. 57, no. 3-4, pp. 277–281, 2002.

[34] Louisiana, S. o. Louisiana Board of Pharmacy, Laws and Regulations (40) L. Legislature. Section 989.1, C. (3) (kk), April 2013.

[35] K. Simonienko, N. Waszkiewicz, and A. Szulc, "Psychoactive plant species—actual list of plants prohibited in Poland," *Psychiatria Polska*, vol. 47, no. 3, pp. 499–510, 2013.

[36] F. Zucco, I. De Angelis, E. Testai, and A. Stammati, "Toxicology investigations with cell culture systems: 20 Years after," *Toxicology in Vitro*, vol. 18, no. 2, pp. 153–163, 2004.

[37] C. L. Broadhead and R. D. Combes, "The current status of food additives toxicity testing and the potential for application of the three Rs," *ATLA Alternatives to Laboratory Animals*, vol. 29, no. 4, pp. 471–485, 2001.

[38] M. A. Perazella, "Renal vulnerability to drug toxicity," *Clinical Journal of the American Society of Nephrology*, vol. 4, no. 7, pp. 1275–1283, 2009.

[39] M. Schetz, J. Dasta, S. Goldstein, and T. Golper, "Drug-induced acute kidney injury," *Current Opinion in Critical Care*, vol. 11, no. 6, pp. 555–565, 2005.

[40] R. C. Harris and E. G. Neilson, "Toward a unified theory of renal progression," *Annual Review of Medicine*, vol. 57, pp. 365–380, 2006.

[41] M. J. Ryan, G. Johnson, J. Kirk, S. M. Fuerstenberg, R. A. Zager, and B. Torok-Storb, "HK-2: an immortalized proximal tubule epithelial cell line from normal adult human kidney," *Kidney International*, vol. 45, no. 1, pp. 48–57, 1994.

[42] K. Vlasakova, Z. Erdos, S. P. Troth et al., "Evaluation of the relative performance of 12 urinary biomarkers for renal safety across 22 rat sensitivity and specificity studies," *Toxicological Sciences*, vol. 138, no. 1, pp. 3–20, 2014.

[43] H. Venegas-Flores, D. Segura-Cobos, and B. Vázquez-Cruz, "Antiinflammatory activity of the aqueous extract of Calea zacatechichi," *Proceedings of the Western Pharmacology Society*, vol. 45, pp. 110–111, 2002.

[44] L. Mayagoitia, J.-L. Díaz, and C. M. Contreras, "Psychopharmacologic analysis of an alleged oneirogenic plant: *Calea zacatechichi*," *Journal of Ethnopharmacology*, vol. 18, no. 3, pp. 229–243, 1986.

[45] M. J. Lenardo and D. Baltimore, "NF-κB: a pleiotropic mediator of inducible and tissue-specific gene control," *Cell*, vol. 58, no. 2, pp. 227–229, 1989.

[46] Z. Sun and R. Andersson, "NF-κB activation and inhibition: a review," *Shock*, vol. 18, no. 2, pp. 99–106, 2002.

[47] A. M. do Nascimento, M. J. Salvador, R. C. Candido, I. Y. Ito, and D. C. R. de Oliveira, "Antimicrobial activity of extracts and some compounds from *Calea platylepis*," *Fitoterapia*, vol. 75, no. 5, pp. 514–519, 2004.

[48] A. M. do Nascimento, M. J. Salvador, R. C. Candido, S. de Albuquerque, and D. C. R. de Oliveira, "Trypanocidal and anti-fungal activities of p-hydroxyacetophenone derivatives from Calea uniflora (Heliantheae, Asteraceae)," *Journal of Pharmacy and Pharmacology*, vol. 56, no. 5, pp. 663–669, 2004.

[49] V. L. S. Ribeiro, J. C. dos Santos, J. R. Martins et al., "Acaricidal properties of the essential oil and precocene II obtained from *Calea serrata* (Asteraceae) on the cattle tick *Rhipicephalus (Boophilus) microplus* (Acari: Ixodidae)," *Veterinary Parasitology*, vol. 179, no. 1–3, pp. 195–198, 2011.

[50] G. M. Marchetti, K. A. Silva, A. N. Santos et al., "The anticancer activity of dichloromethane crude extract obtained from *Calea pinnatifida*," *Journal of Experimental Pharmacology*, vol. 4, pp. 157–162, 2012.

[51] N. Matsuura, M. Yamada, H. Suzuki et al., "Inhibition of preadipocyte differentiation by germacranolides from *Calea urticifolia* in 3T3-L1 cells," *Bioscience, Biotechnology and Biochemistry*, vol. 69, no. 12, pp. 2470–2474, 2005.

[52] A. Rivero, J. Quintana, J. L. Eiroa et al., "Potent induction of apoptosis by germacranolide sesquiterpene lactones on human myeloid leukemia cells," *European Journal of Pharmacology*, vol. 482, no. 1–3, pp. 77–84, 2003.

[53] Y. Nakagawa, M. Iinuma, N. Matsuura et al., "A potent apoptosis-inducing activity of a sesquiterpene lactone, arucanolide, in HL60 cells: a crucial role of apoptosis-inducing factor," *Journal of Pharmacological Sciences*, vol. 97, no. 2, pp. 242–252, 2005.

Permissions

List of Contributors

Shivangi Goyal, Nidhi Gupta and Sreemoyee Chatterjee
Department of Biotechnology,The IIS University, Gurukul Marg, SFS, Mansarovar, Jaipur, Rajasthan 302020, India

Idalia Jazmin Castañeda-Yslas and María Evarista Arellano-García
Facultad de Ciencias, Universidad Aut´onoma de Baja California, 22800 Ensenada, BC,Mexico

Marco Antonio García-Zarate
Centro de Investigaci´on Cient´ıfica y de Educaci´on Superior de Ensenada, 22800 Ensenada, BC, Mexico

Balam Ruíz-Ruíz
Escuela de Ciencias de la Salud, Universidad Aut´onoma de Baja California, 22800 Ensenada, BC, Mexico

María Guadalupe Zavala-Cerna and Olivia Torres-Bugarín
School of Medicine, Universidad Aut´onoma de Guadalajara, 44100 Guadalajara, JAL, Mexico

Claudia Leticia Moreno Ávila, Jorge H. Limón-Pacheco, Magda Giordano and VerónicaM. Rodríguez
Departamento de Neurobiología Conductual y Cognitiva, Instituto de Neurobiología, Universidad Nacional Autónoma de México, Boulevard Juriquilla 3001, 76230 Querétaro, QRO, Mexico

Egbe Edmund Richard, Nsonwu-Anyanwu Augusta Chinyere, Offor Sunday Jeremaiah Usoro Chinyere Adanna Opara, EtukudoMaise Henrieta and Egbe Deborah Ifunanya
Department of Medical Laboratory Science, Faculty of Allied Medical Sciences, College of Medical Sciences, University of Calabar, Calabar 543000, Nigeria

Star Khoza and Ishmael Moyo
Department of Clinical Pharmacology, College of Health Sciences, University of Zimbabwe, Harare, Zimbabwe

Denver Ncube
Department of Anatomy, College of Health Sciences, University of Zimbabwe, Harare, Zimbabwe

Said Said Elshama
Department of ForensicMedicine and Clinical Toxicology,College ofMedicine, Suez Canal University, P.O. Box 3457, Ismailia, Egypt Taif University, Taif, Saudi Arabia

Ayman El-Meghawry EL-Kenawy
Taif University, Taif, Saudi Arabia
Department of Molecular Biology, GEBRI, University of Sadat City, P.O. Box 79, Sadat City, Egypt

Hosam-Eldin Hussein Osman
Taif University, Taif, Saudi Arabia
Department of Anatomy, College of Medicine, Al-Azhar University, P.O. Box 345, Cairo, Egypt

Yaqoob Lone,Mangla Bhide and Raj Kumar Koiri
Department of Zoology, Dr. Harisingh Gour Central University, Sagar, Madhya Pradesh 470003, India

Amy Clewell, Philip A. Palmer, John R. Endres, Timothy S.Murbach and Tennille Marx
AIBMR Life Sciences, Inc., 2800 East Madison Street, Suite 202, Seattle,WA 98112, USA

Gábor Hirka, Róbert Glávits and Ilona Pasics Szakonyiné
Toxi-Coop Zrt., Magyar Jakobinusok tere 4/B, Budapest 1122, Hungary

Binbing Ling, Bosong Gao and Jian Yang
Drug Discovery and Development Research Group, College of Pharmacy and Nutrition, University of Saskatchewan, 107Wiggins Road, Saskatoon, SK, Canada S7N 5E5

Isaac Julius Asiedu-Gyekye, Benoit Banga N'guessan and Paul Osei-Prempeh
Department of Pharmacology and Toxicology, University of Ghana School of Pharmacy, College of Health Sciences, Legon, Ghana

Samuel Frimpong-Manso
Department of Pharmaceutical Chemistry, University of Ghana School of Pharmacy, College of Health Sciences, Legon, Ghana

Mahmood Abdulai Seidu
Department of Medical Laboratory Sciences (Pathology), School of Biomedical and Allied Health Sciences, University of Ghana, Legon, Ghana

Daniel Kwaku Boamah
Geological Survey Department, Accra, Ghana

Jessica Paken, Cyril D. Govender and Mershen Pillay
Discipline of Audiology, School of Health Sciences, University of KwaZulu-Natal, Private Bag X54001, Durban 4000, South Africa

Vikash Sewram
Discipline of Audiology, School of Health Sciences, University of KwaZulu-Natal, Private Bag X54001, Durban 4000, South Africa
African Cancer Institute, Faculty of Medicine and Health Sciences, Stellenbosch University, P.O. Box 241, Cape Town 8000, South Africa
Division of Community Health, Faculty of Medicine and Health Sciences, Stellenbosch University, P.O. Box 241, Cape Town 8000, South Africa

Bhupesh Patel and Manorama Patri
Department of Zoology, School of Life Sciences, Ravenshaw University, Cuttack, Odisha 753003, India

Saroj Kumar Das
Department of Zoology, School of Life Sciences, Ravenshaw University, Cuttack, Odisha 753003, India
Department of High Altitude Physiology, Defence Institute of High Altitude Research, Leh 901205, India

Rasha Abdel-Ghany, Ebaa Mohammed and Shimaa Anis
Department of Pharmacology & Toxicology, Faculty of Pharmacy, Zagazig University, Zagazig, Egypt

Waleed Barakat
Department of Pharmacology & Toxicology, Faculty of Pharmacy, Zagazig University, Zagazig, Egypt
Department of Pharmacology & Toxicology, Faculty of Pharmacy, Tabuk University, Tabuk, Saudi Arabia

Masahiro Okamoto
Graduate School of Bioresource and Bioenvironmental Sciences, Kyushu University, Higashi-ku, Fukuoka 812-8582, Japan

Ryuta Saito
Graduate School of Bioresource and Bioenvironmental Sciences, Kyushu University, Higashi-ku, Fukuoka 812-8582, Japan
Biology Research Laboratories, Mitsubishi Tanabe Pharma Corporation, Toda-shi, Saitama 335-8505, Japan
DMPK Research Laboratories, Mitsubishi Tanabe Pharma Corporation, Toda-shi, Saitama 335-8505, Japan

Makoto Yamazaki
DMPK Research Laboratories, Mitsubishi Tanabe Pharma Corporation, Toda-shi, Saitama 335-8505, Japan

Natsuko Terasaki, Naoya Masutomi and Naohisa Tsutsui
Safety Research Laboratories, Mitsubishi Tanabe Pharma Corporation, Kisarazu-shi, Chiba 292-0818, Japan

Manik Das and Kuntal Manna
Department of Pharmacy, Tripura University (A Central University), Suryamaninagar, Tripura 799022, India

Naofumi Bunya and Keigo Sawamoto
Sapporo Medical University, Sapporo 060-8556, Japan

Hanif Benoit and Steven B. Bird
Department of Emergency Medicine, University of Massachusetts Medical School,Worcester, MA 01655, USA

Dexter Tagwireyi and Patience Chingombe
Drug and Toxicology Information Service (DaTIS), School of Pharmacy, College of Health Sciences, University of Zimbabwe, P.O. Box A178, Avondale, Harare, Zimbabwe

Star Khoza
Department of Clinical Pharmacology, College of Health Sciences, University of Zimbabwe, P.O. Box A178, Avondale, Harare, Zimbabwe

Mandy Maredza
School of Public Health, Faculty of Health Sciences, University ofWitwatersrand, Johannesburg, South Africa

MarwaM.M. Refaie, Entesar F. Amin and Aly M. Abdelrahman
Department of Pharmacology, Faculty of Medicine, El-Minia University, El-Minia 61111, Egypt

Nashwa F. El-Tahawy
Department of Histology, Faculty of Medicine, El-Minia University, El-Minia 61111, Egypt

Miriam E. Mossoba, Thomas J. Flynn, Sanah Vohra, Paddy Wiesenfeld and Robert L. Sprando
Center for Food Safety and Applied Nutrition (CFSAN), Office of Applied Research and Safety Assessment (OARSA)
Division of Toxicology (DOT), US Food and Drug Administration (US FDA)
Neurotoxicology and In Vitro Toxicology Branch (NIVTB), 8301 Muirkirk Road, Laurel, MD 20708, USA

Index